CULTURE AND HEALTH
Applying Medical Anthropology

CULTURE AND HEALTH

Applying Medical Anthropology

MICHAEL WINKELMAN

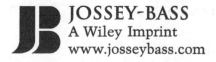

JOSSEY-BASS
A Wiley Imprint
www.josseybass.com

Published by Jossey-Bass
A Wiley Imprint
989 Market Street, San Francisco, CA 94103-1741—www.josseybass.com

Jossey-Bass books and products are available through most bookstores. To contact Jossey-Bass directly call our Customer Care Department within the U.S. at 800-956-7739, outside the U.S. at 317-572-3986, or fax 317-572-4002.

Jossey-Bass also publishes its books in a variety of electronic formats. Some content that appears in print may not be available in electronic books.

Library of Congress Cataloging-in-Publication Data has been applied for.

ISBN 13: 978-0-4702-8355-4
ISBN 10: 0-4702-8355-6

Printed in the United States of America
FIRST EDITION

PB Printing   SKY10031109_110121

CONTENTS

FIGURES, TABLES, AND EXHIBITS

FIGURES

TABLES

EXHIBITS

SPECIAL FEATURES

APPLICATIONS

BIOCULTURAL INTERACTIONS

CASE STUDIES

CULTURE AND HEALTH

PRACTITIONER PROFILES

PREFACE

Cultural factors are central issues in the health problems that confront the world today. When reading newspapers and magazines, I find a barrage of information about cultural, social, economic, and political factors that impact the health of people around the world. Culture and health interactions are involved in cardiovascular deaths due to lifestyle; in soft-drink bans in public schools; in the epidemics spreading around the globe; and in deaths due to pesticides, infant diarrhea and dehydration, cigarette smoking, and the side effects of drugs such as Vioxx. Cultural factors are central to health issues of obesity, accidents, problems of the homeless and medically uninsured, child sexual abuse, and drug addiction. Social, economic, and cultural factors underlie major international health problems, including the spread of the acquired immunodeficiency syndrome (AIDS) epidemic, infant mortality due to preventable disease, the prohibitive cost of pharmaceuticals, diseases from environmental contamination, and social pathologies such as mental illness and violent assault.

In examining these health problems, I see that these are not simply medical problems with established clinical or pharmacological solutions but societal problems with complex cultural dimensions. These health conditions are generally not directly caused by biology—genetics, viruses, or bacteria—but, rather, by the effects of individual and collective cultural behaviors such as diet and resource allocation. How can we as a society come to understand and manage the social and cultural conditions that affect health?

I wrote this text on culture and health to present basic anthropological perspectives for understanding disease and illness and promoting healing and health. The text has two main audiences: health science students, particularly those in medical anthropology, nursing, and public health, and health care professionals, including physicians, nurses, psychologists and counselors, and public health and social workers. Both students and professionals need to understand how cultural perspectives can enhance the management of disease, assist in the promotion of health behavior, and provide a basis for culturally responsive care. This requires an understanding of the perspectives of medical anthropology.

MEDICAL ANTHROPOLOGY'S PERSPECTIVES

Medical anthropology's biocultural approach expands the biomedical perspective that views health as basically a biological issue. Human health and disease derive from the interaction of humans' biological potentials with numerous environments through culturally, socially, and individually mediated experiences that have effects on biological processes. Understanding how culture affects health enhances providers' understanding of health problems and the needed care. The cultural and social effects on health and health care also mean that "we the patients" need to understand these effects, empowering consumers to manage health care interactions with greater awareness of the cultural, social, and institutional factors affecting health and treatment access. Cultural models provide frameworks for consideration of the impacts on health through culturally mediated inter-actions of human biology with the environment.

Cultural Competence and Responsiveness

This text provides perspectives and knowledge of medical anthropology that help health professionals provide culturally sensitive, responsive, and competent health care. I share perspectives acquired across two decades of teaching nursing, public health, and anthropology students, and learning from them as well, about the roles of culture in provider-client interactions. Education about cultural patterning of health and health care is a fundamental aspect of the preparation of health care professionals. It is also part of the broader roles of medical anthropologists as cultural brokers mediating between cultures, professional groups, institutions, and conceptual frameworks. Anthropologists' roles as intermediaries in relationship to biomedicine, the dominant paradigm of Western medicine, includes (1) explaining the cultural dimensions of biomedicine and other healing processes to providers and patients, (2) explaining healing processes that lie outside the current understandings of biomedicine, and (3) providing education to facilitate mediation across these different conceptions of health and care.

Cultural Systems Models

Many factors affect health: personal behaviors; nutrition; environmental conditions; exposure to infectious or noxious agents; and availability of health care resources, social support, and material assistance. The ability to avoid and resist diseases derives from effects of many cultural beliefs and practices on health behaviors and physiological responses. Cultural systems models provide tools for organizing our understanding of the many factors that have effects on health. This integrative cultural perspective is reflected in models developed in medical anthropology, biomedicine, nursing, and public health to address cultural effects on health conditions, behaviors, and outcomes. These models show how diverse aspects of environment, society, and culture shape health and responses to disease. These interactions are illustrated throughout the book in essays that examine the factors relevant to the elevated levels of cardiovascular disease among African Americans.

Cultural Effects on Biology

Medical anthropology addresses the interrelations between biology and culture to show how culture has effects on health and disease. Cultural factors engage symbols with biology in a mind-body dynamics manifested in traditional healing practices, psychosomatic illness, "spontaneous remission of diseases," and other ways in which beliefs affect our health. Perspectives of "psychophysiological symbolism" address how cultural meanings—symbols—have effects on human physiology. Consequently, traditional cultural beliefs regarding causes of illness—spirit aggression, witchcraft, and possession—have effects on psychophysiological processes, including inducing both healing and stress responses. Cultural rituals evoke physiological, emotional, and psychological healing processes and engage social support and elicit group bonding that provokes the release of neurotrans-mitters. These kinds of cultural effects on biological processes underlie the efficacy of traditional healing practices as well as the high incidence of some diseases, such as cardiovascular disease among African Americans.

Ethnomedicine and Alternative Medicine

My studies of ethnomedicine, the healing traditions found in every culture, have shown me that ritual healing practices have effects at physiological, psychological, emotional, symbolic, and social levels, providing many healing mechanisms. Ethnomedical practices can make important contributions to future health care, just as herbs contributed to the development of the biomedical pharmacopoeia. An "anthropological medicine" derived from cross-cultural health practices, exhibited in the alternative and complementary medicine used by people around the world, contributes new possibilities for physicians by expanding perspectives on health resources. Readers of this book have undoubtedly seen, and probably used, one or more of the many alternative medicine treatments available today: herbal teas, special diets, healing crystals, acupuncture, hypnosis, and spiritual and energy healers. So-called alternative and complementary treatments are a health treatment industry serving more than a hundred million Americans and producing an economy valued at billions of dollars annually in the United States. Medical anthropology helps us understand why these treatments are so popular and their roles in relationship to biomedical care.

Understanding Health Activities as Cultural Practices

Medical anthropology can help you, whether practitioner or consumer, become more aware of the cultural dimensions of health and disease and how they are affected by behaviors, beliefs, societal institutions, and the social relations involved in treatment. Health care always involves many aspects of culture, and health institutions function as cultural systems influenced by values, beliefs, and other biases. This text helps demystify biomedicine and its cultural aspects. Awareness of the social, economic, and political dimensions of health make both providers and consumers better prepared to address health needs and options effectively.

CHAPTER OVERVIEWS

The chapters address major cultural perspectives in understanding health and facilitating health care. The first five chapters introduce perspectives of medical anthropology and cultural systems analysis that illustrate a wide range of health concerns in which cultural factors have important roles. These chapters introduce approaches for the development of cultural competence that are applicable across the helping professions. They illustrate the roles of medical anthropology and cultural knowledge in enhancing the quality of services provided by professionals and in empowering clients to better understand the cultural context of their health and care. This requires an understanding of the systemic nature of cultural and environmental interactions through cultural systems models. These models detail the range of factors in the physical and social environments and the cultural behaviors, beliefs, and practices that affect health. Self-assessments at the end of each chapter direct readers to examine these relationships in their personal life, other cultures, and society. Chapters Six through Ten examine anthropological approaches that illustrate mechanisms through which cultural, ecological, political, and mental processes affect physiological responses and health. Each chapter addresses one of the major anthropological paradigms for studying health: transcultural psychiatry, medical ecology, political economy, and symbolic and shamanic perspectives.

Chapter One illustrates the importance of cultural perspectives in health care by showing that health involves broader cultural and personal concerns than addressed by Western medicine. Contemporary community health approaches require an understanding of the diverse cultural groups in society to develop appropriate public health programs. Cultural diversity requires that health care providers ascertain patients' perspectives and develop the cultural competence to address their care needs effectively. The relationship of health to biological and cultural influences illustrates the necessity of a "biopsychosocial" perspective. Cultural systems models are introduced as frameworks for the analysis of health problems and the diverse impacts of culture on health. These perspectives illustrate how both the physical and cultural environment and other forces in society affect health and disease. This provides a range of areas of application for medical anthropology. Readers' levels of cross-cultural competence are assessed in Self-Assessment 1.4.

Chapter Two addresses the fundamental importance of cultural issues in different concepts of health maladies—disease, illness, sickness, and the sick role—and the relationships of cultural and biological processes in producing them. Cultural influences on disease illustrate the limitations in the biomedical model and the socially constructed nature of health maladies. Culture is shown to influence biomedical conceptualizations of health maladies and treatments. Similar social and cultural effects shape the personal experience of illness and the social response to the diseases that produce sickness: socially induced suffering. This chapter introduces the health belief and explanatory models as tools for assessing culture and health relationships and determining the health and disease beliefs that guide patients' health behaviors and responses to health care providers. Self-Assessment 2.1 provides direction for examining the personal and cultural bases of one's own and others' health beliefs and behaviors, providing the self-awareness necessary for adapting to cultural effects on health practices.

Chapter Three focuses on the general dynamics of cross-cultural adaptation and the development of cultural competency, applying its principles and skills for improving client-provider relations and enhancing the well-being of health practitioners. Cultural competence is achieved through employing anthropological perspectives and developing personal, interpersonal, and professional skills. These perspectives emphasize the recognition of, respect for, and accommodation to patients' beliefs and preferences and the development of appropriate communication skills, social relationships, and negotiation approaches to engage patients in their treatment. These roles of cultural perspectives and anthropology in clinical practice and public health are illustrated in mediation, advocacy, education, program development, research, administration, and consultation functions of applied anthropologists. Clinically applied anthropology provides approaches for overcoming cultural problems in doctor-patient relations and enhancing care through cultural competence. The importance of culture in clinical assessment and care is illustrated, as is the role of culture in improving the care of both patients and providers. Medical anthropology also addresses the needs of biomedical practitioners by providing cultural knowledge that facilitates effective clinical practice in reducing cultural conflict and misunderstandings.

Chapter Four illustrates diverse areas of cultures' effects on health through applying cultural systems perspectives. Examples are provided in the areas of diet, reproduction, pregnancy, and family organization. Health care providers and consumers can acquire broader perspectives on the nature of care by being aware of the therapeutic approaches of other cultures' ethnomedical practices and cross-cultural patterns of health practices. This "witch doctor's legacy" and anthropological medicine provide guidelines for the modifications of physicians' styles to enhance patient and community relationships. A significant feature of cultural approaches is their ability to provide healing as opposed to a cure. Community involvement in health can be achieved through ethnographic approaches. Guidelines are provided for implementing policy approaches and programs sensitive to community needs through assuring their involvement and empowerment. The anthropological rapid ethnographic assessment, response, and evaluation models are ideals for incorporating communities into health care assessment, planning, development, and delivery.

Chapter Five examines the major sectors of health care resources: the popular, folk, and professional sectors. Popular culture's health beliefs and practices have important implications for biomedicine; they are the context for decision making and the first line of resources for the care of health problems that often replace biomedical care. Popular culture involves social and personal factors that affect the recognition of symptoms, expression of pain, care-seeking behaviors, and access to health resources. Folk medicine and other alternative medicines are also frequently used in conjunction with biomedical care, potentially causing treatment complications. I review principal aspects of the complementary and alternative ethnomedical traditions found in the United States. Cultural factors also affect the professional sector of biomedicine, particularly the interpersonal dynamics of clinical relations. Recognition of these cross-cultural dynamics can make providers more effective in patient care and patients more effective in managing their clinical visits.

Chapter Six introduces psychiatric anthropology and transcultural psychiatry. These areas are concerned with the nature of humans and the manifestations of physical and psychological maladies in cross-cultural perspectives. Cultural programming of concepts of self and psychology provides the basis for cultural definitions of conditions of normalcy and abnormality and deciding whether behavior constitutes psychopathology or a normal cultural response. These perspectives are illustrated in the assessment of cultural factors that can be confused as psychopathologies. The concept of indigenous psychologies is presented as a cultural framework for understanding the nature of self and others. These cultural adaptations to biological universals, such as gender conceptions of male-female differences, are examined within the context of psychocultural models. Psychocultural models provide a framework for describing cultural psychologies and their environmental, social, and cultural effects on universal human potentials. These psychocultural systems perspectives provide characterizations of ethnicity in the cultural shaping of personal and social identity. The cultural shaping of self is illustrated in the phenomenon of "possession," where spirits are thought to take over the personality of an individual. These conditions and other culture-bound syndromes (folk illnesses) are analyzed according to their relationships to biomedical classifications, cultural conceptions, psychosocial dynamics, and the manifestation of specific biological responses. Cross-cultural perspectives identify both universals of ethnomedical theories derived from human nature and culturally specific illnesses derived from particular cultural dynamics and social conditions. The relation of these ethnomedical conceptions to biologically based response patterns illustrates culturally specific adaptations to and shaping of innate physiological responses.

Chapter Seven presents the medical anthropological perspectives of medical ecology and biocultural perspectives on evolutionary adaptations affecting health. These interactions are illustrated in evolutionary medicine, nutrition, reproduction, emotions, and the evolution of human healing responses in the capacities for caring and empathy. Interactions of biological potentials and cultural influences include individual and group adjustments (acclimatization) and evolutionary adaptations that produce both susceptibility to and resistance to disease. Classic epidemiological perspectives on morbidity and mortality are presented, illustrated with U.S. ethnic differences in rates of death from specific causes of disease. These ethnicity and disease relations are explained with a cultural-epidemiological approach that assesses the causal and contributory sociocultural and behavioral factors in disease exposure and susceptibility. Consideration of the concept of "race" is used to illustrate human similarities and differences and the limitations of biological explanations in understanding human differences, including susceptibility to disease. An evolutionary basis for culture and health interactions is provided by the model of the triune brain and its different components, which provide a basis for understanding the symbolic cultural effects on emotions and stress responses. The relations among these major functional units of the brain provide a framework for understanding the factors shaping the evolution of human sickness and healing responses. These biocultural interactions are also illustrated in cross-cultural differences in emotions and the cultural shaping of emotional responses.

Chapter Eight describes critical medical anthropological approaches to health, introducing political-economic perspectives that illustrate how political and economic forces produce disease and differentially distribute risk and health resources. The impact of social class and economic factors on clinical interactions and patient care is illustrated in physician-patient behavior and the effects of poverty on the sick role. I show the importance of community building for health assurance by the evidence that social networks and support are significant mechanisms through which social relations have effects on health. Advocacy, policy development, and community empowerment approaches are tools through which anthropologists address societal discrepancies in health and work to ensure collective health and well-being.

Chapter Nine describes models of healing based in the interactions between symbols and physiological responses that provide mechanisms for ritual, religion, and belief to affect biological responses. The universal role of religion in cultural healing practices derives from its power to affect belief, motivation, and symbolic and social processes through which culture elicits endogenous biological mechanisms involved in adaptations to stress, anxiety, fear, and other emotions. Mechanisms of cultural healing involve symbolic manipulations of bodily responses through the associations established during socialization processes. Ritual activation of the autonomic nervous system provides bases for the mechanisms of placebo effects, hex death, and symbolic healing rituals. Understanding the relationship of the neurophysiology of stress to psychological and cultural processes provides a basis for understanding ritual effects on health through its symbolic effects on stress, anxiety, and fear. The placebo phenomena are examined as meaning-based symbolic cultural processes that have effects on physiological activity, providing an expanded view of disease and healing processes. These symbolic and social effects are further illustrated in the use of metaphors and myths to manipulate healing responses.

Chapter Ten introduces the most primordial of all ethnomedical practices, those associated with the shaman and shamanistic healing using altered states of consciousness (ASCs). Cross-cultural studies illustrate the commonalities and variation in shamanistic healers, magicoreligious practitioners who use ASCs in therapeutic activities. These universals of shamanistic healing involve neurological structures that provide the basis for therapeutic processes. ASCs represent universal psychobiological features of healing derived from an enhanced integration of brain functions. Variation found cross-culturally in shamanistic healing practices is related to social influences on physiological conditions. I review the psychobiological bases of ASCs, their psychophysiological effects, and the clinical evidence for their therapeutic efficacy. Therapeutic aspects of ASCs are examined in terms of their general physiological effects and through clinical and laboratory studies on specific procedures (e.g., drumming, meditation, music, and hallucinogens). Shamanic ritual mechanisms produce a range of psychosocial, cognitive-emotional, and psychophysiological transformations. The persistence of shamanic dynamics in contemporary illness and healing is illustrated. Shamanistic perspectives can contribute to modern medicine as therapies operating through socioemotional and psychophysiological mechanisms.

SPECIAL FEATURES OF THE TEXT

Medical anthropology's integration of cultural and biological perspectives helps us better understand health problems and their solutions. The relevance of medical anthropology and cultural perspectives to biomedicine, and the interactions of culture and health, is illustrated in special features organized around Biocultural Interactions, Applications, Practitioner Profiles, Self-Assessments, Culture and Health, and Case Studies.

- *Biocultural Interactions* illustrate the effects of culture on biological processes, exemplifying a central point of this book: culture has direct effects on physiology.

- *Applications* present examples of how anthropology's tools and perspectives can assist health professionals in understanding and resolving health problems.

- *Practitioner Profiles* are biographical sketches of some leading medical anthropologists and illustrate how they use cultural perspectives to address health problems.

- *Self-Assessments* have been provided at the end of each chapter to engage readers in the material discussed through a process of self-examination designed to help understand how cultural, social, and ecological factors affect health.

- *Culture and Health* essays present examples of cultural concepts in health, health care, and the expressions of illness.

■ *Case Studies,* a classic teaching approach of biomedicine, are presented to illustrate the relevance of cultural information for health care by showing how it affects health behaviors and health care utilization and how anthropological approaches and cultural knowledge can assist in resolving health problems. Throughout the book, I have used examples of American ethnic groups to illustrate these cultural and health relations.

■ *Glossary* items **bolded** in the text and compiled with definitions at the end of the book are provided to facilitate learning of specialized concepts from medical anthropology.

Case Study: A Clash of Spirits and Biomedicine

Throughout the book, a case study on a Hmong family is included to illustrate the cultural conflicts this ethnic group has experienced with biomedicine. I selected the Hmong because they became widely known to health care providers through Anne Fadiman's (1997) award-winning book, *The Spirit Catches You and You Fall Down.* This "classic of medical anthropology" written by a journalist presents a tragic account of encounters between a Hmong family and their daughter's physician and dramatically illustrates why medicine needs cultural and anthropological understandings. Fadiman's account reveals how cultural conflicts and misunderstandings produced disastrous consequences: a brain-dead child in a permanent vegetative state.

Fadiman analyzes conflicts between staff in the Merced County Hospital and their Hmong patients through the tragedy that befell Lia Lee, daughter of mother Foua Lee and father Nao Kao Lee. The Hmong, who constituted a secret CIA army in wars in Southeast Asia, fled for their lives following the collapse of U.S.-supported South Vietnam. A people perpetually without a country of their own, many Hmong were relocated to rural California and other parts of the United States.

The Lees went to the hospital because of their infant daughter's seizures but always arrived after the seizures had ended. Because of the lack of any translators, Lia Lee's condition and its complications went undiagnosed for five months, leading to consequences that could have been avoided with an earlier diagnosis.

Conflict between biomedicine and Hmong culture regarding Lia Lee's treatment led to her being removed from her family by court orders obtained by her physician. Although eventually returned to her parents, she suffered a major seizure that left her brain-dead at age three. One cause of her demise was an infection acquired in the course of her hospital treatments. Fadiman concludes that Lia's life was ruined by cross-cultural misunderstandings that could have been prevented by anthropological approaches.

These case studies illustrate some crucial cultural issues that impede effective health care and that medical anthropological perspectives can resolve. The problems raised by Fadiman can be addressed by providing culturally responsive care for the Hmong, as described in *Healing by Heart: Clinical and Ethical Case Stories of Hmong Families and Western Providers* by Kathleen Culhane-Pera and coauthors (2003). The arrival of thousands of additional Hmong in 2004 illustrates the continued importance of understanding and effectively addressing the role of culture in health.

Audiences

This book addresses the roles of anthropology in developing cultural competency and cultural perspectives in health sciences and medicine. The intended audiences are students in the health sciences, particularly medical anthropology, medical sociology, nursing, counseling, social work, medicine, and public health, and the same fields of health professionals. My more than twenty years of providing cross-cultural training and teaching in medical anthropology and medical, nursing, and public health programs have shown me that the fundamental perspectives regarding cultural competency are relevant to all the health professions and medical social sciences. This book can be useful to diverse students and professionals because the underlying issues of culture and health interactions are the same for everyone: providers, support staff, and students, whether in nursing, anthropology, public health, psychology, or biomedicine.

How This Book Should Be Used

The dual audiences of the book—medical anthropology and health sciences—may suggest different strategies in using the text material. Students or practitioners of nursing, medicine, or public health are best served by reading the book as organized by chapters. Those who have a focus on medical anthropology may want to first read the Preface and Chapters One and Two, then skip to Chapters Six through Ten where classic paradigms of medical anthropology are covered: transcultural psychiatry, medical ecology, political and economic anthropology, symbolic healing, and shamanistic healing practices. Chapters Three through Five, which cover cultural competence, cultural systems analysis, and the sectors of health care, can be addressed last as specialty topics.

This book also has an audience in health care consumers. Fadiman tells us that she was transformed as a patient by learning of Lia Lee's experiences. You, too, can be transformed as a consumer and patient by understanding the ways in which culture and its manifestations in the environment, power, and resources affect human health. Cultural and power perspectives can enable individuals to renegotiate the intercultural relations that are always part of medical encounters. Anthropological perspectives situate health in relationship to numerous environments where ecological, political, and symbolic factors have effects on health and care. A greater awareness of social and cultural contexts affecting health and health care make us better-informed providers and consumers.

"To future generations of health care professionals and medical social scientists—that they may better understand the roles of culture in health and well-being, and in the care of patients and prevention of disease."

THE AUTHOR

Michael Winkelman, Ph.D. (University of California-Irvine), M.P.H. (University of Arizona), is an associate professor in the School of Human Evolution and Social Change at Arizona State University and former head of Sociocultural Anthropology. For sixteen years, he directed the Ethnographic Field School in Ensenada, Baja California, Mexico. He taught for sixteen years in the California State University Statewide Nursing Program and currently teaches in the Arizona State University School of Nursing and Innovative Health Care. He was cofounder of the Arizona State University M.A. degree program in Cultural and Behavioral Dimensions of Health and served as director of the M.P.H. degree program. He served as president of the Anthropology of Consciousness section of the American Anthropological Association and was the founding president of its Anthropology of Religion section.

Winkelman has engaged in cross-cultural and interdisciplinary research on shamanism for the past thirty years, focusing principally on the cross-cultural patterns of shamanism and identifying the associated biological bases of shamanic universals and altered states of consciousness. His principal books on shamanism include *Shamans, Priests and Witches* (1992) and *Shamanism: The Neural Ecology of Consciousness and Healing* (2000). His textbooks for cross-cultural classes include *American Ethnic History* (2005) and *Cultural Awareness, Sensitivity and Competence* (2006). His recent work includes edited books on various aspects of healing: *Pilgrimages and Healing* (Dubisch and Winkelman, 2005), *Divination and Healing: Potent Vision* (Winkelman and Peek, 2004), and *Psychedelic Medicine: New Evidence for Hallucinogen Substances as Treatments* (Winkelman and Roberts, 2007). He has also explored the applications of shamanism to contemporary health problems of addiction ("Alternative and Complementary Medicine Approaches for Substance Abuse Programs: A Shamanic Perspective," *International Journal of Drug Policy* (2001); and "Complementary Therapy for Addiction: 'Drumming Out Drugs.'" *American Journal of Public Health* (2003). His forthcoming book with John Baker, *Supernatural as Natural,* addresses the biological bases of religion. He can be contacted at michael.winkelman@asu.edu.

ACKNOWLEDGMENTS

I have benefited from the experiences with several groups of students whose sharing has assisted me in writing this text. These include particularly the nursing students of the California State University Statewide Nursing Program, whose papers exposed me to many practical dimensions of cultural knowledge in nursing care, and the Medicine, Culture and Healing Learning Community students at Arizona State University, who read an earlier version of this book and let me know where they did not understand what I was saying. I have also benefited from the papers and perspectives of the medical anthropology students at Arizona State University and the public health students in the University of Arizona-Arizona State University-Northern Arizona University Public Health Program. I particularly want to thank Sue, Cindy, and Eileen Winkelman for their assistance in the final preparation of the manuscript.

CULTURE AND HEALTH
Applying Medical Anthropology

CHAPTER

1

APPLIED MEDICAL ANTHROPOLOGY AND HEALTH CARE

In improving patient satisfaction . . . administrators' attention
is being directed to the impact of culture—of organization, roles,
and values—upon overall quality of care and outcomes
—PRESS, 1997, P. 6

LEARNING OBJECTIVES

- Introduce how culture affects health
- Illustrate how anthropological perspectives can facilitate effective health care
- Introduce the nature of cultural competence in health care
- Illustrate medical anthropology's major applications in addressing cultures' impacts on health
- Illustrate the broad range of concerns people have with respect to their health
- Introduce the biopsychosocial framework for understanding diverse effects on health
- Present a cultural systems model for addressing factors that affect health
- Illustrate principal mechanisms of culture's effects on health

CULTURE AND HEALTH

Have you ever felt when you went to the doctor that your problem wasn't understood or that your treatment was not relevant to your health problem? Cultural differences between physicians and their diverse clients make cross-cultural misunderstandings inevitable. Culture affects patients' and providers' perceptions of health conditions and appropriate treatments. Culture also affects behaviors that expose us to disease and the reasons prompting us to seek care, how we describe our symptoms, and our compliance with treatments. This makes culture central to diagnosis and an important issue for all of the health professions.

Patients and providers need knowledge of the relationships of culture to health because culture is the foundation of everyone's health concerns and practices. Improving health care requires attention to cultural influences on health concerns, conditions, beliefs, and practices. People's health occurs within cultural systems that are concerned with broader issues of well-being than addressed by physicians' concerns with disease and injury; we are also concerned with psychological, social, emotional, mental, and spiritual well-being. As biomedicine turns from a disease-focused approach to concepts with health and well-being, cultural perspectives and cultural competency emerge as central frameworks for improving care.

Medical anthropology is the primary discipline addressing the interfaces of medicine, culture, and **health behavior** and incorporating cultural perspectives into clinical settings and public health programs. Health professionals need knowledge of culture and cross-cultural relationship skills because health services are more effective when responsive to cultural needs. Cross-cultural skills also are important in relationships among providers of different cultures when, for example, African American and Filipino nurses interact with each other or with Anglo, Hispanic, or Hindu physicians. A knowledge of culture is also necessary for work in community settings, such as collaborating with diverse groups and organizations to develop culturally relevant public health programs. Health care providers and patients are more effective in managing their health and care with cultural awareness and the ability to manage the numerous factors that affect well-being.

What do health professionals—providers, researchers, social service personnel, educators, and other "helping professionals"—need to know about the effects of culture on health? They all need systematic ways of studying cultural effects on health and developing cultural competence. Cultural responsiveness is necessary for providers, researchers, and educators if they are to be effective in relating to others across the barriers of cultural differences. The cultural perspectives of medical anthropology are essential for providing competent care, effective community health programs, and patient education. For biomedicine to be effective, providers need to know whether a patient views the physician as believable and trustworthy, the diagnosis as acceptable, the symptoms as problematic, and the treatment as accessible and effective.

The concept of culture is fundamental to understanding health and medicine because personal health behaviors and professional practices of medicine are deeply influenced by culture. **Culture** involves the learned patterns of shared group behavior. These learned shared behaviors are the framework for understanding and explaining all human behavior. This includes health behaviors, particularly intergroup differences in health behaviors and beliefs. Culture is a principal determinant of health conditions, particularly in exposing us to or protecting us from diseases through structuring our interactions with the physical and social environments: for example, through producing environmental contamination, work activities, contact with animals, sexual practices, diet, clothing, hygienic practices, and others. Culture also defines the kinds of health problems that exist and the resources for responding to health concerns, defining our perceptions, and producing the resources for responding to them.

Cultural knowledge is also essential for addressing public health mandates to assess communities' health needs, develop appropriate health policies and programs, and ensure adequate and culturally competent health services. The health needs of communities vary widely, requiring an understanding of each community's perceptions of health and illness to develop appropriate services. Public health initiatives require knowledge of culture to change the behaviors and lifestyles associated with an increased incidence of disease. Addressing the effects of culture on health is an important issue for everyone, not just physicians, because disease in any group impacts society as a whole. According to Durch, Bailey, and Stoto (1997), "Improving health is a shared responsibility of health care providers, public health officials, and a variety of other actors in the community." This requires people with an ability to engage communities in a culturally appropriate manner and understanding of their cultural systems, health beliefs, and practices.

Perspectives for addressing culture and health relations are provided by medical anthropology and the **cultural systems model**s used within nursing, public health, and medicine to understand systemic ecological and social effects on health. The foci on principal factors affecting health reflect the major traditions of medical anthropology:

- Medical ecology, which examines culture's mediation of health through the physical, biological, and material relationships with the environment

- Political economy and critical approaches that address how health is affected by economic resources, power, and social activities that produce risks and distribute resources

- Symbolic approaches that examine how cultural meanings create the socially legitimated healing processes and link beliefs to physiological processes

This book helps you understand how cultural effects occur across a wide range of health concerns, ranging from clinical care to prevention programs and the funding priorities of health care. Hundreds of factors can have effects on our health, ranging from social conditions producing or reducing exposures to germs and noxious agents to the cultural, economic, and political factors that enable a person's access to quality care.

CASE STUDY

Cultural Conflicts in Health Care

The potentially tragic consequences of conflicts between biomedical culture and the culture of patients became more widely known to providers and the general public through the accounts provided by Anne Fadiman (1997) in *The Spirit Catches You and You Fall Down*. Numerous factors produced a disastrous outcome in infant Lia Lee's interaction with her doctors, factors that derived as much from the Hmong culture as from that of biomedicine and its efforts to control the Hmong and ignore their beliefs. The result was a brain-dead child; physicians blamed the parents and their failure to adhere to the prescribed medications.

In trying to explain why Hmong patients did not accept the physician's point of view, Fadiman recounts the Hmong history of resistance to the Chinese and other outside invaders and authorities: fighting rather than surrendering and standing up to intimidation. Fadiman suggests that their history of resistance is the root of their opposition to the doctor's orders. But the Hmong are not some static culture caught in the past; rather, they have continually adapted and changed in the face of many dominant cultural groups that have attempted to control, tax, assimilate, militarize, and profit from them. The Hmong have changed in many ways, adopting influences from other cultures that have served them well. This is manifested in their Christianization, U.S. military service, education, and acculturation.

Lia's family had undergone acculturation and accepted the value of biomedicine, taking her repeatedly to emergency departments and doctors' appointments. Nevertheless, they often resisted visiting hospitals, which they believed were haunted by spirits of the dead. And they resisted treatments imposed by physicians, viewing them as coercion rather than gifts of healing. The Hmong view of health was a mixture of religion, economics, lost souls, and spirits, a balance of virtually all aspects of life. To the Hmong, many basic aspects of medicine were taboo or horrifying—blood specimens for tests, autopsies to study diseased organs, and invasive procedures including spinal taps, surgery, and vaginal exams. Their doctor's orders for the constant drawing of blood, sometimes as often as three times a week for Lia, increased her parents' concern about the vital fluids being taken from their child. Experimental procedures and treatments unrelated to her complaints reinforced many of the Hmong's worst fears: that doctors would eat the liver, kidneys, and brains of their patients. They had seen the doctor's offices with body pieces cut up and stored in jars, preserved like food.

Lia's parents often resisted her treatment, not understanding why she was restrained to her bed in the hospital, why boards were attached to her arms to hold intravenous lines in place, or why the doctors changed her medicine so frequently. The frequent changes in Lia's prescriptions made it impossible for her nonliterate parents to medicate their daughter effectively. This contributed to her seizures and the repeated visits to the emergency department that evoked frustration and anger in Lia's physicians. So exasperated were the physicians in their relations with the Hmong that a standard joke among them was that the preferred method of treating the Hmong was "high-velocity transcortical lead therapy"—a bullet to the head.

CULTURE, ETHNOMEDICINES, AND BIOMEDICINE

Culture is at the foundation of all medicine, the **biomedicine** of physicians (M.D.s) as well as all other **ethnomedicines,** the health care practices of a culture. Medical systems are intimately intertwined with a culture's economic, social, political, and philosophical systems; this is illustrated in the United States in biomedicine's control of governmental resources, its successful lobbying in Congress, and its powerful economic position in society, including government.

Culture affects health behavior in many ways:

- Conceptualizing health maladies (disease, illness, and sickness) and their significance

- Affecting the distribution of causes of disease and illness

- Creating risk behaviors and disease exposure

- Informing symptom recognition and care-seeking behavior

- Creating health providers' and their institutions' responses to health care needs

- Shaping utilization of the popular, folk, and professional sectors of health care

- Producing social, economic, and political impacts on health and health care

- Creating emotional and psychodynamic influences on health and well-being

- Providing psychodynamic, symbolic, and social mechanisms of healing relationships

Culture mediates our responses to health maladies through ethnomedicines, cultural practices for addressing health problems. The term ethnomedicine typically distinguishes other cultures' health practices from biomedicine, the dominant ethnomedical system of the United States, which is also referred to as Western medicine, scientific medicine, and allopathic medicine. Biomedicine is also an ethnomedicine, reflecting the culture where it is practiced (see Chapter Five).

Ethnomedical studies (see Bannerman, Burton, and Wen-Chieh, 1983) reveal that health problems and treatments are conceptualized within cultural frameworks. Culture directly affects the manifestations of conditions, their assessment and social implications, and processes of treatment. Ethnomedical analyses show the importance of understanding healing from the cultural perspective of the group, their social dynamics, the social roles of healers, and the conceptual and cosmological systems (Rubel and Hass, 1990).

Many contemporary U.S. health issues illustrate underlying cultural dynamics:

- Death due to lifestyle (e.g., poor diet and alcohol and cigarette use)

- Political decisions that leave major segments of the population without health services

- The spread of infectious diseases through immigration and lifestyles

- Pharmaceutical companies and physicians' groups lobbying Congress for legislation to deny U.S. citizens access to foreign medicines

Health concerns often feature prominently in the most important institutions of the culture from birth to death. In the United States, virtually all social institutions interface with biomedical practices that regulate our lives at all stages:

■ With preconception management of birth through prescriptions for contraceptives

■ In birthing processes, with legally mandated neonatal treatments and birth certificates

■ In required school immunizations and health exams

■ Through required marriage screening (e.g., blood type, Rh factor, and AIDS tests)

■ Via validation of work absences and workers' compensation

■ In the management of terminal illness and issuance of death certificates

Most Americans probably think of biomedicine as the normal resources for health problems. Health choices in the United States are strongly influenced by biomedicine, but people around the world, including many in this country, also use other ethnomedical systems. These include numerous forms of self-care and medication, ethnic healing traditions, and other professionals (e.g., chiropractors, homeopaths, naturopaths, herbalists). Personal expenditures in the United States for "unconventional" medicine—complementary and alternative medicine—are at twice the level of out-of-pocket expenses for biomedical care (Eisenberg, Kessler, Foster, Norlock, Calkins, and Delbanco, 1993). These resources are also used by many patients who also see physicians. This constitutes a medical pluralism that illustrates the need for biomedical providers to understand the ethnomedical resources used by patients.

Biomedicine characterizes its approach as scientific, contrasting itself with other ethnomedical systems that it accuses of being religions, superstitions, quackery, or fraud. Other ethnomedical practices are not, however, lacking in empirical content and have often provided agents for modern medicine, such as biomedicine's use of derivatives from the plant digitalis for the treatment of cardiac conditions. Although ethnomedical practices involve religious rituals, these activities may have social, psychological, and even physiological effects (see Chapter Nine). Rituals such as white coats and rigidly scheduled temperature and blood pressure measurements are also widespread in biomedicine, which has many practices not substantiated by scientific methods. These *cultural* traditions of biomedicine have led to a recent emphasis on developing criteria to reveal "evidence-based practice."

Cultural perspectives are essential for understanding the nature of biomedicine (Sargent and Johnson, 1996). Cross-cultural perspectives clarify the nature of biomedicine: one of many sources of knowledge about health treatments but not an exclusive, exhaustive, or infallible source. Effective techniques for health are not exclusive to any one ethnomedical system. The relevance of ethnomedicine to scientific medicine was recognized in the World Health Organization's programs of *Health for All by the Year 2000* and the continuing emphasis for the future. These programs emphasize that ethnomedical traditions are essential for the health care of most of the world because of the prohibitive cost of pharmaceuticals. Consequently, if scientific medicine is to be widely available, it requires establishing the scientific basis for traditional ethnomedical practices.

Cultural approaches help explain why other ethnomedical practices persist. The greater use of alternative therapies in the United States among those with higher economic and educational status reflects reasoned considerations, rather than desperate efforts of those lacking access to biomedicine. Ethnomedical traditions engage cultural and symbolic healing processes that involve influences of mental, psychological, and social levels on the physical body (e.g., the experiences of physiological stress when thinking about a problem). The biological effects of social and mental factors constitute a fundamental revision of the biomedical paradigm, as seen in fields such as **psychoneuro-immunology**, which reconceptualizes healing as the causal effects of symbolic processes on physiological responses.

Different health systems can be compared using some key distinctions provided by anthropology. These include **emic** (the definitions of the world that are particular to a specific culture) and **etic** (universal models of human behavior applicable to all cultures). For instance, some cultures' beliefs (emic) consider that the failure to do rituals for one's ancestors can cause nightmares and death (see "Nightmare Deaths" in Chapter Six). Biomedical approaches consider a universal etic sleep paralysis response to be responsible for these and similar cases found around the world. Biocultural approaches ask questions about how emic beliefs elicit etic physiological responses, how our expectations may influence the biological responses of our bodies.

Anthropology illustrates the importance of emic perspectives for health, how a particular culture views health concerns and shapes people's health behaviors. Anthropology also contributes to establishing an etic system that recognizes the mechanisms of efficacy found in other groups' practices as well. Anthropology shows the limitations of biomedicine's claims as a universally applicable etic framework in illustrating cultural differences in health needs. Physicians have often presumed that they alone have scientific and legitimate healing procedures and that these are equally applicable for everybody. Anthropological studies show important cross-cultural differences in concepts of health and effective treatment.

Ethnomedicines as Subcultures

The concept of culture is important for understanding biomedicine because its practices are shaped by cultural systems. All healing occurs within a cultural system, but health providers also have different subcultures (e.g., doctors versus nurses; see Chapter Five). Biomedicine shares with all ethnomedicines three major interrelated cultural functions (Kleinman, 1973b):

■ Providing meaning and efficacy: the construction and organization of the illness experience

■ Creating cognitive categories for naming, classifying, ordering, and explaining illness

■ Performing acts of healing

Kleinman (1973b, 1980) characterizes all ethnomedicines as systems that are "social and cultural in origin, structure, function and significance . . . [and can be analyzed] . . . in the same way that political systems, religious systems, kinship systems, language and other symbolic systems" are analyzed (1980, pp. 27, 33). The social realities of medical systems are created through culturally ascribed relationships and meanings. For instance, biomedicine has the power to determine which medicines you can have access to or, in their capacity as public health officials, to have a person quarantined because of contagious disease.

Beliefs about the causes of maladies and appropriate treatments are related to social power and political ideologies, such as when the Congress passes legislation (e.g., Americans with Disabilities Act) that explicitly excludes people with addictions as disabled. Instead, it heightens their difficulties with legislation, increasing the penalties for their biological addictions (e.g., the highly punitive crack cocaine versus powder cocaine laws that were only recently given some relief through judicial review).

Religious beliefs also affect care: for instance, when providers express their disapproval of patients who have sexually transmitted diseases (STDs) caused by promiscuous sexual relations. The clinical interactions between providers and clients are created through broader cultural and social relations that provide content and structure for clinical relations. For example, the poor, who are considered beneficiaries of "free" public assistance in their health care, often fail to use it. Their reasons for refusing such free care generally involve the demeaning way in which they feel they are treated at these facilities by an unsympathetic staff. Social analyses might also point to the tendencies of lower-class people to delay care seeking until their condition reaches a critical stage, at which point it may be beyond treatment.

Cultural analyses of medical practices need to consider both **microlevel** approaches, where the interpersonal dynamics of care occur in the interactions between doctor and patient, and **macrolevel** approaches, the societal institutions that affect care through the ways in which it is provided (e.g., **socialized medicine**, where care is provided by the government, versus **capitalist medicine**, where care is purchased by consumers). All ethnomedical systems have characteristics related to the cultural systems that produce them. Consequently, a society's total medical system must be studied to understand how health is produced through a number of interpenetrating realities: biological, personal, psychological, cultural, and social.

Knowledge of ethnomedical conceptual systems can also be an essential aspect of providing correct diagnoses and appropriate care. Cultural conceptions of health problems may not be accepted by biomedicine but may nonetheless be important in terms of care needs, as illustrated in the case of the Mexican *caida de mollera*.

CULTURAL COMPETENCE IN THE HEALTH PROFESSIONS

Health service professionals face common concerns in addressing how culture affects relations with individual clients and how their well-being is produced in interaction with many aspects of the environment. Effectively addressing these concerns requires

BIOCULTURAL INTERACTIONS

Clinical Significance of Mexican Illness Beliefs

The illness concept *caida de mollera* is important for medical practice because associated conditions require medical attention and can provide information about symptoms useful in diagnoses (Baer and Bustillo, 1993, 1998). Caida de mollera refers to a depressed, sunken, or fallen fontanel. A common belief is that it is caused by pulling the baby away from the breast or bottle too quickly or by falls, tossing the baby, or otherwise bumping the baby's head. Caida de mollera is all too often viewed as just a cultural belief by health care providers. This emic cultural concept, however, reflects something real: an entity with etic status and reflecting life-threatening conditions. The sunken fontanel likely reflects severe dehydration. Cultural treatments for it are not likely to be adequate, but a parent's diagnosis of caida de mollera can indicate recent dehydration in the child. Physicians presented with the symptoms associated with caida de mollera typically consider them to be life threatening and requiring medical attention.

In the vast majority of cases, however, mothers of the children with these illnesses do not present them for medical care unless symptoms persist for a long time and do not respond to ethnomedical remedies. Most patients never receive biomedical attention. Reporting these conditions to physicians is increasingly rare because of their negative and critical reactions. Given that these conditions reflect symptoms that physicians consider to be worthy of biomedical attention, the importance of the ability to communicate about these conditions is apparent. Culturally sensitive communication between mothers and physicians can provide patient education as to the necessity of bringing specific conditions for treatment. If health care providers continue to view these folk illnesses as superstitions, their ignorance will contribute to increased morbidity and mortality from treatable life-threatening conditions that Mexican Americans recognize (Baer and Bustillo, 1993). Appropriate care requires the development of cultural competence.

cultural competence, which includes both individual and organizational capacities, behaviors, attitudes, and policies that effectively address cultural differences through the use of cultural knowledge and intercultural skills. Cultural competence involves the ability to address a range of cultural factors. These include cultural knowledge and personal awareness, as illustrated in the classic assessments of areas of cultural knowledge required in social work practice (Bartlett, 2003):

- Cultural systems, including work organization and culture

   The internal processes of communities, including their social resources

   Health service resources and their access organization and procedures

■   **—Socialization** processes

Economic, social, cultural, and interpersonal influences on human development

The effects of group processes and influences on individual health behavior

The effects on health of religious and spiritual beliefs

■   Personal, interpersonal, and group dynamics

How the interactional processes between groups affect health behaviors

The culture's social psychology of providing and receiving help

Patterns of expression, especially feelings and nonverbal communication

The practitioner's awareness of how emotions and attitudes affect healing relations

Overcoming cultural barriers to clinical competence requires several distinct approaches:

■   A systems approach to understanding the nature of culture

■   Knowledge of the other cultures' health perspectives

■   Assessment of the effects of socialization processes on health and health behaviors

■   Cultural self-awareness, especially regarding health and care values

■   Skills in managing intercultural dynamics

Knowledge of cultural systems and organizational culture is part of the ability to address clients' problems by recognizing economic, political, and other social factors that have effects on well-being and health behaviors. Effectively adapting to others' health behaviors requires knowledge of both their cultural influences and the effects of the provider's culture. These differences can produce conflicts that impede effective cross-cultural relations and clinical communication. Cultural knowledge and intercultural skills together can help overcome these barriers through an accommodation to the cross-cultural realities of clinical care and public health.

Cultural competence levels range from destructiveness (ethnocentrism), incapacity, and blindness through varying degrees of skill represented in the concepts of **cultural awareness, sensitivity, responsiveness, competence**, and **proficiency**. Awareness of cultural differences may be followed by sensitivity in response to them. Competence involves the capability to deal effectively with cultural differences. Proficiency involves the ability to transfer this knowledge and these skills to others. Cultural awareness and sensitivity assist in adapting to other cultures through a knowledge of specific cultural information and the ability to provide culturally responsive care by addressing general barriers to effective cross-cultural relations. The ability to deal with cultural differences begins with overcoming ethnocentrism and developing an awareness of other cultures that leads to an understanding of the more sophisticated skills necessary to adapt effectively to cultural differences and intercultural processes.

Enhancing cultural competence requires the assessment of an individual's level of development and needed skills. A self-assessment is provided here (see Self-Assessment 1.4. Cross-Cultural Development) to help readers to assess their intercultural attitudes, beliefs, behaviors, and accomplishments. Cultural competence requires personal cultural awareness and an understanding of one's own professional culture and its unconscious assumptions, values, and motivations that affect patient relations (see Chapter Three). Learning about the effects of one's culture on health expectations and the medical encounter provides the basis for understanding intercultural conflicts in provider-patient relations and enhancing patient care by providing caregivers and consumers greater knowledge of one another.

Areas of Applied Medical Anthropology

The many different areas of medical anthropology reflect a growing trend of applying cultural knowledge to resolve health problems; a variety of aspects are listed below in "Applications: Areas of Medical Anthropology." Cultural knowledge and intercultural perspectives help facilitate relations among provider cultures, patient cultures, and institutional cultures. Cultural perspectives inform providers regarding how patients, families, and significant others conceptualize health problems and will respond to proposed care. Cultural perspectives enhance effectiveness in clinical practice and community health by enabling changes in professional style, institutional practices, and community behaviors where appropriate. Understanding a patient's personal and social life in relationship to the treatment plan helps ensure effective communication, appropriate resource utilization, and the success of treatments. Culturally sensitive approaches also help patients by helping providers accommodate to patients' concerns with alienation, powerlessness, distress, and despair (Kleinman and Good, 1985). Cultural approaches empower health care consumers by providing perspectives that enable them to respond to interpersonal and institutional aspects of health care.

Medical anthropology addresses interfaces between culture and health in the following ways:

- Training health care providers in cultural sensitivity and competency
- Mediating among the different community segments and between providers and clients
- Researching health threats and responses in a community
- Developing policies and programs to create culturally responsive health programs
- Participating in advocacy and community empowerment to ensure the development of responsive programs

Areas of Medical Anthropology

Public Health

Design primary health care programs and coordinate community development
Develop immunization, family planning, and infant and maternal health programs
Introduce oral rehydration and immunization programs
Develop culturally based drug abuse rehabilitation and prevention programs
Perform health education and preventive medicine
Perform epidemiological studies and community assessments
Provide health policy analysis and advocacy
Supply international health and international medical relief (aid)
Perform health systems integration (traditional and modern)

Physical and Biological Areas

Provide nutritional anthropology: diet, culture, and infant nutrition
Peform genetic anthropology and human genome studies
Perform forensic anthropology, skeletal analysis, and medical examiner work
Study ethnopharmacology and traditional healing practices
Study evolution of the body in relation to disease and healing responses
Create cross-cultural human development
Study culture, drug use, and drug reactions

Clinically Applied Anthropology

As cultural consultants and advisors, and sometimes as therapists, engage in mediation
Serve as advocates, reformers, institutional change agents
Serve as policymakers and program developers
Perform program needs assessment and evaluation
Teach **transcultural** nursing and transcultural psychiatry
Identify culture-based mental disorders and "culture-bound syndromes"
Identify or develop "cultural healing": psychological, social, and mental healing processes
Study cultural anthropology of ethnic health practices
Develop alternative or complementary medicine traditions in the United States

Institutional Analysis and Culture Change

Mediate between different groups and conceptual systems (patients and providers)
Facilitate relations among staff (doctors, nurses, therapists, administrators).
Represent community groups, organizers, advocates, and social reformers
Perform research, assessment, and evaluation
Develop programs and educate staff
Serve as omsbudpersons (patient advocates)
Provide institutional assessment and organizational culture studies
Assess politics and economy of medicine
Enhance provider-client relations

PRACTITIONER PROFILE

Linda M. Whiteford

Linda M. Whiteford, Ph.D., M.P.H., is professor of the Department of Anthropology, University of South Florida. What follows are some of the things a medical anthropologist might do. Whiteford's research has centered on questions of equity and equality, access to resources, health behaviors, and health care policies and, most important, how they intersect.

In the 1980s, Whiteford participated in a nationwide project for the Children's Defense Fund on access to health care for poor children in Tampa, Florida. The research showed that, due to reduced federal funding for health care, no pediatricians would see Medicaid children in their private practices and that poor children were being denied access to health care. Policy was then changed to increase children's access to health programs. The medical anthropological approach of on-site observations, patient and practitioner interviews, and a community-based research team generated both the data and the community support necessary to change access to health care for poor children in Tampa Bay.

For the past ten years, Whiteford has conducted research on health care systems in Cuba and the Dominican Republic, which share geography, environment, history, and populations. But since the Cuban revolution, their health care systems have differed in important ways. Cuban political will translated into successful community-based health care programs, with radical reductions in infant and maternal mortality rates, rates of infectious disease, and the control of outbreaks of dengue fever. The Dominican Republic initially developed an extensive and effective primary health care system in the early 1960s and then, as politics in both the United States and the Dominican Republic changed, that community-based primary health care system was allowed to be replaced with a hospital-based system (see Whiteford and Nixon, 1999).

In 1989 Whiteford coedited (with Poland) *New Approaches to Human Reproduction*, discussing social and ethical issues around the evolving reproductive technologies. In 2000 Whiteford coedited a book on international health in which medical anthropologists from various countries addressed the question of how anthropologists can help level the playing field in international health, a field unleveled by history, geography, and economics. The authors document how anthropological methods and theoretical approaches help us understand what happens when local needs and realities conflict with international health care policies, such as the availability of "super" antibiotics.

CONCEPTS OF HEALTH

Cultural concepts underlie people's health concerns, which involve broader issues than physical disease, including vague sensations; sharp, dull, or punishing pains; a lack of energy; and a loss of harmony involving personal, emotional, social, and spiritual dimensions. From the early work of anthropologists on spirit illness, witchcraft, and other supernatural causes of disease to the later-twentieth-century work on supernatural theories of illness (e.g., Murdock, 1980), cultural beliefs are illustrated as central concerns of healing systems. Cultural perspectives on health as well as contemporary concepts used in public health and community medicine involve broader issues than physical disease.

What Is Health?

Conceptions of what constitutes health vary widely. This book takes Durch and colleagues' (1997) perspective that health involves not only physical, mental, and social well-being but also the ability to participate in everyday activities in family, community, and work, commanding the personal and social resources necessary to adapt to changing circumstances.

Ancient meanings of health implicating the sacred (holy, hallowed) illustrate a broad range of concerns still attested to in contemporary ethnomedical systems: wholeness, morality, wickedness, spiritual crises, soul loss, possession, bewitchment, and other maladies that afflict humans. To some people, health is a general sense of well-being, "feeling good." For others, health includes the expectations that they will not become ill or will be able to recover quickly. For most, health involves the ability to do what they want to do, with one's body not presenting difficulty in normal activities. For some, health has moral connotations, with disease the consequence of immorality. People's prominent concerns

CULTURE AND HEALTH

Etymological Views of Health

These wider concerns of **health** are reflected in ancient root meanings of "heal," "disease," "sickness," and "illness." **Heal** means "To restore to health . . . to set right, amend. . . . To rid of sin, anxiety or the like. . . . To become whole and sound" (*American Heritage Dictionary,* Morris, 1981, p. 607). *Heal* is derived from the Indo-European root *kailo-,* which means "whole," "holy," and "good omen"; Old English derivative forms include "holy," "hallowed," and "whole." *Disease* has its root meaning in "ease" and means a reversal of ease. *Sick,* meaning "ailing, ill, unwell," "mentally ill or disturbed," also refers to suffering or deeply affected by emotions, mental affliction, or corruption. *Sick* is derived from the Indo-European root *seug-,* meaning "troubled" or "sad." The linguistic roots of *ill* in the Middle English *ill(e)* mean "bad" or "sickness of body or mind"; older meanings emphasized evil and wickedness (Morris, 1981, pp. 655–656), still reflected in its use to refer to evil, hostile intentions, wrongdoing, wickedness, sin, and disaster. The responses to health maladies represented in the concepts of medicine and care also reflect broader concerns. *Medicine* derives from the Latin *medicina* and the Indo-European root *med-,* which means "to take appropriate measures." *Cure* means "restoration of health" from the Indo-European root *cûra,* "care" (Morris, 1981, p. 1510). *Cure* also has ecclesiastical or religious significance, meaning "spiritual charge or care of souls, as of a priest for his congregation," from the Medieval Latin *curatus,* "one having spiritual cure or charge" (Morris, 1981, p. 323).

with health generally encompass physical, psychological, emotional, and spiritual dimensions of well-being.

Biomedical concerns with health focused on biological diseases often clash with patients' conceptions, so much so that effective care is impeded. Even doctors and patients from the same culture have different views of health because professional education socializes doctors into a worldview that patients generally do not share. Health is generally poorly understood by physicians because their medical education emphasizes detection, diagnosis, and treatment of disease, rather than health and well-being.

Biomedical Measures of Population Health Standard biomedical measures of health include mortality, the incidence of causes of death, and morbidity, the frequency of disease. There are also positive measures based on population statistics, such as

- *Life expectancy*: The average length of life for members of a specific group

- *Span of healthy life*: Adjusted average life expectancy by subtracting years of poor health

- *Health behaviors*: Acts, activities, and lifestyles that may improve health

- *Reserve health*: Capacity to resist disease and stressors

- *Social support*: Relationships providing physical and emotional support

- *Overall birth rate*: Number of children born per year

- *Population growth rate*: Birth rate divided by death rate

The numbers alone, however, do not directly reveal a population's health. Health implications of fertility must be assessed in relation to the ecological system, the population's resources, and cultural priorities (e.g., population growth, stability, or reduction). A birth rate may be excessive if it will outstrip available resources. A low birth rate may be evidence of poor overall health if the culture values large families.

World Health Organization's Concept of Health The World Health Organization (WHO) characterized health as complete physical, mental, and social well-being and the capability to function in the face of changing circumstances. The WHO also emphasized the "highest possible level of health" that allows people to participate in social life and work productively (World Health Organization, 1992). Health involves social and personal resources in addition to physical conditions; a sense of overall well-being derived from work, family, and community; and other relations, including psychosocial and spiritual (Durch et al., 1997). Some consider the WHO definition to also have problems. Can people be healthy when others suffer from inequality and a lack of resources? What about emotional, spiritual, moral, and metaphysical effects on one's sense of well-being? What about one's sense of ill health from environmental circumstances, war, injustice, and violence? Would it make you feel sick to know that children were being massacred and tortured in a nearby country by extremists? Others' pain can be our own.

Critical Medical Anthropology Concepts of Health Critical medical anthropology adopts perspectives on health that emphasize the importance of access to resources (material and nonmaterial) necessary for sustaining life at a high level of satisfaction. Health is analyzed from the perspectives of the societal factors that affect the distribution of health resources and threats to health (e.g., environmental contamination). Health conditions are affected by political decisions regarding resources for immunizations provided for care, access to care and nutrition, and exposure to environmental conditions and socially produced risks such as poverty and crime. The recognition of health effects in social, economic, and environmental factors force attention to be paid to the interactions of biological and social conditions. Multiple environmental interactions, including a range of economic, social, political, and ideological influences, mold the interactions at the microlevel of interpersonal dynamics of community and family that consequently shape an individual person's physiological conditions.

Public Health Concepts of Health Public health models (see *Healthy Communities 2000: Model Standards* [American Public Health Association, 1991] and the Assessment Protocol for Excellence in Public Health [see Durch et al., 1997]) emphasize community involvement as key to a conceptualization of health. Healthy communities have health institutions that are accountable, incorporating community involvement from planning stages through implementation and evaluation activities (see Chapter Four). Community involvement facilitates incorporation of diverse cultural perspectives on health and the services required. Community health includes services provided (treatment, immunizations) and standard performance measures. Because availability of care is a major aspect of community health, health includes the capacity of the community's health institutions to respond to potential health problems. Responsiveness requires that health institutions understand cultural and social effects on health, incorporate community perspectives on needs and desired services, and assess perceptions of the quality of services.

Cultural and Organizational Concepts of Health The revolution in health care promoted by health maintenance organizations (HMOs) in the United States since the 1980s has emphasized assessment and monitoring of health and perceptions of quality of care. This has required an expansion of the concept of health from the "absence of disease" to views reflecting culturally valued functional abilities and conceptions of well-being. Quality of care is an experience based in patients' personal, social, and cultural expectations and has become a legitimate criterion in the health industry for assessing patient satisfaction and determining how to improve health care (Press, 1997). The organization, values, and roles of providers are cultural phenomena central to the overall quality of care that a patient experiences. The focus on quality and patient experiences provides roles for anthropologists in improving health care by the following measures:

- Determining the culturally based conceptions of what constitutes quality care

- Creating organizational change in health institutions to enhance their ability to provide culturally responsive care

■ Instituting community assessment and organization to guide the development of institutional and personal resources to ensure health

■ Providing staff training in cultural dynamics of interpersonal relations

Improving the quality of care requires the development of cultural measures that reflect community priorities for health and perceptions of well-being. Culture is central to health assessments because culture affects the interpretation of experiences, criteria for normalcy, social expectations, and expectations regarding quality of life. Cultural health concepts include

■ Concepts of desirable physical abilities

■ Views of ideal, normal, and problematic bodily conditions

■ Preferred psychological dynamics, emotional states, and social relations

■ Illness concepts and perceptions of symptoms

■ Spiritual or metaphysical conditions and relations

CULTURE AND HEALTH

Native American Religious Health Beliefs

Religion is important in the traditional indigenous health care systems of Native Americans and their conceptual frameworks of disease. Health issues are not merely biological but are spiritual and religious issues as well. Native American concepts of health as situated in a balance of forces are expressed through the four aspects of the medicine wheel, involving the physical (body), mental (mind), spiritual (soul), and emotional (heart). Illness is the consequence of disharmony and imbalance, rather than just disease; even disease may be the consequence of imbalance. Consequently, healing must address not only symptoms of disease but also the root causes, healing the mind, spirit, and emotions. This religious view of health does not reject the views of biomedicine. Some diseases are considered to be "white man's diseases" and require treatment by physicians. Even disease, however, may require treatment by traditional ceremonies that address the ultimate causes that placed one at risk of disease, taking spiritual actions to restore the personal and social harmony that permits good health. A Native American may receive healing of an illness (spiritual dimension) and experience enhanced health, even if the disease (biological problem) is not cured. This is the power of traditional healing ceremonies that make life more meaningful and balanced, as illustrated in Hammerschlag's (1988) *The Dancing Healers*. In his book *Indian Healing* (1982), the psychiatrist Jilek suggests spiritual concepts as key to indigenous healing rituals and vital to Native Americans' health. These health practices reintegrate their identities, addressing the split in self and the conflicts from being caught in between Native American and European American models of self and well-being. Jilek discusses "spirit illness" as a manifestation of anomic depression, depressive experiences resulting from anomie—the breakdown of societal norms.

Assessing Personal Concepts to Improve Health Health is not merely the absence of disease or distress; it is also a positive state of physical, emotional, mental, personal, and spiritual well-being and a balance with nature and the social world. This notion of health as a relationship between the individual and his or her environment illustrates that what constitutes health differs from person to person and culture to culture. In some cultures, obesity is viewed as unhealthy and low body fat as healthy; for other cultures, it is the reverse: obese people are viewed as healthy and skinny people as sickly. Because perceptions of health are functional and related to the ability to carry out everyday activities, there is both cross-cultural and intracultural (within-culture) variation in the concept of health. People of different educational levels, social classes, and occupations (e.g., warehouse workers versus clerks) have different everyday activities and expectations about well-being. Self-assessments (see Self-Assessment 1.1 for examples) of health beliefs and behaviors provide an enhanced awareness of health concerns that facilitate the work of providers and empower patients. Differences in health conceptions affect the medical consultation process, but providers are often unaware of or ignore these differences, assuming that patients accept the medical view. Ignoring patients' perceptions undermines providers' ability to relate to patients to understand their concerns and to get them to accept treatments. Effective health care requires that practitioners understand patients' perceptions of health so that they can be integrated into treatment. Patients' perspectives are essential for developing prevention services because the recognition of conditions and the use of resources depend on people's perceptions of what constitutes a threat to health.

Awareness of the cultural basis of one's own health beliefs can facilitate relations of providers with patients and vice versa. Awareness by providers that their self-care practices often fall outside the biomedical paradigm can facilitate insight into clients' behaviors and promote empathy between provider and patient. If providers do not conform to the biomedical paradigm—agreeing that there is only biological cause of disease and depending on physicians for care—there is little reason to expect that their clients will. Health concerns can be best understood in relationship to culture. Biomedical views of health based strictly on biology impair understanding of underlying causes of disease that result from social conditions.

SYSTEMS APPROACHES TO HEALTH

Blum (1983) proposed that we need to recognize somatic, social, and psychic dimensions of health. *Somatic health* is based primarily on the functions of a person's bodily systems, *social health* derives from the appropriateness of one's behavior from perspectives of family and social others, and *psychic health* reflects a balance in sociocultural demands and perceptions. Somatic, social, and psychic health may be affected by perturbations in any aspect of the system: by national decisions (such as war), interpersonal relations (such as conflicts), and biological levels (such as bacterial infections). These levels interact, such as when bacterial infections increase because wars destabilize and contaminate ecological systems, or conflict in interpersonal relations causes stress responses and compromised immune systems. The "Practitioner Profile" of Whiteford (above) illustrates how government policies lead to poor children's lack of access to pediatricians. These interactions among many parts of the natural systems are mediated by culture; the complex aspects of these interactions are illustrated through cultural systems models, which detail the many aspects of the physical, social, and cultural environments that affect health and well-being.

Biopsychosocial Model of Health

A **biopsychosocial model** was introduced by Engel (1977, 1980) as a corrective to the biomedical focus on disease as basically a physiological condition. The biopsychosocial model (see Figure 1.1) portrays health as related to both natural and cultural environments,

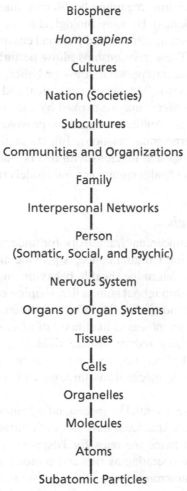

Biosphere

Homo sapiens

Cultures

Nation (Societies)

Subcultures

Communities and Organizations

Family

Interpersonal Networks

Person
(Somatic, Social, and Psychic)

Nervous System

Organs or Organ Systems

Tissues

Cells

Organelles

Molecules

Atoms

Subatomic Particles

FIGURE 1.1. *Biocultural Interactions: Hierarchy of Natural Systems*

Source: Adapted from Engel, 1980, and Brody, 1973.

involving biological as well as psychological, social, and cultural contributions to patients' psychosocial factors and relationships to the health care system. A more inclusive scientific approach to the study of health requires addressing biological, psychological, social, and other cultural determinants that affect health and the physical environment. The biopsychosocial model presupposes many influences on health, including a number of aspects of culture—society, nation, community, and family—that affect biological processes. Addressing psychosocial dynamics also improves provider-patient relations and communication because understanding patients' complaints requires a perspective that links the individual to the social and cultural environments within which conditions are experienced and interpreted.

Human functioning within physical environments, cultural influences, and hierarchical physiological systems enables our health to be affected through influences at levels above us (e.g., political decisions regarding health care funding) or below us (e.g., contaminants absorbed by our lungs). Humans' biological processes operate in relationship to many influences from the social, cultural, and physical environments, causing disruptions of homeostasis (balance). These relationships allow perturbations induced at one level (e.g., discrimination-induced interpersonal stress or beliefs about exposure to germs or threats about terrorist attacks) to affect our psychological and biological well-being. Social stress and its physiological effects may be evoked by social or psychological factors and affect our organs and tissues. Political events may provoke psychological distress—for instance, stress in our interpersonal relations. Effects in the environment, such as the weather, can affect our moods and relations with others—and make our joints hurt! The numerous factors that impact health require general models to organize our considerations of the diverse inputs.

Cultural Systems Models

Culture provides the core conceptual framework for understanding all of human behavior, including health behavior. Cultural concepts provide an important corrective to the prevalent view that biology determines health, behavior, and intergroup differences. The effects of culture are found throughout human life, shaping even biologically based needs such as reproduction, diet, and elimination. Culture affects health through **risk factors**, conditions associated with an increased likelihood of diseases (e.g., smoking), and **protective factors**, behaviors that reduce disease risks (e.g., sexual restrictions such as monogamy). These cultural effects occur within a system of material, social, and mental (belief) relations that provide mechanisms through which cultural effects are basic to health conditions.

Cultural perspectives are essential to understanding ethnic differences in health status. Why, for instance, do African Americans have rates of mortality due to cardiovascular disease (CVD) that are about twice the rates for Hispanic Americans? These differences reflect influences of culture operating as risk and protective factors. African Americans face risks that come from numerous aspects of the environment—physical, social, and cultural. In this book, we explore these cultural dynamics of CVD for African Americans, summarizing at the end of each chapter some of the principal implications derived from the material covered.

Cultural effects on health are part of a system linking the physical environment, social institutions, and biology. Although they also include the physical environment, I refer to these systems as cultural systems models out of recognition that culture shapes our understandings of and interactions with the physical environment, including having effects on the physical environment. Similar cultural systems models have been proposed by physicians, nurses, and public and community health practitioners (Brody, 1973; Engel, 1977, 1980; Blum, 1983; Leininger, 1991, 1995; Baer, Singer, and Johnsen, 1986; Sallis and Owen, 1998), who use cultural systems approaches as conceptual frameworks for addressing health, disease, and care in relationship to the **ecology,** the total physical and social environment. These models also incorporate demographic, technological, economic, political, and other social conditions that affect the physical environment.

To understand the relationships of organisms to their physical environments, cultural systems models are essential because they are mediated through sociocultural systems. Cultural models direct attention to the many conditions that affect health. Cultural systems approaches expand the biopsychosocial perspective in recognizing social factors as fundamental causes of disease. The biopsychosocial approach called attention to the *individual* psychosocial determinants while neglecting the broader *social* factors that are fundamental causes of disease and necessary concerns in prevention efforts.

Cultural systems models help explain the many factors that affect health by illustrating conditions affecting the causes and distributions of disease and the responses of individuals and health care systems. Economic, political, and other social conditions, as well as cultural values, beliefs, and meanings, have active roles in the causation of disease and the allocation of remedies. Cultural beliefs and resources, sickness and healing roles, and the distribution of resources affect an individual's experience of a condition. Cultural beliefs and technological, economic, and political priorities are reflected in treatment. Effectively addressing health requires understanding the structural components of cultural systems and their influences on health. Cultural systems approaches to health examine the interaction of the physical and sociocultural environments. The "environment" is not merely physical but fundamentally cultural, which includes economic, familial, community, class, political, and religious dimensions and their effects on the physical environment.

Physicians, nurses, and public and community health practitioners (Brody, 1973; Engel, 1977, 1980; Blum, 1983; Leininger, 1984; Baer, Singer, and Johnsen, 1986; Sallis and Owen, 1998) have proposed similar systems approaches as conceptual frameworks for addressing health, disease, and care in relationship to the ecology. These models also incorporate demographic, technological, economic, political, and other social conditions that affect the physical environment. Cultural systems perspectives prominent in community health include the "environment of health" or "force-field paradigm" (Blum, 1983; Evans and Stoddart, 1994), which views health as a product of the relationships among many subsystems or fields:

- The physical environment, including sanitation, housing, environmental toxicity, and the physical infrastructure of health care
- The social environment, including family, work, class, education, and social networks

- Persons' individual behavior, especially lifestyle, that links them to the environment
- Medical care services, part of the social environment with a special role in health
- The genetic and biological level

These interdependent fields (or subsystems) affect one another, operating through natural resources, the population and its ecological balance, and cultural systems mediating human interaction with all of the fields: for example, resources, social networks, and medical services. Environmental influences include the reciprocal influences of human impacts on the environment (such as contaminants) and stressors produced by social conditions (such as crime). Lifestyle and behavioral factors affecting health involve many cultural and social dimensions, including risk behaviors, social support, and individual activities. The multiple determinants of health and their dynamic relationships illustrate that health is not strictly a function of disease, biology, or genetics but rather their complex interaction with social, economic, political, and other cultural conditions that produce the individual's behavior and biological conditions. Blum (1983) emphasized hereditary forces as last in order of relative importance for health and the environment, including physical, economic, and social dimensions, as having the greatest impacts on health.

Public health models of health (Sallis and Owen, 1998) emphasize the need to address interrelated levels, including the intrapersonal (psychological), interpersonal (primary groups, especially family), and institutions in community and society. For example, effective programs for improving health must address a spectrum of levels, going beyond personal and interpersonal approaches in identifying how cultural and ecological factors interact in producing influences on health.

Systems perspectives are important because health behavior is not merely a function of microlevel interpersonal interactions of family and community; they are also affected by our mesosystems linkages between our microlevel interpersonal relations and the macrolevel resources such as political power and societal resources that affect health. Does your family know how to obtain welfare, disability payments, or food assistance? These are mesolevel linkages to resources provided at the macrolevel by governments. Do you know how to obtain scholarships and grants to pay for medical school? These, too, are mesolevel linkages. Cultural approaches to health emphasize the necessity to direct interventions at the various environments that influence health and risk behaviors. Health problems created by ecological conditions such as air pollution and poverty cannot be eradicated in the clinical setting but only by altering those macrosystem conditions.

Clinical services are not passive agents affecting health but resources mediated by economic and political factors, especially health policies (e.g., who gets to receive federal funding for health services: individuals or only local governments and hospitals?). When there is government funding for public health, who are the real beneficiaries, the poor who receive free immunizations or the stockholders of the companies who may receive millions or even billions of dollars for providing the vaccines? Political effects on health are revealed in the enormously greater public investment in hospitals and biomedicine versus public health activities and community health centers that can more directly affect the occurrence of disease. Public health approaches are more cost-effective in preventing disease, with systemic interventions such as public service announcements or free clinics affecting a large population, rather than the individuals seen in clinical treatment. Public health interventions directed at groups and communities require culturally informed approaches that use information on the environment, community dynamics, health resources, and social networks.

Sociocultural Theories of Disease

How does culture produce health consequences? In medical anthropology, explanations of the cultural effects on health have emphasized three basic theoretical approaches that supplement the biomedical approach:

- Medical ecology theories concerned with interactions with the ecology, the total environment affecting human adaptation, using human genetics and group behavior as principal levels of explanation

- Political economy and critical medical anthropology approaches that show how social relations, economic resources, and power are determinants of disease and disease outcomes through producing risks and distributing resources

- Cultural theories concerned with how beliefs, values, and customs are determinants of disease, operating through symbolic processes that have effects on biological levels

These three approaches are all concerned with the impacts of culture on biology, as illustrated in Hahn's (1995) discussion of mediation, production, and construction models of sociocultural disease causation.

Mediation Mediation approaches reflect perspectives similar to the biopsychosocial approach, emphasizing how sociocultural factors affect people's exposure to pathogens. Mediation models of sociocultural influences on health are partially recognized in biomedicine, manifested in the concern with health influences of lifestyle and personal habits (e.g., effects of diet, drugs, and sex on health). Mediation models view sociocultural effects on health as the differential distribution of the population with respect to the environment, risk factors, economic resources, occupational hazards, social activities, and other conditions that produce diseases and provide resources to ameliorate their effects. Cultural behaviors and social conditions affect exposure to pathogens and access to treatments, differentially affecting the well-being of different segments of the population (e.g., poor versus rich). These medical anthropology approaches are exemplified in the medical ecology perspectives presented in Chapter Seven.

Production Production perspectives emphasize how social conditions produce health maladies through the distribution of risks and resources and by social and symbolic effects on biology. Production perspectives recognize a stronger cultural determination of health in its potential to cause biological disorder. Cultural practices such as contamination, work conditions, drug use, and unsafe sex directly cause disease. Culture directly affects biological processes through psychosomatic reactions, social stress precipitating the disruption of cardiac function, and social conditions (e.g., industrial waste, traffic, and labor accidents). Hahn suggests that the "production" model is ridiculed in biomedicine because it is seriously misunderstood and contradicts biomedicine's model of biological determinism. Production perspectives challenge the traditional biomedical paradigm by showing the social and mental effects on physiological processes. Cultural influences provide more than just mediation of people with respect to risks: "sociocultural effects are causal in the same way that environmental carcinogens, toxins, and bacterial and viral pathogens are" (Hahn, 1995, p. 76). The placebo phenomena exemplify the cultural production of biological responses (see Chapter Eight).

Construction   Construction approaches elucidate that a culture constructs how its members think about health conditions and their social, moral, and cosmological implications and, consequently, constructs their experience of health maladies. Construction perspectives emphasize that culture affects health, illustrated in the relationship of symptom recognition to cultural values and social norms. Cultural criteria determine whether a given condition is construed as a disease or is viewed as falling within normal human variation. This cultural determination also occurs in the activities of biomedical practitioners who define relevant symptoms and interpret them. Culture is the basis of this "social labeling," where diagnosis involves a social process in which individuals are given disease labels. Ethnomedicines produce cultural realities of health by providing models of what diseases exist and their significance, causes, and available treatments. Construction approaches may also present models similar to production perspectives, noting that people's beliefs can have physiological consequences, as discussed in Chapter Nine.

The different approaches to the relationship of culture to health also reflect theoretical and practical differences among medical anthropology. Should health be primarily concerned with addressing biological conditions? Or should we address the political and economic forces that produce contamination, food shortages, and available services, conditions that affect health? Should alternative medicine practices be accepted as equal in efficacy to biomedicine, or should they be opposed as outdated superstitions? Should medical anthropology help physicians with cross-cultural competency skills, or should they help patients develop an understanding of the politics of medicine to better resist medicine's political control? Despite their differences, the various approaches all use concepts of cultural systems and systems models with multiple domains to assess the many factors affecting disease and health.

SUMMARY

Cultural systems models provide integrative cross-disciplinary approaches to understanding the multiple factors affecting health. These synthetic approaches are used in all health professions. Cultural systems models that detail the many factors affecting health are discussed in Chapter Four. An extensive model focusing on the more specific dynamics of specific health problems is provided in Chapter Four's "Rapid Assessment, Response,

BIOCULTURAL INTERACTIONS

African American CVD in System Perspective

The higher CVD risks of African Americans can be seen as the outcome of all of the sociocultural models of disease. Environmental factors mediate CVD through increased high-risk behaviors such as stress, poor diet, alcoholism, and cigarette smoking. Racism, discrimination, and poverty produce CVD through stress, unequal distribution of health resources, and the fast-food industry that saturates inner-city areas. Cultural beliefs construct health beliefs and illness behaviors that affect how CVD is recognized and addressed through traditional ethnomedical systems. To use the force-field model, although genetics may play an important role in African Americans' higher rates of CVD, there are important influences in the physical environment and ecology, socially and culturally induced lifestyle patterns, influences in the social environment, and the quality and nature of medical care services.

When the multiple factors contributing to high levels of CVD in African Americans are examined, it quickly becomes clear why a cultural systems model is necessary. Factors affecting the manifestation of CVD begin with the general ecological system, where a dangerous inner-city environment increases stress and inhibits exercise, an important protective factor in CVD. There are further risk factors derived from diet, both traditional "soul food" and fast foods. Treatment utilization is affected by family, community, and religious self-care practices, which often preclude timely care. The lack of care caused by poverty, lack of education, and insufficient public care facilities all contribute to increased risks. Political factors further compound risks by neglecting public education programs, reinforcing feelings of racism that increase stress. The health beliefs may also complicate CVD problems, with the concepts about dietary treatment of "high-pertension" conflicting with medical advice regarding diet. We will explore these and other interacting factors further in the following chapters.

and Evaluation (RARE)" modules. Additional models are also provided in Chapter Six in the coverage of the psychocultural model. Effective adaptations to cultural differences require more than understandings of the structural models of culture.

CHAPTER SUMMARY

This book provides the basis for developing a cultural competency approach to health and health care. Health care providers, helping professionals, anthropology students, and consumers can all benefit from the basic understanding of how cultural processes affect health. Medical anthropology contributes to biomedicine and the study of health through an integrative study of humans across their physical, behavioral, social, and cultural dimensions. Anthropology's interdisciplinary biological and cultural approaches have practical applications in medicine, nursing, public health, community health, psychology,

PRACTITIONER PROFILE

Edward C. Green

Edward C. Green, Ph.D., is director of the AIDS Prevention Research Project at the Harvard Center for Population and Development Studies. He has worked for a number of international development or health organizations or agencies over the past thirty years, much of the time as an independent consultant based in Washington, D.C. Most of his work has been in Africa, but assignments or research have also taken him to Asia, Latin America and the Caribbean, eastern Europe, and the Middle East, adding up to about forty countries. He worked as an applied medical anthropologist for the ministries of health in both Mozambique and Swaziland. Much of his work since the 1980s has been in AIDS and STDs. He is currently involved in AIDS-related behavioral studies in Uganda and South Africa. Green has been a pioneer in integrating indigenous African and Western biomedical health systems and in promoting evidence-based AIDS prevention.

In addition, Green has worked in family planning including contraceptive social marketing, primary health care, maternal and child health, psychosocial issues of children affected by war, child nutrition, potable water and sanitation programs, environmental health, U.S. minority health issues, and biodiversity conservation. He believes that anthropologists are able to move among specialties and cultural areas more easily than those trained in other disciplines due largely to the holistic nature of anthropology and the steady demand for qualitative and survey research skills and experience.

Of Green's six books, *Rethinking AIDS Prevention* (2003) has had the most impact on global AIDS policy. He argues that the "generalized" epidemics of Africa are fundamentally different from all other HIV epidemics and that prevention requires reduction in multiple and concurrent sexual partnerships and cannot be left to technology transfer alone. He has debated this issue in Congress, on radio and television, in public debates, op-eds in leading newspapers, and on advisory councils (Presidential and National Institutes of Health).

and other disciplines. Health professionals need cultural perspectives because of multicultural societies' diverse health practices and the cultural differences between providers and the population at large. Cultural approaches contribute to the scientific concerns of biomedicine by providing culturally specific knowledge and cross-cultural perspectives. The basic ethnographic methods of cultural anthropology provide the "other's" perspective and a basis for understanding health beliefs and behaviors and their consequences for health. Anthropology also provides cross-cultural approaches that help establish perspectives, exemplified in transcultural psychiatry and nursing, that apply to all humans.

Health care practitioners need to understand cultural effects on health to improve relations between providers and clients. A major challenge facing biomedicine is people's behavior—compliance or patient adoption of medical recommendations—whether it involves changing risk behaviors, acceptance of public health directives, or adherence to treatment plans. To address biomedicine's alarmingly high rate of nonadoption by patients of doctors' clinical recommendations (20 percent to more than 80 percent), effective relationships and communication need to be established between providers and clients. This requires an understanding of the patients' models of health and skills in negotiating between doctor and patient perspectives. Anthropology can enhance the effectiveness of biomedicine in helping to address patients' cultural concerns, perspectives that providers need to understand to achieve patient satisfaction and ensure treatment compliance. Cultural perspectives provide a range of clinical benefits, including accurate assessment, appropriate communications, and institutional goals such as reduced patient alienation and litigation and increased satisfaction.

Medical anthropology addresses concerns of the public, enhancing patients' care by improving providers' ability to provide effective care. Medical anthropology also increases the public's understanding of the cultural and political dynamics of health and engages in advocacy on behalf of those less able to secure needed resources and in regard to encouraging society to adopt educational approaches to empower consumers. Medical anthropology's studies of health and healing give both providers and patients an enhanced understanding of healing processes. A principal anthropological insight involves the effects of culture on physiological processes. Anthropology illustrates culture's role in shaping the organism's response to disease, providing a new paradigm for health that is more encompassing than the biomedical paradigm's emphasis on physiological causation. Medical anthropology integrates environmental, biological, interpersonal, political-economic, and symbolic perspectives in a cultural systems model that helps explain health effects and behavior.

Knowledge of cultural systems' effects on health and health care enhances the effectiveness of providers and empowers patients because culture provides the foundation for all health and health behaviors. Recognition of those cultural dynamics enables practitioners to enhance relations with diverse client groups, reducing the difficulties presented by cultural differences and enhancing the well-being of both providers and clients. Knowledge of the cultural, social, and political dimensions of health and health care can empower both professionals and consumers. These models allow them to address the systemic cultural effects on health; in addition, they provide cultural perspectives in training, research, community empowerment, and organizational change. Anthropology's perspectives provide a basis from which to understand

- Cultural effects on the conceptualization of health problems (Chapter Two)

- Cross-cultural relationship and communication skills for clinical consultation (Chapter Three)

- Cultural systems models for addressing diverse impacts on health (Chapter Four)

- Cultural effects on health behaviors and utilization (Chapter Five)

- Cultural effects on psychological normalcy, development, and identity (Chapter Six)

- Cultural-ecological perspectives on the evolutionary basis of health problems in interaction with the current environment (Chapter Seven)

■ Critical social perspectives on the ways in which economic and political factors affect health (Chapter Eight)

■ Interdisciplinary understanding of the ways in which cultural beliefs have effects on physiological processes (Chapter Nine)

■ Ethnomedical models of healing processes, such as shamanism, that expand our conceptual frameworks beyond the mechanisms typically addressed in biomedicine (Chapter Ten)

KEY TERMS

Biomedicine	Emic
Biopsychosocial model	Ethnography
Capitalist medicine	Ethnomedicine
Competence	Etic
Culture	Macrolevel
Cultural awareness	Microlevel
Cultural competence	Morbidity
Cultural proficiency	Mortality
Cultural sensitivity	Protective factors
Cultural systems model	Psychoneuroimmunology
Culture	Risk factors
Ecology	Socialized medicine

SELF-ASSESSMENT 1.1. PERSONAL HEALTH ASSESSMENT

How do you personally define health?

What does it mean to you to be healthy?

What do you do to maintain your health?

What are some of the values you associate with health?

What personal values or failures do you associate with having health problems?

How are your health values related to your culture's values in general?

Do your values help or hurt your health?

Are there specific diseases that have a moral quality to them?

What are some of the things you do to reestablish your health when you have problems?

Have you ever used an alternative or complementary treatment? What was it and for what condition? What was the outcome?

SELF-ASSESSMENT 1.2. MINORITY HEALTH CULTURE ASSESSMENT

Using the above questions, interview one or more people from a minority, ethnic, or foreign culture, preferably someone with a traditional cultural orientation.

How is their cultural background reflected in their responses?
What are major differences in their responses from your own?
How could their health culture affect relationships with biomedical practitioners?

SELF-ASSESSMENT 1.3. CULTURAL DYNAMICS OF HEALTH

What are some of the physical and environmental conditions in your community that affect health status? For the better? For the worse?

What are some of the social conditions in your community that affect health status? For the better? For the worse?

What are some of the ideological conditions (beliefs and attitudes) in your community that affect health status? For the better? For the worse?

SELF-ASSESSMENT 1.4. CROSS-CULTURAL DEVELOPMENT

Respond to how you feel about each of the following statements by circling **No** (=0) or **Yes** (=1). See Exhibit 1.1 for the scoring. After you have assessed your responses on the scales provided, read more about them in Chapter Three.

1. **No Yes**   I am just a normal person, without any special cultural identity or characteristics.

2. **No Yes**   My principal characteristics as a person reflect basic aspects of human nature.

3. **No Yes**   Immigrants to the United States should be expected to keep their own values and customs.

4. **No Yes**   People of a racial group are generally all basically the same.

5. **No Yes**   True Americans are all basically the same.

6. **No Yes**   My cultural group is superior to most other cultures.

7. **No Yes**   My basic values and beliefs are based in ethnocentrism and prejudice.

8. **No Yes**   The government should control minority groups for their own good.

9. **No Yes**   There is only one correct way to behave if you are going to live in the United States.

10. **No Yes**   Cultures that do not have Christian values are basically immoral.

11. **No Yes**   It would be better if people of different ethnic groups kept to themselves.

12. **No Yes**   I would prefer to live in a community where foreigners are not allowed.

13. **No Yes**   I think that we should treat everybody the same.

14. **No Yes**   Minority groups would be better off if they "melted in" like everybody else.

15.   **No**   Yes   I feel that we would be better off if we practiced color blindness.

16.   **No**   Yes   People from minority groups are poorer because of societal prejudice and discrimination.

17.   **No**   Yes   People of specific races are all basically the same.

18.   **No**   Yes   Differences in personal success generally result from different opportunities in life.

19.   **No**   Yes   I think that religious punishments should be outlawed everywhere.

20.   **No**   Yes   Cultural background basically determines the way that people behave.

21.   **No**   Yes   Cultural differences are less important than humans' biological commonalities.

22.   **No**   Yes   Despite cultural differences, all human behavior is governed by the same principles.

23.   **No**   Yes   There is only one true god who evaluates the morality of humans' behavior.

24.   **No**   Yes   I am comfortable attending religious services of faiths other than my own.

25.   **No**   Yes   What is normal behavior differs from one culture to another.

26.   **No**   Yes   Other cultures' ways of behaving are as valid and legitimate as my own.

27.   **No**   Yes   Politicians need to pass laws to help ensure that foreigners do not change our country.

28.   **No**   Yes   It is dishonest when ethnic minorities try to act as if they are like other Americans.

29.   **No**   Yes   Everyone should have to learn about the cultures of American minority groups.

30.   **No**   Yes   I behave in different ways depending on whom I am with.

31.   **No**   Yes   Islam is just as moral as Christianity or Buddhism.

32.   **No**   Yes   People who practice animal sacrifice as part of their religion should be put in jail.

33.   **No**   Yes   Cultures in which people eat dogs and cats are really evil.

34.   **No**   Yes   Other cultures' values are as worthy of respect and tolerance as my own values.

35.   **No**   Yes   There are no universal standards for evaluating what is right or wrong.

36.   **No**   Yes   Americans would be better off if we adopted some practices from other cultural groups.

37. **No Yes** In Muslim cultures, women should generally appear in public only with their faces covered.

38. **No Yes** I have been able to show that I can view reality from the perspective of another culture.

39. **No Yes** There are many different cultural definitions of reality and morality that are equally valid.

40. **No Yes** It is important to me to be able to speak more than one language.

41. **No Yes** I have incorporated aspects of other cultures into my life and behavior.

42. **No Yes** I have established close friendships with people from other cultures.

43. **No Yes** You can relate better if you know a person's age, racial identity, education, and social class.

44. **No Yes** My culture makes me really different from the people with whom I regularly associate.

45. **No Yes** I do not identify with the traditions of my parents and grandparents.

46. **No Yes** I would be embarrassed if my friends found out about the cultural background of my family.

47. **No Yes** I feel like I have a split personality, that I am a different person at home than I am at work or school.

48. **No Yes** Some aspects of my parents' or grandparents' culture embarrass me.

49. **No Yes** Sometimes I feel like there are two different cultures fighting inside me.

50. **No Yes** I sometimes feel like I am putting on an act to fit in with others.

51. **No Yes** I feel more comfortable when I am with people from a culture different from my own.

52. **No Yes** I use the language and cultural behaviors in everyday life of groups other than my birth culture.

53. **No Yes** People in another cultural group have adopted me, considering me to be their own.

54. **No Yes** I can feel totally comfortable being in a culture different from my birth culture.

55. **No Yes** I can feel like a totally different person when I am with people of a different culture.

56. **No Yes** The way in which I evaluate a situation and behave depends on who is involved.

57. **No Yes** There is no objectivity; I create my own reality.

58.   **No   Yes**   I do not adhere to the values and beliefs of any one culture.

59.   **No   Yes**   Whether or not something is immoral depends on the situation and who does it.

60.   **No   Yes**   Who I am depends on whom I am with.

61.   **No   Yes**   Clients should be required to use English when seeking social services.

62.   **No   Yes**   Services provided by employees of public agencies should always be provided in English only.

63.   **No   Yes**   I am able to work effectively with clients from a cultural group different from my own.

64.   **No   Yes**   Policies of social work agencies ought to reflect the expectations of the cultural groups they serve.

65.   **No   Yes**   Public agencies should use the same procedures for dealing with clients of all ethnic groups.

66.   **No   Yes**   Public service organizations should be required to hire personnel at all levels of the organization that reflect the ethnicity and culture of the community.

67.   **No   Yes**   I have solicited suggestions from community groups on how to improve my professional practice.

68.   **No   Yes**   Public agencies should support the alternative health services in their communities.

69.   **No   Yes**   Community groups ought to have a say in the policy and practices of social service organizations.

70.   **No   Yes**   Social service agencies should have advisory and review boards that include representatives from all of the major ethnic groups in their service area.

71.   **No   Yes**   Public agencies should translate written materials into the major languages of their community.

72.   **No   Yes**   Social service agencies should provide services in the language most comfortable to their clients.

73.   **No   Yes**   I engage in activities to make sure the rights of minority groups are protected from discrimination.

74.   **No   Yes**   Developing cultural sensitivity in staff is the responsibility of government organizations.

75.   **No   Yes**   I have trained people to use knowledge of culture to understand others, communicate empathy, and use relevant skills in working with people from another culture.

EXHIBIT 1.1. **Self-Assessment 1.4 Scoring: Cross-Cultural Development**

For each answer on your self-assessment, assign the value of 0 for **No** and 1 for **Yes**. Write the answer (0 or 1) to each question in the space beside the question number. Add up the totals of your answers for each line, convert your answers where instructed, and add the subtotals for an overall score for each scale.

Scale N = N1 + N2 = _____ (range 0 to 12) **Normal/Ethnocentric:** higher values indicate higher levels of ethnocentrism

N1 = 1. ___ + 2. ___ + 4. ___ + 5. ___ + 6. ___ + 8. ___ + 9. ___ + 10. ___ + 11. ___ + 12. ___ = _____ (N1)
N2 = 3. ___ + 7. ___ = ___*   *If 0, N2 = 2; if 1, N2 = 1; if 2, N2 = 0   + _____ (N2)
                                                                          = _____ N

Scale U = U1 + U2 = _____ (range 0 to 11) **Universalism:** higher values indicate universalist assumptions rather than recognition of the importance of cultural principles

U1 = 13. ___ + 14. ___ + 15. ___ + 17. ___ + 19. ___ + 21. ___ + 22. ___ + 23. ___   = _____ (U1)
U2 = 16. ___ + 18. ___ + 20. ___ = ___   *If 0, U2 = 3; if 1, U2 = 2; if 2, U2 = 1; If 3, U2 = 0
                                                                          + _____ (U2)
                                                                          = _____ U

Scale AC = B + V = _____ (range 0 to 12) **Acceptance:** higher values indicate higher levels of acceptance of other cultures

B1 = 24. ___ + 25. ___ + 26. ___ + 29. ___ + 30. ___   = _____ (B1)
B2 = 27. ___ + 28. ___*   *If 0, B2 = 2; if 1, B2 = 1; if 2, B2 = 0   + _____ (B2)
V1 = 31. ___ + 34. ___ + 35. ___ =   + _____ (V1)
V2 = −32. ___ + 33. ___*   *If 0, V2 = 2; if 1, V2 = 1; if 2, V2 = 0   + _____ (V2)
                                                                          = _____ AC

Scale AD = E + P = _____ (range 0 to 8) **Adaptation:** higher values indicate higher levels of adaptation to other cultures

E = 36. ___ + 37. ___ + 38. ___ + 39. ___   = _____ E
P = 40. ___ + 41. ___ + 42. ___ + 43. ___   + _____ P
                                                                          = _____ AD

Scale C = C1 + C2 + I = _____ (range 0 to 10) **Cultural Competence:** higher values indicate higher levels of cultural competence

C1 = 63. ___ + 64. ___   = _____ (C1)
C2 = 61. ___ + 62. ___ + 65. ___*   *If 0, C2 = 3; if 1, C2 = 2; if 2, C2 = 1; if 3, C2 = 0 + _____ (C2)
                                                                          + _____ (I)
                                                                          = _____ C

Scale M = _____ (range 0 to 8) **Marginalized:** higher values indicate higher levels of experiencing a *marginalized* biculturalism

M = 44. ___ + 45. ___ + 46. ___ + 47. ___ + 48. ___ + 49. ___ + 50. ___ + 51. ___   = _____ M

Scale B = B1 + M = _____ (range 0 to 12) **Bicultural:** higher values indicate higher levels of biculturalism
B1 = 52. ___ + 53. ___ + 54. ___ + 55.   = _____ (B1)
                                                                          + _____ (M)
                                                                          = _____ B

Scale I = _____ (range 0 to 5) **Integrated:** higher values indicate higher levels of ethnorelativism
I = 56. ___ + 57. ___ + 58. ___ + 59. ___ + 60. ___   = _____ I

Scale P (range 0 to 10) **Cultural Proficiency:** higher values indicate higher levels of cultural proficiency
P = 66. ___ + 67. ___ + 68. ___ + 69. ___ + 70. ___ + 71. ___ + 72. ___ + 73. ___ + 74. ___ + 75. ___
                                                                          = _____ P

ADDITIONAL RESOURCES

Books

Albrecht, G. L., R. Fitzpatrick, S. C. Scrimshaw. 2000. *Handbook of social studies in health and medicine.* London: Sage.

Henderson, G. E., N. M. P. King, R. P. Strauss, S. E. Estroff, and L. R. Churchill. 1997. *The social medicine reader.* Durham, N.C., and London: Duke University Press.

Jamner, M. S., and D. Stokols, eds. 2000. *Promoting human wellness: New frontiers for research, practice, and policy.* Berkeley: University of California Press.

Kahssay, H. M., M. E. Taylor, and P. A. Berman. 1998. *Community health workers: The way forward.* Geneva: World Health Organization.

Reid, R., and S. Traweek, eds. 2000. *Doing science + culture: How cultural and interdisciplinary studies are changing the way we look at science and medicine.* New York/London: Routledge.

Journals

Anthropology and Medicine
Medical Anthropology
Medical Anthropology Quarterly

Web Sites

Medical Anthropology: http://www.medanthro.net
National Institutes of Health (NIH): http://www.nih.gov

CHAPTER 2

DISEASE, ILLNESS, SICKNESS, AND THE SICK ROLE

Illness, an individual's perception of a medical problem, sickness,
the social construction of a condition of illness, [and] disease . . .
what exists from a physical/organic standpoint
—FÁBREGA, 1997, P. 3

LEARNING OBJECTIVES

■ Distinguish concepts of health maladies: disease, illness and sickness, and the sick role
■ Show the limitations of biological explanations and the biomedical concept of disease
■ Illustrate the importance of the concepts of illness as personal experiences of health maladies and sickness as the socially induced aspects of maladies
■ Illustrate sick-role consequences, how social expectations influence the experience as a malady
■ Demonstrate the clinical and public health relevance of cultural illness and sickness concepts
■ Illustrate dimensions of disease, illness, and the sick role with HIV and AIDS
■ Present the health belief and explanatory models as approaches for mediating across different conceptions of health maladies

EXPERIENCE OF MALADIES

There is often a disconnection between the experience of a health problem and the determination of its cause and appropriate treatment. Perhaps you have felt ill, but your doctor couldn't find any recognized disease. Or perhaps someone has told you that you are "not really sick," refusing to validate that you truly felt bad. Maybe you know someone who often misses work because of a previous injury, even though they recovered some time ago. Feeling bad, having others accept our claims, and having a doctor's diagnosis of a disease do not always co-occur. This is because of fundamentally different ways of conceptualizing the nature of threats to our health and well-being.

This chapter looks at different conceptions of the conditions that afflict human health and how to mediate between them. Threats to health are discussed as a **malady**, an umbrella term for unwanted health conditions that encompasses many concerns about compromised well-being. Many things cause health maladies: "germs" such as bacteria, virus, and fungi; our behaviors, such as smoking, drinking, and overeating; our psychological concerns, such as worries, depression, and anxiety; and even others' behaviors, such as assaults or vehicular manslaughter. Different kinds of maladies such as **disease, illness,** and **sickness** are considered synonyms in English, but there are important distinctions among them in medical anthropology. Biomedicine views *disease* as a biological problem involving abnormality in the body's structure, chemistry, or functions. *Illness* refers to a patient's experience of something wrong, a sense of disruption in well-being that may be the result of disease or caused by cultural beliefs (such as feeling that you are "too fat" or being persecuted by witches, UFOs, or the CIA). The distinction of *sickness* focuses on consequences of social responses to a person, for instance, his or her personal experiences when shunned for having AIDS or being obese. The *sick role* focuses on social expectations for the behaviors of a person diagnosed as suffering from a malady, for instance, being excused from work or school.

Concepts of disease, illness, and sickness reflect differences among medical, personal, and social realities. These differences illustrate the importance of cross-cultural perspectives in understanding health concerns. Biomedicine tends to view our health problems as primarily based in biology. The perspectives of medical anthropology illustrate the health effects of personal, cultural, and social influences. These influences place limitations on the biological assumptions associated with disease, as illustrated in case studies of leprosy, cardiac arrest, epilepsy, depression, and mental retardation that reveal the fundamental roles of culture in their causes and consequences.

Medical anthropology emphasizes social constructivist approaches to understanding health problems, illustrating the roles of social and cultural processes in defining, interpreting, and responding to maladies. Illness and sickness concepts show the importance of understanding personal experiences of malady and the consequences of social responses for our sense of well-being. Illness—the personal experience of a problem in well-being—involves much more than disease. Even biologically based diseases such as leprosy have their impacts largely shaped through social responses. Experiences of disease are manifested through culturally based concepts because they shape the perceptions of the significance of a condition that affect an individual's treatment-seeking and responses to diagnosis and treatment. The consequences of culture for disease are also seen in the social responses to health problems that are represented in the concept of the sick role: social expectations about how a person with a specific malady should be treated.

CASE STUDY

Disease and Illness

The problems that occurred in the case of infant Lia Lee resulted from differences between biomedicine and Hmong culture in the understanding of Lia's health condition. Differences between what doctors recognize as disease and what people recognize as illness often underlie miscommunication and lack of compliance with medical recommendations. Lia's doctors were trying to treat a disease they called epilepsy, while her family was concerned with an illness resulting from a "lost soul."

The Hmong believe the life-soul, particularly that of babies, can be stolen by the spirits, wander off, or become separated by being startled by a loud noise or through anger, grief, or fear. Loss of the life-soul can lead to loss of consciousness. Lia's parents believed she lost her soul when it was startled and fled when her sister loudly slammed the door. Jerking and twitching with her eyes rolled back, Lia had fainted, symptoms of a condition the Hmong call *quab dab peg*, its meaning giving the title to Anne Fadiman's book: "the spirit catches you, and you fall down."

The Hmong-English dictionary translates quab dab peg as epilepsy, but to the Hmong it is interpreted as a divine calling, that a spirit with healing potentials has taken up an abode in the person. Lia evidenced this in her increasingly lengthy convulsions and periods of unconsciousness. Such symptoms indicate that one has a call to follow the vocation of a healer who can control the spirits that affect health. Thus, the condition that afflicted Lia, while a source of concern, was also something that bestowed honor and distinction, potentially a blessing that could lead to her becoming a respected healer. But to the doctors, it was a severe medical condition, one that could be seen in the abnormal electrical activity that spread across her brain with increasing frequency. Their efforts to identify its "real" cause left the physicians frustrated, a seizure without known etiology (cause). Ultimately, one of her physicians offered that the final near-fatal convulsion that left her in a vegetative state was septic shock caused by a bacillus she was infected with in the hospital. The drugs that treated her epilepsy had the side effect of compromising her immune system, thus increasing her susceptibility to infection.

The ways in which Lia's parents and the Hmong community viewed her condition (a potential blessing of spirit powers) and her medications (something that caused her problems) were never recognized by the physicians. Consequently, there were serious problems in convincing her parents to provide her with the medications her doctors thought were essential for her recovery. An effort to apply state-of-the-art medical treatment—a complex combination of changing medicines—was beyond the capacity of Lia's illiterate parents. Disease could not be treated because the distance between the doctor's conceptions and the family's beliefs and understandings was too great.

This case illustrates the consequences of differences in biomedical and cultural views of a malady. A coma-inducing seizure was not the necessary outcome of the cultural differences between the physicians and the Hmong. Medical anthropology offers tools that could have enabled providers to recognize the differences and negotiate between worldviews by eliciting the explanatory model of Lia's family. A mediator could have helped identify her problems in ways that would have ensured Lia's adequate care and well-being, instead of leading to misunderstanding that left her in a comatose state.

The conditions of AIDS and a positive status for the human immunodeficiency virus (HIV) are used to illustrate these dimensions of disease, illness, and sickness and the role of social factors in the transmission and control of HIV. These distinctions enable providers to better address the range of patients' health conditions and manage their concerns with effective and culturally sensitive health care. The **health belief model** and **explanatory model** are introduced as frameworks for health providers to use in discovering patients' illness beliefs and their cultural expectations regarding the malady and its treatment. Self-assessment tools at the end of this chapter provide you the opportunity to examine your personal and cultural health and illness beliefs.

BIOMEDICAL ASSUMPTIONS ABOUT DISEASE

Biomedicine, also referred to as allopathic ("against symptoms"), Western, and scientific medicine, views maladies primarily as disease, which is understood as biological abnormalities in the body's structures, chemistry, or functions (Eisenberg, 1977; Hahn, 1995). Some specialties within biomedicine, such as psychiatry, do use psychological, behavioral, and social models of maladies. However, biology is the dominant model embodied in both the *Diagnostic and Statistical Manual of Mental Disorders* (DSM) (American Psychiatric Association, 1994), the official diagnostic manual of psychiatry and psychology, and the International Classification of Disease (ICD; World Health Organization, 2000), the official diagnostic manual of physical medicine. Most of the DSM models have assumed that mental health problems are primarily the consequences of abnormalities in biology, particularly neurotransmitter levels, which biomedicine attempts to modify with medications. This assumption of biological disease is so deeply engrained in the thinking of most health professionals that they consider the biomedical views to encompass the valid perspectives on the causation of human maladies.

Basic biomedical assumptions regarding disease include the following:

- Diseases are basically biological and are indicated in the departure from normal measures of biological functioning

- The generic conception of diseases is reflected in a universally valid system of classification

- The belief that each disease derives from a specific physical cause or etiology

- The belief that medical practice is culture-free and scientifically neutral and objective

However, an examination of specific diseases and their associated consequences illustrates the limitations of these assumptions and reveals the fundamental roles of culture even in the biological consequences of diseases.

Biological and Cultural Aspects of Disease

Biomedicine has accustomed us to thinking of health problems as involving basically diseases or genetic problems for which medicines and surgeries are the most appropriate responses. When we examine the actual causes of death (mortality) in the United States, we find that the data point not to biology but to culture, patterns of human behavior, as the fundamental factor underlying the leading causes of death. Table 2.1 illustrates the leading causes of mortality for the United States as a whole by gender and for the different major ethnic groups used by the U.S. government to categorize cultural differences in the population. It shows that the five leading causes of death for all Americans in 2004 were heart diseases, cancers, CVDs (strokes), chronic respiratory tract diseases, and unintentional injuries (accidents).

These principal causes of mortality are not strictly biological diseases in the sense of bacteria or viruses or genetically caused physiological dysfunctions. Rather, these conditions are the result of many social influences on normal biological development, including some that have fundamental causal roles in producing the pathology. Conditions such as lung cancer, CVD, automobile accidents, and liver disease may be considered as caused by behavioral problems, such as overeating, cigarette smoking, and excessive alcohol use. The predominant causes of death in the contemporary United States—CVD, cancers, respiratory tract diseases, and vehicular accidents—are called **sociogenic diseases** in recognition that the problems are generated (produced) by social factors. For example, although CVD produces physiological abnormalities, the causes are largely from lifestyle: poor diet, inactivity, and drug use (alcohol and tobacco). Likewise, many cancers have a strong association with behavioral factors such as stressful life changes and exposure to air pollution and cigarette smoke, the principal causes of respiratory tract diseases. Death from vehicular trauma is also a direct reflection of cultural activities, such as fast driving and alcohol use. These conditions reflect our behaviors, that is, our cultural lifestyles. Men are about twice as likely as women to die of liver diseases or accidents and have four times higher rates of death due to suicide and homicide. The differences in mortality for men and women are not something determined by biology but by lifestyle differences.

The biomedical model views disease as a deviation from biological norms and assumes that biology is more basic and significant than psychological or cultural issues in the nature of maladies. The biological emphasis on abnormal physiological conditions results in a neglect of other factors responsible for patients' maladies and concerns. Social and emotional factors may be recognized as complicating some diseases by increasing stress or encouraging nonadaptive behaviors (such as poor diet). Biomedical treatment approaches nonetheless primarily focus on physiological conditions and ignore the social factors that may cause disease (e.g., giving diazepam [such as Valium] to reduce stress rather than having a patient focus on changing the conditions that cause stress). Understanding the impact of maladies, including diseases, requires consideration of the cultural context of a patient. When health providers ignore psychological and social factors, the care of patients is limited because biology represents only part of the consequences of a malady. For example, the treatment needs of AIDS patients are from more than the effects of the virus. Because HIV infection is socially stigmatized and implies an early death, it affects an individual's experience, with personal illness effects and social sickness consequences that go beyond the immediate biological effects of the disease.

Not only may mortality be primarily a function of cultural patterns of behavior, the consequences of biological diseases may be largely determined by cultural and social responses.

TABLE 2.1. Age-Adjusted Death Rates (per 10,000) for Selected Causes of Death in the United States, 2004

Age-Adjusted Death Rates (per 10,000)

	Total Population	Male	Female	White	Black or African American	American Indian or Alaska Native	Asian or Pacific Islander	Hispanic or Latino
All causes	800.8	955.7	679.2	797.1	1,027.3	650.0	443.9	586.7
Diseases of heart	217.0	267.9	177.3	216.3	280.6	148.0	117.8	158.4
Cerebrovascular diseases (strokes)	50.0	50.4	48.9	48.3	69.9	35.3	41.3	38.2
Malignant neoplasms (cancers)	185.8	227.7	157.4	188.6	227.2	124.9	110.5	121.9
Chronic lower respiratory tract diseases	41.1	49.5	36.0	44.9	28.2	28.5	14.7	18.4
Influenza and pneumonia	19.8	23.7	17.3	19.6	22.3	17.6	16.0	17.1
Chronic liver disease and cirrhosis	9.0	12.5	5.8	8.7	7.9	22.7	3.2	14.0
Diabetes mellitus	24.5	28.2	21.7	21.5	48.0	39.2	16.6	32.1
HIV infection	4.5	6.6	2.4	1.9	20.4	2.9	0.7	5.3
Unintentional injuries	37.7	52.1	24.5	39.7	36.3	53.1	16.7	29.8
Motor vehicle-related injuries	15.2	21.4	9.3	15.6	14.8	26.0	7.8	14.4
Suicide	10.9	18.0	4.5	12.9	5.3	12.2	5.8	5.9
Homicide	5.9	9.2	2.5	2.7	20.1	7.0	2.5	7.2

Source: Compiled from U.S. Department of Health and Human Services data on the Centers for Disease Control and Prevention (CDC) Web site.

BIOCULTURAL INTERACTIONS

Leprosy and Social Stigma

The disease of leprosy, currently referred to as Hansen's disease, has been recognized for thousands of years. Leprosy is the consequence of a bacillus, *Mycobacterium leprae,* that produces skin lesions, nerve damage, and deformity of the extremities. Leprosy exemplifies how social consequences of a disease can be far more devastating than the biological effects (Pearson, 1988; Waxler, 1981), affecting patients' well-being and longevity more than the physical conditions. Leprosy appears only mildly communicable or infectious and usually requires long-term contact (ten to fifteen years) for transmission. Common early symptoms of leprosy (minor lesions, skin patches, or ulcers) are often unrecognized and may go untreated for years; most people exposed to the bacillus develop only subclinical (unapparent) infections because of their effective immune systems. Typical patients with leprosy are unlikely to have spread it before diagnosis, early treatment with sulfone drugs apparently eliminates its communicability within months, and the symptoms are likely to disappear.

Societies such as traditional Tanzanians viewed leprosy as relatively innocuous, allowing people to eat and sleep with and even marry lepers. But where there are strong moral associations with leprosy, the consequences for a patient's life can be devastating. In India, for example, leprosy is grounds for divorce, expelling patients from their villages, and even excluding them from family inheritance. Socially rejected and banned from their homes, lepers migrate to cities and become beggars. There they are shunned, despised, and subject to isolation and legal segregation. It is social reactions, rather than direct biological effects of the bacillus, that create the most important aspects of patients' experience of the disease. Exclusion from village and family and the lifestyle of a street beggar create many additional impacts on health (dietary, hygienic) that allow the bacillus to ravage a patient.

In the United States, historical (late nineteenth- and early twentieth-century) treatment of leprosy involved lifetime isolation in asylums such as the Catholic Church's Louisiana Home for the Lepers (later the U.S. Public Health Service Hospital) in Carville, Louisiana. Even though untrue, these institutions maintained the belief that leprosy was highly contagious out of interest in institutional survival: raising funds to support the organizations and providing a means of fulfilling religious needs to engage in "saintly" work with the diseased. Patients internalized these beliefs about the necessity of segregation, and many preferred to live out their lives in these institutions rather than attempt to return to society.

Waxler (1981) showed that the moral definition of leprosy emerged from cultural, social, economic, and historical circumstances that largely determined the experiences of those afflicted. This is illustrated in dramatic differences in life experiences of leprosy patients in different cultures, depending on whether the disease was conceived of as being highly contagious. In some societies, stigmatization occurred when medical models were introduced to control the disease, and health providers emphasized avoiding contact with infected persons. Cultural effects on patients' treatment decisions are illustrated in travel to distant facilities where anonymity could be assured and social ostracism within one's own community avoided (Pearson, 1988). Cultural reactions to and social expectations of the leper are the primary determinants of the individual's experience of leprosy. The powerful cultural determinants of the experiences of leprosy require that appropriate medical care address these influences as well. Treating the bacillus is not enough; the social impacts on patients' well-being also need to be addressed.

Biomedicine tends to address health problems in isolation from the social context that affects a patient's condition (e.g., how social factors affect nutrition, stress, and access to medicine). Considering a patient's malady strictly in terms of biology fails to address its broader consequences for the patient's experiences and outcomes. The social relations within which the malady occurs affect the consequences of disease, as illustrated in leprosy.

Deviation from Normal Biological Functioning

In defining the presence of disease, biomedicine tends to focus on the results of laboratory tests, neglecting the patient's experiences. For example, if you think you have intestinal parasites indicated by specific symptoms and signs (such as rectal itching, bloating, and gas), your physician will probably refuse to treat you unless this is confirmed by laboratory tests (which are notoriously unreliable in detecting these problems!). Biomedicine favors what is viewed as objective confirmation from the numerical "facts" from laboratory results or an indication of deviation from "norms," a range of expected measurements, over patient reports. However, there are several mathematical concepts of normal— average, mode, median—that must be understood within the patterns of variation within a population. Biomedicine presumes that numbers are "objective," but what is normal may be culturally specific. For example, the normal size of thyroid glands varies as a function of diet. Thyroid enlargement, normally considered a clinical symptom of goiter, is a normal adaptation to high levels of iodine in the diet and not evidence of disease in such populations. Specifying normal and normal range of variation requires reference to a specific population and even to different groups within the population—for instance, normal weight for men versus women. Because criteria for normal, such as weight and height, are culturally specific, the concept of "normal" is problematic.

Cultural influences on normal may be seen in diagnoses of type 2 diabetes mellitus, which encompasses a variety of metabolic conditions characterized by hyperglycemia (high levels of blood glucose or sugar). Most clinical diagnoses of diabetes are not made on the basis of patients' complaints or overt symptoms (such as thirst, frequent urination, weight loss, hunger) but from results of routine lab tests. These provide the basis for diagnoses of subclinical diabetes because it is not apparent in a clinical examination, only on the basis of laboratory results indicating deviation from what medicine presumes to be normal blood glucose levels. Although high blood glucose levels are taken as indicative of diabetes, such measurements can be unreliable indicators because many symptoms of diabetes are also characteristic reactions to psychological distress. There is no strong correlation between blood glucose levels and the severity of diabetic complications (Engel, 1977; Mishler, 1981). Blood glucose levels and insulin insufficiency have to be understood in reference to other metabolic processes and in relation to psychosocial and cultural factors (Engel, 1977). "Normal" glucose levels vary by population and individuals. For example, I have been with physicians measuring blood glucose levels in indigenous (Indian) populations of Mexico. Some levels were so low that the physician declared, "This person should be unconscious," but they obviously were not and appeared to function normally. The biological condition is not the sole determinant of a disease but, rather, how the conditions relate to the social context, illustrated in the special feature on epilepsy as an induced spiritual condition.

CULTURE AND HEALTH

Epilepsy as an Induced Spiritual Condition

Lia Lee's family and the Hmong culture viewed her seizures as evidence of spirit **possession**, a belief reported in many areas of the world. Seizures may also be induced by ritual activities. Seizures and ritual activities are linked in India, where traditional rituals use a rapidly alternating bath of hot water followed by cold water poured over the individual's head. This results in a variety of symptoms of generalized seizures in the ritual participants, who are without evidence of neurological disorder. Seizurelike characteristics may also be used as criteria for selecting people, such as mediums, for specialized magicoreligious functions. Cross-cultural research reports a significant clustering of amnesia, convulsions, and uncontrolled flailing of the body in religious practitioners such as especially mediums, who are characterized as having altered states of consciousness involving spirit possession. These mediums are initially recruited as patients suffering from spirit possession, a condition that is considered to be an illness. As the mediums become adept in managing their spirit possession, the spontaneously occurring seizures disappear (Winkelman, 1992a).

Epilepsy is often considered a disease but actually refers to a wide variety of symptoms indicative of electrical discharge patterns in the brain. Epileptic seizures range from partial seizures with limited effects on consciousness to major seizures resulting in convulsions and loss of consciousness. In either case, they may be associated with déjà vu and paranormal experiences, hallucinations, motor activities, and changes in personality involving sexuality, aggression, and religiosity. A typical brain characteristic of epileptic seizures involves synchronous slow-frequency brain-wave patterns. Rituals used for healing can also provoke these brain discharge patterns but without apparent pathology. There are numerous causes of the discharges that are labeled as epileptic, including genetic factors, injury, diet, drugs, metabolic imbalances, central nervous system diseases, and trauma. Such diversity of causes confronts a basic assumption of biomedicine, that of generic disease.

Assumption of Generic Disease

A basic assumption of the biomedical model is that there are universal diseases found across cultures characterized by identical specific and distinguishing features, symptoms, causes, and processes. These classification systems such as the DSM (American Psychiatric Association, 1994, 2000) and the ICD (World Health Organization, 2000) provide lists of mental health conditions presumed to be universal (e.g., schizophrenia, psychosis, depression). These systems of classification, called **nosologies**, claim to offer universally valid criteria for determining disease.

Cross-cultural approaches challenge this presumed universality of mental illnesses. Although some diagnostic categories are universally valid (e.g., anxiety, depressive

BIOCULTURAL INTERACTIONS

Depersonalization and Depression from Yogic Perspectives

The values attached to symptoms of depression vary; the "generalization of hopelessness" central to Western diagnostic categories of depression is viewed as characteristic of a good Buddhist (Castillo, 1991a). "Given their willing participation in an accepted practice at the heart of Buddhist ways of thought, it would be perverse to describe successful practitioners as sick, or, more particularly, depressed" (Hahn, 1995, p. 34). Richard Castillo illustrates the necessity of characterizing a malady in relationship to desired cultural conditions and values. The development of Hindu yogis leads to the creation of co-conscious selves, ones that participate in and are engaged with the physical world. Castillo calls this co-conscious **self** "the personal self" (participating self, or *jiva*), and the one that is an uninvolved observing self, the transpersonal self (observing self, atman or *purusha*). The personal self performs actions in accordance with social norms and experiences sensations, thoughts, and emotions, whereas the transpersonal self observes but is uninvolved in experiences (Castillo, 1991a). The goals of yoga meditation are the separation of these two aspects of self and consciousness. This is accomplished by restraining the personal self, an achievement referred to as *moksha*, meaning "liberation." Liberation is achieved by a new awareness: witnessing events but not participating in them and becoming freed from the suffering that comes from identification with the things of the personal self and its attachments in the external world.

disorders, schizophrenia, organic dysfunctions), it is doubtful that many other categories are (Kleinman, 1988a). There are difficulties in assessing mental disorders across cultures because even biological conditions are experienced and evaluated differently by different groups (e.g., dyslexia in nonliterate societies). Cross-cultural perspectives reveal that Western psychiatric categories are not universally applicable but reflect Western cultural concepts of impairment and psychosocial dysfunction. Cultural differences in what is considered normal mean that the same conditions may be conceptualized and treated in different ways in different cultures—and with different consequences. The symptoms associated with the Western category of schizophrenia seem to be recognized as mental illness around the world, but responses to such symptoms vary considerably. In Western cultures, schizophrenia has a poor prognosis, with permanent disability the frequent outcome, but in non-Western cultures, prognosis is generally good (Castillo, 1997a). But even diagnosing schizophrenia is problematic. The World Health Organization found that only 37 percent of patients manifested all relevant diagnostic criteria for schizophrenia, illustrating how cultural differences affect how conditions are conceptualized.

Castillo (1997a) reviews the DSM criteria for schizophrenia to illustrate the cultural assumptions. Hearing voices could be considered a symptom indicative of schizophrenia, but this makes judgments about normal experience; in some places, hearing voices is considered normal, even saintly. Kleinman (1988b) suggests that schizophrenia is not

This yogic practice of detachment has been analyzed as a flight from worldly life because of failure and despair, a renunciation based on frustration and depression. This depression and hopelessness are not seen as pathological in this cultural context but rather as the characteristics of a "good Buddhist." The yogis' cognitive models, which view the world as consisting of suffering and pain, enable the experience to be seen as the achievement of great spiritual insight. This sets the stage for meditation as a tool to escape emotional distress, anxiety, and problems, allowing the individual to accept the conditions of life (suffering) without experiencing them.

This type of experience is viewed in Western psychiatry as **depersonalization**. DSM definitions emphasize the experience of being detached from one's own body and mind, a sense of being an outside observer of one's self. There is a sense of false reality, emotional detachment, even of being dead. Descriptions of these experiences by Western psychiatric patients parallel accounts of yogis, but Western patients feel panic and anxiety whereas the yogic practitioners view these experiences positively because they confirm their worldview. Failure to understand an experience in its cultural context misses the fundamental meaning for the person and consequently the nature of the experience. This problem plagues the diagnostic approaches of the DSM based on behavioral "symptoms" divorced from the cultural context of their production and personal experience. This problem is illustrated in the cross-cultural examination of the DSM diagnostic category of **somatoform disorders**.

found in all cultures, and Castillo indicates that in nonindustrialized societies, the symptoms are less severe and prognosis for successful treatment is much better (e.g., traditional care in Africa). What is relevant is not merely some generic disease or condition but how it is related to the broader social context. A universal nosology is possible only if it describes the variation in disease found in different cultural settings, the conditions reported in other cultural settings, contextual variation in sickness conditions, and the factors that modify their manifestations (Hahn, 1995). Subsequent examinations of **somatization**, the physical expression of psychological conditions, as well as depression in cross-cultural perspectives help to illustrate the fundamental role of cultural context in determining the nature of a malady or whether a condition even constitutes a malady. Different cultures value different conditions, making one culture's pathology another's paradise, as illustrated in "Biocultural Interactions: Depersonalization and Depression from Yogic Perspectives," where ignoring cultural context and values confuses enlightenment with depression.

Doctrine of Specific Etiology

Biomedical assumptions about causes of diseases attribute the primary etiology to *specific* biological factors. This doctrine of specific etiology is derived from historical developments in biomedicine related to infectious diseases, which were shown to result from

BIOCULTURAL INTERACTIONS

Somatoform Disorders in Cross-Cultural Perspective

Somatoform disorder is a general term, a broad diagnostic category used to include a wide range of conditions characterized by prominent somatic or bodily symptoms or experience of pain in a specific organ (or part of the body) but without an organic cause. For example, the physical symptoms may include paralyses of limbs or the entire body, anesthesia in specific body areas, or hysterical blindness that is without medical explanation or neurological basis. These conditions are generally considered to be of a psychosomatic nature, with the body area or organ unconsciously symbolizing a psychological conflict. Formal diagnostic criteria include the presence of pain, sexual dysfunction, gastrointestinal disorders, and pseudoneurological distress not related to organic dysfunctions. Typical symptoms include chronic fatigue; diffuse, vague bodily aches and pains; headaches; nausea and diarrhea; loss of appetite; depression; dizziness; and tiredness, all without a biological explanation (Castillo, 1997a). Fainting and dissociation may also occur. Specific subcategories of somatoform disorders include conditions of hysteria (conversion disorder), somatization, hypochondria, pain disorders, and an unspecified category.

Somatization is viewed in various ways (Kirmayer, Dao, and Smith, 1998):

- As a group (family) of somatoform disorders (disorders with body-based symptoms)
- As a process by which psychological conflict is transformed into bodily symptoms
- As a clinical presentation emphasizing symptoms of somatic conditions rather than emotional or psychological concerns

Rather than a biological problem, the specific focal symptoms of somatization represent a cultural idiom for communicating distress and conflict (Kirmayer et al., 1998). Somatization reflects psychosocial and psychodynamic problems and stress communicated through the symptoms, which provide a cultural medium for communicating distress and social conflicts. For instance, Chaplin (1997) discusses the symptom presentation of a Chinese woman who complained about sleeplessness for excessive fire in her liver and a weakness of her heart. Chaplin notes that her actual symptoms suggested depression but that she did not understand her situation as involving depression. He suggested that these symptom presentations reflected a cultural system of expressing bodily sensations through reference to the organ systems, which are understood as metaphors for emotions. These physical terms are more socially acceptable than the expression of anger or aggression. The people, however, understand reference to a weak heart as a reference to a poor mood and the reference to fire in the liver as indicating anger or irritation.

Castillo (1997a) argues that cross-cultural assessments of the cases illustrate the inappropriateness of the DSM category of somatoform disorders. In China and India, psychiatrists take cases that could be classified as somatoform disorders and instead diagnose them as different forms of mental illness, neurasthenia, or hysteria. These somatoform disorders are referred to with terms used in earlier periods of psychiatry (hysteria, neurasthenia) but now subsumed within the category of somatoform disorders. The concept of hysteria originated in Western psychiatry but is no longer recognized in the DSM. Neurasthenia, referring to "tired nerves," also originated in the

United States but is not currently in the DSM; it has remained a common diagnosis in China because it fits well with cultural forms of expression (Castillo, 1997a).

Somatization in China: Neurasthenia

Because the Chinese give little attention to depressive symptoms, patients are more likely to emphasize somatic symptoms, leading to a clinical diagnosis of neurasthenia, involving somatic complaints, fatigue, and anxiety (Kleinman, 1980). The Chinese cultural emphasis on physical symptoms as a means of expressing emotional distress somatization is extremely common due in part to a lack of words for describing psychological states. This leads to their expression in terms of organs whose referents and functions are thought to affect psychological conditions. Chinese culture inhibits introspection and open expression of emotion, shaping the presentation of psychosocial stress as somatic complaints, without mention of emotional problems, distress, or depression. Physical symptoms are understood as metaphors through which emotional states and psychological problems are expressed. For instance, complaints about physical conditions such as liver disease are understood as an emotional message; rather than actual liver problems, they were really communications about anger. Nonetheless, the liver may be treated with herbs to harmonize it with other bodily functions and eliminate anger.

Somatization in India: Hysteria

Castillo (1997a) compares cases diagnosed as hysteria in patients in India, where the emphasis is on symptoms of anxiety, dissociation, depression, and somatic complaints. Symptoms of hysteria are also found in cases that the traditional ethnomedical system diagnoses as spirit possession, but this diagnosis is not appealing to modern women in India. Hysteria, however, does provide a meaningful labeling of the symptoms for modern patients. Recommended treatments of hysteria are similar to the traditional healing of spirit possession (increased attention to the patient, protection from stress and insult, enhancement of status) but with different explanatory models and treatment processes consistent with patient identities and expectations.

Somatic distress is normal in all mental and physical disorders, a universal, but more predominant in some cultural groups (Kirmayer et al., 1998). Somatization is a common medium for the expression of emotional distress and personal and social conflict and may also be used to avoid the presentation of more stigmatizing psychiatric symptoms. In somatization, the physical symptoms involve a culturally meaningful "language of distress" in which a specific focal organ and symptoms represent a particular psychodynamic constellation of symbolic and metaphoric significance of broader cultural concern. For instance, when Chinese speak of liver problems, it is in reference to beliefs about the liver as a cause of anger. When suffering from somatization, patients are generally not aware of the relation of their physical complaints to their psychological and social dynamics. Patients may nonetheless be aware that interpersonal relations give rise to their affective (mood) reactions and that their responses (such as repression of feelings) can lead to illness.

Continued

BIOCULTURAL INTERACTIONS   *Continued*

The diagnosis of somatization is complicated by

- Culturally specific presentations of somatic syndromes
- Its more general use as culturally based codes or **"idioms of distress"**
- The overlap of anxiety states with somatic and affective disorders

The association of symbolic and somatic conditions, however, conflicts with the notion of discrete disorders implied by DSM categories. Hence, somatic disorders remain as a category that places the symptoms into a diagnostic system but lacks conceptual rigor because the standard categories fail to capture the culturally significant features (Castillo, 1997a). The concept of somatization is employed in diverse ways with a multitude of meanings (Kirmayer et al., 1998). The somatoform category implies a mind-body dualism or separation not found in most cultures and a separation of mind, body, and emotion in ways inconsistent with the actual occurrence of suffering. Consequently, the diagnostic category provides little usefulness in clarifying individual conditions.

specific microorganisms. Biomedicine has generally assumed that biological factors *alone* (such as bacteria) produce specific diseases, but biological conditions are generally only one of many factors necessary for the occurrence of disease. Exposure to microorganisms and their presence in one's body may not result in disease if one's immune system and antibodies can resist infection. For example, tuberculosis occurs primarily in the lower social classes because infection also requires contributory factors such as poor nutrition and hygiene and crowded living conditions, which compromise the immune system and increase contagion. Even where genetic influences operate, such as with diabetes, CVD, and schizophrenia, the social environment—dietary and behavioral conditions (such as hygiene, housing, and interpersonal relations)—generally play a more significant role.

The case of Lia Lee's epilepsy illustrates that it is not merely the physical condition that is at issue but a variety of contributory factors (such as diet, toxins, and stress) and conditions that inhibit treatment and appropriate medication (misdiagnosis) or further complicate a condition (hospital-induced infections). It is necessary to distinguish among levels of causality and contributing factors to diseases. A **necessary cause** is one that must be present—for example, a germ—but it is seldom a **sufficient cause**, one that alone makes the disease occur. Bacteria in the body are not sufficient to produce disease. In addition to these remote or **distal causes**, which can initiate a disease, there are **contributory factors** or causes: for example, when poor nutrition, stress, or lack of adequate housing can weaken one's immune system or where lack of access to treatment of a simple infection can lead to a fatal case of gangrene (also see the section in Chapter Seven, "Identifying Causes of Disease").

CASE STUDY

Cardiac Arrest

Cardiac pathology has biological contributions, but its onset, presentation, course, and outcome involve the interaction of behavioral, psychological, and social factors in the patient's life, as illustrated in the case of a patient, "Mr. Glover" (Engel, 1980). Mr. Glover had a previous cardiac arrest, and symptoms experienced at work reminded him of that event. Fortunately, the insistence of his employer led him to seek immediate care and induced a calm and confident state. He was without symptoms or discomfort when he arrived at the emergency department of the hospital. His previous heart attack and report of the symptoms experienced earlier in the day at work led the physician to an easy diagnosis of myocardial infarction and the recommendation of routine coronary care.

Despite Mr. Glover's stable condition on admission, he experienced a cardiac arrest within a half hour and lost consciousness. Why did this happen? Events following admission involving interpersonal processes led to the cardiac arrest. During his workup for routine coronary care, hospital physicians spent ten minutes trying to insert an intravenous line and failing and then left Mr. Glover alone as they sought help. This undermined Mr. Glover's confidence in the doctors, making him feel as if incompetent beginners were victimizing him. "[T]he patient found himself getting hot and flushed. Chest pain recurred and quickly became . . . severe . . . [and] culminated in his passing out as ventricular fibrillation supervened" (Engel, 1980, p. 540). Medical staff viewed the problem as strictly physiological, but the immediate precipitation of the cardiac arrest in the hospital was more psychodynamic: stress caused by incompetent care.

Disease only rarely results just because of the presence of infectious agents but, rather, occurs in interaction with contributory psychophysiological and sociocultural factors that affect the body's response to the agent. Social conditions such as nutrition, environmental exposure, emotional reactions, social responses of others, and interpersonal stress can undermine the body's balance, as illustrated in the special feature, "Case Study: Cardiac Arrest."

What is referred to as cardiovascular disease does not pertain to a single condition or disease but is a general category that includes many different kinds of problems related to the heart and circulatory system. The associated symptoms, such as hypertension, high cholesterol levels, and arteriosclerosis, are also not diseases, even though they may be referred to as diseases; rather, they are conditions or symptoms that may contribute to— and result from—a variety of diseases (CVD, stroke, diabetes). Fatalities of the heart are generally associated with the progressive weakening of the muscle of the heart that leads it to miss beats (arrhythmias) and eventually stop. The cessation of the heartbeat— a "heart attack"—is a malfunction that results from the cumulative effects of many different types of conditions.

Heart problems can derive from many factors in the circulatory system, the blood vessels that are conduits for the blood that the heart pumps. Damage to these blood vessels, such as atherosclerosis (deposits on the arteries that occlude blood flow), can affect the heart in many ways, including raising the blood pressure, which contributes to hypertension, commonly referred to as high blood pressure. This reflects that the heart is having to work harder, and greater pressure is exerted on the blood vessels, which may cause other diseases such as stroke. The plaque on the walls of the arteries not only constricts the flow of blood but can rupture with a thrombus that is large enough to completely block the flow of blood through an artery.

The rupture of a thrombus can be triggered by many factors: "emotional or physical stress or trauma, exposure to certain drugs, exposure to cold, and acute infections" (Papademetriou, 2004, p. S33). Heart attacks do not occur just because of the presence of certain necessary conditions (weakened heart) or distal causes (factors causing atherosclerosis and high blood pressure). Heart attacks also require proximal factors and triggering events in daily life, including psychological and physical stress. People die of heart attacks while shoveling snow; if they had stayed inside tranquilly, the likelihood of a heart attack that day would have been minimal.

Scientific Presumptions of Medicine

Biomedical practitioners generally presume that their professional practice standards produce scientific, morally neutral, and objective "culture-free" treatment approaches (Gaines and Davis-Floyd, 2004). Although the practitioners see themselves as scientists, biomedicine is not consistently scientific but instead influenced by social and political conditions and ideological assumptions.

Biomedicine is not consistently scientific in basing its practice on findings established by clinical trials (Hahn, 1995). Many commonly accepted clinical practices are not based on strict scientific criteria (**double-blind clinical trials**) or scientific evaluation. For instance, although the Food and Drug Administration (FDA) must approve new drugs based on controlled studies, many pharmaceuticals that were used before the laws were established remain in use. Drugs approved for one use are often marketed for other unapproved uses ("off-label" treatments). Doctors often prescribe several drugs at once, although such uses have never been tested, resulting in drug-drug interactions that kill tens of thousands of people annually.

Many physicians are starting to recognize that their treatment practices are not strictly scientific, leading to the development of an evidence-based approach to clinical practice that aims to augment traditional professional assumptions with a new, critical appraisal of their practices. Much of clinical practice is based on conventional wisdom and traditional beliefs, not on systematic evidence from controlled laboratory or clinical studies (see the section in Chapter Five, "Evaluating Biomedicine and Alternative Medicine," for further discussion). Social and political biases of biomedicine are illustrated in many areas: for example, the long-held opposition of the American Medical Association (AMA) to Congress's efforts to pass legislation that provides basic health care for all Americans. The AMA was not opposed, however, to the government providing billions of dollars in federal funds to privately owned medical schools, hospitals, and physician groups.

BIOCULTURAL INTERACTIONS

Mental Retardation as Social Classification

Political functions of medicine are illustrated in the social processes of the diagnosis of mental retardation. The Western concept of intellectual disability reflects concerns with mental processes that are not as important in other societies, particularly nonliterate cultures. The biomedical model assumes that mental retardation reflects underlying brain pathology, but the formal determination of mental retardation involves social and practical adaptive skills related to how people function in specific settings in contemporary modern society. This reveals that social and cultural conditions, rather than biology, determine what is considered normal and adaptive. Mental retardation is a cultural construct that is socially defined in specific contexts and in relationship to local expectations.

Mercer's (1973) studies show how Hispanics and African Americans were differentially impacted by the social processes used in channeling individuals into the category of mentally retarded. The role of a teacher in holding a student back a grade was a crucial step in the process of diagnosing mental retardation. Psychological testing, applied without consideration of cultural biases (such as English-language ability), constituted another step. Intelligence testing explains only part of the recommendation process because only 49 percent of Anglo students who fail the test are recommended for placement in special classes compared with 70 percent of the Mexican and African American youth who fail. Nearly all these minority children are placed in remedial classes whereas Anglos are more likely to remain in regular classes.

Mercer's work revealed what she referred to as "six-hour mental retardation." During the school day, children were in classes for the mentally retarded, with school performance reflecting the designation. When the children were in the home and community, their social and personal behaviors were normal for their age. The retardation was with respect only to the social activities found within the context of schooling and not in life in general. Factors such as depression, stress, motivation, and racism all likely reinforced the stereotypes of mental retardation in the school.

When I worked as a consultant for the Regional Center for the Developmentally Disabled in Los Angeles, I interacted with Mexican American children who were diagnosed as mentally retarded and placed in special education programs. I was called in when families had problems with their child's placement, including when they protested what they considered the inappropriate placement of their child in classes for the severely disabled. My job was to evaluate the children's functioning in the context of the home and community environment and sometimes mediate the family relations with schools, counselors, and medical staff. Time and again, I discovered the normal abilities of what had been labeled a mentally retarded child. This was often because of a quiet, timid, fearful, nonassertive, withdrawn demeanor they displayed, compounded by communication barriers created by language differences that affected confidence in self-expression. At home, however, they were outgoing, verbal, expressive, creative, and inquisitive. Their mental condition manifested only during school hours.

Rather than being based strictly on scientific evidence, physicians' activities reflect the values of the dominant economic and political interests of society. Biomedicine is practiced through social institutions that affect who receives what treatment, in what manner, and at what cost. There is nothing value-free about deciding to fund technology-intensive hospitals for cardiovascular surgery for the elite, rather than spending money on primary health care for the poor, pregnant women, and infants. There is a value orientation in bio-medicine's presumption of scientific objectivity by focusing on biological disease while discounting the roles of political, economic, and psychosocial factors as causal agents. Biomedicine has decontextualized medical problems, removing them from the sociocultural contexts within which the health problems occur or are defined. This is exemplified in mental retardation diagnoses, which are applied strongly along ethnic lines.

Meaney (2004) notes the difficulty in defining mental retardation in objective terms because the formal criteria for evaluating mental retardation are with respect to the ability of individuals to function with practical skills in their social and cultural context. An explicit reference to the community, peers' abilities, and practical tasks make mental retardation an inherently cultural assessment. For example, which of the following is a practical skill indicative of intelligence: operating a mobile phone or making a trap with branches to catch a rabbit for dinner? Would you think someone who cannot learn to use a cell phone is mentally retarded? Being unable to learn to use a cell phone is a failure in social competence in New York City but not in the wilderness. Can you make a trap to catch an animal? You might seem mentally retarded if dropped off in the bush.

Cultural conceptions and social contexts and their adaptive demands for locally relevant practical skills, rather than universal standards, are fundamental to what constitutes mental retardation. Cultures can produce different consequences for the physical conditions involved in what are called diseases. For instance, dyslexia (reversal of letters in written language) illustrates how biological effects produce conditions, but whether or not they impair mental functioning is in relationship to culture. Dyslexic children face severe obstacles in modern societies, where their reversal of letters presents formidable obstacles to their success in reading, school, and life. Dyslexia presents little problem, however, in societies where writing is not an element of social competence and practical survival skills are based in farming and social relations.

Even when the DSM characterizes maladies with objective criteria that are defined in scientific ways and numerically objective, Hahn (1995) points out that there are nonetheless political and cultural factors that determine what is listed and how it is characterized. Hahn (1997) notes that the effects of political and cultural factors in the DSM are illustrated in the shifts from the early characterization in the DSM of homosexuality as inherently pathological. Later homosexuality was a "sexual orientation disturbance," and currently it is discussed as "ego-dystonic homosexuality," which is a pathological condition only if it is experienced as an unwanted feeling. If a person is OK with being homosexual, it is not pathological, but if a person feels bad about it, it is a disease. Cultural values are further revealed in the lack of a classification of unwanted heterosexual feelings as a pathological condition, only unwanted homosexual ones.

Hahn (1995) notes that the formal classification systems do not explicitly state the criteria for classification or clearly establish the rationale for their use. Many different

CULTURE AND HEALTH

Cultural and Historical Bases of the DSM

Cultural biases in biomedical concepts of mental illness are illustrated in historical changes in the DSM (Castillo, 1997a). Cultural construction of biomedical views is reflected in changes in the ICD and DSM between editions, where diseases disappear or are subsumed into other categories. The DSM was originally derived from the ICD. First published in 1952, DSM-I was based on a biopsychosocial paradigm: it attributed underlying causes of mental disorders to the interaction among biological, psychological, and social factors, with treatment approaches focusing on undoing the psychological causes of mental disease. DSM-II (1968) shifted its emphasis toward the biomedical paradigm of mental illness as biological disease. The treatment of mental illness was based in the use of psychotropic medications and electroconvulsive therapies, and physiological and anatomical disorders, such as neurotransmitter imbalances or dysfunctions in specific brain regions, were viewed as the primary underlying causes of mental illness. This shift was completed in the 1980 version of DSM-III, in which a disease-centered perspective of mental illness became the dominant paradigm, and the psychodynamic paradigm of DSM-I was abandoned. DSM-III also shifted the classification system, emphasizing symptom patterns as the basis for classification of disorders. The assumptions of the disease-centered paradigm of DSM-III were generally not verified by laboratory research because studies of abnormalities in brain structure, function, and process have not revealed specific brain diseases underlying mental disorders (Castillo, 1997a). Studies do show correlations between brain abnormalities and mental disorders, but evidence does not support the conclusion that the physical differences cause the mental disorders, rather than the reverse. To date, there is no laboratory procedure that can reliably identify even the major mental illnesses considered to have a genetic basis (such as schizophrenia or depression) (Castillo, 1997a). The physical abnormalities associated with schizophrenia do not have to be present for schizophrenia to be diagnosed, and they also occur in individuals without schizophrenic symptoms. Abnormalities in neurotransmitter systems are statistically associated with depression, but there is no single simple relationship between neurotransmitter levels and depressive symptoms; moreover, those abnormalities may be consequences of depression rather than their cause (Castillo, 1997a).

Castillo suggests that DSM-IV (1994) involves an emerging paradigm shift that is being driven by the influences of psychiatric anthropology. This has led to an increased emphasis on a client-centered approach more concerned with the effects of cultural meaning on mental illness. Cultural constructions of reality produce effects on the individual at both the psychological and biological levels; hence, culturally specific rather than universal frameworks are central to understanding patients' conditions. The new paradigm recognizes that the causation of mental disorders occurs in interaction with the sociocultural environment. This requires multidisciplinary frameworks that address the complex interactions among biological, behavioral, environmental, and psychological factors in producing mental and physical disorders.

CULTURE AND HEALTH

Ethnomedicine and Evolved Adaptations

Callahan (2006) notes that geophagy—dirt-eating, which is considered a disease (pica) in biomedicine—is considered a therapeutic practice in many cultures. The examination of geophagy cross-culturally and in an evolutionary perspective suggests that it is actually an adaptive behavior with significant health consequences. The biomedical characterization of an adaptive behavior as a disease illustrates the social construction of diseases. The DSM diagnoses the disorder of pica as engaging in eating of nonfood substances over periods of time. Biomedical practices consider this disorder to result from a variety of factors, including environmental deprivation, family dysfunction, brain damage, and malnutrition. Pica is associated with a variety of psychological disorders, but there is no basis for considering it to be a disease other than the assumption that it is abnormal.

The biomedical perspectives consider eating dirt to be fundamentally dysfunctional—a value judgment—instead of recognizing the adaptive effects of these practices. Callahan describes how geophagy fills a variety of nutritional and immunological functions and plays a variety of roles in ethnomedical traditions. The ingestion of clays is a prevalent form of nutritional and medicinal geophagy, adding important minerals to the diet and removing toxins from food. Geophagy is a pattern of behavior noted in pregnant women in cultures around the world, in which it is used as a source of calcium and treatment for a variety of conditions, including nausea. It likely also

criteria are used in the various conditions found in the ICD classifications. Some are based on causal agents or pathological processes, others on vectors or stages of disease, and still others on the body part or organ affected or on changes in the behavior of a patient. There are no explicit criteria for determining why some human problems are included but others are excluded. This cultural basis for the DSM classification system is illustrated by its history and development.

SOCIAL MODELS OF MALADIES AND DIAGNOSES

The limitations of the biomedical perspective that disease is basically physiological and that mental and psychosocial issues are irrelevant led Engel (1977, 1980) to introduce the biopsychosocial model discussed in Chapter One. Understanding the nature of health and addressing maladies require this broader perspective concerned with the psychological, cultural, and social dimensions affecting well-being. Effective assessment requires an understanding of psychological and social aspects of unwanted conditions, linking diseases and symptoms to the cultural context within which the malady is produced and experienced. Constructivist perspectives point out that cultural values produce cross-cultural variation in the recognition of diseases, the significance of symptoms, their treatments, and their consequences. The differences are manifested in the distinction between physicians' concern with disease and patients' experience of illness, differences that affect the diagnostic processes. Cultural criteria determine the meaning of a given set of behaviors provides enhanced immune system responses for both mother and embryo. Callahan proposes that the consumption of dirt in pregnancy and early childhood is an evolutionary adaptation that has a variety of adaptive consequences, including enhancing the development of fetal immunity.

Universally, early childhood (before two years old) is the most prevalent time of geophagy; Callahan notes that the period of intense dirt ingestion corresponds to the time (one year and more after birth) when immunoglobulin levels provided in mother's milk begin to decline. The early exposures to bacteria provide the basis for developments that enable appropriate immune system responses later in life. Eating dirt appears to provide adaptive benefits by stimulating the immune system. The gut is the primary area for the production of immunoglobulin. Exposure to dirt may assist in the development of intestinal flora and provide exposure to germs that strengthen immune responses to later threats. Aluminum salts found in dirt can assist in the immune response by functioning as adjuvants that provide a nonspecific amplification in the immune system response (Callahan, 2006). Thus dirt-eating likely has a variety of health benefits. Although the practice poses risks for exposures to a variety of helminthic (worm) and other parasitic infections, considering it merely a disease makes little empirical sense. Biomedical perspectives reflect a particular cultural viewpoint that in most cases is unrelated to the biological and cultural realities of the behavior.

or symptoms as disease or normal variation in behavior, such as in dyslexia, depression, mental retardation, and "dirt eating."

The facts of biomedicine are based in social processes of the construction of meaning, just as with other ethnomedical systems, and the conditions recognized may be a reflection of values and assumptions rather than evidence of pathology. What is considered pathological and a disease is established by cultural and social conventions, even if they are called by medical and scientific terms. The role of cultural values in determining what is considered a disease was illustrated above in "Biocultural Interactions: Depersonalization and Depression from Yogic Perspectives" and in the following consideration of pica or geophagy—dirt-eating—where what is considered a disease in biomedicine is seen as a healing practice in many cultures.

Social Construction of Disease

Engel's biopsychosocial model (1977, 1980), which views sociocultural conditions as affecting disease through the mediation of risks such as exposures to diseases or other conditions that cause health problems (such as contamination) is extended in **constructivist perspectives.** These perspectives view the conditions in a culture as producing health problems as well as constructing how its members think about disease and its implications, and consequently, how they experience health maladies.

Constructivist perspectives emphasize cultural influences, including social relationships, as fundamental in the causation of biological disorders. For example, politics produces disease through decisions that allow the creation of environmental conditions, such as pollution or toxic waste sites, and the distribution of their risks. The risk of cancer is increased by governmental policies that allow cancer-causing pesticides to be used in agricultural fields or companies to discharge toxic chemicals into waterways. Social determination of disease occurs through political decisions that affect the availability of prevention services and treatment, such as when funding for preschool nutrition programs is cut, increasing nutrition-related disorders among poor children. Stress produced by social conditions reduces resistance to disease, or even produces disease, as when extensive work demands increased blood pressure and levels of hormones that compromise the immune system. Constructivist perspectives place the social dimensions of disease at the principal focus of the inquiry, as described earlier in the discussions of cardiac arrest, depression, and mental retardation.

Different constructions regarding the causes of maladies reflect the power of cultural institutions to select specific worldviews to explaining diseases. For instance, do poor people

CULTURE AND HEALTH

Genital Cutting: Surgery or Mutilation?

Although it is assumed that medical practice is based on scientifically established procedures, there are many exceptions (e.g., lower back surgery, cesarean section, and circumcision). Is having a penile sheath, provided by our genetic code, a "disease" that requires medical treatment? It would seem so today, given the volume of circumcisions performed in the United States. Wallerstein (1980) argues, however, that male circumcision is without medical justification; his points were later extended in examinations of genital mutilations in cross-cultural contexts (Denniston and Milos, 1997). Although female genital mutilation has received the most attention, male circumcision is the most frequently performed and medically unnecessary surgery. A deep cultural bias is illustrated in the use of "mutilation" to refer to cutting female genitalia but not male genitalia.

The historical introduction of male circumcision into the United States (during the nineteenth century) was as a cure for masturbation, immoral behavior and STDs, epilepsy, and cancer. Other arguments such as hygiene have been subsequently proposed, but the health risks of circumcision are considerable and have not been shown to outweigh any presumed advantages. Nonetheless, male circumcision remains a prominent feature of contemporary neonatal care (about 70 percent in this country) and a focus in public health and STD campaigns. Current arguments for adopting circumcision are often with no more justification in medical science than were its original uses for curbing masturbation. The persistence of an unnecessary surgery can be attributed in part to having been integrated into mainstream American culture as well as the economic benefits that physicians receive. The persistence of American opposition to female genital mutilation while ignoring the dynamics of male genital mutilation is increasingly noted by other cultures as a form of gross ethnocentrism. Anthropologists and medical researchers have begun to turn their attention to this medical practice that has little or no justification in science or culture and that has broad but generally unassessed negative health consequences for men (e.g., see Goldman, 1997).

suffer from higher rates of lead poisoning because they are ignorant about such risks or do not care? Or does their higher risk reflect the influences of a capitalist society where impoverished people are more likely to have access restricted to old housing with contaminated paint and plumbing? Do higher levels of toxins in the bodies of inner-city children reflect their parents' neglect or the consequences of business and civic leaders that allow the operation of highly polluting industries in these locations? These different perspectives produce different kinds of approaches to these conditions, one based on blaming the poor for their problems and the other attributing responsibility to broader societal factors, even the criminal neglect by industrialists who cause diseased conditions by polluting the environments.

Constructivist perspectives emphasize that social concepts are more fundamental than biological conditions, that physical effects are produced, mediated, and experienced through human activities and cultural responses. Maladies, including disease, are produced through social relations and in a cultural context that creates risks and the values that frame the experiences and give meanings to maladies. This is not to exclude biology as a causal or contributory factor but to recognize that social context is part of the causation of health problems and that cultural belief and resources not only create the experience and outcome of the conditions but may actually create conditions through beliefs.

The constructivist perspectives reframe the fundamental issue of diagnosing health problems as a discourse that involves ideological constructions, concepts based on cultural ideas regarding which aspects of health problems are most significant in a society. Cultural ideas are central, even in the formulation of biomedical diagnoses and the conceptualization of conditions that need to be treated, as discussed in the special feature "Culture and Health: Genital Cutting: Surgery or Mutilation?"

Diagnoses as Construction

The social construction approach differs from biomedicine's model of generic diseases in emphasizing that cultural processes create the systems within which maladies are defined and produced. Constructivist approaches illustrate that physicians' diagnostic activities selectively predefine relevant symptoms out of a variety of vague conditions presented by patients. Patients express *symptoms,* which refer to their subjective assessment of their condition based on their experience of some unwanted conditions. A physician may derive important ideas from a patient's expression of symptoms but is actually looking for *signs* of disease, what are considered objective data derived from laboratory tests, x-ray exams and other diagnostic procedures, indications revealed by physical examination, and past episodes revealed by the medical history. Physicians may depend on the patient's expressed symptoms to formulate the diagnosis but tend to rely primarily on the signs provided by test results to "fit" a patient's condition within standard diagnostic categories.

Medical diagnosis is a social labeling process whereby individuals are given disease labels that only partially encompass their experience of a malady. For instance, you may complain about fever, a sense of fatigue, bodily aches, coughing, sneezing, and diarrhea, and your physician diagnoses that you have the flu. Sneezing and diarrhea are not flu symptoms, however, and may be ignored in your treatment. For both doctor and patient, social factors affect which symptoms and conditions are selected as relevant. This reflects general cultural norms of what is appropriate (e.g., ignoring habitual back pain if you are a physical laborer or sexual symptoms when complaining about a general sense of "dis-ease").

Differences in diagnoses given to patients occur even when physicians use the same objective criteria as guidelines (Helman, 2001). As reported by Helman, British physicians were more likely to diagnose manic-depressive psychosis whereas American physicians were more likely to note apathy and paranoia in the same patients and diagnose schizophrenia. Hospital staffs in both countries were more likely than research staff to diagnose schizophrenia. Doctors from different cultures come up with different diagnoses because of cultural influences on what is considered most significant.

The underlying assumptions of diagnostic processes are generally not subject to critical questioning and reflection but, rather, are a part of the taken-for-granted assumptions of medicine (Mishler, 1981). Doctors tend to think that they are actually discovering a disease rather than coming up with a culturally relevant classification. Consequently, there is little consideration of what diagnosis involves or actually means because it would involve questioning the whole enterprise of medicine. Problems are recognized in the accuracy of diagnoses, but assumptions of universal generic diseases allow physicians to overlook the uncertainty and ambiguity in their efforts to determine the essential underlying features. The assumption is that the disease is real and that problems in diagnosis reflect a lack of accurate knowledge, rather than unjustified assumptions. To clarify the diagnosis of disease, physicians attempt to isolate what are considered biological features from the social context. But disease is socially constructed, with its consequences in part derived from the social context.

Constructivist approaches illustrate how diagnostic criteria are applied in relation to cultural and institutional factors, as discussed in the diagnosis of mental retardation. Constructivist perspectives portray biomedical knowledge as the product of a particular cultural history and not a permanent empirical reality, as illustrated in the changing criteria used in the DSM.

Rather than merely accepting epidemiological findings about different rates of disease, or **prevalence**, in specific ethnic groups, constructivist approaches examine these findings to ascertain how health care institutions operate. The relationships of ethnic variables to health statistics may not reflect the actual prevalence of disease. Instead, they may reflect ways in which

- Social and economic conditions determine who seeks care for disease and illness: for example, poor people who do not seek care for back pain caused by work conditions

- Cultural factors affect what is perceived as a condition requiring treatment: for example, cultures in which obesity is considered normal or parasitic disease is endemic

- Patients' symptoms are selected by providers in formulating a diagnosis that provides epidemiological data: for example, flu diagnoses rather than gastrointestinal disorders

- Culture dictates preferences for certain appearances: for example, where a drug overdose or suicide is categorized as an accident

A patient's malady is an interpretation within a system of cultural meanings and priorities, making cultural processes central to diagnosis. The social constructivist approach regards diagnoses as data for analysis, rather than objective decisions, as illustrated in a physician diagnosing a viral flu and prescribing ineffective antibiotics for what is more likely an undiagnosed bacterial infection.

CULTURE AND HEALTH

Confusing Disease in "the Flu"

Differences between biomedical concepts of disease and people's concepts of their maladies have important implications for clinical practice and **epidemiology**, the study of factors predicting the distribution patterns of diseases. In her role as a public health investigator, McCombie (1987, 1999) found that popular views of flu affect the diagnosis and treatment. Influenza (flu) has symptoms and causes distinct from popular conceptions of flu. These differences detrimentally influence physicians' judgment, practice, treatment, and consequently, epidemiological studies of the sources and causes of diseases. The biomedical conception of flu refers to a respiratory tract infection caused by viruses, particularly of the Orthomyxoviridae family, and occurring with sudden onset during the late fall and early winter. This viral syndrome produces symptoms of fever, chills, and headache, along with sore throat, congestion, and general bodily pain. Antibiotics do not affect viruses and are not an appropriate treatment for viral conditions.

What the general public often calls "flu" involves symptoms indicative of gastrointestinal conditions: diarrhea, nausea, and vomiting. In McCombie's (1987) study of people who contacted public health offices seeking advice for the treatment of flu, only about 15 percent reported symptoms characteristic of influenza whereas more than 80 percent reported gastrointestinal symptoms not characteristic of flu. McCombie found more callers complaining about so-called flu during periods when influenza was absent. These popular health beliefs about flu present problems for epidemiologists because when people conclude they have the flu, they generally deny the possibility that their condition has anything to do with food contamination. This can result in infectious gastrointestinal conditions going unreported and untreated, obstructing efforts to investigate food-borne diseases because people affected refuse to cooperate in investigations of probable food sources of their illness. If someone got sick after visiting their grandmother's house, they might be offended if an investigator's questions about what they ate suggested that grandmother had less-than-hygienic food preparation practices.

Physicians succumb to the labeling demands, using "viral syndrome" as the initial diagnosis for likely bacterial diseases. McCombie noted that physicians often diagnosed viral syndrome without confirming laboratory tests and even in cases of doubt about a patient's actual condition. This can present serious consequences for a patient because when bacterial diseases are misdiagnosed as viral flu, no treatment may be provided for bacterial disease. Physicians may also accommodate embarrassments about the causes of gastrointestinal problems, failing to communicate to patients that their infection was transmitted by a fecal-oral route. This can contribute to further infection of others because of the failure to adopt appropriate hygiene. Or physicians may prescribe antibiotics for a diagnosis of viral syndrome because patients demand antibiotic treatments, contributing to antibiotic-resistant infections. McCombie suggests that people's self-diagnosis of flu plays important functions in American society, providing socially acceptable excuses that enable people to avoid reporting more socially embarrassing conditions (diarrhea, hangovers, or menses). Illness diagnoses may be more socially acceptable than disease classifications.

ILLNESS AND SICKNESS ACCOUNTS

"Illness" and "sickness" are sometimes used synonymously, reflecting a sufferer's personal accounts, experience, and interpretations: the patient's perspective. In contrast to *illness* as a personal experience of a malady or unwanted condition, there is a distinction emphasizing *sickness* as the socially induced nature of the experiences produced by the responses of socially significant others. Although disease and illness also necessarily have socially induced aspects, the concept of sickness focuses on social effects on a malady. This includes the effects of resource allocation, stigmatization, and consequences of medical treatment on a patient's life experience.

Illness can also reflect some kind of dysfunction or disharmony in interpersonal and social relations. When others' behavior produces distress, depression, anger, fear, or disgust, it can make us ill. The horrors of war, the fear of assault, the grief of loss, and the anger and desire for revenge can all produce unpleasant states and ultimately unwanted conditions. These experiences can also produce illness and a variety of physical symptoms.

Hahn (1995) proposed that instead of beginning with biology, biomedicine should focus on illness, the personal experience of an unwanted state. Illness involves an individual's psychological and subjective response to being unwell or feeling unhealthy; it includes the sensations of the condition, its effects on the individual, and his or her personal and culturally derived beliefs and attitudes about the defined malady (Helman, 2001; Twaddle, 1981). Illness experiences include effects from perceived personal consequences of the condition, such as limitations on abilities to engage in valued activities such as eating certain foods or doing vigorous activities. Illness is generally conceptualized as one's ability to carry out ordinary daily activities. These produce influences from sickness: how significant others respond to one's condition. Cultural beliefs about the causes of the malady affect its evaluation and the responses of others.

Characteristics that define an individual as ill include the following (also see Helman, 2001; Brody, 1987; and Twaddle, 1973, on illness as deviance):

- Changes in bodily functions or their appearance

- Changes in behavioral abilities or interpersonal or social relations

- Unusual sensory experiences or unpleasant symptoms

- Experiences of excessive and disturbing emotional states

Conditions we experience as undesirable come from many sources and conceptual frameworks, in addition to feelings within our bodies. Other undesirable feelings come from aspects of feelings about ourselves derived from our social relations with others (depression, anger), the environment (cleanliness, balance, warmth), and supernatural or religious beliefs (good, bad, deserving, guilty, punished). We may feel ill from overwhelming personal challenges, interpersonal conflicts, or perceptions of a sickening world. Illness will also include the effects of sickness: how significant beliefs about the causes of the condition affect its evaluation and the responses of others.

Illness may also reflect feared impairments or limitations (e.g., permanent disability versus recovery). Cultural beliefs shape the experience of illness. For instance, in cultures where hunting is fundamental to success, failure in hunting may be viewed as illness. Similarly, poverty and unemployment may be regarded as a form of illness, with the unwanted condition increased by social evaluations that affect self-concept and self-esteem. Culturally important or stigmatized bodily conditions (fat, skinny, weak, dark-skinned), personality characteristics, or emotions (aggression, shyness, greed, rage) may also be regarded as unwanted conditions. Even biological aspects of disease are affected by cultural perceptions, which may define as healthy a symptom or condition viewed as evidence of disorder in another culture. For instance, in areas of the Amazon where parasitic skin disease is endemic, the people who are considered abnormal are those whose immune systems provide immunity to the disease. The illness bearer's assessment of conditions as being a threat to oneself may come at any level: body, personality, mind, or connection with the physical, social, or spiritual world.

CULTURE AND HEALTH

Clinical Significance of African American High-Pertension

African American beliefs about hypertension (or "high-pertension") and "high blood" are similar to biomedical concepts of hypertension and high blood pressure and pose risks for misunderstanding in medical contexts. Hypertension is defined from a biomedical perspective as specific systolic and diastolic blood pressures (above 140 and 90 millimeters of mercury, respectively), with high blood pressure increasing the risk for cardiac diseases and strokes, kidney diseases, and other circulatory complications. High-pertension is related to nerves, stress, and excitable emotional reactions. Like high blood, it involves blood rising up to the head but much more rapidly and with the possibility of causing immediate death. African American concepts of high-pertension and high blood express concern with the amount of blood located high in the body, with excessive blood in the brain leading to headaches, disorientation, dizziness, fainting, strokes, and even death. High-pertension is thought to result from a variety of factors: diet (high levels of fat and rich foods and seasonings), stressful events, excessive alcohol consumption, and supernatural causes (evil spirits or hexes). Health beliefs regarding dietary treatments of high blood and high-pertension are important for biomedical practitioners because similar terms (hypertension and high blood pressure) complicate communication about and management of the conditions (Schoenberg, 1997). Clinicians' diagnosis of high blood pressure may lead patients to rely on traditional remedies to produce "low blood" (eating salty foods, vinegar, and pickled food) that directly conflict with what is advisable for high blood pressures. Heurtin-Roberts (1993) illustrates that high-pertension is a mechanism of personal adaptation for addressing problems related to stress, tension, and anxiety. Hypertension is believed to affect the heart and provides a mechanism for manipulating social relations and alleviating demands to be a caretaker for others. Because hypertension can cause death if the person is emotionally excited, it can be used to reduce demands from others and control the emotional tone of social interactions, especially with family and friends.

Popular conceptions of illness are much broader than the clinical concept of disease, involving a balance of the individual with natural, social, and supernatural worlds. Illness and sickness have broader concerns with psychological, social, and moral issues that have implications for the self.

The inability of providers to address clients' culturally based conceptions of their conditions can create a range of problems in the context of clinical consultation. The discussions of *caida de mollera* (Chapter One) and of "high-pertension" show that ignoring clients' conceptual frameworks can lead to the neglect of serious biomedical conditions or contraindicated folk treatments.

Illness Narratives

Frank's (1995a, b) work on illness illustrates the powerful role of the illness accounts that patients provide in restoring their sense of empowerment, agency, and care of the self. These narratives allow them to cast off the stigmas that have been ascribed to them and their condition, rewriting their medical history and recovery in intelligible terms. These narratives may connect them with social networks of similar sufferers who turn their stigmatized condition into a fight for basic human rights (e.g., the AIDS movement). Or their dialogues may reconstruct their situation in honorable terms, alternative histories that characterize the formation of their victim status or their heroic efforts to heal despite dismal odds of success. These stories of success can provide the motivation for overcoming the limitations imposed by a malady or adjusting one's life to cope with the circumstances. In this sense, illness stories may convey the effort to succeed despite medical conditions.

Brody (1987) shows that among physicians, stories are ways of illustrating how general scientific knowledge is applied to individual cases, with anecdotes providing a link between scientific knowledge and particular patient problems. Illness narratives (Loewe, 2004) are also an important source of information for educating providers and consumers about the impacts that disease and diagnosis have on people's lives, addressing the destabilizing effects that maladies—and biomedical treatment—have. These accounts also help contextualize the abstract diagnoses of diabetes or CVD within the context of its effects on day-to-day existence. The importance of addressing patients' experiences of illness and their narratives about them is illustrated in Mattingly's (1998) *Healing Dramas and Clinical Plots* and Mattingly and Garro's (2000) edited book, *Narrative and the Cultural Construction of Illness and Healing*. Narratives help reveal the personal experience of a malady and the broader linkages of sufferers' situations to the cultural environment and social milieu within which they function. These narratives can reveal problems with treatment, complications with patient compliance, and challenges in everyday life posed by both the malady and the treatment.

Illness narratives and stories of sickness that physicians and patients share about maladies address broader social implications of the malady and its explanation: the why, what, when, where, and how that explain the occurrence, treatment, and resolution of a malady.

For patients, stories of sickness involve placing their experiences in the broader social context, the labeling and classification of their experiences for others, thereby linking the individual and social dimensions within a patient's life experience and meanings

CULTURE AND HEALTH

Healing Stories from Jewish Women Saints

Sered's (2005) examination of the curative roles of pilgrimage illustrate how patients' experiences of suffering are framed in the models provided in the stories associated with the mythological "Rachels," the shared name of three Jewish female saints. Their mythical representations provide models of personal suffering and endurance for women's management of grief and loss. Through storytelling, mythological models become entwined with one's self-identity and dynamics, supporting the renouncement of one's personal needs in service to others. The mythical stories provide a tangible presence for modeling one's behaviors, reinforcing an ability to endure personal loss through the mythical models provided for the transcendence of suffering.

Healing takes place by associating women's lives with those of the saints, placing their situations in analogy with the models of myth. This linking of personal circumstances and cosmic order provides **meaning** in a way that unburdens the self by placing its circumstances within the meaningful cosmic patterns of the universe. Sered shows how women are able to invoke their own mythical model of the universe that resonates with their personal experiences, allowing them to heal from the cognitive reinforcement that comes from feeling that one's own experiences and feelings are shared with others. These therapeutic transference and release processes are enacted in a pilgrimage to the shrines of the saints, where women unburden their loss of children, spouses, and parents and their life sufferings.

Healing stories often involve pilgrimage, a journey to a shrine where the sufferer joins with others in a quest for hope. When healing stories are reinforced through pilgrimage, the physical voyage with others provides a broader social context for the transformation of identity and suffering (Winkelman and Dubisch, 2005). Or if successful, the healing process produces a self-transformation, where a resolution of emotional problems, psychological trauma, and other forms of social suffering release one to psychological growth. The social engagement with stories can provide an opportunity for relieving burdens or constructing a new identity as a survivor. Even if physical impairments and disease are not addressed, these social processes may provide important mechanisms for healing as opposed to cure, coming to terms with one's condition, the permanence of one's limitations due to disease.

(Whaley, 2000). Storytelling creates connectedness that provides understanding through linking the sufferer's past and social context, giving an acceptable explanation within the patient's worldview that provides a sense of confidence of eventual mastery over illness. The placement of sickness stories within religious or mythical contexts provides psychological integration by linking the individual's suffering to broader contexts of positive expectations or endurance.

The importance of storytelling in Native American illness experiences is illustrated by Tom-Orme (1988, 2006). These stories express a worldview that links personal and

BIOCULTURAL INTERACTIONS

Stories of Illness as Healing Devices

Brody (1987) examined patients' stories of sickness to understand their roles in healing processes. Healing processes are elicited by social activities of telling stories regarding those processes. Patients use stories to deal with the suffering produced by the meanings they have attached to their experiences and to produce healing or "whole-ing" through attaching particular meanings to their malady and its context within their life.

Pennebaker's (2003) investigations of the effects of stories of illness on sufferers illustrate that they are powerfully healing. His research found that patients who shared their stories of illness showed clinically measurable improvements in immune system functioning. Jewish Americans (holocaust survivors) who took a "let sleeping dogs lie" approach to their internment trauma had poorer immune outcomes than those who expressed their traumatic past in a "confession is good for the soul" approach to reliving these experiences. These confessions provided a narration of life and self that fit with cultural norms regarding the sharing of experiences as a part of the mourning process. The process of telling stories of one's malady provides meaning to life experiences.

The suppression of trauma causes disease, and the sharing and release of trauma are a part of the healing process. Putting traumatizing experiences into words and sharing them with others in a coherent narrative regarding their meaning and significance for people's lives brings them from the margins of consciousness, where they are actively repressed, into an emotional release. The healing power of storytelling, of illness narratives, derives in part from the way in which the stories' expression transforms how we understand the trauma and how we think and respond to it emotionally. The creation of the story of illness provides a narrative that assists in confronting the anxiety produced by trauma.

The story makes the occurrence of illness or trauma and its impact, consequences, outcomes, and implications manageable. Words define maladies in ways controlled and managed within the patient's conceptual frameworks. Stories assist in management of the emotional effects of the traumatic experiences, leading to improvement in both physical and mental health (Pennebaker, 2003). Stories have a coherent narrative, a logic and consistency that allow still-disturbing or anomalous aspects to be ignored or rationalized. Pennebaker suggests that words also have the power to reformulate the experience and definitions of self, empowering by defining the nature of the previously vaguely experienced trauma in reference to a social context.

cultural elements in a holistic perspective that helps to explain why illness happened. Stories articulate relationships between the human and spirit worlds that are essential to balance and harmony. Storytelling can help improve provider-client relationships and communication if they are effectively incorporated into the medical encounter. This requires that providers take worldview differences into consideration with an open mind, create an environment to receive and share stories, and demonstrate patience that allows a trusting relationship to develop (Tom-Orme, 1988, 2006). This means accepting a view of health that is not merely related to biology and disease but one in which healing includes concepts of balance among the physical and social worlds, one's emotions, social relations, mental state, and spiritual relations. Religious views often play an important role in determining how individuals relate to their malady and significant others.

THE SICK ROLE AND SICKNESS CAREER

When ill, one may feel treated differently by others and even behave differently. The changes in social behaviors and relationships with others that are adopted when ill or diseased are referred to as the sick role. The **sick role** involves cultural, social, and interpersonal expectations regarding the ill or diseased person's behavior. These social expectations include reciprocal expectations the patient has of others (family, physicians, nurses, therapists) and the right to avail herself or himself of special considerations from others that may remedy the malady or assist in coping with it.

Expansion of the Sick Role

Parsons (1951) popularized the notion of the sick role and social analysis of illness behaviors. The *sick role* is based on the concept of the expectations of certain behaviors, rights, and responsibilities associated with occupying a specific position. The *patient role* is a specialized form of the sick role that occurs when the ill person interacts with physicians or other designated healers or health care personnel. The sick role more broadly encompasses the social consequences of being labeled as ill or diseased. Biomedicine's validation of disease can result in changes in social expectations, allowing the individual to reduce ordinary expectations and obligations. Parsons suggested that the sick role resulted in exemptions from responsibilities and certain obligations or responsibilities:

- Exemption from performing certain normal social obligations or responsibilities

- Release, to a certain degree, from responsibility for one's condition and only peripheral responsibility for recovery if medical advice is followed

- A temporary legitimization of the sick role and the expectation that the sick person has the obligation to recover and leave the sick role status as rapidly as possible

- An obligation to comply and cooperate with medical orders

The sick role and its exemptions provide coping mechanisms. These exemptions make it likely that the individual will be relieved of certain expectations by others. For instance, a homemaker may no longer be expected to cook and clean, and a breadwinner may be allowed the luxury of not going to work. But not everyone can avail themselves of these coping mechanisms: a mother may feel a responsibility to take care of her family no matter what the condition, and a father may feel obliged to work to support his family, even when he is sick.

CULTURE AND HEALTH

Sick Role in Mexican American Culture

There are potential conflicts of Mexican American illness beliefs and sick role behaviors with those espoused by Western medicine, which emphasizes responsibility of the individual for his or her illness. In Hispanic disease theory, an individual is not responsible for being ill but is an innocent victim of external forces such as poverty, exposure, and supernatural causes. Approaches that blame the person for his or her condition, even if failure to seek care is contributory, alienate patients. For many Mexican Americans, illness is borne with dignity, and normal activities are continued. The sick role and the excuses from ordinary responsibilities it can provide may not be accepted because endurance of difficulties with stoicism is an ideal value; both male and female roles encourage silent suffering. Men also reject the sick role because of machismo, which emphasizes tolerance of pain to work and support the family. A woman may not accept the sick role and seek medical care because of the expectation that she be strong and fulfill her obligations to her family. This is referred to as *marianismo,* a reference to the Virgin Mary and the ideals that she represents as a servant to her family. Consequently, religious ideals mean that a woman should not complain or take off from her responsibilities but instead persist in her service to others despite her own suffering and need for treatment. The silent suffering demanded by the ideals of the sick role may persist in the context of labor and delivery, where women may silently endure contractions. Many an obstetric nurse has noted a woman's rapid change to a dramatic wailing and crying when the woman's husband arrives. Such is the power of social context to affect our expressions of suffering.

This classic notion of the sick role is too limited to encompass all of the social consequences of suffering from some malady. Many sick roles differ from the "ideal" sick role. Parson's classic (1951) conceptualization of the sick role is most appropriate in people suffering from diseases that are temporary and for which it is normal to expect full recovery. In patients with chronic degenerative diseases, there is no realistic expectation of recovery and relinquishing of the sick role. In many cases of chronic disease, there may not be a release from normal role obligations, although activities may be restricted. Parson's conceptualization of the sick role excludes the expectations in many cases of mental illness, where the patient may not be exempt from social responsibilities. Rather, treatment of the mentally ill may involve expectations that they assume personal and social responsibilities previously neglected, and extension of sick-role exemptions may be far more limited.

The view that patients are not responsible once a physician has validated their disease is also only partially correct, especially for diseases for which it is believed that immoral behavior is responsible for the condition (see the section on AIDS below). Rather than being an inherent condition of the disease, the moral responsibility is culturally defined. In earlier periods, society viewed tuberculosis, epilepsy, and cancer as "shameful diseases" in which people were responsible for succumbing to the condition. In contemporary

American society, addiction, venereal disease, and AIDS are often viewed as the result of moral transgression and, hence, fitting punishments (see Singer, 1997, 2006). Consequently, the patient is not removed from responsibility, even though the sick role is ascribed. Even when personal responsibility is not viewed as a contributing factor, diseases are still often discussed as if we were responsible for our condition. Foster and Anderson (1978) discuss a number of common expressions that attribute this responsibility to the patient, such as

"What did you do to yourself?"

"You cut yourself, broke your leg, sprained your ankle, etc."

"You caught a cold (or other disease)."

Sequences in Sickness Experiences

The experience of sickness, the social response to one's experience of illness, has been suggested to follow distinguishable stages. Spector (1991) suggested that onset, diagnosis, patient status, and recovery were sufficiently general to apply to any culture. These idealized conceptions do not do justice to the diverse experience of maladies. The concept of onset is useless in patients with asymptomatic conditions. Not all ethnomedical systems offer diagnoses, as exemplified in Finkler's (1985a, 1994a) study of Mexican spiritualist healers. Just as an ill person may acquire the sick role without medical legitimization, not all people with medically validated disease will accept the sick role. The recovery phase is absent in patients with terminal illness or persistent pain. Even where there are similarities in major stages (Suchman, 1965), the stages are affected by cultural and social factors, producing cross-cultural variation in the experiences.

Experience of Symptoms The individual experience of changes, pain, discomfort, or other conditions that indicate that something is wrong varies in expectations and interpretations. It evokes varying emotional responses, including in some cultures ignoring or discounting symptoms. The behavior and opinions of others are important factors in seeking or postponing care and making selections among available options.

Assumption of the Sick Role As a person begins to share concerns about his or her health with others, there begins a provisional validation of the sick role that involves social support, exemption from certain habitual social expectations, and the direction of the person toward health care resources. Cultures differ in the conditions for which the sick role will be validated (e.g., is "fright" an acceptable disease to everyone?). Cultures also differ with regard to which exemptions from normal role expectations are allowed.

Medical Care Contact The medical contact stage involves efforts to validate the illness claim as disease and receive proper treatment. Decisions made at this stage vary considerably, even within the same society, where ethnic and class differences affect responses by both the ill person and the healer. Social and cultural norms frame whether appropriate responses to the ill person involve self-medication or professional treatment. Economic factors can make illness not merely a personal condition but a fiscal crisis involving others (e.g., family members) who may need to agree to treatment. For many, the search

CULTURE AND HEALTH

African Americans and the Sick Role

The sick role may not be easily available to poor African Americans. A lack of resources for medical care and a fatalistic acceptance of conditions may preclude active intervention or preventive efforts and contribute to a tendency to endure discomfort. Utilization of self-care practices, prayer for religious intervention, lack of resources for health care, and fear of racist treatment in health care institutions often lead to delays in seeking treatment. Consequently, medical care is more commonly sought in emergency departments when crises occur. Even African Americans not actively involved in religious organizations may rely on religious coping in times of stress. Religion may give hope and positive expectations or may "spiritualize" difficulties, viewing problems as part of God's plan and passively trusting God to take care of them. Seeking psychotherapy departs from African Americans' traditional reliance on coping and management of difficulties within one's family. Consequently, entering into therapy and accepting the sick role as a psychiatric patient is a strong statement about perceived needs for help.

for resources is not with biomedicine but with family or ethnomedical traditions (see Chapter Five).

Dependent-Patient Stage   Once under the care of a provider, patients enter a dependent stage in which they are expected to comply with recommendations and treatment. Whether the condition is remediable or terminal determines whether the patient role is a temporary condition or a permanent condition of the self. The social consequences of diagnoses have effects on the experience of the condition.

Recovery or Rehabilitation Stage   In remediable illness, the patient role is to be relinquished on recovery and rehabilitation. Societies have rituals, ceremonies, and activities that indicate termination of the patient role. However, in some cultures, particular illnesses carry a social stigma that a person cannot escape (e.g., mental illness, cancer, and addiction).

Sickness Career

The concept of the sickness career recognizes that a series of interactions with others occurs over time and in definable stages (Twaddle, 1981). Becoming sick is a *social process,* one in which perceptions of and responses to impaired well-being are shaped by the behavior of significant others. Although physicians may be official arbitrators regarding the sick role, it is generally family, friends, and employers who legitimate the sick role, validate changes in an individual's status, and accommodate to their implications.

Cultural, social, and personal factors affect people's willingness to accept the sick role. Some do not want to adopt the sick role, and others liberally use it for sympathy, release from obligations, and assistance. The social benefits of the sick role may make patients ambivalent, wanting to maintain their sickness rather than eliminate it because of beneficial effects such as

■ *Primary* gains, beginning with the relief of symptoms and associated unpleasant feelings, including diverting attention from other problems. The sick role may serve psychosocial needs, providing attention and concern from others, a use employed by those of marginal status and with weak social support.

■ *Secondary* gains of exemption from responsibility, including work, and special consideration from others. The sick role may relieve individuals from ordinary responsibilities and provide an excuse for personal failure and not meeting social expectations. The sick role can alleviate blame for personal shortcomings, placing responsibility on the malady.

■ *Tertiary* gains, benefits others receive from a patient's sickness (e.g., being a helper).

PRACTITIONER PROFILE

Nancy Romero-Daza

Nancy Romero-Daza, Ph.D., from 1994 to 1998 worked at the Hispanic Health Council (HHC) in Hartford, Connecticut, as an ethnographer researching AIDS, violence, and other health issues and coordinating service units. In 1998 she joined the Department of Anthropology at the University of South Florida (USF) where she teaches medical anthropology and does research in HIV/AIDS and substance abuse among Latino and African American populations. She is also interested in traditional healing practices and in women's health issues.

Romero-Daza became interested in HIV/AIDS while conducting research on the use of traditional medicine in Lesotho, Africa, and assisting with data collection on nutrition among women and children. The results of her work there emphasized the need to examine the spread of HIV/AIDS from a political-economic perspective that looks at the impact of social, economic, political, and cultural factors at both the local and international levels.

At the HHC, Romero-Daza was actively involved in various federally funded research projects related to HIV/AIDS prevention among injection drug users. In addition, she conducted several small-scale projects among African American and Latino (mainly Puerto Rican) injection drug users, crack cocaine users, and sex workers. These projects also addressed issues such as violence victimization, cancer prevention, and dietary practices among inner-city drug users.

Since joining USF in 1998, Romero-Daza has participated in various projects related to the health and well-being of Hispanics and African Americans. Besides different research, design, and implementation projects, she has conducted research on HIV/AIDS among Hispanic women who accompany their partners as migrant laborers in rural areas around Tampa. She has also studied the potential impact of tourism on the spread of STDs in rural Costa Rica, where she conducted a project in which she worked with forty women from four towns in creating culturally appropriate AIDS awareness materials for women and their families.

Others, too, may receive benefits from providing care and the social prestige and material rewards it can provide, such as was provided by the care of leprosy. The sick role may enable individuals to manipulate others through obligations imposed on them by the sick role: for example, guilting the public into paying for unnecessary asylums and indirectly to support the Catholic Church. The sick role may serve religious ends in cultures where illness is seen as a consequence of wrongdoing and may serve as a punishment by which guilt is expiated and social consequences atoned. Suffering from illness as payment for past misdeeds may evoke forgiveness from others.

AIDS AS DISEASE, SICKNESS, AND ILLNESS

AIDS and the associated virus HIV illustrate the same malady as involving disease, illness, and sickness. The social and cultural factors associated with AIDS indicate that the consequences are not strictly from biological issues but also involve personal and social dimensions (see Singer, 1997). The spread of HIV is primarily through behavior: sexual intercourse. Whether this is associated with homosexual or heterosexual behavior differs around the world. In the United States, the once-disproportionate association of AIDS with homosexual men was dramatically reduced through prevention programs targeted at this population. Other behaviors also directly contributed to the spread of HIV through the transfer of blood or other bodily secretions, such as injection of drugs and prostitution. The association of AIDS with gay and drug-addict lifestyles and prostitution stigmatized the condition, with moral judgments of these behaviors contributing to illness and sickness.

The spread of AIDS and HIV illustrate the fundamental role of social factors in disease (Feldman, 1986). After a hypothesized origin of AIDS in Central Africa, it was spread primarily through prostitution and other sexual relations. Feldman suggests that it spread from Central Africa to other parts of the world through migrant Haitian workers in Zaire and sexual contact with U.S. homosexual men both in Africa and Haiti in the 1970s and 1980s. International sex tourism contributed to worldwide spread of HIV into gay and heterosexual populations. The gay community responded to the AIDS epidemic with educational programs promoting behavioral changes that reduced risk. Subsequently, new cases of AIDS were increasingly found in impoverished populations: ethnic minorities, the poor, and third-world countries (Singer, 1992). The highest incidence among disadvantaged groups continues to stigmatize the disease and affect societal responses to its prevention, treatment, and care.

AIDS as Disease

AIDS and HIV are interrelated as a complex of symptoms (a syndrome) and a group of retroviruses, respectively. AIDS is not a specific disease but a complex of symptoms that reflect failure of the immune system. HIV destroys cells of the immune system, undermining immune system resistance. AIDS symptoms vary considerably because reduction of the body's resistance increases susceptibility to a wide variety of diseases, primarily rare cancers and pneumonia. HIV is present in people in whom the immune system remains intact and, consequently, there are no symptoms of infection. HIV also has a long latency period, the time between infection and manifestation of symptoms. HIV can be viewed as the cause of AIDS, but differential distribution of HIV and AIDS among ethnic populations illustrates the fundamental importance of sociocultural factors. The disproportionate occurrence of new HIV cases among U.S. ethnic minorities reflects the influences of poverty on access to preventive, educational, and treatment services. Because there is no cure for HIV infection, the only effective response is changing behaviors that contribute to disease transmission. Because the highest incidence is among ethnic populations and isolated social groups (intravenous drug users and sex workers), knowledge of cultural factors involved in these groups' risk behaviors is essential to prevention.

AIDS as Sickness

Experiences of AIDS patients and HIV-positive individuals include consequences of the social perceptions of these conditions. Sickness dimensions of AIDS result from ways that institutions (political, research, and medical) respond to AIDS patients. An association of HIV with socially stigmatized groups has contributed to blaming HIV infection on the victims and their lifestyles, increasing personal suffering. Social responses to AIDS also impact disease-free members of high-risk populations, justifying discrimination against these groups (such as Haitians) in public policy. Family members who do not have HIV but experience sickness and suffering from the associated stigma may share the socially induced suffering.

AIDS as Illness

Cultural attitudes play a significant role in shaping illness experiences of those with HIV and AIDS diagnoses; consequently, appropriate care requires addressing institutional responses and the interpersonal and psychosocial dynamics of discrimination. Significant aspects of the illness experience come from cultural stigmatization and neglect that compound suffering. A patient's experience of HIV and AIDS is affected by the fear others have of the patient, and homophobia, a negative societal attitude toward gay behavior, may induce shame or guilt.

Political and Economic Aspects of AIDS Treatment

The face of AIDS today has been changing and expanding. Its early association in the United States with those with gay and drug-user lifestyles has changed. Now it is minority women and youth of all ethnic backgrounds who are at greatest risk. The early association of AIDS with Haiti is now replaced with the estimated bulk of documented cases in sub-Saharan Africa.

The treatment of AIDS has become a political and economic issue, rather than strictly a medical issue. The "AIDS cocktails" used by patients with HIV are sold by pharmaceutical companies at very high prices, with some doses running into hundreds of dollars a day. The "cocktails" of antiretroviral drugs can suppress HIV and other side effects, but millions of

APPLICATIONS

Anthropological Approaches to AIDS Prevention

Anthropology has played an important role in AIDS prevention research (see Singer, 1992; Bowser, Quimby, and Singer, 2007). The social dynamics of AIDS transmission and its social evaluation illustrate why it must be addressed not only as a disease but also as sickness and illness. Cultural perspectives are essential for addressing the spread of HIV infection because, without a cure, the only effective response is prevention, which requires changes in people's behavior. Cultural perspectives are necessary for determining

- Factors predisposing high-risk populations
- Risk behaviors in the general population
- Relatively secretive and hidden aspects of high-risk behaviors
- Social responses affecting the perception of AIDS
- Medical, political, and economic policies that affect AIDS research and treatment

Behavioral and community-based efforts are necessary to assist populations in avoiding exposure, based on knowledge regarding the immediate contextual influences on risk behavior. High rates of HIV/AIDS in minority populations in part reflect failures of prevention programs to provide culturally appropriate interventions. What leads people to engage in behaviors that expose them to HIV? When is exposure most likely to occur? The ability to change relevant behaviors is complicated by the primary mode of transmission—sex—that constitutes a tabooed area in all cultures. The need to alter sexual behaviors not ordinarily discussed makes it of utmost importance to understand the social and cultural factors affecting risk-related behaviors. Cultural approaches provide understandings of the context and motivation of high-risk behaviors that must be addressed for effective risk-reduction programs.

Because risk behaviors contributing to transmission are generally private or stigmatized forms of conduct, ethnography and **participant observation**, observations that take place in the normal context of these activities, are necessary to identify relevant behaviors and contexts. The specific cultural contexts within which high-risk behaviors occur need to be understood to change those behaviors. Immersion in the context of high-risk behaviors provides data not available through structured surveys, which often produce socially appropriate responses rather than actual behaviors. Also of relevance are sexual values, interpersonal dynamics, and social interaction patterns that contribute to what are often spontaneous, rather than deliberate, behaviors. People may intend to engage in appropriate risk-reduction behaviors (e.g., using a condom) but instead engage in contextually motivated high-risk behaviors (e.g., from peer pressure). These behaviors can best be identified through the participant observation approach. Formal surveys cannot inquire about relevant behaviors unless these contextually manifested activities are previously identified through participant observation.

Assessments of changes in high-risk behaviors among communities receiving AIDS prevention programs show that education alone is not sufficient to eradicate high-risk behaviors. Cultural approaches are necessary to identify factors that inhibit the adoption of safe-sex techniques and contribute to the continuation of unsafe sexual practices. Because behavior is typically reinforced in social networks and interpersonal contact, knowledge of the norms, beliefs, and influences within a community is essential for understanding how to prevent the spread of HIV.

Anthropologists have also made contributions to the study of AIDS in directing attention to the specific issues involved in various ethnic and cultural groups. Cultural aspects of AIDS prevention programs are illustrated in Singer's (1992) approach to the AIDS epidemic in U.S. ethnic minorities. He shows that anthropologically informed research is necessary for project design, implementation of project structure and content, and evaluation of project effectiveness. Anthropological methods are particularly effective in acquiring in-depth understandings that provide a basis for culturally sensitive approaches. Implementing culturally sensitive approaches also requires community liaison skills, producing partnerships among community and health care organizations by engaging community participation. Culturally sensitive, socially relevant, and locally grounded information needs to be obtained before program development. Ideal methods for obtaining these data include the anthropological methods of participant observation, informal and unstructured interviews, and focus groups made up of relevant participants (e.g., sex workers or injection drug users). These methods accommodate to natural social environments in ways that facilitate disclosure, allow group dynamics to contribute insights, and express variability within the target group.

Interventions with culturally sensitive content produce far higher levels of program participation. Culturally relevant interventions require culturally appropriate project structures (e.g., location, context, scheduling). Cultural sensitivity includes accessibility, culturally appropriate groupings (e.g., single sex), scheduling, appropriate language or idiomatic formats, and other cultural aspects affecting interpersonal relations and disclosure. Anthropological approaches have been effective in ascertaining the resistance to safe-sex practices found in the cultural dynamics of specific groups.

Community collaboration helps ensure the appropriate management of issues such as gender roles, community differentiation, interpersonal and social dynamics, and other local conditions affecting participation. This requires that interventions be tailored for each population based on the risk behaviors and social factors affecting each specific subculture (e.g., women versus men, ethnic differences, generational differences). Natural social networks provide invaluable assistance in the diffusion of AIDS prevention programs, helping to ensure that educational messages are provided in linguistically, culturally, and socially appropriate formats. These networks also provide the peer support necessary to produce community-level behavioral change necessary for AIDS prevention. Prevention programs should use peer educators and culturally knowledgeable consultants as role models. Anthropology has also made contributions to AIDS care in areas of understanding sickness, the stigma produced by the HIV/AIDS diagnosis.

Waterston (1997) argues that the popular prevention theories based on educational interventions and behavioral change, while helpful in reducing the spread of HIV, are inadequate because they focus attention on the individual, obscuring the social and economic factors that contribute to HIV infection. Waterston explores an anthropologically informed alternative based on principles of social responsibility and advocacy for social justice through humane social programs, principles engaged by critical and political economy approaches discussed in Chapter Eight.

AIDS patients around the world cannot afford these drugs. Who has precedence, the share-holders of these multinational corporations or the millions of impoverished AIDS patients whose only hope of longer survival depends on these medications, which their own countries could produce cheaply? Here we see how political-economic priorities—capitalism or socialism and nationalism—affect decisions about what is fair treatment of disease.

Third-world countries are resisting these exorbitant prices and threatening to produce their own generic versions of these drugs. For instance, Brazil has attempted to get the Swiss pharmaceutical giant Roche to reduce the prices or allow the government to manufacture the anti-AIDS drug nelfinavir. Some countries have attempted to produce these drugs themselves but find their efforts blocked by the legal actions of the pharmaceutical companies, which want to assert exclusive rights to these medicines. Brazilian law allows the government to produce the drug in the case of national emergency and when the companies engage in an abuse of their economic situation. Having decided that the law applied to the case of the AIDS cocktails, Brazil obtained the support of the World Trade Organization in its legal struggle to break the patent of American pharmaceutical companies and to produce low-cost generic versions of other AIDS treatments. Negotiated settlements allow the Brazilian state company Far-Manguinhos to produce brand-name AIDS drugs, dramatically reducing costs while still paying the pharmaceutical companies royalties for their patent rights. Here national rights to access to medications are taking precedence over the unbridled economic rights of companies. This strategy has also compelled some drug manufacturers to reduce their prices rather than face the prospect of the national laboratories producing generic versions.

There are significant social and cultural dimensions to AIDS, particularly the behaviors that contribute to transmission and the social responses that produce sickness and illness. Because biomedicine does not have a cure for AIDS, the primary means of addressing the spread of HIV infection is through changing the behaviors that lead to exposure and the social conditions that increase the possibility of infection. Consequently, anthropology has played a significant role in addressing the AIDS epidemic (see the special feature "Applications: Anthropological Approaches to AIDS Prevention").

HEALTH BELIEFS AND EXPLANATORY MODELS

An understanding of the perspectives of disease, illness, and sickness can better meet the health needs and concerns of consumer-patients and the treatment goals of providers. The recognition of the importance of patients' personal views of the health problem has led to the development of models for inquiry into patients' beliefs about their malady and treatment. Principal models are the Health Beliefs Model (Becker, 1974) and the Explanatory Model (Kleinman, 1980, 1988b). Peoples' understandings and conceptual frameworks regarding their malady and its relevant sensations and symptoms provide information for physicians to make sense of patients' conditions. An understanding of patients' conceptions of their maladies is vital for biomedical care because different physician and patient vocabularies and conceptual frameworks can undermine care. Because of different frameworks of understanding, miscommunication will likely occur, even if provider and patient are from the same cultural group. This can lead to misdiagnosis and inappropriate treatment.

The challenge of cultural competency is to understand culture, language, and conceptual systems to help ensure effective care despite differences. The effects of poverty, lack of education, unemployment, children out of wedlock, welfare, drug abuse, and other social problems on daily life and world conceptions generally fall outside the personal experience of providers. Consequently, they are unable to understand the problems of clients, the complicating factors in keeping appointments or adhering to care plans, or patients' unwillingness or inability to accept the medical regimen. Patient compliance is fostered through an informed response to the ways culture affects care by incorporating client perspectives into treatment plans and public health programs.

Clinical Adaptations to Illness

Clinical adaptations to addressing illness and sickness along with disease are based in the approaches of health beliefs and explanatory models, which elicit patients' personal and cultural knowledge and expectations as a basis for bridging the differences between patients' and biomedicine's worldviews. Helman (1985, 1994, 2001) suggests the following interrelated strategies for dealing with clinical problems created by differences in biomedical and **lay** perspectives of disease and illness:

- Understand "illness"

- Improve communication

- Increase cultural self-awareness

- Assess cultural context

- Treat illness and disease

Understanding illness involves discovering how a patient and important figures in the patient's life view the origin of the illness, its significance for him or her, its prognosis (outcome), and its implications for other aspects of his or her life (Helman, 1985). To determine these patient perceptions, it is necessary to obtain information on cultural, religious, social, and economic backgrounds and the patient's **health beliefs model** and **explanatory model** (see below).

Improving communication requires that clinicians learn patients' cultural illness conceptions and make clinical diagnosis and treatment intelligible to patients through their views of health and illness. To accomplish this, clinicians must understand patients' experiences and interpretations. It requires the development of cross-cultural adaptation skills, presented in Chapter Three.

Increased cultural self-awareness, or reflexivity, in the clinical encounter is an awareness of how providers' cultural beliefs affect care. Providers' social and cultural backgrounds structure their behavior and affect perceptions of patients, their symptoms, and their health care. Awareness of the cultural dimensions of what seems normal can be developed through the kinds of self-assessments provided at the end of each chapter.

Assessing cultural context is crucial for effective medical care. Socioeconomic factors—economic status, discrimination, unemployment, and social roles—have implications for illness, presentation for care, and treatment compliance. Cultural systems models and community assessment protocols are provided in Chapter Four as frameworks for assessing the broader social and cultural contexts that affect health behaviors.

Treating illness and disease means that medical treatment must deal with the dimensions of illness that affect patients' emotional, social, and behavioral well-being, not merely their physical conditions. These personal aspects of illness management are described in Chapter Five. Physicians may also address these dimensions through collaboration with social workers or traditional healers and by educating themselves to address the broader psychological, ecological, political, and symbolic contexts of disease and illness addressed in Chapters Six through Nine.

Health Beliefs Model

The Health Beliefs Model was developed by many contributors (Strecher and Rosenstock, 1997; Becker, 1974). It originated in public health after the recognition that decision-making models shape patients' preventive actions and treatment responses. This model is based in theories regarding seeking health or avoidance of illness (value) and the perceived benefits of certain actions (expectancy) (Strecher and Rosenstock, 1997), focusing on patients' perceived susceptibility to disease, likelihood of contracting a condition, severity of that condition, benefits of action, and barriers to care.

The original cognitive orientation was expanded to emphasize perceptions about

- Availability of services and cost-benefit analyses of changing behaviors or accessing services

- "Cues to action," information such as billboards or public service announcements that stimulate people's thinking about needed health behaviors

- Self-efficacy, an individual's belief in his or her ability to take actions to achieve changes

Self-efficacy is an important component of engaging in treatment, particularly where conditions are part of lifestyle, such as excessive eating and drug addictions. People have to feel threatened by conditions and believe they can benefit from changes; they also have to be motivated to alter their behaviors. Even with these extensions, the health beliefs model's "rationalistic" approach does not address all of the factors affecting patients' decisions, such as emotions and interpersonal relations. Economic, political, and institutional factors play important roles in influencing health behavior, particularly in regard to accessing services and indicating preventive behaviors.

The health beliefs model makes important contributions to understanding health behavior and improving compliance by addressing the client's framework. Personal conceptions of risks, illnesses, sick-role behaviors, and treatment options shape responses. Decisions about health behaviors occur within cultural frameworks of beliefs about desired health conditions; individual beliefs about personal susceptibility, severity, and risks; and perceptions of costs and availability of treatment.

Explanatory Model

Physician-anthropologist Kleinman (1980, 1988a, 1995) articulated the explanatory model, which examines how patients interpret the causes and progress of a malady and how they think it should be treated. The explanatory model elicits the patient's view of

- The cause of the condition, that is, what has happened and how or why
- The timing of symptom onset: why this has occurred now
- Pathophysiological processes: what the condition does to the body
- The natural history of the malady: its anticipated course and effects if left untreated
- Appropriate treatments: what the patient thinks should be done

The explanatory model provides a format for eliciting how a malady is interpreted by both patient and provider, making explicit the models used by both to interpret and explain a malady and decide among possible therapies. Because explanatory models may not be explicit, the process is useful in formulating the different clinical realities of the various participants, particularly giving voice to patients and their families. Explanatory models also give providers a mechanism for developing self-awareness and identifying

APPLICATIONS

Eliciting an Explanatory Model

I participated as a staff member in a free community clinic in Mexico run by U.S. physicians and medical students. My role was that of translator and consultant. One patient had recently received eye surgery elsewhere, with the eye still bandaged. He was complaining about gastrointestinal problems (diarrhea and vomiting), nervousness, chills, and an inability to sleep. The presenting complaints appeared to have nothing to do with the recent surgery or complications and did not fit together in a diagnosis. The physician was frustrated, unable to determine the nature of the malady, and felt that another issue was going on with the patient. He called on me in a translator role to interview the patient.

I began to elicit the explanatory model—What do you think is the cause of your condition?—which the patient initially resisted. But on prodding, the patient reported that he had a stomach condition previously treated in a clinic. The physician rejected that diagnosis, based on the patient's present symptoms and conditions. I continued with the elicitation of the patient's explanatory model, asking what he thinks is the appropriate treatment. Although he initially evaded response, his wife eventually offered that he wanted a renewal of a previous prescription. The physician indicated that it was a powerful sedative for calming the stomach and nerves. His interpretation was that the patient, distressed by the eye surgery and subsequent incapacitation, was attempting to obtain a controlled substance that he had previously used and felt applicable to his present malady because it would reduce tension. Symptoms were being presented to justify the prescription.

CULTURE AND HEALTH

African American CVD and Illness Beliefs

In addressing the higher incidence of CVD among African Americans, the health beliefs model points to questions regarding the awareness they have about their risks and risk factors. Have adequate public health campaigns for raising awareness of CVD been directed at the African American population? For those who recognize their elevated risk of CVD, do they feel that resources are available that are effective in countering the disease, and do they have the sense of self-efficacy that they can successfully seek the necessary care? The explanatory model approaches reveal that there are significant differences between disease and illness, reflected in the easily confused distinctions between the biomedical disease hypertension and the African American cultural illness called "high-pertension." These differences can lead to complications for African American cardiovascular patients. Patients confusing the biomedical diagnosis of hypertension with their own similar-sounding "high-pertension" may resort to traditional remedies for the latter that can increase blood pressure. "High-pertension" treatments include the use of salty and pickled foods that can exacerbate blood pressure problems. African Americans may also believe that "high-pertension" can be controlled through these dietary changes and changes in stress levels (Schlomann and Schmitke, 2007), leading to the erroneous conclusion that they no longer require their medication for treatment of CVD. The explanatory model is an ideal tool for determining patients' perceptions of their conditions, their expectations regarding treatment or nontreatment, and their likely responses to proposed medication and dietary treatment. As such, the explanatory model becomes a significant tool for overcoming barriers to effective treatment produced by different conceptualizations of disease and illness.

sources of clinical miscommunication. Kleinman (1988a) states that patients' explanatory models tend to be context- or illness-specific and reflect patients' individual psychocultural dynamics, assumptions, and preconscious beliefs. Social, economic, or religious factors may also be important determinants of the explanatory model, which may not be scientifically correct but, nonetheless, have an internal logic and guide health behavior. Patient explanatory models play an important role in diagnosis because they provide the conceptual framework within which patients interpret, assess, and express maladies. These models may reveal that a patient has taken particular remedies or experienced conditions of relevance to biomedical diagnosis. They may also reveal patients' "hidden agendas," as illustrated in "Applications: Eliciting an Explanatory Model."

To effectively bridge different perceptions, providers must incorporate patients' explanatory model. Kleinman (1988a) notes that patients may resist unless the physician shows genuine interest and explains how the questions may help to tailor the treatment plan. Providers must understand patients' explanatory models to adapt treatment plans to patient beliefs and expectations and achieve a consensus about the nature of the malady and the treatment to be implemented. Consensus is achieved through negotiation between explanatory models, but noncompliance is the likely result when the provider's explanatory model is too discrepant for the patient, and the gap between them is not effectively bridged in the clinical consultation. The provider needs to work with the patient's explanatory model, even if the provider considers it wrong, because it represents how the patient understands the situation.

In summary, the health beliefs and explanatory models provide complementary perspectives for understanding the relationship of an individual to a malady and that person's likely responses to the condition and proposed treatment. The health beliefs model provides a focus on the broader societal factors affecting exposure to causes as well as preventive messages and information about relevant health resources that affect care-seeking behaviors. The explanatory model provides a focus on the immediate context of treatment, the factors affecting the likelihood that the patient will do what the doctor prescribes. Together they provide an understanding of the sociocultural factors affecting exposure and treatment.

CHAPTER SUMMARY

Distinguishing the disease, illness, and sickness concepts provides a focus on the biological, personal, and social dimensions of health maladies. Responses to these maladies involve learned patterns of thought and behavior acquired through socialization and cultural patterning of expression and responses to conditions. These influences must be recognized for accurate assessment and treatment of conditions because they affect the importance of symptoms and their disclosure to providers. Patients' perspectives on their malady and intended responses to treatment are important because they determine whether they follow medical advice. Acquiring the patient's perspective facilitates diagnosis and follow-up by ensuring that the physician acquires full access to the patient's knowledge of his or her condition. Explanatory models reveal their perceptions and anticipated behaviors and can establish the need for negotiation between different views. A major challenge to medicine is compliance; understanding patients' beliefs and expectations regarding maladies helps gauge patients' intended compliance, permitting communication and negotiation to achieve successful treatment. The next chapter introduces the foundations for achieving such cultural understandings.

KEY TERMS

Biopsychosocial model
Constructivist perspective
Contributory factors or cause
Disease
Double-blind clinical trial
Epidemiology
Explanatory model
Health beliefs model
Illness
Malady

Meaning
Necessary cause
Nosology
Remote distal cause
Sickness
Sick role
Sociogenic diseases
Somatoform disorders
Sufficient cause

SELF-ASSESSMENT 2.1. DISEASE, ILLNESS, AND SICK-ROLE EXPERIENCES

What diseases are most prevalent in your ethnic or social group?

Why are these diseases the most prevalent in your group?

Is there a genetic basis, or are these diseases a function of cultural lifestyle and behaviors? Relationships with other groups?

How are these diseases viewed within your culture?

Is there a moral evaluation associated with them?

Have you ever been ill but unable to find a medical explanation for your condition?

Have you ever had illnesses that physicians did not accept as real?

What are your personal attitudes toward the sick role?

Which of the following behaviors do you feel are appropriate for a sick person?

Withdrawal

Complaining

Crying

Moaning

Anger

Irritability

Pain medication

Silent suffering

Missing work or school

Are there typical attitudes toward the sick role that are part of your family traditions?

Are there typical attitudes toward the sick role that are part of your culture? Subculture?

What sick-role behaviors do you tend to adopt when you are ill?

How does being sick affect your personality?

When you are ill, do you want frequent visits from family and friends? Or would you prefer to be left alone?

When you are sick, do you expect to take care of yourself, or do you expect others to care for you?

What expectations do you have of family members when you are sick? Are they different for your mother versus your father? Brothers versus sisters? Sons versus daughters? Your spouse?

Are there people you know who appear to use the sick role excessively? How do you respond to them?

Do you feel that some illnesses and diseases have a moral or ethical component? Which ones, and why?

Are there diseases or illness for which people deserve our compassion, understanding, and assistance?

Are there diseases or illness for which people deserve to be sick?

Are there some diseases that have a moral implication in a patient's responsibility for his or her condition? Does this affect how he or she is treated?

How do your sick-role behaviors and attitudes reflect your cultural and social background?

How do you obtain your medical services? Do you have a prepaid health plan (e.g., an HMO)? How does that affect your willingness to seek out health services?

ADDITIONAL RESOURCES

Book

Royer, A. 1998. *Life with chronic illness: Social and psychological dimensions.* Westport, Conn./London: Praeger.

Journal

Health: An Interdisciplinary Journal for the Social Study of Health, Illness and Medicine.

CHAPTER

3

CULTURAL COMPETENCE IN HEALTH CARE

[Quality care depends on] 1) respect for patient's values, preferences and expressed needs; 2) communication and education; 3) coordination and integration of care; 4) physical comfort; 5) emotional support and alleviation of fears; 6) involvement of family and friends; and 7) continuity and transition

—DELBANCO, 1992, P. 414

LEARNING OBJECTIVES

- Characterize the bases for developing cultural competence in health care
- Illustrate the major levels of intercultural competence
- Present anthropological perspectives that facilitate development of cross-cultural competence
- Present personal and interpersonal strategies for adaptation to intercultural relations
- Illustrate medical anthropologists' use of cultural competence in health settings
- Illustrate the applications of cultural frameworks in clinical settings to enhance well-being of patients and providers

CROSS-CULTURAL ADAPTATIONS IN HEALTH CARE

Differences between providers and their clients interfere with clinical consultation and treatment, program development, and disease prevention. This is true not only in health beliefs and behaviors but also in styles of communication, social expectations, world-views, and other aspects of culture. This chapter illustrates how the barriers and problems produced by differences can be addressed with the development of cultural competence, based in the abilities to apply cultural knowledge and intercultural skills to effectively address the impacts of culture on social relations.

Effective adaptation to other cultures' health realities requires several areas of personal development of new cognitive orientations by

- Developing awareness of the impact of cultural values and social processes on personal characteristics, including health care preferences

- Improving intercultural interactions by acquiring strategies for enhancing understanding and reducing conflict and noncompliance through intercultural relations and negotiation skills

- Acquiring models of culture for analysis of culture and health relations

This chapter describes personal and interpersonal skills relevant to intercultural encounters. Personal cultural awareness is a prerequisite for effectively managing cross-cultural differences and overcoming conflicts. The values assessment exercise at the end of the chapter (see Exhibit 3.1) provides an understanding of how your own health values relate to your health behaviors and preferences for care. Intercultural skills help overcome cultural communication gaps and facilitate adaptations to cultural factors that affect clients' reality. Perspectives from anthropology and intercultural communication indicate specific ways of facilitating the effectiveness of medical encounters in bridging the cultural differences between providers and clients. Social and cultural factors are relevant to all aspects of clinical relations, not just communication. Competence also requires awareness of how social factors external to a client's culture (e.g., other cultural groups in the broader society) affect clients' health opportunities, attitudes, beliefs, and behaviors. Knowledge of these specific aspects of culture is important in making clinical consultations more effective as providers understand the significance of the malady and its consequences within the life circumstances of a client.

Anthropologists are involved in a range of areas related to the effectiveness and quality of care. This begins with their roles as trainers and mediators, instructing health care providers in more effective ways of dealing with people from other cultures. Anthropologists also have roles in culturally sensitive research approaches, facilitator roles in the formation of community coalitions, and research and public advocacy roles on behalf of underprivileged groups. Anthropologists may also undertake the development of cultural change programs for health institutions as well as other mediator activities in the relationships between health care institutions and communities. Anthropologists may also be cross-trained in other professions, such as psychology, nursing, or social work, and play a more direct role in patient care. The concepts of clinically applied anthropology are introduced to illustrate the range of roles that anthropologists may play in enhancing the quality of care. Anthropologists also have important roles in community and public health programs. Accurate assessment, interpretation, and intervention require that concern about symptoms and responses available to care be understood in the cultural life context of clients. Frameworks are presented for the assessment of the effects of culture in clinical interactions, developing culturally sensitive approaches to client care, and using the concepts of culture to provide care for practitioners, thus reducing the stress of their jobs.

CASE STUDY

Lost Without Translation

Serious challenges are presented when patients do not speak English, the situation faced by Lia Lee's parents. The hospital did not fund translators, instead relying on bilingual employees—janitors, ambulance drivers, and lab technicians—to translate when they were free from their job responsibilities. They were generally unavailable, such as when Lia's parents went to the hospital emergency department because of concern about her seizures. But the symptoms were no longer present when she was seen, and with no translator, the physician was not informed about her seizure. Her chest x-rays showed congestion; he misdiagnosed it as bronchopneumonia rather than recognizing that it was caused by her having swallowed vomit during the seizure. Her parents were given a prescription for an antibiotic and signed a paper acknowledging they had received instructions for her care. But they understood nothing of what they were told to do, including to return to the hospital in ten days.

Lia's medical treatment came to involve a large number of medications given in different combinations and at different times of the day. In addition to anticonvulsants, there were antibiotics, bronchodilators, antifever medications, and vitamins. Her family was utterly confused by the vast amount of information regarding her medications. Being illiterate, they were unable to keep track of the information relevant to medicating their child. The attending physicians were initially unaware that her parents did not understand the instructions and were not properly medicating their daughter.

When the Hmong visit hospitals, the lack of translators means that bilingual adolescent family members are often called on to translate. This could result in ten-year-old girls being the first to advise their family members that their elder relative is dying or teen-aged boys having to discuss their mother's gynecological conditions with doctors. Translators are often ineffective because the Hmong language does not have terms for many of the concepts used by physicians. Long explanations have to be used to express simple concepts like "parasite," "pancreas," and "chromosome," and accurate translation is often incomprehensible to patients, who lack the conceptual framework to make the information intelligible. And when medical consent and release forms have to be signed, the complicated legal language is a challenge for even bilingual educated Hmong. The decision-making processes of the Hmong community also challenge the providers. Hospitals are seldom prepared to address chain-of-command issues in making medical decisions, where the father or husband consults with "elder brother" and a hierarchy of clan leaders.

CULTURAL COMPETENCE

The need for people to effectively deal with cultural differences is widely recognized in the concepts of cultural awareness, sensitivity, and competence, which involve knowledge of intercultural skills necessary to manage cultural differences effectively. *Cultural awareness* involves an understanding of the importance of cultural differences. *Cultural sensitivity* goes beyond awareness to provide an appropriate response to cultural differences: for instance, knowing that people from some cultures do not like to look directly into another's eyes. *Cultural competence* refers to having further capabilities to deal with differences effectively, generally implying the ability to function effectively in the context of everyday life of a culture. *Cultural responsiveness* falls between sensitivity and competence; in nursing care, it is conceptualized as the ability to respond to a patient's care needs in a way that is congruent with the patient's cultural expectations. *Cultural proficiency* involves the ability to transfer cultural knowledge and skills to others, providing others with the skills to effectively manage cultural differences. Cultural competence involves personal, interpersonal, and organizational skills, including behaviors, attitudes, and policies that enable people to work effectively with the various cultural groups they serve.

Cultural competence has several major dimensions:

- Knowledge of the general dynamics of culture and of cross-cultural relations

- Skills in intercultural adaptation and relations

- Specialty-specific skills for professional relations

- Culture-specific knowledge of behaviors and beliefs of specific groups

The ability to deal effectively with cultural issues in clinical settings can be conceptualized as three major factors: capacity level, specialty area, and specific cultural groups (Castro, 1998). There is a range of cultural capacity levels such as awareness, sensitivity, and competence. An individual's cultural competency varies across different ethnic groups as well as specialty areas (e.g., mediation, assessment, treatment, research, community intervention, policy formation). An individual's cultural capacities can even differ across segments of a specific ethnic group. One may be culturally proficient in relations with elderly Mexican Americans but lack understanding of and empathy for younger Mexican Americans or monolingual Spanish-speaking Mexican immigrants.

Cultural competence in clinical care also involves professional attitudes and clinical skills, combining them with a knowledge of cultural systems and their effects on behavior and opportunities (Chrisman and Zimmer, 2000). The professional attitudes necessary for effective cross-cultural clinical relations begin with an awareness and acknowledgment of the effects of culture on one's self and clinical practice, combined with the knowledge of how to adapt to these influences in self and others in the context of intercultural relations. These include the ability to adapt to the effects of prejudice, ethnocentrism, cognitive attribution, culture shock, transference, and discrimination. A culturally skilled clinician can respond to the feelings of discrimination and prejudice that clients may harbor, preventing these normal but nonproductive intercultural dynamics from impeding clinical care. These reactions can be countered with skills that include anthropological approaches discussed below that facilitate the understanding of clients' cultures and their health behaviors and beliefs.

Clinical skills depend on intercultural abilities for carrying out culturally competent assessments. Cultural competency is embodied in the elicitation of the explanatory model to obtain clients' concerns, enabling the negotiation of an acceptable treatment plan that incorporates both clients' and providers' perspectives. This **general cultural competence** involves knowledge of the ways culture in general affects intergroup interactions and an ability to apply cultural knowledge, cultural resources (translators, interpreters), and intercultural skills to resolve the difficulties presented by cultural differences. General cultural competency includes an awareness of the dynamics of cross-cultural interactions and the ability to adopt perspectives that facilitate those interactions, including cultural awareness, **cultural relativism**, conflict resolution, and cross-cultural negotiation.

Specific cultural competencies refer to abilities in relating to *particular* cultures (e.g., Mexican Americans or Hmong immigrants; see Winkelman 1998, 2006a). Specific cultural competencies require a long time to develop and are generally beyond the reach of providers unless they are native members of that culture or spend long periods engaged with the culture in both the clinic and everyday life. Providers are more likely to learn how to incorporate aspects of cultural knowledge into culturally aware, sensitive, or responsive care than to develop true cultural competency.

Even achieving culturally responsive care requires a development of cultural competency (Culhane-Pera et al., 2003). Providers require knowledge of cultural beliefs, values, and attitudes for an appropriate understanding of patients. Acquiring cultural competence involves several major areas of development (see Hogan-Garcia, 2003; Chrisman and Zimmer, 2000):

- Self-awareness of personal cultural features and level of personal cultural competency development

- Personal and interpersonal skills for managing the dynamics of intercultural relations

- Knowledge of cultural systems and specific cultures

To facilitate that learning and development, the next sections describe

1. The general levels of cultural competence that were assessed in Chapter One

2. A range of skills for intercultural adaptation. Chapter Four provides additional models for understanding culture and psychocultural development.

Levels of Cross-Cultural Competence

Cross-cultural effectiveness ranges from a dislike and misunderstanding of out-groups through varying levels of appreciation of the nature and significance of cultural differences. This learning may culminate in multicultural competencies and bicultural identities (Bennett, 1993; Bandlamudi, 1994; Winkelman, 1999, 2001c). These involve increasing degrees of awareness of cultural influences on the self and the abilities to adapt effectively to cultural differences. The following categories explain the scales presented in Chapter One in Self-Assessment 1.4. Cross-Cultural Development.

Ethnocentrism People begin in an ethnocentric condition, ignorant of the relation of culture to behavior and self, lacking competency in understanding cross-cultural issues, and lacking appreciation of the effects of historical and contemporary racism. An exaggerated sense of cultural superiority impairs relations with other groups and limits awareness of cultural differences. Attitudes may be characterized by a belief that other people behave differently because they are stupid or inferior. Bennett (1993) considers the purest form of ethnocentrism to involve denial and ignorance of differences, normally maintained through separation from others who are different. The ethnocentrism phase suffers from a lack of awareness of cultural differences and their relevance. Others are unreflectively evaluated from one's own cultural perspective. One's cultural perspective is not recognized as such; rather, it is seen as a universally valid system of evaluation. For instance, a physician might believe that only biomedicine is established as effective in treating diseases and dismiss the possibility that other ethnomedical systems have general effectiveness and validity.

Universalism Universalism involves minimization, a perspective that rejects fundamental differences across cultures and, instead, emphasizes human similarities. Cultural differences are trivialized, manifested in the idea that "everybody's basically the same" and that you should "treat everybody the same." This perspective is naïve regarding the importance of cultural differences, ignorant to the fact that one's perspectives about human universality and sameness are based in one's own cultural assumptions. In the minimization stage, people often assume that being one's "natural self" and expressing genuineness can achieve success in intercultural relations. This attitude emphasizes the appropriateness of one's own cultural behavior in intercultural contexts, an ethnocentrism that reduces the ability to recognize and incorporate an understanding of cultural differences. The minimization process may be manifested in a physical universalism, where human physical and biological commonalities are emphasized while the culturally unique aspects that direct behavior are ignored or discounted. In transcendental universalism, despite behavioral differences, one believes that all humans conform to some single transcendental principle. This is often embodied in religious universalism in which a single god is believed to have created all humans and demands their adherence to the associated religion. Universalistic perspectives in biomedicine include ideas of standard dosages by body weight or normal ranges of weight or laboratory results.

Cultural Awareness and Acceptance Awareness of the importance of cultural differences and knowledge of their influences on behavior are the beginning of intercultural adaptation and effectiveness. This awareness includes self-awareness of cultural values and how they affect one's behavior. Awareness of cultural influences on beliefs, behavior, and interpersonal relations helps reduce cross-cultural misunderstandings and provides a basis for developing appropriate approaches to culturally different others. For instance, knowing that most Hispanics have two last names can provide an understanding of why a person might give a last name that is different from that given on the previous visit if you only ask for one of them or ask for the mother's versus the father's last name. Such awareness can facilitate record keeping.

Adaptation (Cultural Sensitivity) Cultural sensitivity involves the ability to accommodate to cultural differences through appropriate adaptations. Adaptation involves making appropriate adjustments for interactions with people from other cultures by adjusting behavior and communication to cultural differences. This development of cultural sensitivity is acquired through using knowledge about differences to direct the development of new kinds of behavior and communications in relationships with members of other cultures, leading to culturally appropriate behaviors. Cultural sensitivity leads to questioning one's own assumptions and replacing them with assumptions from other cultures to appropriately interpret their members' behaviors. Cultural sensitivity recognizes both specific cultural characteristics and intracultural (within-group) differences. *Empathy* develops as one learns how to view reality from the other person's perspective, a consequence of the intentional shift of interpretative and evaluative frameworks. The abandonment of one's habitual cultural frames of reference enables the recognition of many valid cultural forms and behaviors, creating a philosophical commitment to accept many different cultural definitions and constructions of reality (pluralism). General intercultural sensitivity engages a commitment to maintain positive attitudes toward all cultural differences and an attitude of learning to adapt to them constructively.

Cultural Competence Cultural competence involves an ability to work effectively with clients from a cultural group based on an understanding of cultural values, beliefs, and behaviors. Culturally competent individuals are capable of using knowledge of cultural patterns to understand priorities, communicate empathy and acceptance, be responsive to individual and community needs, and work effectively with cultural groups to develop culturally relevant interventions. Cultural competence includes the ability to use culturally relevant communication skills, motivational strategies, and organizational approaches (Castro, 1998). Cultural competence generally implicates a personal bicultural development as one acquires the ability to identify with and relate effectively to another cultural group based on their expectations and perspectives. Cultural competence generally develops through relationships with members of other cultures that produce personal growth, leading to a transformation of self-identification.

Marginalization and Biculturalism Biculturalism involves developments where an individual has internalized two or more different cultures' expectations. This may or may not involve the ability to function effectively in those different cultures. Some bicultural persons are marginalized, feeling a lack of identity and acceptance in either cultural group. Some are intermediaries, functioning effectively in two cultural groups but keeping those cultural lives separate. Bicultural people have skills and perspectives that allow them to adapt effectively to people from different cultural groups and mediate effectively between the cultures.

Integration Integration involves transcending the limitations of the previous cultural self, producing a new identity that incorporates the other culture. Integration produces a person who defines his or her identity in relationship to specific cultural contexts. Contextual evaluation emerges as a skill for managing choice in the problematic contexts produced by ethnorelativism, to shift cultural context in evaluating situations using a variety of cultural perspectives. The evaluation of context is key to decisions about whether a certain behavior is moral. Personal identity is also contextual, shifting as a function of the situation, the context created by others, and personal goals. Constructive marginality may provide a subsequent stage of development, one where the individual attempts to suspend the use of cultural frames of reference. This person constantly questions assumptions and rejects absolute norms of what is right and wrong, operating outside the framework of any specific reference group. Bennett (1993) considers constructive marginality a powerful position from which to serve as a mediator without unreflective adherence to any reference group and capable of restraining excesses of ethnocentrism and value-based conflict.

Cultural Proficiency   Cultural proficiency involves the ability to teach and direct others effectively in their development of culturally sensitive and competent approaches. Cultural proficiency extends cultural competence in a social activist approach that involves the community in developmental projects that enhance health resources. This proactive approach engages the cultural group, health organizations, and the broader community in the design, development, and delivery of culturally relevant services. Cultural proficiency uses a "strengths" approach that recognizes community health and helping resources and strengthens them by incorporating them in community health programs. Individuals and health organizations need to acquire proficiency to engage in a proactive stance of training and preparation for managing cultural differences.

Organizational Cultural Competence

The Office of Minority Health of the U.S. Department of Health and Human Services has issued *National Standards for Culturally and Linguistically Appropriate Services (CLAS) in Health Care* (Office of Minority Health, 2000). These indicate areas of organizational competence (also see items 61 through 75 in Self-Assessment 1.4. Cross-Cultural Development). Principal aspects of organizational cultural and linguistic competence are embodied in the following principles:

- Continuing organizational assessment to integrate throughout programs culturally sensitive and linguistically competent services and assessments

- Inclusion in client records of pertinent information regarding cultural background and language preference

- Provision of understandable health care that is respectful of and compatible with clients' cultural health beliefs

- A culturally diverse staff, representative of the community, at all levels of the organization

- Language services needed by the community that are provided by bilingual staff and professional translators

- Provision of written materials and signs in the languages used by the local community

- Educational services that train staff in providing services that are culturally sensitive and linguistically appropriate

- A strategic plan with clear goals and policies that support culturally appropriate services

- Performance of needs assessments of local communities and engagement of local communities in collaborative partnerships in developing appropriate services

- Provision of culturally sensitive grievance and conflict resolution services for clients

- Provision of information to the public about cultural competency standards of the organization and efforts to implement them

Other aspects of organizational cultural competence are discussed in Chapter Four regarding assessment processes and community involvement and in Chapter Eight regarding the activist role of anthropology, an advocacy approach that engages with health and political institutions to change them in ways to enhance the quality of services provided.

PRACTITIONER PROFILE

Mikel Hogan

Mikel Hogan, Ph.D., during the late 1970s coordinated a program funded by the California State Department of Education that implemented desegregation plans for twenty-six school districts. From 1982 to 1993, she was field director for the Office of Civil Rights and the Department of Education, which conducted civil rights evaluations of school districts throughout the state. In 1989 she designed and implemented a cultural competence training program offered as a thirty-four-hour certificate program through the Office of Extended Education at California State University, Fullerton (CSUF). Successful graduates received certificates in cultural competence training in such work sectors as health, business, education, government, nonprofit, and human services. Since 1983 she has taught courses in anthropology and human services, which is an applied bachelor of science degree that integrates theory and practice in the delivery of services. She is currently a professor and chair of the Human Services Department at CSUF. As an applied anthropologist, Hogan has taught courses in human services; medical anthropology; educational anthropology; applied and urban anthropology; and race, ethnic, and gender relations for more than twenty years.

Hogan's work in various applied anthropology projects in education, civil rights, and cultural competence provided the field experience that culminated in the publication of *Four Skills of Cultural Diversity Competence* (Hogan, 2007). Her knowledge of how to implement cultural awareness, understanding, and skills grew to include a direct and highly specific problem identification and problem-solving approach to cultural diversity issues in medical (and nonmedical) work organizations.

Her ethnographic research on cultural issues and problems in medical facilities and the intervention programs she designed to address them integrate the lessons of medical anthropology into the health care delivery system, resulting in better care for everyone. At another level, the data from her research promote the articulation of a theory of effective medical practice.

ANTHROPOLOGICAL PERSPECTIVES ON CROSS-CULTURAL ADAPTATION

Anthropological principles address barriers to cultural competency at personal, interpersonal, and organizational levels through the concepts of culture and emic (insider) perspectives, cultural relativism, cross-cultural (etic) perspectives, cultural characterizations and intracultural variation, racial categories as social concepts, and distinguishing social from cultural effects.

CONCEPTS OF CULTURE

Culture and Emic Perspectives Culture is a fundamental tool for understanding cross-cultural relations, providing the perspective that individuals' behaviors are shaped by the patterns of their group. A fundamental tool for overcoming intercultural conflicts is the emic perspective: understandings that members of a culture have about themselves. This insider's view—a culture's perspective, worldview, values, assumptions, and motivations—provides the basis for cross-cultural understandings. For example, you would recognize eating dirt as possibly an effective ethnomedical practice rather than being bizarre or a sign of illness.

Cultural Relativism The emic perspective empowers a methodological approach to cultural differences—cultural relativism—which understands behavior as relative to an actor's culture, the context in which that behavior is meaningful and rational. Knowledge of cultural patterns and values enables providers to transform problems, conflicts, and paradoxes into meaningful behavior. Cultural relativism requires "reflective judgment" (Fitzgerald, 2000), the ability to identify one's own assumptions, reevaluate their validity for a situation, and formulate new assumptions based on another culture's perspectives.

Cross-Cultural or Etic Perspectives Cross-cultural (etic) perspectives understand specific patterns of human behavior as general patterns of cross-cultural variation. These cross-cultural patterns are embodied in cultural system perspectives such as the cultural-ecological and psychocultural models. Etic models understand the cultural particulars of health behavior in the comparative cross-cultural framework of differences and universals of human behavior. For example, we recognize specific cultural behaviors such as possession as the cultural manifestation of illness behavior and the sick role, rather than a psychotic delusion.

Cultural Characterizations Versus Stereotypes Some resist the attribution of cultural features to members of specific groups because it risks stereotyping, that is, viewing everybody in a culture as being the same. Cultural characterizations based on normative behaviors provide an understanding of typical patterns and variation within a culture. Cultures produce both common patterns of behavior that characterize their members and intracultural (within-culture) variation in self, personality, and social roles. Cultural competence includes an ability to respond to the culturally patterned differences reflected in age, generation, **acculturation**, class, gender, family roles, economics, and other aspects of intercultural variation. Complex societies have even greater variation—occupational specialization, political position, education—and different subcultures. Intracultural variation does not eliminate the importance of culture but, instead, requires a complex understanding of cultural influences. Acculturation produces change and differentiation among members of ethnic groups, creating intracultural variation.

Racial Concepts The application of the concept of **race** to intergroup differences is misleading if erroneously presumed to reflect biological differences (see Chapter Seven). Racial concepts reflect racist traditions rather than genetic differences that distinguish members of groups. But the concept of race is important in clinical assessment as a statistically significant marker for both genetic predispositions (high blood pressure) and socially induced health conditions (high blood pressure). We should not confuse individuals' racial identity as reflecting biological determinants. Racial concepts have clinical significance because beliefs about races are reflected in societal patterns of prejudice and discrimination affecting prenatal care, diet, exposure to diseases, diagnosis of conditions, and treatment.

Social Versus Cultural Effects Patterns of health behavior found in a culture may occur as a consequence of effects from institutions or groups external to the culture. These are *social,* as opposed to *cultural,* influences. Characteristics of minority groups in a multicultural society may be the consequence of economic and political relationships with other groups and societal institutions that have effects on their culture. Ethnic groups' utilization of emergency services, lack of immunizations, and lack of preventive care may reflect social class-related influences. This confusion is found in the concept of the so-called culture of poverty, considered to be learned behaviors of the poor. But the culture of poverty may represent the social structure of poverty: characteristics that occur as a consequence of being a subordinated group. This includes relationships with health institutions and providers where experiences of discrimination shape health behaviors and interactions with providers, for instance, and lead to the avoidance of prenatal care.

Effective Cross-Cultural Adaptations

Cultural competency requires a range of learning experiences and personal adaptations. A variety of methods need to be employed as a basis for cross-cultural training, combining the teaching of general principles and cultural specifics with experiences and activities that promote self-awareness, behavioral adaptations, and emotional transformations. Cross-cultural training procedures are available to learn how to adapt personally to situations one is likely to encounter (see Weeks, Pedersen, and Brislin, 1986; Kohls and Knight, 1994; Kohls and Brussow, 1995; Gropper, 1996; Seelye, 1996; Fowler and Mumford, 1999). Cognitive learning must add interactions with people in other cultures in everyday life, learning new behaviors. Personal changes include the development of cultural self-awareness, an attitude of willingness to change, the acquisition of skills for managing culture shock and associated emotional distress, and restraint of cultural projection tendencies.

Culture Shock Adaptation Cross-cultural contact produces stress, emotional reactions, and resistance to learning about and accepting cultural differences. Culture shock, a negative reaction to being exposed to another culture, is a major threat to intercultural success. Culture shock produces a dislike of another culture and a desire to leave it or even psychological disorders such as transient neurosis, paranoia, and acute psychotic breakdowns. Effectiveness in cross-cultural relations requires the recognition of culture shock and taking steps to manage it by developing a sense of self-efficacy through cognitive and behavioral coping strategies (Winkelman, 1994). Adaptation to culture shock requires the management of these emotional reactions and stress, suspension of ethnocentric attitudes about one's own culture, and acceptance of others' perspectives. Physical stress management and maintenance of one's physical well-being are important for cross-cultural adaptation. Culture shock management requires a knowledge of likely provocative and distressing situations and the means of reducing stress and conflicts through cultural adaptations and maintaining self (Winkelman, 1994).

Personal Change and Transformation Developing cultural competence requires an effort to change personally, facilitated by an awareness of the benefits. Cross-cultural contact produces strong emotional reactions and resistance to learning about and accepting cultural differences. Developing cultural competency requires adopting a positive attitude about working through the difficult personal challenges of intercultural adaptation. Developing cross-cultural competency requires a deep personal passion and commitment that is shared with others and implemented in actions that interrupt oppression through proactive responses (Fukuyama and Sevig, 1999). Cross-cultural development produces changes in the self, a transformation process that leads to increasing identification with and internalization of others' points of view.

Cultural Self-Awareness Cultural competence requires the recognition of one's own cultural characteristics and influences, particularly one's values, prejudices, and beliefs and their effects on behaviors and attitudes (see Exhibit 3.1.). Cultural self-awareness begins with the knowledge of one's own culture and its effects on one's self, identity, preferences, patterns of behavior, and the characteristics of one's professional practice (e.g., see Chapter Five on biomedical and nursing professional cultures). Knowledge of one's culture is most important because it underlies all of one's behavior, personal and professional. Self-awareness needs to include consideration of the nature and sources of one's attitudes toward other ethnic groups. Values assessments (see the self-assessment exercises at the end of this chapter) are an essential part of developing cultural self-awareness and cultural competence, understanding how one's cultural orientation affects relations with others. Cultural self-awareness provides a basis for anticipating the conflicts to be encountered with a foreign culture and managing potentially conflictive situations. Awareness of one's cultural values helps suspension of the habitual tendencies to judge others, based unconsciously on our cultural assumptions, and facilitates acceptance and understanding of other cultures.

Cognitive Reorganization Cross-cultural effectiveness requires cognitive changes, that we suspend our habitual cultural assumptions about what is normal, reducing the normal cultural attribution or projection of values and assumptions. These "self-reference criteria" involving the use of our own culture for understanding others' behavior must be limited to reduce the judgmental intrusion of our culturally based values and beliefs. Instead, one consciously adopts the perceptual framework of *cultural attribution* (or cultural relativism), using the emic perspectives of the culture of the people one is trying to understand. These interactions require a knowledge of other cultures and interpersonal intercultural skills.

INTERPERSONAL SKILLS FOR INTERCULTURAL RELATIONS

Culture-sensitive care requires the abilities to communicate effectively, especially in regard to interviewing; utilize translators, interpreters, and mediators; express respect with a culturally appropriate social interaction style; manage conflict; and negotiate differences. Specific interpersonal skills for cross-cultural competence include language and communication capabilities; appropriate relational, communication, and management styles; and conflict management and negotiation skills. Cross-cultural adaptation also requires social support: people we rely on for affiliation, affirmation, learning, emotional caring, instrumental aid, and information. Specific skills that enhance the effectiveness of cross-cultural adaptations include

- Achieving communication competence
- Adjusting to another culture's behavioral expectations
- Developing and maintaining interpersonal relationships
- Developing interpersonal skills for expressing empathy and cultural understanding

Language Barriers

Cultural competence requires a management of language barriers. Culturally sensitive interactions may require interpreters, but they also require skills in their effective management, particularly a differentiation of translator and interpreter roles. Cultural knowledge is key to interpretation, which goes beyond translation in placing a client's communication in cultural context to reveal its full meaning. For instance, if a patient verbally denies pain but winces when touched, an interpreter would point out cultural reasons to accept the nonverbal indications rather than the verbal statement. Low rates of **compliance** with medical advice are partially produced by communication problems. Even when providers and clients share a common language, communication problems may nonetheless interfere with clinical relations and therapy. Medical terminology is often incomprehensible to patients, and common terms are often used to mean different things (e.g., stomach) or imply different processes (e.g., hypertension; see Chapter Five). Patients are often confused by providers' professional terms, which allow them to communicate within their profession but not with their clients. Effective communication requires the expression of medical concepts into terms intelligible to patients. Because most patients do not have the language to express their experiences within the medical purview, providers must acquire patients' health models and vocabularies to communicate effectively.

Faulty communication also results from a misinterpretation of clients' symptoms, which may be misunderstood if not viewed in relation to their worldview, values, health beliefs, and body metaphors for expressing distress. Competence requires an ability to express understandings and communicate respectfully in a culturally sensitive manner, based in a knowledge of cultural preferences, including manners of addressing people and asking questions. Chrisman and Zimmer (2000) suggest that an important way of eliciting respect involves using the explanatory model interview to determine how clients and their families perceive problems. This provides the basis for negotiating an appropriate treatment plan that incorporates their concerns and perspectives. Using the explanatory model requires a culturally appropriate communication style and active listening skills.

Listening and Attending

Active listening is a primary tool through which anthropologists learn about the perspectives of other cultures; it involves attention to the speakers and an effort to place what they say in the broader context of their life. To be an effective listener, one has to refrain from judgment, using cultural relativism to understand communications in the context—personal, social, and cultural—of the communicator. In provider-client relations, active listening can occur only with the acquisition of the patient's perspective. Cultural competence requires active listening: an effort to grasp the meaning of the range of messages and feelings communicated by others. Physical attending uses the body to enhance receptivity to communications and to show others that one is focusing attention on them. This requires a knowledge of social interaction rules of the culture, including appropriate social distance and personal space, touching, culturally appropriate eye contact, and other social dynamics. See Self-Assessment 3.4. Group Exercise at the end of this chapter, which illustrates the consequences of different styles of relating.

Behavioral and Social Relations

Intercultural effectiveness requires adopting a variety of *social interaction rules* that involve behavioral and nonverbal communication forms such as gestures, gaze, and postures; emotional communication rules and patterns; space and touch rules (proxemics and kinesics); and patterns of social reasoning. The list shown in the sidebar ("Interpersonal Differences in Social Interaction Rules") illustrates some of these differences. These differences are key to acquiring cultural competence because this competence requires developing appropriate social relationships. These culturally shaped dynamics of interaction are important in getting patients to agree to implement their treatment plans. The changes in perspective necessary for incorporating cultural competence into physicians' clinical behaviors are inhibited by the biomedical belief that the profession naturally selects for people with interpersonal sensitivity. This is manifested in the belief that cultural sensitivity is represented in concepts such as *bedside manner, good will,* and *compassion* (Press, 1982). The traditional white upper-middle-class cultural background of physicians contributes to their lack of awareness of how their characteristics differ from the populations they serve. Their perceptions from their upper-middle-class views of family life, social behavior, norms, and worldviews are distant from the realities of most Americans; this produces problems in doctor-patient consultation that are worsened by the relational and communication styles of the biomedical culture. This is changing with the fairly recent large influx of women, ethnic minorities, and foreign-born people into the rolls of physicians in America.

Cultural Communication Style

Appropriate communication with others involves stylistic and nonverbal cultural norms regarding social and informational priorities and aspects of interaction involving posture, spacing, gestures, physical and eye contact, interpersonal space, tone of voice, and timing.

Health care providers need a heightened awareness of how their culturally and profession-ally based relational patterns affect patients' perceptions and, consequently, health care. For instance, a direct communication style is offensive in cultures where social pleasantries and indirect reference to embarrassing situations are preferred. For many cultures, a lack of a personal relationship may impede effective clinical consultation. Biomedical interpersonal relations styles exemplify the European American impersonal task orientation.

Major cultural differences in communication priorities regarding how messages are delivered contrast technical approaches with relational approaches. Technical styles empha-size information and speaking directly, openly, and honestly. Relational styles are concerned with harmony and respect, avoiding offense to dignity and reputation or disturbing others' harmony. In relational cultures, communication serves the need to maintain appropriate human relationships. Verbal communication is frequently suppressed and emphasis placed on maintaining socially appropriate moods, emotions, and relations. Communication takes place through nonverbal mediums (such as gesture and facial expressions) that carry the bulk of information. European American preferences for direct, verbally explicit messages may lead them to miss significant communication.

This biomedical focus on information relevant for diagnoses, a "doctor-centered" rather than "patient-centered" approach, contributes to patients' dissatisfaction. The biomedical doctor-centered interactional style is authoritarian, dictatorial, self-protective, and largely unskilled in counseling and communication techniques and is intended to control the inter-action with the patient. Implementation of most treatment depends on cooperative relations between provider and client. More effective communication can be achieved by adapting

 SIDEBAR 3.1. Interpersonal Differences in Social Interaction Rules

Language dialects and jargon	Contextual communication
Paralinguistic cues	Metalinguistic messages
Communication style	Relational styles
Greetings and formalities	Formality of relations
Family roles	Gender roles
Expressions of respect	Personal relations
Presentation of self ("face")	Self-disclosure
Emotional communication	Proxemics (space)
Kinesics (touch)	Facial expressions
Eye contact	Gestures and signs
Body posture	Time orientation
Learning styles	Authority relations
Decision-making processes	Persuasion or argument styles
Negotiation approaches	Conflict management
Power distance	Work values and attitudes

BIOCULTURAL INTERACTIONS

Social Interaction in Hmong Medical Relations

The Hmong generally believe that they deserve government services, a promise made to them because of their extreme sacrifices for the U.S. Army and the Central Intelligence Agency (CIA) in Southeast Asia. They are often disappointed with the inconsiderate care that they receive. The Hmong expect their providers to be respectful and trustworthy and express compassion in their relationships with patients' families. Direct eye contact is viewed as disrespectful, especially when directed to elders or members of the opposite sex. Respect is communicated in many ways: polite formality, respecting their decisions, and conveying an attitude of service. A personal connection is necessary for a trusting relationship, so providers should share personal information as part of relationship-building preliminaries. When lacking interpreters, physicians often focus on bilingual adolescents, ignoring parents and other important adults. Doctors often compound their unintended disrespect by looking people in the eye, touching them on the head, and appearing in informal attire and blue jeans. Sincerity may be communicated by brief eye contact followed by looking away. The Hmong may look at the floor to communicate that they are listening.

The family, not the physician, is viewed as the decision maker in the care of a patient. The elder men of the patient's paternal side of the family are viewed as the most important people in negotiating patient care. The best interests of a patient are considered in relationship to the family's needs, and decisions are made collectively to avoid blame in case of adverse outcomes. Physicians are not viewed as having the right to make decisions for the family. Sick-role behavior is usually passive, with patients not expected to care for themselves; instead, family members will care for the sick and make their health care decisions.

If patients are not fluent in English, a translator should be used and communication directed to the appropriate elders present. The communication style should incorporate using a soft voice,

different styles; providers can reduce their image as uncaring, insensitive, and arrogant by adopting client-sensitive styles of communication and using nonverbal mediums to assure and encourage patients. Most cultures' rules of communication and social behavior affect medical communication because questioning authority figures is considered inappropriate. Consequently, providers need to encourage clients to ask questions (Press, 1982).

SPECIALTY CROSS-CULTURAL APPLICATIONS OF MEDICAL ANTHROPOLOGY

Rush (1996) considers *clinical anthropology* to involve the application of anthropological concepts in clinical settings. Johnson (1991), however, uses the term *clinically applied anthropology* for such activities, using clinical anthropology to refer to the activities of anthropologists cross-trained in a clinical discipline (such as psychology, psychiatry, social work). I follow Rush's use of clinical anthropology to refer to many other contexts avoiding prolonged eye contact, and communicating respect by asking for permission to touch patients. The head nod may convey assent or agreement but may also be a respectful encouragement to continue speaking so that the communication may be understood. Agreement should be ascertained rather than assumed. Physicians are slow to learn that even when tHmong patients politely answer "Yes" to a doctor's many instructions, they are not understanding, much less agreeing, but merely being polite, an acknowledgment that they have been spoken to! Even when they disagree, a polite "yes" rather than challenging the authority of the doctor is a standard behavior.

Emotional communication in the form of laughter may not communicate assent but may reflect discomfort, embarrassment, fear, or confusion. Facial expressions are generally controlled to convey neutrality and a calm and collected disposition. The expression of anger or a displeased countenance is considered to be disrespectful. Touch is a sensitive issue and should be done only with permission. Touching the head is generally taboo, and women are generally disinclined to have pelvic or breast exams by male physicians.

Recommended treatments should be provided as advice rather than coercion. To obtain compliance, it is necessary to develop a treatment plan in conjunction with the family network of elders and clan and offer options rather than force courses of action on them. Sensitive matters and disturbing news should be presented indirectly, and the patient's condition should be discussed in a manner that encourages hope and positive expectations. Questions about sensitive issues should be addressed indirectly, using stories or asking about people (or Hmong) in general rather than the patient in particular. Death and other bad news may be communicated through metaphor or allusion instead of directly conveying disturbing prognoses, which may be viewed as threats or curses. Physicians should encourage and facilitate the use of cultural healing practices for conditions with spiritual causes, contributions, or consequences.

besides hospitals and clinics, including criminal justice settings, governmental policy development venues, and other situations involving cross-cultural adaptation to issues that have positive effects on health. Medical anthropologists address cross-cultural issues in a variety of contexts that affect health care, including

- Teaching, training, and mediation activities to enhance cross-cultural sensitivity and responsiveness in interactions between diverse cultural groups

- Research activities, particularly involving community participation and coalitions

- Advocacy for community health development and provision of health education

- Administrative functions to change organizational cultures of health institutions

- Applications in community and public health programs

- Roles in clinical settings to enhance therapeutic outcomes as consultants

PRACTITIONER PROFILE

M. Jean Gilbert

M. Jean Gilbert, Ph.D., consults on cultural and linguistic issues in health care. Current projects include participation on a team that is assessing the cultural and linguistic best practices in MediCal (California's Medicaid) HMOs and work on a U.S.-Mexico border drug and alcohol prevention program. She has been a visiting professor in the Department of Anthropology, California State University, Long Beach, and director of Cultural Competence for Kaiser Permanente, California, where she provided expert consulting to the organization in the design of services to diverse populations and conducted training in cultural medicine to health care professionals. Before that, she was a National Institute on Alcohol Abuse and Alcoholism Scholar in Latino Alcohol Studies at the Spanish-Speaking Mental Health Research Center, University of California, Los Angeles. From 1978 to 1984, she was associated with the Social Process Research Institute, University of California, Santa Barbara, where she conducted research on Mexican American family dynamics and cross-cultural research on maternal and child health, alcoholism, and health care services utilization. Her interests in medical anthropology are primarily in the application of research information and anthropological knowledge for the creation of health care policy and the delivery of services to diverse patient populations.

During the time Dr. Gilbert worked at Kaiser Permanente, she served on various government-related policymaking bodies to help bring about organizational change that she felt was important in serving diverse patients. She served on the MediCal Managed Care Cultural and Linguistics Task Force, which sought to make policy that would guide culturally sensitive services for culturally diverse and limited-English speakers.

In another cross-disciplinary team effort, Dr. Gilbert convened an expert panel of medical anthropologists, physicians, nurses, and health educators to set standards for the teaching of cultural competency to health care professionals. This collaborative work resulted in the document, *The Principles and Recommended Standards for the Cultural Competence Education of Health Care Professionals* (2002), which is widely used in curriculum planning in colleges and universities.

Cross-Cultural Training and Mediation

Culture affects health care quality through effects on interactions between patients and providers. Anthropologists' applications of cultural perspectives in health generally involve intercultural education and training. Training providers in cultural knowledge and cross-cultural perspectives and skills enhances the quality of biomedical practice by facilitating an understanding of patients' language and worldview and using intercultural communication skills to elicit relevant information. Cross-cultural competence facilitates the resolution of a primary clinical problem—noncompliance—through teaching negotiation skills. Providers' and clients' different cultural conceptualizations of health interfere with communication, diagnosis, treatment, compliance, and satisfaction with care. Providing physicians with an awareness of the cultural influences on both clients' and providers' care behaviors can contribute to patient care by providing perspectives linking their different health views. Mediation between diverse perspectives underlies basic medical anthropology applications in health, including dispute resolution, education, research, advocacy, community development, and institutional cultural change. Mediator functions involve facilitating communication between different cultural and professional groups and translating between conceptual systems. Cross-cultural orientations can contribute to more satisfactory patient care by helping providers develop cultural skills in adapting to the diverse client cultures they encounter. Major aspects of clinically applied medical anthropology involve assisting providers in learning the principles for culturally sensitive and competent care (Chrisman and Zimmer, 2000). Anthropological perspectives and cultural knowledge involved in preparing health professionals for cultural competency include

- Teaching skills for cross-cultural relations, communication, and negotiation
- Understanding ethnomedical conceptions of illness and approaches to treatment
- Assessing cultural impacts on health and responses to health problems
- Recognizing, assessing, and responding to community health needs

Researcher

Public mandates to ensure culturally relevant health services provide anthropologists with roles in determining health problems and needs, developing programs, administering their implementation, and evaluating their quality and effectiveness. Anthropologists' professional responsibility for the well-being of those studied has produced research focused on responses that can result in direct benefits to communities. Anthropologists' community health research has expanded traditional needs assessments to focus on community strengths, perspectives that emphasize how cultural practices contribute to well-being. Strengths approaches can play an important role in indicating cultural resources to be utilized in developing community health programs: for instance, incorporating midwives into campaigns to encourage breast-feeding.

Research on culture and health provides essential data for public health and clinical medicine. Anthropology's ethnographic and participant observation approaches are the tools of choice for the investigation of the cultural bases of high-risk behaviors. Participant observation involves a direct engagement with people's ethnomedical systems, providing information about cultural illness beliefs and behaviors that affect care through patients' conceptualization of and responses to health problems.

Anthropology's multimethod research approach dovetails with the interdisciplinary nature of health research (Sargent and Johnson, 1996). Anthropologists collaborate with a variety of professionals in ensuring the cultural appropriateness of research, using ethnography and participant observation to understand health behaviors. Anthropology's culture-specific approaches are fundamental across the human services in developing research proposals, implementing studies, evaluating results, and institutionalizing programmatic changes (Poland, 1985). Anthropology's holistic perspectives communicate to others the interacting economic, political, and social effects on health (Chrisman and Johnson, 1990). Anthropologists use their ability to translate across perspectives to demystify the researcher role and data collection techniques and to explain analyses and value of the research to those studied. Observations of staff behavior at research sites help determine the effectiveness of the implementation of interventions (process evaluation; see Chapter Four). Assessing staff perspectives helps ensure that they feel benefits from the project, understand its contributions, and are not resistant in ways that undermine the project.

Cultural perspectives are also essential to epidemiology: research into the factors associated with the incidence of diseases (see Chapter Seven). Because behavior brings people into contact with disease or injury, understanding cultural dynamics of behavior is fundamental to public health and prevention programs. An important cultural focus in epidemiological research is the community morbidity study, which uses community-based (as opposed to clinical) data to reveal the actually experienced incidence of illness, rather than just those conditions presented to physicians. People may not present illness to physicians for a variety of reasons, including the prohibitive cost of services; inaccessibility of treatment; the cultural acceptance of their symptoms; the inability to leave work, family, or other responsibilities; or self-treatment. Community morbidity studies based on studies of health problems from the perspectives of the public help provide a more accurate picture of the actual incidence of health conditions.

Community morbidity surveys, based in interviewing a sample of the population, provide approaches for assessing unreported conditions and, hence, the actual maladies experienced, including diseases. Accurately assessing the incidence of disease requires a community morbidity study based on assessment of a general population rather than a clinical population. This approach also faces methodological challenges, including verification of self-reported diseases and assessments of determinants of disease that occur over long periods. The usefulness of community morbidity studies is exemplified in Kleinman's (1980) assessment of the illness reported in a study of Chinese family-based popular health care. Kleinman's method used the interviews to determine illness episodes, treatment decisions, all treatments applied, and the outcome of illness episodes. Interviews are generally conducted in the home, including as informants all household members and assessing illness episodes experienced by the household. In community-based interviews, household groups can be asked to report other health care beliefs and practices, particularly cultural remedies, medicinal plants, folk practitioners, and popular mental health resources.

Community Advocacy and Empowerment

Anthropology has a long history of involvement in public health community advocacy and empowerment. These involvements include community development and self-help programs, leadership training, consciousness raising, health education, and health partnering. Nutrition issues provided a basis for early anthropological involvement in international public health (Ritenbaugh, 1982; Quandt, 1996). Recognition of social causes of malnutrition led anthropologists to advocacy, addressing the funding and development of community resources and health programs to ensure access to food.

A primary role of anthropologists in international health programs has involved overcoming cultural barriers to adaptation of modern health practices to local conditions (Chambers, 1985). More political roles have been necessary, however. Primary causes of disease in impoverished third-world communities are due to the failure to allocate resources to support public health programs and the development of **infrastructure** (such as clean water, sanitation and sewer systems, prenatal care, nutrition, and education) necessary for healthy life (Rubinstein and Lane, 1990). Recognition of macrolevel effects of the capitalist economy on health produced by economic, social, and political processes spurred the development of an advocacy role reflected in critical medical anthropology (Baer, Singer, and Johnsen, 1986) and political economy orientations (Morsy, 1996) (see Chapter Eight).

These approaches emphasize empowering communities to achieve changes by altering the distribution of health resources. Community empowerment begins with enlisting the participation of relevant community members and a variety of public and private organizations involved in community health: schools, public health education and prevention programs, advocacy groups, and government. Anthropologists work as mediators in ensuring effective collaboration among many entities, integrating their different values, goals, and perspectives using organizational and conflict-resolution skills. Planning effective health programs requires the formation of participatory research teams that include the local community (Nichter, 1984). This helps ensure understanding of the community's needs, facilitates acquisition of sociocultural data required by planners, and helps ensure that programs address issues relevant to the community. This requires an understanding of the local community's health conditions, their communication networks, and local social and political structures.

Anthropologists may assist community leaders in effecting broader political processes and decision making. Community empowerment emphasizes the development of community capacities to access resources, participate in political processes, and form community organizations to address needs. These approaches also take prevention perspectives and emphasize the creation of sustainable community programs. This is achieved through changes in community institutions and governmental organizations to affect fiscal and political processes that allocate health resources. Training community research teams creates a community resource that can monitor community health problems and program successes, a fundamental aspect of health.

Applications in Public Health Prevention Programs

The ultimate goal of removing preventable determinants of disease requires changes in lifestyle and behaviors, not just of individuals but also of communities. Cultural perspectives are therefore essential for effective implementation of the basic goals of public health: reduction of disease through public health planning, policy development, and program implementation. Understanding how groups of people behave in ways that increase disease is fundamental to developing culturally appropriate programs to change those high-risk behaviors. Effective prevention requires understanding the roles culture plays in placing entire groups at risk. Cultural perspectives facilitate primary prevention by identifying the behavioral and social conditions that may lead to disease. Secondary prevention strategies

Cultural Defense as Advocacy in the Courtroom

Anthropologists can contribute to health justice through roles as expert witnesses in which they explain the cultural relativity of normal personality, assumptions, beliefs, and behaviors. One aspect involves the **cultural defense** in criminal law, where aspects of culture that create a person's state of mind and reasonable assumptions are examined to determine whether a person is guilty of crime or acting under normal cultural assumptions. For instance, did the defendant willfully kill his or her neighbor or did he or she really believe that it was a dangerous witch that they saw in the light of the moon?

Cultures distinguish behaviors that are wrong or criminal from those that result from mistakes of fact or mental illness that make individuals not responsible for their actions. Awareness of right and wrong and the notion of intent are central to issues many cultures address in determining responsibility and in the determination of criminal guilt in the United States. A person's *mens rea*—"state of mind"—is considered in determining guilt in most crimes. An individual's culturally based perceptions are part of the legal concepts of responsibility and reasonableness (normalcy) that determine legal culpability in criminal cases. These are underlying issues in the cultural defense in criminal law, which involves presenting cultural factors to establish extenuating or mitigating circumstances and the reduction of charges (Winkelman, 1996b; Dundes-Renteln, 2004).

Cultural defenses function through traditional defenses such as mistake of fact, diminished capacity, nonresponsibility, and insanity where mens rea determines the intent that defines culpability. The mental state of a defendant at the time of a crime is a cultural construction and is key to establishing a category of legal defenses called excuses: personal characteristics that establish mitigating circumstances that reduce the severity of actions. Consideration is given to a defendant's state of mind in degrees of culpability in homicide (e.g., first-degree murder versus negligent homicide or self-defense) and in excuses such as extreme duress, defects of knowledge, reasonable deficiency, and nonresponsibility. The cultural defense examines personal and cultural circumstances to determine an actor's state of mind. The mind at fault, a guilty state of mind, is the mental condition generally needed for criminal guilt (Sheybani, 1987). A key concern is reasonableness, "determined from the point of view of a person in the actor's situation under the circumstances as he [or she] believes them to be" (Sheybani, 1987, p. 759). Cultural assessments are necessary to appraise an actor's situation, which is interpreted from the actor's point of view. Cultural factors affect one's state of mind, with cultural norms, beliefs, customs, and upbringing potentially leading an individual to a condition of "diminished responsibility," which may make them guilty of a lesser offense.

Cultural factors determine what constitutes provocative conduct. If the defendant perceives the victim's behavior as a threat, this may establish that the crime resulted from provocation and reasonable actions based on the defendant's cultural background. A crime of passion based on perceptions of provocation or threat might mitigate or excuse a crime if it was reasonable and expected for someone in the defendant's situation. A victim's violation of cultural norms can arouse passions and obscure reason in an ordinarily reasonable person. There is an absence of malice if an act is committed under extreme emotional or mental duress resulting from provocation as determined by cultural traditions and personal perceptions.

These excuses, a category of defenses long recognized in criminal law, seek forgiveness based on involuntariness, reasonable deficiency, and nonresponsibility (Kadish, 1987). Central concerns are the person's capacity to choose. A person's "choice" is not blamable when ignorant with respect to significant features of the situation or when circumstances would lead "a reasonable normally law-abiding person to act in the same way" (Kadish, 1987, p. 266). Exculpation is based on the concept of the "ordinarily law-abiding person" acting under constraints of knowledge or defects of will. Defects of knowledge undermine intentionality, the mental state necessary for a crime to have occurred. Cultural factors can negate criminal intent because the defendant's subjective state of mind, resulting from cultural beliefs and norms, can produce a reasonable (mis)understanding of the situation and consequences of one's action. "People from a foreign culture may perceive reality so differently from those raised in the majority culture that their assessment of a situation may be tantamount to a mistake of fact" (*Harvard Law Review*, 1986, p. 1294). Legal systems have found acquittal, absolution, or insanity in cases where defendants killed devils, witches, or supernatural beings—in human form. The mistake of fact argues that the client lacked the requisite mental state: intention and knowledge of consequences of acts. Because criminal liability requires intent, cultural factors affecting behavior in terms of purpose, or recklessness or negligence, may negate the presence of the necessary state of mind and intent (Lyman, 1986, p. 94).

Nonresponsibility is an excuse based on extenuating circumstances, an inadequate capacity for making judgments as exemplified in the legal insanity defense. Legal insanity is a situation where "mental disease prevented the defendant from conforming his conduct to the requirements of the law . . . incapable of making choices that count as such because of impaired reasoning and judgment" (Kadish, 1987, pp. 261–262). Because the person no longer acts as a rational agent, it is not fair to hold the person liable because he or she lacks the normal capacity for judgment and reason. The cultural defense may be used in an insanity plea, but it strains the definition of mental disease to the point unlikely to be accepted by the courts (*Harvard Law Review*, 1986; Kadish, 1987). This is particularly true when the determination of mental disease is limited to those defined by earlier versions of the DSM (but see DSM-IV-TR, 2000). A broader view of mental illness incorporating the concept of *culture-bound syndromes* is necessary to effectively incorporate cultural factors within the traditional insanity defenses.

Elsewhere I have reviewed the use of cultural factors at the pretrial, guilt, and penalty phases (Winkelman, 1996b). A primary role of the anthropologist as an expert witness involves informal factors, including being a "bargaining chip" for defense lawyers in the negotiation of charges. Charges carrying the death penalty obligate the state to extensive support of the defense, including expert witnesses, but lesser charges do not. Cultural information may be used in the guilt phase of trials, but the penalty phase, where mitigating circumstances are assessed, is a more likely context for introducing information regarding character and background circumstances. Wright (1992) suggests that anthropologists' testimony establishing mitigating cultural factors involves the defendant's socialization in informal and formal social institutions and groups, including effects of economic and political institutions, social services, and the justice system. The cultural aspects of mitigating and extenuating circumstances may involve any aspect of a defendant's background, particularly cultural values and their effects on behavior, socialization regarding aggression and violence, beliefs regarding what constitutes provocation, family and kinship roles and expectations and their relationship to coping and mental health, political and social obligations, and religious beliefs and practices (Winkelman, 1996b).

are based on an early detection of diseases, requiring that programs be tailored to help ensure their cultural congruence so that relevant risk groups take advantage of screening and identification processes. Tertiary prevention, involving the reduction of disease consequences, requires an understanding of how disease affects activities of daily living and compromises the ability to reestablish healthy functioning within a social context.

Public health requires a multilevel ecological paradigm and cultural methodologies for understanding the linkages of risk factors and diseases (McKinlay and Marceau, 2000). Cultural approaches consider the numerous relationships between humans and their environments that affect the distribution of disease risks. Genetic and physiological influences are manifested within a broader context that includes

■ Lifestyle influences from culture that shape individual behaviors

■ Social, environmental, economic, and political influences on material resources affecting health

■ Macrosocial influences from social class, race, and ethnicity

■ The impacts of culture, economics, and politics on public health policies and programs

Identifying the sociocultural dynamics that affect individual risk behaviors requires the implementation of qualitative research designs. These include the classic ethnographic approaches of interviews, participant observation, and key informants as well as more recently developed approaches that focus on specific relevant groups (see Schensul and LeCompte, 1999). Qualitative approaches develop indicators appropriate for assessing organizations, communities, and cultures and identifying cultural behaviors that determine risks and exposure. Cultural approaches are fundamental to the construction of measures that assess the interactive biological and social causes of illness.

Cultural perspectives provide the linkages of social structural factors, environment, and lifestyle, calling attention to the need for interventions at multiple levels rather than simply at the most proximate level to disease outcomes (e.g., changing diet and exercise levels to reduce heart disease rather than just treating high blood pressure or cholesterol levels with medication). Cultural approaches shift the prevention focus "upstream" (earlier causal factors) to the "real or underlying determinants" that cause disease (see McKinlay and Marceau, 2000).

Cultural perspectives play a role in prevention by focusing on the modification of risk behavior at the community level and in the social and cultural contexts that structure and elicit individual behavior. Changing exposure to risks may involve social and political activities, such as the legal actions taken to reduce public smoking and exposure to secondary smoke. Risk behavior occurs within the context of community norms and expectations, and changes must be focused at the level of the social ecology, where interventions impact a spectrum of people and reinforce changes in risk-associated behaviors. Efforts to change individual behavior are likely ineffective without consideration of the social context and cultural influences supporting or undermining the desired behaviors. For instance, AIDS reduction programs must address how using condoms is affected by cultural beliefs about condom use (such as their association with prostitutes in Mexican culture).

Intervention strategies must target the arenas influencing behavior, requiring multiple interventions targeted at all levels of the social ecology: personal, interpersonal, organizational, community, and government. Changing risk behaviors requires a simultaneous focus on

■   Individual risk and coping behaviors

■   Family and other interpersonal influences

■   Interfaces with relevant health education and services

■   Supportive and risk-inducing community influences

■   Policy and administrative activities affecting risk and health

Prevention programs require an understanding of the cultural conceptions of diseases that increase risk as well as the actual disease risks. Cultural approaches are essential for getting at the real incidence of disease rather than just that reported to and by physicians and other biomedical and public health agencies, which miss assessments of health conditions for which treatment is not sought, such as

■   Psychiatric disorders, for which some people may never obtain medical services

■   Conditions commonly treated by household and ethnomedical resources

■   Ethnomedical syndromes not considered in public health and biomedical assessments

Administrative and Organizational Change

One of the roles of medical anthropologists involves institutional change directed toward the provision of a more humane medicine through adaptations of services and organizations. Knowledge of organizational culture is crucial in addressing the bureaucratic processes necessary to develop and implement programs. This may involve mediating between different resource bases to acquire the support necessary for providing services or training. New management models provide a variety of opportunities for anthropologists to participate.

Cultural approaches are integral to addressing the focus on patient satisfaction as a fundamental measure of quality. Quality of care is a patient-based experience, making patients' experiences of care fundamental to improving patient satisfaction. This involves major changes in the organizational culture of health care delivery systems (Chassin, Galvin, and the National Roundtable on Health Care Quality, 1998), applying total quality management (TQM) to produce systematic changes in organizational culture. The TQM perspective requires a consideration of the system of interrelated roles and responsibilities that makes cultural systems approaches appropriate tools to refashion corporate health cultures. Anthropologists are well suited for addressing these changes in institutional cultures of health care organizations, moving beyond concerns with clinician sensitivity to minority groups by focusing on the health institutions. Concerns about malpractice and risk management require a systems perspective in which organizations, rather than individuals, are key determinants. These issues require changes in the organizational culture and its value orientations.

Press (1997) emphasizes that anthropological approaches are well suited for changing the complex social organization of hospitals. Short-term research projects based on observation, key interviews, and focus groups can provide important insights into an organizational culture and its problems. Systemic views of culture enable better understanding of conflicts between the various functional systems of hospital organizations. Barriers between units are typically created by cultural differences, and conflicts are often exacerbated by the inability of participants to understand others' perspectives, needs, and limitations. Old hospital culture and social structure prevent effective communication and collaboration, affecting patients' perceptions of the quality of care.

Anthropologists can shift institutional cultures to a participatory perspective and a more humane and democratic environment (Wiedman, 1990b, 1992, 1998, 2000a, 2000b). The anthropologist may be the lead person in introducing cognitive and organizational changes, initiating processes of learning and self-examination, and engaging people to change personally. These leadership functions often depend on brokering among groups, professions, and conceptual systems and drawing others into programs for organizational change through adopting roles of mediator, facilitator, idea broker, educator, and organizer.

Increases in the power and control of clinical administrators in developing health policy and education programs and monitoring health professionals make administrators important players in incorporating cultural perspectives into health care settings (Press, 1985). Anthropologists can use administrative concerns about risk, quality, and patient satisfaction to integrate cultural perspectives in

- *Quality assurance:* institutional studies of medical errors to prevent their repetition

- *Liability management:* identifying sources of potential malpractice claims

- *Institutional assessment:* training staff in data collection protocols

- *Patient representation:* resolving problems and training employees to enhance patient satisfaction

- *Patient and community relations:* getting and keeping happy customers and a satisfied community through activities that enhance the institutional image

- *Disability management:* reducing worker and patient injury by identifying and remedying problems

Clinically Applied Anthropology

Although most medical anthropologists are not involved in therapy, some roles of anthropology in clinical practice may involve an anthropologist as a member of a therapeutic team (see Shiloh, 1977; Rush, 1996; Chrisman and Johnson, 1990; Johnson, 1991). Anthropologists contribute to therapeutic activities by explaining behaviors, mediating between physicians and patients, and ultimately, teaching clinicians how to understand patients' behaviors in cultural context and in their social and personal lives. Responsiveness to others' needs and mediation among diverse groups and perspectives are key features of the anthropologist's role in clinical settings.

The primary clinical consultant role for anthropologists involves applying cultural data and anthropological methods and theory to clinical concerns (Chrisman and Johnson,

1990). This generally involves assistance in the management of psychosocial concomitants of disease, including social and economic influences on the family system and resolution of conflicts between staff and patients. Anthropologists help address social consequences of disease and sickness and problems that result from cultural differences between biomedicine and patients. Cultural perspectives provide practical solutions to problems of conflicts in treatment settings and therapeutic relationships. Anthropology's ethnographic approaches provide practical solutions for problems in patient care by focusing on the effects of sickness and treatment on everyday life. Cultural information is useful in making diagnoses and suggesting courses of treatment and in educating about social constraints on compliance (such as work obligations) and sociocultural features affecting the clinical intervention. By providing information about patients' cultural help-seeking, illness behaviors, and communication approaches and using the explanatory model to grasp patients' understandings, anthropologists help providers bridge the gap between their conceptual worlds and those of their patients. Cultural information may be used to address problems between patients and staff. For example, appropriate at-home care for a discharged patient might not be assigned if there was a failure to understand cultural patterns of in-law avoidance, where a daughter-in-law is not supposed to directly interact with her father-in-law, or the son-in-law with his mother-in-law.

Kleinman (1982) suggests that the principal clinical strategies for the integration of cultural perspectives into medical practice involve negotiation between providers and patients to address the difference between biomedicine's diseases and the patients' experiences of illness. A focus on the sociocultural dimensions of their disease requires the use of the explanatory model, an assessment of clients' perspective on the nature of a health problem. Kleinman (1982) considers clinically applied anthropology to deal primarily with

- Bureaucratic and structural constraints on care
- Providers' expectations regarding patient behavior
- Psychosocial problems and burdens caused by disease stigma and treatment effects
- Problems involving communication and relationships in clinical settings

USING CULTURE TO CARE FOR PATIENTS AND PROVIDERS

Training providers in culturally responsive and competent care enhances the quality of patients' experiences and produces care for providers, which enhances work satisfaction by reducing conflict and stress. Addressing these issues requires that anthropologists have ethnographic immersion in the health care setting to familiarize themselves with clinical aspects of physicians' consultation, diagnosis, and therapeutic activities. These experiences sensitize anthropologists to medicine's stresses, limitations, and burdens and provide perspectives necessary for communicating with physicians in their accustomed language and conceptual frameworks.

To be successful in clinical settings, anthropologists must understand and adapt to biomedical culture. Johnson (1991) outlines a variety of strategies for such adaptation, providing perspectives from which to bridge physician and patient models to accommodate the effects of cultural factors on illness and healing.

APPLICATIONS

Guidelines for Working in Clinical Settings

Johnson (1991) provides a number of guidelines to assist social scientists in preparing for work in clinical settings. These are based on the perspectives of consultation-liaison psychiatry, which provides services to other physicians in managing the psychosocial problems associated with patient care. Anthropology contributes to clinical care through explanations provided by systems approaches, emic perspectives based in participant observation, use of the explanatory model, and cultural relativism. An awareness of the culture of medicine and its sensitivities is important. An appreciation of institutional patterns and providers' perspectives is essential for the development of programs of change that do not violate the local cultural systems and their norms. Anthropologists' history of criticism of biomedicine makes it important to adopt a nonjudgmental approach.

As in all field work, a familiarity with the overall clinical culture and socialization process is important. Cross-training in another health discipline obviously enhances access. A knowledge of medical cultures can derive from a review of material on medical education and professional socialization, familiarization with the language of medicine, and immersion in clinical settings to acclimate to the culture. Participation in the "attending rounds," particularly those at challenging early morning hours, exposes one to a basic aspect of medical activity and shows a commitment to professional concerns.

Anthropologists can contribute to medical care by teaching providers how to use systems perspectives to understand clients' behavior, placing individual actions and concerns within their sociocultural context. Anthropology's systems perspectives also lend themselves to addressing the institutional dynamics that affect patient care. Anthropologists can make contributions to care through the role of a cultural broker in mediating between different subsystems (professional or organizational). The biopsychosocial perspective and general systems theory are the frameworks within which patient and clinician behaviors are addressed. Understanding a patient begins with family systems and community perspectives and extends into the broader bureaucratic and political systems. This situation-oriented consultation examines the factors in a patient's life milieu that contribute to the patient's health problems, particularly compliance with treatment. Physician behavior is similarly approached in a systems perspective that considers the different professional cultures (physicians, nurses, administrators, etc.) and subcultural systems within the hospital. Following the consultation-liaison psychiatry approach, patient problems are also analyzed through a physician-oriented approach that looks at the contribution of treatment providers and their institutional settings to patient problems. Analysis of the hospital as a cultural system can contribute to an understanding of the systemic dysfunctions that produce difficulties for patients and physicians, including conflicts among providers or different divisions of health care institutions.

Fadiman (1997) suggests that the explanatory model could have provided a tool to prevent the disaster that occurred in the case of Lia Lee. Eliciting patients' perspectives reveals the psychosocial and cultural dimensions of their responses to treatment and how the condition and treatment relate to a patient's life. Consideration of patients' perspectives reveals disagreements and helps resolve noncompliance. The quality of patient care can be enhanced by assessing dimensions of care concerned with ensuring physical comfort and well-being; respecting patients' values, preferences, and communication styles; providing emotional support and addressing fears; ensuring the involvement of family and friends; and coordinating and integrating different care services and ensuring continuity and appropriate transition (Delbanco, 1992). Kleinman (1980) points to the importance of also considering the macrosocial economic, political, and other structural factors affecting the microsocial clinical views of illness behavior and patient-doctor interactions. Culture is a vital aspect of health because it is fundamental to the health behaviors of patients and providers.

Patient-Provider Relationship Building

Importance of Medical Interview The medical interview is important for obtaining information needed for diagnosis; it is also important as a means for developing the doctor-patient relationship within which the patient's collaboration with the proposed treatment is achieved. Aldrich (1999) emphasizes the role of the medical interview in establishing the provider's interest in the patient, communicating an empathic response on the part of the provider that, in turn, helps establish a relationship in which the patient feels comfortable communicating health concerns.

Aldrich (1999) emphasizes medical interviewing needs to focus on patients' concepts of illness and their views regarding their condition; these concerns are elicited by the explanatory model (discussed in Chapter Two). Interviewing must be sensitive to cultural communication styles, including global aspects related to directness, disclosure, and other dimensions exemplified under social interaction rules. To encourage disclosure, the interviewer needs to adopt a nonjudgmental attitude and give feedback to indicate understanding of the patient's concerns.

Differences between providers' and clients' explanatory models need to be addressed without judgment or ridicule of clients' perspectives. If the differences in clients' explanatory models are significant blockages with respect to the adoption of a provider's recommendations, those differences need to be carefully examined. Providers should explain their own views and the reasons they have for a particular diagnosis and treatment recommendations. If the conflicting explanatory models do not interfere with treatment and compliance, the differences may not need to be addressed. If providers feel they need to understand these differences, further elicitation of the client's beliefs and placing those beliefs in cultural context are recommended.

If clients' beliefs and explanations do interfere with medical treatment, an explanation of the basis for those beliefs, their justification, and patient education regarding biomedical knowledge may be an appropriate part of treatment. O'Connor (1995) suggests addressing conflicts between client and provider explanatory models in terms of beliefs systems and values and with respect to

■ Cultural evaluations of the significance of the illness

■ Concerns regarding the social implications of treatments

■ Religious beliefs regarding the nature of the condition

■ Impacts on lifestyle created by the condition or treatment

■ Means for negotiating between provider and client models

Intercultural contact inevitably produces conflicts and misunderstandings because of cultural differences; consequently, an active approach to minimizing and resolving conflict is necessary for cultural competence. Conflict is worsened by typical personal and cultural approaches of attributing conflict to personal failings of others. This normal tendency to engage in assigning blame (or attribution) needs to be replaced by a conscious decision to understand the other's behavior as culturally reasonable, seeing the situation from the other's point of view and his or her personal and cultural definition of the situation. Cross-cultural problem resolution can be achieved by identifying, describing, and analyzing the problem from both cultures' points of view to negotiate a solution that combines both cultures' concerns and perspectives.

Negotiation Negotiation is necessary to provide culturally competent care. Negotiation provides the mechanism for resolving differences in perceptions, desired treatment processes, and goals of treatment. Without negotiation, the likely outcome is an effort at ethnocentric imposition of the biomedical culture and values. Effective negotiation requires both specific cultural knowledge and generic cross-cultural negotiation and conflict resolution skills. Negotiating linkages between the medical culture and the culture of patients involves a brokering process that enables a conceptual sharing of provider and patient explanatory models. "Managing professional and patient models requires providers' awareness of impacts of personal and professional values, shared cultural biases, and conventional metaphors of self, others, the body, and emotions on clinical assessment and decision making" (Kleinman, 1982, pp. 87–88). This cultural self-awareness and other cultural awareness provide a basis for recognizing the sources of difference and mediation between these two cultural perspectives. Kleinman's model uses "genuine negotiation" to make a patient ultimately responsible for final decisions. Kleinman suggests that it requires a determination of who (patient, family) should make decisions and the culturally appropriate forms and contexts for negotiation.

Kleinman (1982) outlines an eight-stage negotiation approach (which may be expanded or contracted as needed) as a basis for achieving patient compliance:

■ Physician elicits explanatory model and illness problems from patient's perspective

■ Physician presents own explanatory model and proposed treatments in lay terms

■ Patient or physician shift models to form working alliance

■ Physician acknowledges and clarifies physician and patient discrepancies

■ Patient and physician negotiate changes to reach a mutually agreeable treatment

■ Physician offers compromises to conflicts and attempts to implement them

■ Physician acts as expert adviser, patient as final arbiter

■ Physician and patient plan for ongoing monitoring of agreement and participation

O'Connor (1995) suggests the following approaches to support the negotiation of an agreed-on treatment plan:

■ Express an attitude of openness and the willingness to cooperate

■ Explain in everyday language the providers' recommendations

■ Explicate the reasons for disagreement with the patient's beliefs or preferences

■ Accept preferred treatments not in conflict with patient's interests

■ Engage in shared decision making

■ Compromise on issues regarding religious beliefs

■ Adopt cultural behaviors that communicate trust and respect

■ Understand the patient's goals in treatment

These approaches require an ability to place the patient in the context of the cultural system that shapes his or her illness behaviors and healing responses. Anthropologists use a variety of perspectives for contextualizing patients' concerns.

Cultural Effects on Care

A basic role of clinically applied anthropology is to facilitate understanding between clients and physicians and as patient advocates and advocates for broader health concerns that facilitate institutional operations and enhance the well-being of clients and providers. This provides a context for an activist role for medical anthropology. Clinicians need to be aware of the sociopolitical context affecting practice and clients and to facilitate that adaptation proactively. Traditionally, the primary role of cultural information in clinical medicine and public health was indicating areas in which to change the behavior and lifestyle of cultural groups. Cultural perspectives are also needed to understand and change behavior of providers and institutions to provide more appropriate services. Culture has important influences on who will use services, under what conditions, and for what problems. The adaptation of health services to clients' perceptions and expectations is essential for their success.

Anthropological contributions to clinical medicine are based on conveying an understanding of patients' cultural backgrounds, their illness beliefs, and health-seeking behaviors and motivations, which can play an important role in understanding their complaints and the care they want. This enables providers to incorporate the patient into the overall treatment plan that addresses not only disease but illness and sickness as well. Cultural understandings that can enhance clinical relations by addressing factors affecting access to and presentation for biomedical treatment include such features as (Harwood, 1981; Kleinman, 1988a, 1988b)

- Meaning of symptoms
- Factors affecting the recognition of symptoms and disease
- Concepts of disease or illness and theories of its causes and cures
- Conceptions of body and bodily functions and their meanings
- Expressions (language, metaphor) of dysphoria, pain, and sick-role behavior
- Emotional reactions to illness, sickness, disease, and symptoms
- Social networks for managing illness
- Contributions of culture, family, and community to causation of disorders
- Impacts of sickness on social life, roles, behavior, work, and family relations
- Descriptive data on how culture and social organizations affect health
- Effects of government, social policy, and health bureaucracies on health care access
- Relation of morals and religious systems to conceptions of health
- Syncretic approaches and simultaneous multiple-sector use patterns
- Potentially dangerous popular or folk-sector practices
- Patient expectations of the clinical encounter
- Patient communication processes and disclosure norms
- Client group familiarity with clinical language and procedures
- Interactional norms and intercultural conflicts
- Decision-making processes
- Issues affecting compliance, expectations, obligations, family dynamics
- Cultural dietary and drug use patterns
- Client group's everyday activities
- Client's psychocultural dynamics
- Cultural dynamics of clinical communication
- Enhancement of diagnostic interview processes with ethnographic knowledge
- Effects of clinician's culture on diagnostic processes
- Effects of professional biases on clinical encounters

Using Culture to Care for Biomedical Practitioners

A crisis for biomedicine derives from the loss of faith and trust by patients and problems with biomedicine's delivery that together produce dissatisfaction for both patients and providers (Hahn, 1995; Press, 1982). Resolving providers' burnout can be addressed by making their job easier using the perspectives of anthropological medicine to facilitate their care of patients. Resolving patients' alienation requires addressing patients' perspectives and adopting an advocacy approach to remedy the ineffective distribution of health care. Biomedicine faces challenges that can be addressed by understanding cultural effects on health behavior. Challenges range from patients' dissatisfaction and loss of respect for physicians to physicians' dissatisfaction with their profession and the control over them exercised by government, administrative bureaucracies, and health organizations. Physicians suffer from high levels of stress-related conditions (e.g., suicide, depression, and addiction). Physicians face alienation in relations with their patients and the systems that control their practice. Physicians need help, and the crisis that biomedicine faces calls for changes, but physicians do not want change imposed on them.

The alternative is that physicians attempt to change their own practices using guidance from medical anthropology. Central problems facing biomedicine involve interpersonal style, community relations, professional image, and communication competence (Press, 1982). These problems result from class and cultural differences and medical theories alienated from the communities that physicians serve. These problems that confront medicine can be addressed by integrating *anthropological medicine* into biomedical practice (Hahn, 1995).

A basic problem is the challenge to professional competence caused by the variety of cultures for which physicians provide care. Cultural knowledge and cross-cultural skills can facilitate providers' tasks with information and perspectives that reduce ambiguity, uncertainty, conflict, and misunderstanding. Understanding the social and cultural dimensions of health and health behavior facilitates a cultural and psychosocial analysis of illness and healing that can guide providers' adaptations. These promote the well-being of providers by addressing uncertainties through information and interpersonal capabilities. Cultural information about clients and biomedical culture can help improve physicians' understandings of themselves and their work by identifying unconscious assumptions, values, and motivations that underlie their practice and the behavior of their patients. For example, Johnson (1991) suggests that physicians need to be aware of their unconscious desires to control their patients. Cultural knowledge can contribute to more effective ways of meeting this need by permitting more accurate predictions of patient behavior, skills in negotiating compliance, and greater flexibility in the care of patients.

Part of providing healing for practitioners involves processes that change their community image and client relationships. The social image of physicians is affected by their lack of connection with the life-worlds of their clients and their clients' lack of accessibility to their services. Changing physicians' images requires that they take activist roles in community health development and policy formation and serve as mediators and facilitators in public health and clinical contexts. The development of family practice and the neighborhood decentralization of medical resources are partial solutions to accessibility (Press, 1982). Paying more attention to the effects of illness and treatment on everyday life and adjusting medical procedures and schedules to accommodate actual life conditions is important to enhancing sensitivity of services. Physicians can change their relationships with patients through a social advocacy approach in which health care providers accept a broader social responsibility to address the structural constraints that affect health and well-being. A more equitable allocation of health resources is making physicians' care more accessible. Service to communities is a part of healing, a relationship that can provide personal benefits to health providers, a "helper's high," a "sense of well-being, satisfaction, and self-esteem that may bathe helpers after their good works" (Walsh, 1990, pp. 210–211).

Providers are further challenged by clients' dissatisfaction with the impersonal aspects of biomedical care and the inability of biomedicine to address many of the social causes and contributory factors to disease. Use of the explanatory model helps bridge the conceptual gap between providers and patients, enhancing an understanding of patients' illness and sickness behavior, and consequently enabling providers to be more responsive. Anthropologists can also assist overall care by facilitating management of the psychocultural dynamics of illness. A central need is sensitivity to the impact of illness and treatment on patients' everyday lives, addressing the psychosocial concomitants of disease, the social burdens of sickness and treatments, and their effects on the family. Medical anthropologists facilitate physicians' challenges to provide appropriate treatment responses, guiding

BIOCULTURAL INTERACTIONS

African Americans' Cross-Cultural Interactions with Biomedicine

African Americans are often suspicious of doctors and the medical system to such extreme degrees that effective clinical communication and disclosure may be seriously impaired. Various historical factors have contributed to the distrust of doctors (Bailey, 2004), including their use of African Americans in medical experiments. This has often been done without their knowledge or consent and has actually contributed to the spread of disease in the African American community. The infamous Tuskegee study left African American men with syphilis untreated for decades even though antibiotics were available. The study was proposed in the scientific interest of determining if blacks and whites responded to syphilis differently; its continuation for decades suggests that other racist elements were involved in the decisions. This has led to a general distrust of government health initiatives and treatment programs. Providers are more likely to be effective in working with African American patients if they recognize that there is a likelihood of a serious distrust of the doctor. Cross-cultural communication skills become tools at establishing more effective relations and overcoming the burdens of history.

A significant feature of the intercultural relations of African Americans with biomedicine is the feeling of a lack of respect from doctors. Doctors in the United States often try to put their patients at ease (or in their place?) by using first names: "Hi, I am Dr. Jones, how are you doing, Mary?" This might make some people feel more comfortable, but to African Americans, this is often seen as reinforcing a power relationship. Respect can be shown by addressing adults as "Mister" or "Mrs." unless told otherwise by the patient.

clinical practice by accommodating structural constraints on clinical care (e.g., constraints on accessing care produced by work or child care responsibility, transportation issues, or economic resources). The cultural-historical perspectives can also help practitioners understand and respond to some of the problems that patients have with trusting doctors, exemplified in African (Americans') well-founded distrust of biomedicine.

CHAPTER SUMMARY

The effective provision of care requires an understanding of the impacts of cross-cultural dif-ferences and ethnomedical beliefs and practices on clinical relations. Effective cross-cultural adaptation requires self-knowledge and personal management, an ability to understand cultural systems, and knowledge of the dynamics of intercultural relations and an ability to adapt to them. Cross-cultural training in relational, communication, and negotiation abilities is necessary for effective conflict resolution and avoidance. Effective accommodation of biomedicine to client realities requires cross-cultural adaptation and accommodation, the major determinant of whether ethnomedical beliefs derail biomedicine or are complementary approaches that reinforce the biomedical treatment plan. Anthropologists provide cultural knowledge and cross-cultural skills in a range of medical contexts, enhancing the quality of care for patients and the quality of work for providers. This is based on an understanding of the everyday life experience of patients and the broader social conditions that affect their well-being. This requires assessments from perspectives of cultural systems models and community assessments, presented in the next chapter.

KEY TERMS

Acculturation

Clinically applied anthropology

Compliance

Cultural awareness

Cultural competence

Cultural defense

Cultural proficiency

Cultural relativism

Cultural responsiveness

Cultural sensitivity

General cultural competence

Medicalization

Specialty areas

SELF-ASSESSMENT 3.1. CULTURAL COMPETENCE ASSESSMENT

What did your cultural competence assessment in Chapter One reveal about your skill level?

What have been the major factors affecting your development of cultural competence?

What are the principal areas in which you need to work to enhance your level of cultural competence?

EXHIBIT 3.1. Values Assessment Exercise

Assess how important each of the following factors is to you on the following scale:
1 = Very important 2 = Important 3 = Little importance 4 = Not important

	Importance of Values			
	High			Low
Cleanliness	1	2	3	4
Satisfying others' needs	1	2	3	4
Respect for elderly	1	2	3	4
Past traditions	1	2	3	4
Premarital virginity	1	2	3	4
Social equality	1	2	3	4
Family honor	1	2	3	4
Education	1	2	3	4
Self-interest	1	2	3	4
Independence from authority	1	2	3	4
Personal relationships	1	2	3	4
Directness in communication	1	2	3	4
Having many children	1	2	3	4
Punctuality	1	2	3	4
Being loyal to my manager	1	2	3	4
Being given orders by managers	1	2	3	4
Close friendships with coworkers	1	2	3	4
Having independent responsibility	1	2	3	4
Being liked by subordinates	1	2	3	4
Planning well in advance	1	2	3	4
Noncompetitive work environment	1	2	3	4
Sharing ideas with superiors	1	2	3	4
Separate roles for men and women	1	2	3	4
Formal standards for behavior	1	2	3	4
Improving social status	1	2	3	4

Which of these values produce conflict for you at work? Why?
Which of these values are emphasized in your workplace?
Which of these values are rejected in your workplace?
Which of these values do you associate with specific cultural groups?
How do values affect health and health behaviors?
How do values affect the way providers interact with clients?

SELF-ASSESSMENT 3.2. SPECIFIC CULTURAL COMPETENCY

Select one group with which you have important work interactions but for which you lack cultural proficiency. Plan a learning program based on library research, interviews, or both, that will enhance your level of competency. Answer the following questions:

What do you think are important aspects of this group's culture?

How does their culture affect their behavior in ways different from your culture?

What are significant areas of social interaction rules you need to learn to be more effective in relating to this group?

How does this group view health processes and treatments?

SELF-ASSESSMENT 3.3. CULTURALLY RESPONSIVE CARE

Now try to answer the questions in Exhibit 3.1 with respect to another cultural group (e.g., the one you examined in Self-Assessment 3.2. Specific Cultural Competency).

What makes you feel trust in your health care provider?

What interpersonal qualities do you expect your health providers to portray?

What role should emotions play in the relationships of providers with their patients?

How do your ideas about appropriate patient care relate to your cultural values?

What can health providers do to help reduce institutional discrimination in the care of patients?

How should patients behave to receive respect from their health providers?

What roles should a group's cultural values and morals play in the health care treatment they receive?

SELF-ASSESSMENT 3.4. GROUP EXERCISE

Divide your class up into three groups: A, B, and C. *Each group should read only their own assigned role (Role A, Role B, or Role C) defined below.* Then form triads of students, with one member each from groups A, B, and C. All participants in the triad have the same assignment, carried out through the manners described in their roles.

Assignment 1: All of the groups: Develop a consensus plan regarding how to prioritize and implement cross-cultural communication training in your workplace, classroom, or dorm.

Assignment 2: After twenty minutes, discuss the difficulties you had in your group in completing your assignment. Do these difficulties also emerge in cross-cultural interactions? How can they be addressed?

Role A

Your role is to make sure your group stays focused on the assignment of developing strategies for implementing cross-cultural training in your workplace. Keep the group focused on the job; avoid trivialities and personal issues. Maintain a professional, formal atmosphere, and discourage distractions and digressions. Take charge of the group, if necessary, and ensure that everyone makes a contribution to your consensus statement on strategies. You have ten minutes to complete your task, including prioritizing your group's strategies.

Role B

Your role is to warm up the group, making sure that everybody knows each other. Find out about each participant's personal and cultural background and his or her personal experiences in cross-cultural relations. The purpose of this exercise is to see how much the members of the group know about each other's personal experiences of cross-cultural communication. Make sure that everybody in the group contributes, and keep individuals from dominating or withdrawing. Don't let people manipulate you personally or invade your space, but if necessary, use teasing and humor to loosen them up or draw them out.

Role C

You are the support person in the group. You keep your personal business to yourself. You follow the group's consensus rather than lead but encourage the ideas proposed by others. To support the points that other people make, provide examples by telling stories about cross-cultural incidents that you have witnessed (or make them up). Support suggestions made by others, but don't let them make you responsible for proposing ideas. Show your support nonverbally, using close interpersonal distance, smiles, and reassuring touches.

ADDITIONAL RESOURCES

Books

Ainsworth-Vaughn, N. 1998. *Claiming power in doctor-patient talk.* New York: Oxford University Press.

Aldrich, C. K. 1999. *The medical interview: Gateway to the doctor-patient relationship.* 2nd ed. New York: Parthenon.

Bonder, B., L. Martin, and A. Miracle. 2002. *Culture in clinical care.* Thorofare, N.J.: SLACK.

Brislin, R., and T. Yoshida. 1994. *Improving intercultural interactions: Modules for cross-cultural training programs.* Thousand Oaks, Calif.: Sage.

Budrys, G. 2001. *Our unsystematic health care system.* Lanham, Md.: Rowman & Littlefield.

Fowler, S. M., and M. G. Mumford, eds. 1995–1999. *Intercultural sourcebook: Cross-cultural training methods.* Vols. 1 and 2. Yarmouth, Me.: Intercultural Press.

Gropper, R. C. 1996. *Culture and the clinical encounter: An intercultural sensitizer for the health professions.* Yarmouth, Me.: Intercultural Press.

Kohls, R. L., and H. L. Brussow. 1995. *Training know-how for cross-cultural and diversity trainers.* Portland, Ore.: Adult Learning Systems.

Kohls, R. L., and J. M. Knight. 1994. *Developing intercultural awareness: A cross-cultural training handbook.* 2nd ed. Yarmouth, Me.: Intercultural Press.

Seelye, N. H., ed. 1996. *Experiential activities for intercultural learning.* Yarmouth, Me.: Intercultural Press.

Whaley, B. B., ed. 2000. *Explaining illness: Research theory and strategies.* Mahwah, N.J.: Erlbaum.

CHAPTER

4

CULTURAL SYSTEMS MODELS

[F]eedback loops link social environment, genetic endowment, an individual's behavioral and biologic responses, health care, disease, health and function, well-being, and prosperity
—DURCH ET AL., 1997, P. 56

LEARNING OBJECTIVES

■ Present cultural systems models as bases for understanding cultural influences on health

■ Differentiate aspects of cultural systems to emphasize material, social, and mental influences on health

■ Illustrate cultural effects of health in nutrition, reproductive activities, gender, and family activities

■ Present different ideological aspects of culture that can be used to enhance health, particularly religious healing approaches that provide healing and care

■ Introduce evaluation procedures for ascertaining health needs and program effectiveness

■ Present the ethnographic rapid assessment, response, and evaluation protocols for assessing cultural dimensions of health and creating community-responsive health care

BIOCULTURAL INTERACTIONS

Managing Culture, Not Biology

Cultural differences make even putatively biological events such as pregnancy a challenge to providers. Pregnancy has considerable importance in treating the Hmong, who have a fertility rate of nearly ten children per woman. Reproduction is highly valued—a survival of an agrarian past when children were needed to work in the fields—and an immediate concern, given the great mortality from the war and the flight to refugee camps. Birth control pills might be accepted but are more likely used to fertilize home gardens than to be taken! Physicians' and family planners' contempt is often openly expressed in disgust and condemnation of people who "breed like flies." Such hostile attitudes contribute to an avoidance of prenatal care by the Hmong, who are further distressed by pelvic exams. So extensive has been the avoidance of obstetricians that many births occur in hospital parking lots, elevators, and "Hmong birthing chairs": the wheelchairs used to transport them to the delivery ward. The women show up primarily to have the births registered to guarantee their children U.S. citizenship.

Hmong cultural practices surrounding the management of pregnancy conflict with biomedical practices. A woman in delivery is expected to labor in silence, her pain muffled and often unrecognized. Episiotomies are refused even though physicians feel the women risk tearing and that the consequently delayed birth could cause cardiac distress for the newborn. Such concerns may be unwarranted: the Hmong have thousands of years of births in the mountains without medical assistance, and women incapable of birthing without medical assistance did not pass on their genes to the next generation. Circumstances have changed in the hospitals. A traditional avoidance of cold drinks following delivery makes the only available liquids—ice chips and cold water—a

CULTURAL MODELS FOR HEALTH ASSESSMENT

Cultural competence requires an overall understanding of culture because health problems disrupt personal, family, and social life, intimate behavior, and self-image and place additional demands on family and friends. Medical treatment can produce further disruptions and reduce a patient's motivation and ability to comply. Providers can reduce these difficulties by understanding the impacts of maladies and treatments on patients' lives and managing these disruptions as part of the total care of patients. This requires an assessment of the relationship of patients to their cultural context. Appropriate treatment planning requires an understanding of the client's sociocultural environment. Social and cultural factors such as economic resources, unemployment, social roles, and community organization and those of acculturation, education, occupation, class, values, discrimination, and religion affect maladies and patients' treatment.

Culturally responsive care requires attention to many cultural effects on health. Medical anthropology, medicine, transcultural nursing, public health, and social work address culture through similar approaches that involve cultural systems models. While sharing core elements, these models also have variation reflecting context- and task-specific differences in the particular aspects of health on which they focus. For instance, nurses are concerned with source of consternation and anxiety. Hospital food replaces the traditional diet of rice and chicken with herbs that provide vital treatment to help in postpartum recovery. The traditional ritual care of the baby's placenta is a challenging situation for those who live in apartments and cannot follow the tradition of burying it beneath their house.

Family and kinship roles are important in relationship to the staff. The Hmong patriarchal kinship systems and patrilineal residence (newlyweds live with husband's family) give men central roles in decision making. Heads of lineages, rather than patients, may be the focal decision makers regarding health care, but they consult extensively with family members and relatives in reaching a decision and today often consult the wife's side of the family as well. Collective agreement about the course of treatment relieves any individual, including the head of the family, from blame in the event of a poor outcome.

Unlike the respect they traditionally received, Hmong elders in America are culturally and personally traumatized, reduced to menial jobs or dependence on government support. Changing gender roles and the increased independence of women produce further conflicts and stress. Their once tight-knit communities and generational structure have disintegrated, producing alienated youth with mental health problems. The clan systems that helped ensure that marriages remained successful are weak in the United States, contributing to escalating domestic conflicts in isolated nuclear families. Grandparents, once considered authorities in raising their grandchildren, today find their views ignored. Acculturation has produced role reversals where the elderly now depend on their grandchildren for their translation assistance with doctors.

factors that affect the physical assessment of patients whereas public health workers are concerned with behaviors that contribute to the spread of disease. Consequently, diverse models are necessary for organizing learning about and research into the myriad influences on health and addressing the multiple areas of culture. Aspects of the cultural systems models that are discussed in this chapter focus on nutrition, reproductive behaviors, family structures, and ideological culture. The principles of religious healing and traditional ethnomedical practices—the "witch-doctor's legacy"—are addressed as part of anthropological medicine. Anthropological medicine elicits the sociocultural dimensions of healing processes, those that address the personal, social, and cosmological dimensions of health concerns. Culture may not be able to cure disease, but it has many mechanisms for healing illness and providing care for all maladies. Leininger's (1991) concept of culture care is presented to illustrate the cultural dimensions of addressing basic human needs when confronting health problems.

A key issue in developing culturally responsive care and health services is an assessment of community health needs. These approaches incorporate communities into health care planning, development, delivery, and assessment. The basic processes of community health assessment are outlined, beginning with the involvement of community in determining priorities for health planning and programs. Community health assessment approaches are provided in the processes of ethnographic rapid assessment, response, and evaluation, which are tools for creating community-responsive health care programs and extending cultural systems models in context- and foci-specific assessments that guide inquiry into culture and health relationships.

CULTURAL SYSTEMS APPROACHES TO HEALTH

Culture, the patterns of shared group behavior transmitted between generations through learning, provides the core conceptual framework for understanding all of human behavior, including health behavior. Culture is a metatheory for explaining human behavior, particularly differences among groups. All human behavior is shaped by it. Recognizing culture as the principal determinant of behavior is necessary for understanding how it affects health. The effects of culture are found throughout human life, beginning with basic survival functions and structuring of interactions with the physical environment. Cultural learning shapes even biologically based needs: defense, reproduction, sex, eating, defecation, and attachment.

Culture affects health through what we eat, how we protect and expose ourselves, patterns of sex and procreation, our hygienic practices, how we bond together, and lifestyle behaviors. Culture produces risk factors, conditions associated with an increased likelihood of diseases, such as smoking cigarettes or eating poorly cooked meats or the blood of animals. Culture also provides systems that humans use as protective factors that reduce disease risks, such as hygienic rituals of bathing and purification and prohibitions of sex outside of marriage. Cultural conditions are basic to producing the health problems and what we do about them.

Culture guides the experience and management of health conditions through the classification of the condition and treatments available. For example, biomedicine might diagnose a cold and provide you with a decongestant, whereas an ethnomedical healer might consider you to have excess dampness and prescribe a tea to heat up your lungs. Culture's classification of the world shapes the effects and experiences of naturally occurring conditions, as illustrated in Chapter Two in "Biocultural Interactions: Leprosy and Social Stigma." Culture defines our perceptions of problems and produces the social organizations and policies that allocate resources for health.

To examine the ways that culture affects health, medical anthropologists, physicians, nurses, and public and community health practitioners (e.g., Brody, 1973; Engel, 1977, 1980; Blum, 1983; Leininger, 1991, 1995; Baer et al., 1986; Sallis and Owen, 1998) have proposed similar conceptual frameworks. These systems models address health and disease in relationship to the ecology, the total physical and social environments. These models incorporate demographic, technological, economic, political, and other social conditions that affect the physical environment. They also describe specific areas of cultural systems affecting health.

Cultural systems perspectives prominent in community health include the "environment of health" or "force-field paradigm" (Blum, 1983; Evans and Stoddart, 1994) that views health as a product of the relationships among many subsystems or fields, emphasizing

■ *The physical environment,* including sanitation, housing, environmental toxicity, and the physical infrastructure (roads, water, transportation)

- *The social environment,* including family, work, class, education, and social networks

- *Individual behavior,* especially aspects of lifestyle that link people to the environment

- *Medical care services,* part of the social environment with a special role in health

- The genetic and biological levels

These interdependent subsystems affect one another, operating through natural resources, the population and its ecological balance, and cultural systems mediating human interaction with all of the force fields: resources, social networks, and medical services. Environmental influences on health include human effects such as pollutants and contaminants and stressors produced by social conditions of dilapidated housing and rampant crime. The social environment of family and its material and intellectual resources are significant features of health, especially when parents care for their ill children or call on relatives for assistance. Lifestyle and behavioral factors affecting health involve many cultural influences, including high-risk behaviors such as unprotected sex, drug consumption, and tattooing. Medical care services may provide care to all or restrict it to those who can pay substantial fees to providers, resulting in the poor suffering more from easily preventable diseases. Genetic and biological levels are also implicated in health problems, but from public health perspectives, the importance of disease is far less than the other factors that permit it to spread and go untreated.

The multiple determinants of health and their dynamic relationships illustrate that health is not strictly a function of disease, biology, or genetics; rather, health is derived from the complex interaction of physical determinants with social, economic, political, and other cultural conditions that produce an individual's behavior and biological conditions. The specific conditions and factors being investigated vary for different settings and professions. For instance, several cultural systems models have been used in nursing, most notably Leininger's (1991, 1995) "Sunrise Model" and Purnell's cultural competence model (Purnell and Paulanka, 2003). In the nursing models, classic anthropological foci—environment, migration history, economics, societal relations, education, and family structures—are examined as important features affecting health. Nursing practice also pays attention to how skin color may affect physiological assessment, issues related to culture care preferences, life-cycle events affecting health, and cultural factors affecting clinical interactions.

This chapter and others in this book present assessments of culture necessary for culturally competent health care: evaluation, intervention, promotion, and disease prevention programs. The effects of health practices and beliefs, especially as illustrated in illness beliefs and sickness behaviors, were addressed in Chapter Two. This chapter provides an overview of the cultural system features of infrastructure, structure, and **superstructure,** with a focus on the microlevel cultural dynamics of individual interactions, addressing health effects of

- Infrastructure, particularly nutrition and reproduction

- Family and kinship

- The mental level, specifically worldviews regarding illness and healing

Subsequent chapters address other aspects of cultural assessment:

■ Lay and folk-sector health activities (Chapter Five)

■ Specific cultural characteristics, including identity, self-concepts, social norms, and behavioral and communication patterns, illustrated in the psychocultural model and indigenous psychology (Chapter Six)

■ Environmental influences, morbidity and mortality risks, dietary practices, and exposure patterns (Chapter Seven)

■ Structural organization of health practices and the political dynamics of health care (Chapter Eight)

CULTURAL INFRASTRUCTURE, STRUCTURE, AND SUPERSTRUCTURE

Systems models help reveal the regularly occurring features of cultural and social life by providing a metatheoretical perspective for examining group influences on individual behavior. Harris (1988) characterized the cultural system as entailing three major aspects (Table 4.1):

■ Infrastructure: institutions that mediate relations to the physical environment such as roads, sanitary water, and housing

■ Structure: social relations with others such as families and community networks

■ Superstructure: behaviors and ideas or mental representations, such as beliefs about the causes of diseases and the best means of treating them

Cultural systems approaches traditionally emphasized the determining and limiting influences of the infrastructure: for example, the material, technological, and economic factors. Physical energy is necessary for existence, making material conditions necessary for cultural life and crucial determinants of health. Nonetheless, infrastructure may reflect the social and ideological levels of culture, where social practices and beliefs determine the nature of the physical adaptations.

TABLE 4.1.   **Major Aspects of Cultural Systems**

Cultural System	Level	Function	Activity
Superstructure	Mental	Ideology, beliefs, meaning	Communication
Structure	Social	Social organization	Interpersonal relations
Infrastructure	Material	Technology, economy	Behavior

The infrastructure has two main divisions:

- Material production: the energy extraction at the bases of the cultural system

- Reproduction: the population, how it replicates itself and its ecological dynamics

Production is concerned with work, the processes for the acquisition of energy. Reproductive patterns and practices produce the population, another part of the environment that also affects health, producing risks and disease transmission factors (e.g., the rapid spread of diseases in closely confined groups).

Social organization has two main domains:

- Domestic sphere: family, gender roles, and family-based division of labor

- Political sphere: economy, division of labor, class systems, and political structures

Family provides the context for many aspects of health and disease, ranging from genetic inheritance to high-risk behaviors acquired through socialization. Social structure interfaces with the infrastructure through work and resources, affecting the nature and distribution of health care resources and risks, and directly affecting individual and group health status.

Superstructure is the abstract essence of culture, the mental and symbolic forms manifested in ideas and behaviors. A central aspect of superstructure is the worldview, the broad organizing frameworks of values, beliefs, and principles that provide guidelines for understanding the universe and social behavior, including health practices. Superstructure provides meanings that link social and material structures and provide the priorities for behavior at the levels of structure and infrastructure. Superstructure beliefs and knowledge shape beliefs about desirable health conditions and behavioral responses to disease.

Understanding health requires situating it in the interrelated systems of cultural practices and institutions that organize human behavior in the material, social, and ideological dimensions and relating them to the physical environment. A detailed example of a cultural system model is provided in Exhibit 4.1. The cultural systems models emphasize the relationships to the environment as an additional level distinct from culture that involves the physical earth and biotic and abiotic systems that impinge on humans (see Chapter Seven).

INFRASTRUCTURE

Infrastructure is the interface of a culture with the physical environment; it includes both a population's biological reproductive patterns that result in births and its material production system (technoeconomic system) that produces goods such as food and housing. Population relations with the environment provide energy and resources to sustain human life but that also create exposure to disease. Consequently, cultural-environmental relations affect many aspects of health.

Basic aspects of the infrastructure include food production technologies, transportation facilities, communication systems, utilities (water, electricity, gas, and sewage), industries, and economic systems for the distribution of resources. Human work is basic to infrastructure and economic systems, providing the resources that support existence.

EXHIBIT 4.1. Conceptual Framework for Cultural System Health Assessments

Ecological Assessments

Physical boundaries (mapping)

Environmental conditions and risks; EPA standards compliance

Contamination and sanitation

Demography and population structures

Ethnic composition and distribution

Migration, migrants, homelessness

Medical and social epidemiology: principal morbidity, mortality

At-risk groups

Immunization, vaccination rates, and programs

Recreational facilities

Nutritional Practices and the Body

Concepts of food, diet, and ideal body type

Dietary patterns and restrictions

Low-income food support

Low-birth-weight incidence

Drug-use patterns

Reproduction

Biocultural profiles: ethnic risk factors, especially social and genetic

Reproductive rates and patterns

Sexual practices and prostitution; STD risks and rates

Birth control attitudes and practices; beliefs about pregnancy

Birth practices and breast-feeding

Principal mortality and morbidity rates for women and children

Developmental norms and ideals; sexual surgery

Infrastructure

Material goods and economic well-being

Land and property ownership

Housing and housing assistance

Transportation and communication systems

Industry, markets, and exchange

Emergency resources

Economics and Work

Median household income

Work activities and work risks

Informal economies and undocumented workers

Unemployment rates

Welfare resources

Percentage of families, children, and infants below poverty level

Proportion of individuals without health insurance

Household economies and businesses

Family Structures and Roles

Gender roles; social relationships

Attachment patterns

Single-parent prevalence

Adolescent birth rates

Kinship networks

Domestic violence rates; child abuse cases

Adult transition patterns

Marriage and divorce patterns

Care-provision roles and patterns

Community Organization

Group definitions; intracommunity group divisions

Informal networks

Community associations

Community expertise

Community structures and groups

Community leaders

Political dynamics

Police and criminal justice system activities

Social services

Youth organizations and gangs

Community groups with health interests

Extracommunity relations

Health Organization and Infrastructure

Clinics, hospitals, and emergency departments

Ambulance services

Public health facilities

Public health education and outreach

Health coalitions, alliances, and organizations

Organizational Analysis of Health Institutions

Business environment

Values and heroes

Rites and rituals

Structural networks

Management style and decision making

Group Social Psychology

Socialization processes

Acculturation and intercultural conflict

Self-representations; in-group versus out-group status

Values and norms

Cross-gender relations

Emotions

Spirituality and religion, especially health implications and support systems

Cultural event analysis: purposes, activities, and actors

Psychocultural dynamics

Education

Health education needs and programs

School health programs

Learning styles

School quality

High school graduation and dropout rates

Literacy rates; illiterate segments

Communication

Home language and dominant language competence

Nonverbal communication; social interaction rules

Social communication: signs, gestures, styles

Media services

Health Beliefs and Practices

History of relations with biomedicine

Perceived accessibility of health providers

Health and illness concepts

Lay medical beliefs and practices

Folk professional sectors and activities

Explanatory Model; Health Beliefs Model

Stress management practices

Consequently, work influences diverse cultural institutions and health. Work provides resources for purchasing health care and, in the United States, is the primary source of health benefits. Work obligations may preclude seeking health care. Work often constitutes a hazardous place, producing many physical, social, and psychological factors that can compromise health.

Reproductive practices structure population dynamics through fertility rates, which affect group size, health conditions, and population growth. Culture influences demographic structure and population characteristics: sex ratio, age-distributed mortality, fertility and birth rates, morbidity, mortality, population density, and distribution. These factors, in turn, affect many other aspects of health.

Diet and Nutrition

Diet is a primary context of human relationships to the environment and a fundamental determinant of health and disease. Culture shapes what is eaten, by whom, when, where, with whom, and how. Food can be a contributory factor in the development of disease, such as coronary artery disease, diabetes, and some cancers. Eating is a social event with many health implications. The use of food in social activities expresses relations between individuals and groups. Consequently, food sharing has a variety of implications for health: positive ones such as social support, bonding, and resource sharing and negative ones such as disease risks through shared utensils or unhealthy foods. Cultural conceptions of foods have a wide range of implications integrated throughout social life. These include interpersonal obligations (e.g., wedding feasts), life events (e.g., birthdays), social rituals (e.g., drinking), and religious and moral judgments regarding permissible diet (e.g., kosher foods).

Because ideas about food are integrated within cultural systems, it is difficult to change diet, even when it interferes with health care. To propose therapeutic changes to a diet that will be acceptable requires a knowledge of cultural food practices. Recommended diets for the treatment of conditions are generally based on European American concepts of normal diet and customary foods and seldom include foods in the typical diets of immigrant and minority ethnic groups. Consequently, recommended diets are often not adopted. When cultural food preferences are unknown or not considered, individuals may become undernourished because of distaste for hospital food. An effective therapeutic dietary change requires an understanding of cultural patterns of food preparation and consumption and the significance of food. Food can have significance as a marker of status, a means of self-gratification, and a compensatory mechanism for psychodynamic conditions. Such social and personal meanings may lead to various forms of malnutrition, manifested in overeating or undereating to meet some secondary or tertiary social goals (e.g., thinness for attraction, obesity as a form of personal protection, or alcohol consumption as a social lubricant).

Foods may be viewed as medicine and are often part of lay treatments of illness. The hot-cold system of illness and healing incorporates foods to balance illnesses, external conditions, or other treatments. Natural products, particularly plant beverages, constitute self-medication. For example, a number of herbal teas used as beverages among Native Americans of the Southwest have been shown to have a variety of anti-diabetogenic properties (Winkelman, 1992b).

Foods are used as medicine in pregnancy and lactation. Restrictions on diet during pregnancy may favor maternal and neonatal well-being or may prejudice them by restricting the intake of nutrients they need. Infant nutrition is affected by a variety of factors:

■ Those indigenous to the culture and its patterns of resource use and distribution

■ Cultural norms regarding the nature, frequency, and content of foods provided for infants

■ Governmental or market influences that affect the availability of foods

■ Marketing campaigns encouraging bottle-feeding instead of breast-feeding

Sex, Conception, and Pregnancy

Sexual behavior is biologically based, socially elicited, and culturally shaped; it has many health implications, ranging from the spread of disease to the health of young mothers and their offspring. STDs are associated with promiscuity, extramarital sexual behavior, prostitution, and lower socioeconomic status. Norms affecting premarital sex, homosexuality, marriage, extramarital sex, and particular sex practices all have important health implications. So does the process of delivery of babies in the modern world, where biomedicine has managed to acquire a virtual monopolistic control over legal rights to deliver babies (see the special feature, "Practitioner Profile: Robbie Davis-Floyd").

Birth Control All societies regulate conception through diverse means: mores, law, marriage, diet, work, medications, and many other cultural practices. When a woman conceives is not merely a matter of individual choice but a product of many influences: biological, nutritional, familial, economic, and the cultural value placed on having children. Dietary factors that influence the onset of first menses are economic and ecological influences on fertility. Cultural concepts about appropriate family size and birth spacing influence conception. Pregnancy often signals the end of breast-feeding, with dietary implications for the previous child's health. The acceptability of birth control methods varies cross-culturally, affected by cultural attitudes toward the personal significance of pregnancy. Cultural norms about contact with one's genitals affect the acceptability of procedures like diaphragms. People's desire for large families or a man's assertion of virility through many children can make control of fertility unwanted. Knowledge of these cultural beliefs is important in directing appropriate birth control methods. Religious beliefs affect birth control attitudes and are a necessary component of culturally sensitive and relevant fertility counseling.

Reproductive Behaviors Pregnancy and birth are profoundly shaped by culture. Cultural responses to pregnancy may produce support, risk factors for mother and child, or conflicts with providers. Knowledge of these practices is necessary for bridging patient and biomedical realities through patient and provider education. Biomedical pregnancy practices in the United States involve procedures not customary in other cultures: prenatal examinations, childbirth classes, ultrasonography and fetal monitoring with other obstetrical technologies, induction of labor, lithotomy position, and so forth. Ethnomedical models of pregnancy are important for biomedicine and public health because they constitute the

CULTURE AND HEALTH

Cultural Issues in Mexican American Pregnancy and Prenatal Care

For many women of Mexican origin, beliefs about pregnancy have centered on the traditions of *parteras* (midwives). Parteras' ideas about pregnancy and childbirth include food taboos and restrictions on activities that are often followed as part of the management of pregnancy. Ideas of "hot" and "cold" conditions and treatments are also important: conditions must be balanced to restore health. Pregnant women are "hot" and must avoid hot foods and hot treatment conditions or neutralize these conditions by taking cool substances. The postpartum woman is in a cold state and must be maintained in a warm state and fed hot (or temperate) foods to ensure the flow of milk; if the milk becomes cold, it could harm the baby. Restrictions for forty days of convalescence are also derived from parteras' traditional practices.

Cultural values affect teen pregnancy rates and prenatal care. About half of all Hispanics born in the United States in recent decades were to single mothers, a phenomenon reflecting cultural values and social circumstances. The relevance of cultural factors in addressing pregnancy risks among Mexican Americans include cultural values concerning children; negative attitudes toward and an ignorance of contraception; the value and status of parenthood; low levels of parental communication with children regarding sex, pregnancy, and contraception; low levels of the use of contraceptives; and social factors affecting access to sex education (Brindis, 1992).

The cultural value placed on children reinforces keeping a pregnancy even outside of marriage. Machismo and high mortality among male youth reinforces a mentality in which having a baby is a sign of manhood or womanhood and a means of intergenerational continuity. The lack of sex education reflects both social and cultural factors. Problems arise in sex education because of low levels of parental communication regarding sex, pregnancy, and contraception and early school dropout. Early school dropout means that sex education is not obtained. Public health information from health service agencies is often ineffective because of language barriers, cultural conflicts in learning and instructional styles, and barriers presented by a lack of legal residency. The avoidance of teenage pregnancy requires the involvement of cultural institutions, especially the family and church. Because many Hispanics drop out before finishing high school, where sex education is provided, parents must be encouraged to take a central role in the sex education processes. This requires a broader education to assist parents in developing communication skills and relevant knowledge through life education programs that are culturally relevant and sensitive (Brindis, 1992). Communication with parents about sexual matters

basis from which people make decisions. Consequently, ethnomedical models are essential to the formulation of culturally relevant programs that address critical divergences from biomedical beliefs. For instance, traditional beliefs about pregnancy and fertility may increase risk during pregnancy (Snow, 1993). Pregnancy taboos—prohibitions on behavior during pregnancy—are found throughout the world. Many cultures view pregnant appears to inhibit teen pregnancy, as does involvement with the church, which tends to delay first sexual intercourse.

Cultural factors affect prenatal care, a significant factor in maternal and neonatal health. The utilization of prenatal health services by Mexican Americans is much lower than that of other groups (Moore and Hepworth, 1994). Mexican Americans were less likely than non-Hispanic whites to initiate first-trimester care, obtain prenatal care, and make postnatal visits for well-baby care. These differences are present even when Mexican Americans have the same access to services. Predictors of service use included satisfaction with care, lack of transportation problems, and higher social support, advice, and assistance. Low use of care is also affected by income, ineligibility for services, and cultural and language barriers to service satisfaction (Brindis, 1992).

Research on the prenatal beliefs, practices, and patterns of health utilization provide a basis from which to develop prenatal care education for low-income Mexican women (Alcalay, Ghee, and Scrimshaw, 1993). Researchers assessed the effectiveness of mass media campaigns in promoting the use of health care services and identified appropriate communication patterns and messages. This provided the basis for designing an intervention that addressed pregnancy-related problems and the appropriate health behaviors. The pregnancy education project used communication interventions based on a variety of persuasion theories that emphasized the personal relevance of messages, attitude changes, and new role models.

A significant barrier to prenatal care is a belief that it is unnecessary if a woman feels well. Women need to know the necessity of prenatal checkups even if they feel well. Information from practitioners does not provide adequate knowledge about appropriate weight gain, the need for iron supplements, the signs of risks during pregnancy, or supplemental dietary needs. Dissatisfaction is a barrier to care. Women's care-seeking behavior is also inhibited by the lack of their husband's approval for leaving the house and the inability of a man to accompany his wife because of having to work. Traditional sex roles and objections by husbands to another man looking at his wife's private areas are barriers to routine gynecological exams. The hospital and clinical situations where many providers examine the women also make them feel uncomfortable, and they avoid care. Because of the socialization for modesty emphasized in Mexican culture, women may feel particularly strong shame and embarrassment during gynecological or obstetrical exams or in discussing sexual or reproductive issues. Examinations that involve nudity or other lack of personal privacy may result in termination of the doctor-patient relationship. Health care providers sensitive to these cultural factors can adapt by providing greater privacy or by using female personnel for interviews and examinations.

women as being in a vulnerable state or posing a threat to others by her so-called abnormal condition. Understanding cultural taboos regarding pregnancy is important in ensuring the well-being of mother and child. Pregnancy taboos can be in a woman's favor (e.g., reducing fatty foods or foods with high risks of disease) or may negatively affect the mother and neonate (e.g., food restrictions that deprive them of protein or vitamins).

Birth and Delivery Processes In modern societies, birth processes are managed by biomedical institutions. But traditional beliefs and practices concerning childbirth persist. Knowledge of these practices is important for pregnancy, labor, and delivery classes because women use their own cultural beliefs in adapting to medical settings. Traditional practices of birthing while squatting lead women to abandon the gurney and stirrups and seek an area to squat; occasionally, women in a biomedical setting who are following their tradition's norms by seeking a private area in which to squat are discovered in custodians' closets or in stairwells. Cultural norms regarding the expression of pain are relevant to understanding delivering mothers, their expressions during labor, and the relevance of pain medication or other interventions.

Cultural elements of the biomedical obstetrical practices may conflict with cultural norms about modesty. Perineal shaving and routine episiotomies reflect cultural practices of biomedicine rather than scientifically established procedures. Cultural beliefs about who should be the birth attendant may conflict with American norms. Without the recognition of cultural patterns, outreach and marketing strategies may be to no avail (such as recruiting Hispanic men to attend birthing classes to learn to be labor assistants for their wives). Understanding cultural expectations is crucial to the correct assessment of the meaning of others' involvement or lack thereof. A man's failure to participate in the birthing process, or even be at the hospital, may reflect cultural expectations rather than a lack of interest in the mother and child. Support for the mother and her newborn also varies widely, ranging from conditions under which others accept full responsibility for the mother-infant dyad to those where mothers may find little, if any, relief from ordinary responsibilities and little assistance for the care of her newborn.

Differences in delivery expectations between biomedicine and the general culture have contributed to a burgeoning of alternative birthing practices, a popular uprising against biomedicine. The development of modern obstetrical practices led to the adoption of the lithotomic position, with the mother on her back with her feet up in the air in stirrups. While not conducive to natural labor processes, this was convenient for the physician's control. The role of culture in birthing practices is evidenced in the changes in the biomedical approach in the recent development of alternative birth centers and the reintroduction of the nurse-midwife.

Postpartum Taboos Culture shapes a variety of postpartum behaviors affecting the health of newborns and mothers. Cultures have both formal and informal norms regarding the behavior of women following birth, including restrictions on activity and foods to protect the mother and newborn. Seclusion is a frequent source of protection, reducing exposure to infectious disease, providing rest and relief from ordinary work, and encouraging breast-feeding, mother-infant bonding, and healing. Many cultures require new mothers to rest for a month or forty days. Cultural beliefs about activity, diet, seclusion, purification, sex, and protection can favor or prejudice the well-being of mother and newborn. For instance, African Americans often introduce solid food in the first month, a practice considered to be harmful for newborns. Of particular importance are beliefs regarding exposure to temperature extremes, bathing, activity, diet, clothing, and a variety

PRACTITIONER PROFILE

Robbie Davis-Floyd

Robbie Davis-Floyd, Ph.D., a cultural-medical anthropologist, senior research fellow at the University of Texas, Austin, and fellow of the Society for Applied Anthropology, specializes in the anthropology of reproduction (http://www.davis-floyd.com). For her first book, *Birth as an American Rite of Passage* (1992), she interviewed one hundred women about their pregnancy and childbirth experiences. In 1993 she updated and expanded Jordan's classic *Birth in Four Cultures* and subsequently coedited *Childbirth and Authoritative Knowledge* (1997), a collection of ethnographies on birth in sixteen cultures, and *Cyborg Babies* (1998), a collection of anthropological analyses of the technological reproductive experience. She studied the paradigm shifts of holistic physicians, published in *From Doctor to Healer* (coauthored with G. St. John) (1998).

Davis-Floyd's primary research interests remain grounded in the anthropology of reproduction, specifically childbirth, midwifery, and obstetrics. In 1996 and 1998, she received consecutive Wenner-Gren grants to study the development of direct-entry midwifery in North America. She has published a number of articles from this research focusing on midwifery education (1998a, 1998b), politics (2000, 2003), and identity articulation (Davis-Floyd and Davis, 1996; Davis-Floyd, 2001; Davis-Floyd, Cosminsky, and Pigg, 2001) in the United States and Mexico and coedited, with C. B. Johnson, *Mainstreaming Midwives: The Politics of Change* (2006). She has served as senior advisor to the Council on Anthropology and Reproduction since 2005.

Davis-Floyd continues her birth activism, helping to form coalitions, speaking at conferences promoting normal birth and breast-feeding, and (since 1994) serving as consumer representative to the board of the North American Registry of Midwives and since 2006 as editor for the International MotherBaby Childbirth Initiative: 10 Steps to Optimal Maternity Services (http://www.imbci.org).

The chapters in the forthcoming collection, *Birth Models That Work* (coedited with L. Barclay, B. A. Daviss, and J. Tritten), describe and promote excellent birth models from twelve different countries in the developed and developing worlds.

of self-care practices. Many cultures believe that women should not be exposed to cold because it will shock or deplete the body of heat, which is thought to lead to illness. Although many taboos may seem unnecessary from biomedical perspectives, there are important reasons why they should be respected when they do not directly prejudice the health of mother or child. Taboos are often deeply embedded in cultural traditions, and their violation may evoke considerable anxiety for the mother. Given the psychophysiological importance of these rituals for relaxation and peace of mind, they should be permitted to support recuperation and healing.

FAMILY INFLUENCES ON HEALTH AND DEVELOPMENT

A family's genetic contribution to health is mediated through socialization and environmental influences. Family mediates sanitation, housing, diet, physical activities, smoking and drinking, and risk exposures. Family is the context in which the sick role is learned and primary care is given. It is also the context for decision making about health care. Family values and norms influence basic health care behavior, including which resources to access (see Chapter Five on health care sectors) and when or whether to seek biomedical services. Family may also impede the utilization of health care. For instance, the shame associated with mental illness makes many Asian American families reluctant to seek care for family members.

Family mediates cultural and social influences on health through the transmission of gender roles, values, emotional behaviors, and identity. Families are universal, but their structures, roles, and influences vary. In all cultures, men and women form conjugal pairs; however, although some of these marriages form new families, other marriages are into existing families, such as when a woman marries into her husband's patrilineal extended family and lives with his relatives. Universal biosocial care roles of the family (Leininger, 1995) are complemented by culturally varying roles and activities of family members in providing care. An assessment of both cultural (group-specific) and social (universal) influences of the family is vital to culturally responsive health care. A knowledge of family health behaviors, preventive practices, and decision making regarding access to care is a basic foundation for understanding patient needs. Knowledge of the family health culture helps providers decide on priorities for intervention, necessary support, and education.

Addressing clients' needs through family systems perspectives helps overcome the dominant biomedical and cultural tendencies to address problems in the reductive perspective of an individual. The particular dynamics of family health behavior are crucial to various aspects of accessing care needs, such as determining the acceptability of proposed care to the patient and other family members, such as grandmothers, and family members' participation in discharge planning and home treatment of the patient.

Family Structures. Family structures are variable. The European American family ideal, the **nuclear family** of parents (husband and wife) and their children, is not typical in most cultures. Indeed, the nuclear family no longer characterizes the living situation of most Americans; more Americans live in a single-parent family, which is typically a female-headed household. The **extended family,** consisting of a three-generational family structure (grandparents, parents, and children), is the more common ideal pattern of family organization found worldwide. The most typical form of the extended family has been the **patrilineal extended family,** where father-son obedience provides the authority structure, and brother loyalty reinforces the male power structure. Some extended family systems may also include other kin: aunts, uncles, cousins, and fictive kin. A **matrilocal family** is an extended family based on women's kinship ties and residence and may consist of all descendants of a woman, including her sons and daughters and the daughters' offspring. Generally neither the daughters' husbands nor the sons' wives and children are considered to be part of the family. In today's world with widespread divorce and remarriage, other family structures have emerged such as the **blended family,** which combines the members of two families united through marriage. A variety of other nontraditional and alternative family structures are also created by gay and lesbian marriages.

Gender and Health

Family is the primary context where biologically determined sex characteristics are formed by culturally ascribed and socialized conditions of gender identity and behavior. The culturally varying ways of managing the differences between men and women have many implications for health status. Helman (2001) suggests four elements of gender:

- Genetic gender
- Somatic gender based on phenotype, physical appearance, and secondary sex characteristics
- Psychological gender based on self-perception
- Social gender based on cultural definitions that define perceptions and behavior.

Social gender is the most susceptible to sociocultural influences, but all aspects of gender are influenced by culture and have health implications. Cultural expectations regarding appropriate gender behaviors often create health problems and barriers to effective care. The relative value of sexes may affect the way newborns are treated or health care provided: for instance, where preference for males may lead to the neglect of female infants. Cultural rules about women's modesty and exposure of her body affect health care interactions. This applies to men as well, affecting examination, bathing, and other procedures.

The expectation in some cultures that women should be subordinate to men can have a variety of effects in health care settings. In health examinations, a man may accompany his wife and answer the physician's questions for her. For many nurses, this directly clashes with their professional expectations that women should be independent. This often produces anger and frustration in female providers, affecting patient care. Providers need to know cultural gender expectations and construct interactions that facilitate achieving health care goals.

Female status is associated with a number of socially induced health conditions and disorders. In European American culture, these include an increased tendency toward anorexia and bulimia, the use of a variety of cosmetic procedures and beautifying agents that prejudice health, stress from the cultural emphasis on appearance, and conflicts women face when professionalization puts them in conflict with traditional norms. Male status is also associated with health risks. These include higher rates of death from most conditions, a shorter life expectancy, higher risks of disease from smoking and alcohol consumption, a greater tendency to a type A personality, and the associated higher rates of heart disease. Men are often less likely to avail themselves of medical care in a timely manner because of the cultural expectations that they should repress emotions and help-seeking behaviors, not complain about pain or discomfort, and downplay their distress and symptoms in ways that contribute to an underevaluation of the severity of their conditions.

Family Roles in Care and Therapy

Different family realities cross-culturally constitute a source of problems in treatment and compliance. Family roles in primary care provision may include physical care, social and emotional support, and performance of a sick person's ordinary responsibilities. Family roles in this support differ from culture to culture and must be considered in the planning of care. Culturally based family expectations regarding care need to be known in order to include family members appropriately in making treatment decisions and supporting discharge plans. Cultural role expectations and norms about interpersonal interactions between different people, particularly in-laws, are relevant to home health care. A knowledge of family roles is essential in assisting a family in making decisions by knowing who are considered to be the decision makers.

Decision-making processes are based in family but may involve certain members and not others or include others within an extended family and kinship system. Different kinship systems consider different family members to be the party responsible for a patient. In contrast to the European American system, where the obligations are with mother and father, matrilineal or patrilineal kinship structures may place legal, financial, or moral responsibility for treatment within the kinship group of father or mother alone. Although laws may require the parents' authorization of medical procedures, understanding the key figures in the cultural patterns of decision making can facilitate providers' efforts to obtain consent. If cultural practices are not understood and respected, relevant decision makers may be excluded, and legally responsible family members may feel that it is inappropriate for them to authorize treatment. The recognition of cultural authority enables health care providers to seek out culturally designated decision makers to ensure compliance with institutional requirements.

The cultural focus on groups supports new trends in the helping professions that focus on family systems and examining family culture (Helman, 2001). Family structure and relations may be protective or pathogenic and enhance or inhibit therapeutic processes. The family system may scapegoat a particular member, resulting in **psychosomatic disorders** for the patient from disturbed family relations and their emotional effects. A resolution of problems for the patient may be inhibited by family processes, such as live-in grandparents refusing to accept the inevitability of acculturation for their children and grandchildren. Treatment needs to be directed at the family and its (dys)functions, rather than just the identified patient.

A knowledge of the normative family relations within a culture helps determine if certain behaviors are normative or deviant. Knowledge of what is normative in the culture is an important corrective to the tendency to evaluate client conditions from the dominant societal norms. The acculturation processes of the wider society are also important for identifying the source of deviant or problematic behavior in outside social forces or the family system itself when its traditional patterns are maladaptive for a bicultural individual.

Kinship Extensions of family structures into broader networks of relations, such as grandparents, uncles and aunts, and cousins, are referred to as kinship or **kin** networks. Kinship involves interpersonal ties that include both biological relationships and social ties produced by marriage and adoption. In contrast to the isolated family units and limited kinship networks typical of Euro-American middle-class families, many cultures have extended kinship structures that play an important role in everyday life. This extended kinship structure often constitutes the network within which health care and the associated social and economic support are provided during illness. Because of their fundamental role in organizing human social systems, kinship expectations have important health functions. Functions of kinship that affect health care include responsibilities for the care of related children and the provision of material assistance and resources to kin. The obligation of kin to support the ill may create institutional problems such as dozens of relatives visiting a patient in a hospital. Different concepts of family member can also cause problems in hospitals where visiting policies are largely structured on the assumptions of the traditional middle-class American family: nuclear structure with few children. The concept of *fictive kin* refers to unrelated individuals who assume kinship roles and terms: for example, a close female friend being called "sister" by another person, whose children refer to her as "auntie." In today's society where there are many families disrupted by divorce, fictive kin often play central roles in family systems. Culturally sensitive providers recognize these relations and extend to them the prerogatives allowed under narrower conceptions of the nuclear family.

UNDERSTANDING WORLDVIEW AND SYMBOLIC RESOURCES

Effective health care requires an understanding of patients' perspectives; their views of their illness; and how the patient and family view the origin, significance, and implication of the condition for their life. Medical treatment must address a patient's concerns and emotional well-being, not merely his or her physical condition. To address these concerns, it is necessary to obtain the patient's explanatory model and integrate this information within the context of the patient's cultural, religious, social, and economic background. Eliciting patients' explanatory models connects with their systems of meaning within which their maladies and treatments are understood. It is necessary for providers to address patients' perspectives deliberately to make their diagnoses and treatments meaningful to the patients and reduce anxiety.

Understanding a person's worldview and beliefs, the ideological level of culture, provides the template for addressing global effects of culture on health behavior. Although health is dependent on what people do, what they think and believe is often the determinant of behavior and healing responses. The impacts of beliefs and expectations have important lessons for providers. Traditional ethnomedical practices have often been criticized as depending on belief and the placebo effect. The consequences of expectations, however, can be real and may be an important addition to the health providers' healing tools, as exemplified in the healing power of religion and the principles of the witch-doctor's legacy.

Religion as an Ideological Cultural Resource

Religion is a major aspect of the ideological resources of a culture for health care. The use of religion as a healing resource is a human universal (Winkelman, 1992a); every culture has religious healing practices. There are universals of religious healing, reflected in what

I have called "shamanistic healers" (Winkelman, 1992a, 2000a). These practices, which take diverse forms cross-culturally, manifest human cultural universals of healing that include

- The use of altered states of consciousness

- An engagement with what is considered to be the spirit world

- Healing provided in the context of a community ritual

- Diagnosis through information provided by the spirit world

- Illness caused by the evil intentions of other humans or spirits

These aspects of our "primitive" past were supposed to disappear as science and biomedicine discovered diseases and their cures. Yet, religious healing remains a dynamic and widely used resource even in postmodern societies, as illustrated in the many examples in Barnes and Sered's (2005) *Religion and Healing in America*. This use of religious healing persists among major religious denominations, across cultural groups, and even among patients of biomedicine. Some might even suggest that religious healing is particularly important among patients of biomedicine because it helps them deal with some of the negative and toxic effects of the interpersonal dimension of biomedical treatment. In any case, health providers need to understand how people's religious beliefs affect their clinical relations and patients' compliance with prescribed care.

Providers need to recognize that most of their patients today think that religious issues have an influence on the outcome of their malady. Religion affects perceptions of causes because maladies may be seen as punishment by god or spirits, a consequence of immorality, or punishment for sins. The acceptability of treatment opportunities may be affected by religious beliefs, for example, in terms of

- Acceptability of birth control, artificial insemination, and abortion

- Preparation of a body for burial

- Use of blood products and animal-derived medicines

- Acceptability of euthanasia or advanced directives

- Dietary products considered acceptable (e.g., food combinations, pork, beef)

- Acceptability of organ donations and autopsy

The scientific training of physicians generally emphasizes atheistic perspectives. The doubt expressed about the power of religion to heal may seem scientific, but even this will be questioned in Chapter Nine. Rather than doubting and challenging a patient's belief that God can help resolve a health problem, a more appropriate approach would be to recognize the important role of such beliefs in managing the broader impacts of maladies.

Curing, Healing, and Care

Assessing a person's health concerns is complicated by the intersecting dimensions of disease, illness, and sickness. Addressing the totality of health, these different but intersecting dimensions of well-being can be enhanced by understanding the different ways in which health maladies are addressed in personal experience and biological reality. It requires a conceptual framework in which the processes of removing the effects of disease from an individual are distinguished from the processes involved in the remission of the problems derived from illness and sickness.

The concept of *cure* has been applied to the removal of disease: one can be cured of pneumonia, diarrhea, syphilis, and the common cold. When bacteria are eliminated by the actions of antibiotics and one's own immune response, we can say that the person is cured. If, however, someone is seriously injured in a brutal physical attack and rape, the person may soon recover from the physical wounds. But is that person all better? Or are there still some psychological wounds, scars of trauma that need to be addressed? Patients may be physically cured of their wounds but still need healing from trauma.

The concept of healing contrasts with cure in embodying a recognition of the need to recover one's well-being in areas other than just the health of the physical body. Healing involves processes of "whole-ing," putting one's psychological and emotional life back into balance. One's physical wounds may have closed, but the emotional trauma and fears may still be present and in need of healing. Religion has played a central role in this process of healing and of maintaining a faith in one's ability to recover in the face of stark medical reality that suggests a poor prognosis for recovery.

Pilgrimage as Social Healing The social healing processes derived from group participation and the telling of stories of illness are described in *Pilgrimages and Healing* (Dubisch and Winkelman, 2005). Pilgrimage is a form of personal and popular empowerment produced by a journey to a site with religious, historic, and mythological significance. The pilgrimage may begin as an individual quest, but it is typically part of a collective physical movement of up to a million people to a site. These bring the social dimension of the pilgrimage to the experience, where one recounts one's story of illness and search for cure with fellow travelers. These connections provide significant personal meaning and emotional release from guilt, shame, and promises. These experiences induce healing through a realignment of self-concept, status, and identity with the other, both cultural and divine. Symbolic healing involves a process by which meaningful explanations provide a sense of relief that is as much physiological as psychological (see Chapter Nine on the stress response and metaphoric healing). The rituals of pilgrimage provide processes through which participants tap into unconscious innate structures and processes underlying the self and sense of identity. These experiences produce a powerful sense of emotional integration with the community. These symbolic healing processes provide meaningful mythological explanations that counteract the stress reaction, allowing the effects of beliefs and the powerful transformative potentials of ritual to heal the self.

Culture Care

Leininger, the "grandmother of transcultural nursing," has championed an understanding of health care needs in terms of cultural preferences and perceptions. Human needs for care are universal, a part of our human nature, but the ways in which care is provided and expected is particular to culture. **Care,** which is the essence of nursing services, is the assistance necessary for recovery from illness and maintaining well-being and health in

CULTURE AND HEALTH

Religion and Healing in Contemporary America

The efficacy of religion in dealing with many aspects of health maladies is not something confined to the poor or people without access to biomedicine; there is a broad range of religious healing in contemporary America, as illustrated in the dozens of articles in Barnes and Sered's (2005) book, *Religion and Healing in America*. Across the spectrum of ethnic and religious groups, religious healing activities have remained an important part of contemporary America. Central aspects of contemporary religious healing in the United States are exemplified in a study of the United Church of Christ (McKay and Musil, 2005). The concerns of spiritual healing were not predominantly in the physical area, in response to disease. However, when disease was involved, its resolution was often a spontaneous event, a miraculous deliverance from disease in response to intense prayer and **spiritual experiences**. Even when disease was not resolved by prayer and faith, there was often a positive outcome, a paradoxical sense of being healed and at peace without being cured. This was explained by the most frequently reported characteristic of spiritual healing, the experience of peace, a transformation of one's habitual state of being. For patients, spiritual healing involved feeling the presence of God, the unexpected discovery of a presence of God in their ordinary lives. The perception of the role of disease in patients' life included a sense of it bringing them into an awareness of God's presence, making the illness a blessing that brought the person to God.

Religious healing through inner transformation is part of a long metaphysical tradition in America that is also manifested in the more secular New Age movement (Fuller, 2005). New Age spiritual healing practices coexist within the framework of Judeo-Christian beliefs in the sacralizing of the self: the transformation of the sense of self into a sacred being through production of a personal experiential encounter with a sacred reality. The American metaphysical traditions involve the personal and experienced dimensions of the spirit world, engaging with subtle energies of the spiritual world and direct encounters with the divine. This has led to an understanding of the intertwined nature of the physical and spiritual that goes beyond contemporary science and religion. For instance, the physical experience of alternate realities and their real-world power is manifested in healing energies that can be sensed and transferred to others. The experiential engagement with subtle energies and realities produces an expansion of consciousness, propelling a spectrum of physical, emotional, social, and cognitive transformations. These assist in the abandonment of dysfunctional identities and the development of a new sense of self derived from the effects of the experiences and insights. The healing power of spirituality, like religion in general, leads to an emotional transformation and new self-identity involving the social relationships and ideology of the group.

culturally meaningful ways. Health is culturally defined and, consequently, so, too, is the care necessary for maintaining and restoring it.

To provide appropriate care, providers must interact with and respond to patients in ways that are consistent with their care expectations. For instance, should a nurse be chatty and friendly, playful and joking, while performing your rectal examination? Or should nurses be serious, quiet, and reserved? The ways in which care is expected to be provided always come with a cultural style: a reflection of cultural norms, values, beliefs, and expectations. An accommodation to the life ways of patients and their accustomed style of social relationships is necessary for the appropriate provision of care. For example, care expectations in the Mexican American community include the notion that a well-mannered person will also ask about the well-being of other family members besides the patient. In most countries of the Middle East, however, in general it would be inappropriate to ask a man about his wife's health unless he was there to answer questions for her in the consultation room.

Leininger (1995) proposed a cultural systems model that she later renamed the "Sunrise Enabler," a cognitive map for discovering multiple embedded cultural factors affecting health and care. This focuses on the environmental context as the totality of the situation affecting life circumstances and health, including environmental factors and cultural meanings, symbols, values, and views. It also includes consideration of generic cultural concepts of care and care expression, cultural values and beliefs regarding care, care patterns for maintenance and re-patterning of health behaviors, and indigenous care practices. Aspects of the culture relevant to such care include technology, economics, family and kinship organization, politics, education, and religion.

Care includes sensitive actions that provide necessary assistance with daily activities and health care, being supportive and enabling in helping to improve a patient's condition. The way in which care is provided is symbolic, conveying a sense of protection and respect by being culturally congruent care: providing a meaningful fit with the cultural values and care expectations of the client. Care also involves how we help a patient's family deal with illness, disability, and death in other family members. So a significant feature of care includes how impending death and poor prognoses are to be communicated to the patient: directly, through the family, or perhaps not at all.

The provision of care in culturally congruent nursing care includes actions that

- Reinforce cultural patterns of care and health preservation or maintenance, reinforcing the retention of beneficial cultural self-care beliefs (strengths perspectives)

- Accommodate to patient needs in providing care that is culturally congruent and effective (cultural responsiveness)

- Engage patients in modifying their self-care patterns to change behavior in ways that attain better health

Witch-Doctor's Legacy

Traditional ethnomedical practices have had a multifaceted effectiveness that is increasingly lacking in interactions between physicians and their clients. Press (1982) illustrates that biomedical care can be enhanced by using the traditional symbolic

CULTURE AND HEALTH

Cult of the Saints in the Care and Management of Medically Induced Sickness

The role of religion in health care can involve the management of negative experiences induced by disease, illness, and sickness, including the adverse effects of a gloomy medical prognosis or physicians' indifference to religious dimensions of health care. Religious faith and focus can be an important ally in managing the depression and fears that disease brings, providing a counter to defeatist attitudes and an effective tool in combating stress.

Osis's (2005) examination of the "cult of the saints" in American Catholicism illustrates the reasons for the persistent use of saints in healing. Saints provide care through symbolizing expectations of healing and curing and linking the patient with the loving feelings of absent family members. The healing power of saints includes their role in the expression of care, support, and assistance. Saints' representations in pictures and objects are a means of expressing care as a gift, with the saints' presence providing the patient assistance with experiences of sickness. The images of saints are particularly important when a patient is isolated in a hospital and dominated by the images of the medical settings. Saints help patients resist the domination of biomedical beliefs and instead respond to the inspiration of faith in their ability to be healed—even cured—by divine intervention. The potential power of the saints and their miracles allow patients and their families and friends to imagine, to construct an alternate scenario of health, and to have hope. The beliefs in the saints' healing powers also may elicit patients' innate healing processes through the hope and positive expectations derived from those beliefs. Saints' potential interventions allow patients to maintain an emotional state of positive expectation rather than succumbing to depression and acceptance of the inevitability of death.

The saints help produce this positive expectation by their immediate presence. The display of saints' images provides a focus of attention, a sense of a protecting companion, and a focus for prayer. The saints come to be experienced as consolers, providing a sense of the presence of others who are there to help. The gifts of saints' images and relics from different friends and family members provide a tangible connection with them that links the isolated patient back into a network of social support, reinforcing the connection with the social networks and their supportive relationships. These memories elicit feelings of love, generosity, and support from family, linking the patient to them emotionally despite the isolation. Osis characterizes the power of the saints as providing patients and their families with solace and the strength to care for their health and resist a feeling of marginalization.

resources of ethnomedical traditions—what he calls the "witch-doctor's legacy"—involving psychosocial and interpersonal dynamics of healing. Central elements of these approaches are

- Accepting clients' presentation of symptoms, worldview, and explanatory model

- Addressing clients' concerns and the personal and social consequences of illness

- Using cultural approaches to enhance client confidence and disclosure

- Developing a personal style that enhances clients' sense of acceptance and positive relations

- Cultivating a charismatic approach that enhances client confidence

- Creating a positive community image

Incorporating folk healers into medical settings is normally impractical, as is having medical practitioners learn all forms of cultural healing relevant to their multicultural patient populations (Press, 1982). Press suggests that biomedical practitioners can, however, adopt folk healers' general practical principles and stylistic characteristics as guidelines for enhancing clinical care and reducing stress. Cultural knowledge and anthropological perspectives can help providers utilize interpersonal and symbolic resources to enhance healing. These are essential for providing culturally responsive care. Physicians' addressing patients' broader concerns counters the alienation that inhibits cultural healing processes. Engel (1977, 1980), himself a physician, suggested that failure to address the psychosocial concerns undermines the dynamics of the patient-healer relationship that elicits and supports healing. Press suggests that the "biomedical health practitioner should be expert in theology, anthropology, psychology, and urban studies" (1982, p. 196) and self-consciously utilize symbolic resources.

An **anthropological medicine** (Helman, 2001; Hahn, 1995) can help providers connect with the interpersonal dynamics of healing through

- Giving primacy to understanding clients' concepts and experiences

- Examining the sociocultural roots of clients' and providers' conceptual frameworks

- Understanding cultural-behavioral relations and intercultural dynamics

- Possessing personal skills for managing intercultural relations and communication

- Possessing knowledge of specific sociocultural norms and health behaviors

- Adapting to the social and cultural aspects of illness and clients' coping resources

- Managing differences in explanatory models to treat both illness and disease

- Eliciting the symbolic, psychocultural, and emotional dynamics of healing

In addition to issues already addressed here and in Chapters Two and Three, these issues of anthropological medicine are addressed throughout this book, particularly

- Cultural presentation of symptoms and clients' conceptual frameworks (Chapter Five)

- General models of cultural-behavioral relations and psychocultural dynamics (Chapter Six)

- Consumer empowerment by understanding the politics of medicine (Chapter Eight)

- The psychosocial dynamics of the placebo healing response (Chapter Nine)

Part of the engagement with patients' cultural influences means an acceptance of their worldview as it pertains to their health concerns. For instance, what if a patient believes that his or her STD is a result of being sinful and that it will only finally be cured if he or she prays for forgiveness? Providers need not agree with or dispute patients' explanatory models and beliefs if they do not directly impede the treatment. Contradicting them will not reduce anxiety nor necessarily lead to compliance or healing. An attitude that does not reject patients' beliefs helps make patients more amenable to biomedical treatments. Unless personal healing practices are known to be harmful, most cultures should be respected and accommodated. This is therapeutic because culture provides important complementary components to biomedicine in addressing illness and sickness.

Acceptance of patients' worldview facilitates accommodating personal concerns in treatment. Traditional healers generally accept symptoms presented by patients and family at face value, permitting some degree of control over formulating diagnoses. This is in contrast to physicians' often selective utilization of symptoms for diagnosis and the tendency to ignore patient complaints not amenable to biomedical diagnostic categories (Press, 1982). Disease is treated, but illness and sickness remain unaddressed, compelling many patients to seek complementary care practices.

Enhancing biomedical healing requires addressing the social and symbolic dimensions of illness and healing. To be more effective in care, health care providers need to recognize that symbolic and social interactions are key aspects of healing processes in all cultures. In many cultures, the processes of healing are integrated throughout social life—economic, familial, religious, mythological, ceremonial, and so forth—and may require the participation of the entire community. The social linkages of therapy are often extended to the deceased and their concerns, represented as ancestor spirits that reflect the values of the society. Ritual healing is often directed at reinforcing this moral order and strengthening social relationships through the resolution of conflicts.

This suggests that biomedicine could benefit by responding more directly to the social dimensions of healing processes, including familial and community healing rituals to help resolve the sick role as well as social tensions and conflicts. The use of social support in preventing and ameliorating maladies is part of the community dynamics of healing and has implications for biomedicine because epidemiological study results have established the relationship of social support and networks to health (see Chapter Nine). Premodern healers were part of the local community and aware of the social dynamics and personal and family histories that affected individuals. Healers could then assess the long-standing anxieties and concerns of a patient and incorporate the family system into healing processes (Press, 1982). Physicians' disconnection with the communities they serve and health providers' lack of awareness of patients' perspectives and the effects of culture on health leave them unable to address these significant determinants of health behaviors. This can be remedied through knowledge about sociocultural factors that affect health and the development of cultural responsiveness to these broader concerns.

Cultural responsiveness is embodied in the concepts of quality patient care and the recognition that treatment outcomes can be enhanced by addressing patients' values and communication styles, providing integration of care and emotional support, and involving family and community (Delbanco, 1992). Engagement with these dimensions of care assists in tailoring care and reducing physicians' judgmental tendencies, instead focusing attention on nontechnical aspects of care that reflect patients' concerns. In addition to the amelioration of pain and their functional problems, patients want to understand their conditions and therapies and need the opportunity to discuss familial and economic effects of sickness (Delbanco, 1992). These concerns need to be understood in the context of their cultural community.

COMMUNITY HEALTH ASSESSMENT

The critical problem of the medical encounter is the interpretation of patients' conditions within sociocultural systems of experience and meaning. Anthropological and community public health approaches contribute to these perspectives, providing the tools to determine the community-based realities of maladies and their detection and treatment. The development of effective health programs requires resources—physical and intellectual—to engage community involvement, beginning with planning stages and continuing through health program implementation and evaluation activities. Community involvement is necessary because effectiveness must be measured in goals specific to the particular community and its circumstances. Because improving the community's perception of its health is part of public health goals, determining community views of desirable improvements in its health is part of an evaluation. The health of a community is a function not only of biological disease rates but also of quality-of-life concerns based on cultural values and expectations. Community approaches are central to health because they reflect social expectations regarding quality of life.

A variety of models exist for community involvement in the implementation of health improvement programs (e.g., *Healthy People, 2010* [National Center for Health Statistics, 2000]; *Healthy Communities, 2000: Model Standards* [American Public Health Association, 1991]; Assessment Protocol for Excellence [in Public Health; APEX]; Planned Approach to Community Health); Community Oriented Primary Care; and Healthy People and Cities programs [see Lasker et al., 1997; Durch et al., 1997]). These provide health departments with guidelines for community-based approaches to identifying local health problems and creating programs to address them. The Institute of Medicine (IOM) developed national health goals and model standards for local communities to use in formulating appropriate public health policy and culturally responsive services. These provide guidelines for evaluating organizational self-assessment capacities; establishing community relations; determining community health status, needs, and priorities; and monitoring success in achieving goals. The APEX model focuses on the following steps:

Community Process Steps

■ Assess organizational capacities for community relations and organization

■ Collect and analyze health data

■ Form community health committee to identify, prioritize, and analyze community health needs

- Inventory community health resources
- Develop and implement community health plan
- Monitor achievement of health goals

Implementing Model Standards

The following steps are critical for implementing model standards:

- Assess agency capacity for community engagement
- Develop agency capacity-building plan
- Assess community organization and structures
- Organize community members in health coalitions
- Assess community health needs
- Determine community priorities and health resources
- Select outcome objectives
- Develop intervention strategies
- Implement intervention strategies
- Conduct continuous monitoring and evaluation

Approaches for achieving collaborative community engagement in health assessments are illustrated in the IOM's Community Health Improvement Process (CHIP), which utilizes interacting cycles of analysis, action, and measurement. CHIP forms community health coalitions, involving community members in the analysis of community health problems, identifying the critical health issues to be addressed, and developing socially and culturally appropriate responses to those problems. Contemporary national and community health agendas all emphasize community assessment and collaboration, which require cultural perspectives and competence in addressing health issues. Cultural perspectives are vital for addressing all three of the core functions of public health: assessing communities and their needs, developing appropriate policies, and ensuring culturally sensitive services. IOM principles for community health improvement all involve cultural dimensions: the WHO definition of health and its broad conceptual model; the community's desired health outcomes; and community coalitions that incorporate the diverse community sectors and **stakeholders,** people and groups with interests and involvements in specific health outcomes.

Measurements of institutional, coalition, and community preparedness for collaboration are key to addressing community health. Key issues are mediating among the varying priorities, goals, and objectives of the numerous stakeholders. The IOM recommends using frameworks like the cultural systems models to develop indicators that incorporate the broad range of factors that impact health. Assessment of health systems depends largely on anthropology's ethnographic approaches: participant observation, unstructured and informal interviewing, use of experts and key informants, archival research, and the development of formal questionnaires where appropriate. These methods may be supplemented by approaches for hard-to-reach groups (Schensul and LeCompte, 1999).

A variety of methods are used to assess and adapt to community and cultural factors in assessing health care issues (Brownlee, 1978):

■ Practicing direct personal involvement in doing the research

■ Building personal relations and involving community members

■ Finding a confidant who can help bridge the culture gap

■ Understanding the other culture, particularly its differences, as normal

■ Utilizing community resources and networks

■ Observing and listening before asking and acting

■ Finding out if any special rules of protocol need to be followed

■ Getting to know local leaders: residents who are widely respected

■ Talking to ordinary workers and community people

■ Getting to know the patients, the recipients of care

■ Learning through participating, observing, and informal conversations

■ Determining cultural attitudes toward questioning and adapting questions to the culture

■ Learning how to interview within the local area

■ Learning when to ask questions and what questions not to ask

Assessing Community Health Involvement Because engagement with the community is a necessary component of effective public health interventions, measuring the stage of development of community coalitions and their input into health intervention projects is fundamental to evaluating the effectiveness of health programs (Goodman, Wandersman, Chinman, Imm, and Morrisey, 1996). Organizational measures assess the extent to which relationships between public health institutions and their communities have been developed (Smithies and Webster, 1998). Dimensions and levels of community participation include the quality and length of participation and effects and outcome from participation processes. The capacity of the community coalition to respond to health needs is a basic aspect of involvement; other measures focus on the implementation of initiatives and their impacts on the community (Goodman et al., 1996). Effective community participation requires sustained coalition function with community participation and leadership and support from health care institutions. Community involvement can be assisted with rapid ethnographic assessment protocols (see "**Rapid Assessment, Response, and Evaluation [RARE]**" below). These approaches facilitate community participation by accommodating to local cultural dynamics and taking direction from the community. Community health coalitions and advisory boards allow community perspectives to be incorporated into the assessment of health problems, development and implementation of health programs, assessment of their effectiveness, and their continued modification to meet community health needs.

Evaluating Community Health

The evaluation and assessment of community health generally include three phases:

■   Formative evaluations (needs assessments)

■   Process assessments of the implementation of interventions

■   Outcome measures evaluating intervention effects on communities

Because interventions can affect many social levels and groups, multiple sources of data are required for effective program evaluation. **Triangulation** (Goodman et al., 1996; Trotter and Needle, 2000a, 2000b; Beebe, 2001) is a method of relying on several sources of information for ascertaining a condition; it is also known as mixed or multiple strategies or combined operationalism. Combining several sources of information improves the validity of assessments by reducing biases inherent in any single approach. For instance, deciding which areas of the community are in most need of teen pregnancy prevention programs might be best determined by consulting school counselors, adoption agencies, social services, and health care providers.

Formative Evaluation

Formative evaluations emphasize needs assessments (or discrepancy analysis) to discover gaps in services and make programs more responsive. A primary focus is the community health profile: determining existing conditions and local programs that may facilitate interventions. Community-based evaluations of health concerns and needed services are performed before intervention programs are implemented to provide a baseline from which to assess program impacts.

Evaluations generally take place at several levels (e.g., targeted populations, the wider community, and political and administrative organizations). Formative assessments clarify project goals and concerns of sponsors and communities regarding needed information, preferred research designs, and the nature of the results needed. They determine the context for proposed interventions; the antecedents and consequences of the problem of concern; resources available to address the problem; and the programs, policies, and attitudes affecting the proposed interventions. Formative evaluations include an understanding of the administrative and organizational structures of health agencies, their delivery systems, and their interactions with other institutions, agencies, and communities.

The starting point for community health assessments is the production of community health profiles. Minimum IOM indicators for community health profiles include sociodemographic characteristics, the health status of the population and its subgroups, principal risk factors in the environment, and the resources and health status of the population. These profiles address the broader economic, social, and political dynamics of the community, particularly those aspects that most directly affect health status and risk factors. Assessing health needs of communities requires consideration of existing conditions, the community's perspectives on what constitutes threats to health, and the perceived needs with respect to those conditions. Formative assessments use general cultural systems models as well as more specific subsystems directly relevant to the health problem and capacities of institutions, communities, health providers, and other stakeholders (see RARE models below for detailed community assessment protocols).

The extent of the formative assessment depends on resources; the nature of the problem; the scope of the project; and the interests of sponsors, institutions, and communities involved. Analysis of health issues, community health resources, and existing health programs provides a basis for the creation of performance and evaluation indicators and the development of new health improvement strategies. This includes knowledge of a community's infrastructural capacity to respond to health needs: government agencies; community leadership; and programs for surveillance, data monitoring, health promotion, service provision, and other activities that maintain health (e.g., sanitation, food quality).

Process Evaluations

Community health improvement requires monitoring of the implementation of programs. *Process evaluations* (or implementation evaluations) ascertain whether interventions were delivered as planned. Programs are generally assessed as to the effectiveness of program implementation and the effects of programs on intended audiences. Process evaluations use many forms of information:

- A chronological narrative of program activities

- Records of project workers

- Objective-based evaluations of progress toward goals

- Evaluation of cost-effectiveness or cost-benefit analysis

- Expert or professional judgments based on various forms of assessment

- Evaluation of program recipients' use of and views of the program

Evaluations use participant observation and derive information from many sources, including community discussions, interviews, examination of critical incidents, and case studies. They also may include more formal evaluations based on structured interviews, surveys, and organizational records. Process evaluation feedback may be incorporated midcourse to modify processes to ensure achievement of desired goals.

Outcome Evaluations

Outcome evaluations are concerned with the effects of programs. The activist role of medical anthropology makes the outcome-focused evaluation, which attempts to ascertain the attainment of desired outcomes, particularly important. Multiple stakeholders mean a variety of assessments are necessary to determine the impact of intervention programs on different segments of the community (e.g., at-risk groups; different ethnicities, providers, administrators, politicians, educators; and so on). These assessments may ascertain

- Community awareness concerning health issues

- Community knowledge of contributory and risk factors

PRACTITIONER PROFILE

Noel J. Chrisman

Noel J. Chrisman, Ph.D., M.P.H., is professor in the Department of Psychosocial and Community Health, School of Nursing, University of Washington, Seattle, with adjunct appointments in anthropology, health services (School of Public Health), and family medicine. Since 1977 he has been teaching in family medicine. He teaches a course cross-listed between anthropology and nursing, "Clinically Applied Anthropology," that explores data and concepts from medical anthropology and then determines ways to use the information to improve clinician practice. A course cross-listed between nursing and health services is "Dynamics of Community Health Practice," which examines the interface between medicine and public health, explicitly to teach primary care practitioners and managers how to work with communities. Also cross-listed between nursing and health services is "Health, Culture, and Community," a course that explores how to construct health promotion and disease prevention projects in multicultural communities. Within nursing, he teaches "Transcultural Nursing Practice," an examination of thirty to forty years of health practice literature to show how to take care of patients in culturally appropriate ways. For undergraduates in nursing, he teaches "Culture, Diversity, and Nursing Practice," a required cultural competence course. In addition, he teaches senior undergraduate nursing students how to do community organizing for health promotion and disease prevention. As part of this effort, he has been working in a small Latino neighborhood with students since 1995, building community through enhancing the capabilities of a neighborhood coalition.

A large proportion of Chrisman's work has been on cultural competence. He discusses, for example, professional attitudes, practice skills, and system savvy for cross-cultural situations using an easy-to-remember set of guidelines called "culture-sensitive care" (knowledge, mutual respect, and negotiation). In addition to these invented concepts, he uses major ideas from medical anthropology such as ethnocentrism and cultural relativism, the illness-disease distinction, variations in health and illness beliefs cross-culturally, the role of value complexes such as time orientation or human-nature relations, and how to work with interpreters.

- Changes in the community members' lifestyles, attitudes, and health-related behaviors
- Modifications in the physical and social environments
- The nature and extent of enhancement of interaction between health organizations and their constituencies
- The level at which institutionalization of needed programs should be targeted

Assessments are also made of coverage—that is, the extent to which the target population was aware of having received the message, understood its intentions, accepted it, and changed its behavior. Assessment of the effectiveness of the intervention in the target population generally requires controlling for confounding effects: for example, changes in the broader social environment in the direction of program intervention changes. These include public occurrences that influence people's behavior in the direction of intervention (e.g., a prominent person's AIDS-related death motivates people to adopt protective behaviors). Assessments of the effects of intervention also focus on political leaders and policymakers who have the potential to produce long-term changes. Long-term success is achieved by securing the necessary resources through influence on public leaders and bureaucrats. Leaders and organizations can produce long-term changes in the behaviors of communities through institutionalization of interventions into permanent programs.

RAPID ASSESSMENT, RESPONSE, AND EVALUATION (RARE)

A format for creating community collaboration and health program development is exemplified in the rapid assessment, response, and evaluation (RARE) processes. This is an adaptation of classic ethnographic community research methods to rapid assessments and evaluations to provide culturally based community health programs. Rapid assessment approaches use intensive team efforts over short periods, are normally focused on specific problems, and are carried out by researchers already familiar with the community being studied.

Rapid assessment methods began in the 1980s as anthropologists were called on to assist national governments and international organizations in responding to health crises (Scrimshaw, Carballo, and Ramos, 1991). Experts in specific cultural areas were brought in to help develop quick and effective responses to health crises. Further development of the rapid assessment approaches included intervention programs and technical assistance to local communities in developing the local infrastructure to assess problems and formulate community-based responses. The core techniques of assessment and programmatic interventions have been extended to assessment or evaluation of the effects of those programs. The RARE approaches (Trotter and Needle, 2000a, 2000b; Beebe, 2001) extended the process through evaluation components of program effectiveness and reiterative phases of program implementation and evaluation.

The RARE approach has features for producing effective community interventions that address critical health problems (Stimson, Fitch, and Rhodes, 1998, 1999). RARE is particularly suited for providing locally relevant responses through community participation and collaboration that creates the ownership of programs, which, in turn, helps ensure the effectiveness and permanence of the programs. Research on locally prioritized problems helps focus on the local contexts and behaviors to be modified, ensuring that problems are understood within their ecological-cultural contexts and addressed with culturally relevant interventions. RARE incorporates the community in the development of interventions that change risk behaviors and address beliefs regarding risks and disease.

RARE takes a pragmatic approach, building on existing programs with multiple strategies to change the risk behavior of individuals, the processes of care delivery, and the political and policy-making environment. The RARE interventions are then "rapidly assessed" to ensure that they have had the intended consequences. The RARE process is interactive to adapt continually to new information and changing local conditions.

RARE is a cost-effective pragmatic approach that uses local resources to provide a multilevel analysis of community conditions, behaviors, and beliefs. It compiles multiple sources of archival data and combines them with up-to-date data to change behaviors with responses adapted to the specific needs of local vulnerable communities. It uses a wide range of methods, including existing information, formal surveys, informal interviewing, observations, focus groups, and cultural experts. Multiple overlapping data sources permit triangulation and enhance validity and reliability of findings. Thus, consensus is more readily apparent. The different sources of data also provide more appealing results and findings for different audiences (e.g., what is convincing to physicians may be different from what convinces political representatives, community members, or patients). A principle of RARE is the representation of cultural variability—that is, different groups in the study area and differences within target subgroups. Individuals with special expertise in the area are recruited for interviews to establish both normative conditions and variation within the community.

RARE Sequences

RARE begins with an invitation from community leaders to address specific health problems and uses community resources, facilitated by outside governmental consultants (e.g., U.S. Department of Health and Human Services entities such as the National Institutes of Health [NIH] and the CDC). Consultants guide the development of group consensus about how to address the issues and train individuals and organizations in design, implementation, assessment, and analysis. Compilation of available data by consultants helps define the problem to be addressed. Community involvement, responsibility, and ownership, which are fundamental aspects of RARE, facilitate the training and empowerment of communities to respond to their health needs. The community concept fundamental to the RARE process includes many stakeholders: political and health leaders, representatives of health organizations, members of targeted or vulnerable populations, and other community representatives and groups. The community provides the necessary information for the program, making decisions about the priorities for intervention and ensuring the cultural acceptability of the interventions. From the inception, the program is developed in collaboration with the community to ensure an accurate assessment of community needs, the community's cooperation and responsiveness, and the relevance of the program to local needs. RARE methods focus on groups at high risk; those suffering from the condition; and the behaviors, beliefs, and values that increase risk and disease.

RARE Community Teams

The RARE approach utilizes forms of community collaboration and involvement. These are illustrated in Exhibits 4.2 and 4.3 and the following sections on the community advisory committee, the field assessment team and methodological approaches, and the assessment modules.

EXHIBIT 4.2. **RARE Phases, Principles, and Advantages***

Major Phases
- Invitation from local political and health leaders
- Creation of a community RARE working group and community forum for elicitation of concerns
- A crises response team's (CRT) rapid evaluation of existing data
- The CRT's proposal to local officials to identify major aspects of a problem and necessary research and interventions
- Local field research team selection and training by consultants
- Local field research team, using
  - Contextual assessment
  - Risk and health consequences assessment
  - Intervention assessment
- Working group preparation of report and action intervention plan

Principles
- Invitation must come from local political and health leaders
- The primary investigator must have prior knowledge of the culture
- Community members must be involved in project development
- A single focus or problem area must be addressed
- Local research teams with cultural competence in the community studied must be included
- Programmatic interventions must be culturally based and relevant
- Programs must be assessed for their effectiveness

Advantages
- Rapid response to pressing problems
- Commitment of communities to assist in the research process
- Use of existing knowledge and resources
- Multimethod approaches to increase validity and reliability
- Community-based orientation to create ownership
- Enhancement of community power by training local research teams
- Quick development of culturally relevant and effective responses
- Assessment of intervention effectiveness
- Use of multiple methods for triangulation and validity

*Adapted from Trotter and Needle (2000a, 2000b) and Stimson, Fitch, and Rhodes (1998).

Community Advisory Committee The principal mechanism for community input is through a community advisory committee that represents elected officials, public (health) employees, and a wide range of constituencies and stakeholders. These may include official and unofficial representatives of community groups, religious organizations, members of at-risk interest groups, and representatives of advocacy organizations. The inclusion of

EXHIBIT 4.3. RARE Assessment Modules*

Initial Consultation Module

- Identify information and gaps regarding scope of problem
- Ascertain existing community knowledge regarding condition
- Gain local perspectives on problem
- Ascertain health and social consequences of condition
- Assess existing treatments for condition and problems with them
- Identify vulnerable populations
- Identify risk behaviors that need to be changed
- Ascertain cultural and community contexts affecting interventions
- Research the different stakeholders and their priorities
- Identify individuals, groups, and organizations to be included
- Establish, orient, and train community advisory committee (CAC)
- Provide database report to CEO, CAC
- Convene CAC to determine priorities and action plan
- Use local knowledge to develop relevant interventions
- Create research team for assessment and intervention
- Ascertain resources available
- Incorporate community in assessment, implementation, and evaluation

Contextual Assessment Module

Study Area Profile

- Productive and reproductive infrastructure
- Domestic, economic, and political structures
- Policy, administrative, and ideological factors
- Locations of vulnerable populations
- Locations conducive to high-risk behaviors

Key Areas or Factors That Increase or Decrease

- Spread of disease
- Health consequences
- Social consequences
- Vulnerability and progress of disease among infected
- Access to treatments
- Successful implementation of treatments
- Success of interventions
- Behaviors associated with each key area or factor
- Contextual factors associated with key area or factors

Key Contextual Assessment Foci

Factors Facilitating or Inhibiting Risks

- Geographical features affecting risks and consequences
- Population movement relevant to spread of disease
- Economic and occupational factors affecting risks
- Particular social or ethnic groups with increased risk
- Effects of laws and criminal justice system on risk behaviors

Factors Ameliorating or Exacerbating Health Consequences
■ Attitudes and reactions of family, government, and society
■ Provision of services by health care system
■ Factors impeding access and utilization
■ Key health problems that affect focal disease
■ Role of social welfare system in addressing those with condition

Factors Facilitating or Inhibiting Development of Interventions
■ Availability of health services
■ Educational services and media utilization
■ Research and evaluation capacity
■ Local groups affecting implementation
■ Ethnic and linguistic populations affecting implementation
■ Governmental and health decision making
■ Alternative or complementary therapies

Risk and Health Consequences Assessment
■ Extent and frequency of individual risk behaviors
■ Individual motivation for risk behaviors
■ Levels of knowledge regarding risks
■ Behavior- and context-specific risks
■ Community norms affecting risk behaviors

Social Settings and Structural Factors Exacerbating Risks
■ Means of reducing risks
■ Risks from individual lifestyle and living conditions
■ Risks from values, beliefs, and norms
■ Barriers to risk reduction
■ Structural influences (e.g., policy, legal, governmental) on risk behavior
■ Protective factors reducing risk
■ Social consequences of condition
■ Effects of social responses on individual
■ Social implications of diagnosis
■ Implication of condition for social relations
■ Financial implications of condition

Interventions Assessment
■ Existing interventions and effectiveness
■ Need for expansion of existing interventions
■ New interventions needed
■ Obstacles to effectiveness of interventions
■ Factors ensuring sustainable interventions
■ Structural changes affecting access to interventions
■ Environmental modifications enhancing access
■ Education needed to influence service utilization
■ Changes in community-based programs and policies
■ Interventions modifying individual risk behaviors

*Adapted from Trotter and Needle (2000a, 2000b) and Stimson, Fitch, and Rhodes (1998).

influential community leaders and trendsetters is important, as is the incorporation of critics of the system and traditionally excluded groups. The community advisory group provides a context for the community's consideration of relevant data and ascertainment of the specific focus of the project. The community advisory committee must decide what research is most important to focus on, who is most vulnerable, and what can be done about it. The priority issue is then used to direct the activities of the field assessment team, which is directly involved with the community advisory committee in carrying out the research and making the recommendations for interventions.

Field Assessment Team Community members and local cultural experts are central to the field assessment team, which is locally recruited, incorporating health professionals and members of the community. These individuals have appropriate language skills, cultural knowledge, and community relations. The field assessment team is knowledgeable about the health consequences of the disease being investigated. They are trained in the implementation of RARE methods, including mapping, observations, key-informant interviews, focus groups, and surveys. They utilize the assessment modules for collecting and analyzing the data and as the basis for organizing the report and recommendations for the intervention.

RARE Assessment Modules

RARE uses four major modules for the evaluation of the local population, determination of the health problems to be addressed, and development of an intervention program (see Exhibit 4.3 and below):

■ Initial Consultation Module

■ Contextual Assessment Module

■ Risk and Health Consequences Assessment Module

■ Intervention Assessment Module

Initial Consultation Module The Initial Consultation Module provides overall direction for field assessments based on prior studies and evaluations. Results of local studies and national data sources are used to identify local conditions, risk profiles and vulnerable populations, the specific locale for study and intervention, the cultural context of risk for the focal disease, and the culturally appropriate interventions in risk behavior. Key community representatives are recruited for the community advisory committee, which uses the data to decide the direction for the assessments, the local groups most in need of intervention, and the types of interventions needed. A community-based RARE field team is developed to implement assessment, intervention, and evaluation processes.

Contextual Assessment Module The Contextual Assessment Module is designed to identify community information that locates the vulnerable populations in greatest need of services. It uses both existing sources of data and additional information acquired through direct observation, individual interviews, and focus groups. A principal aspect is a study area profile focused on the economic, social, and political contexts of the problem. The Contextual Assessment Module is designed to identify the primary cultural, social, and situational factors that affect risk; the utilization of available programs for prevention and treatment; and the conditions needing to be addressed to implement a locally relevant intervention successfully. The community characteristics and dynamics that affect risks, the specific groups affected, and the nature of resources are assessed to ascertain appropriate interventions. Specific focus is placed on the factors that increase or decrease risk and contagion, the social and health consequences of disease, and the adoption of interventions. The structural factors and cultural conditions necessary for effectively implementing the intervention are identified, including the macrolevel factors (physical, geographical, economic, administrative, organizational, political, religious) (see Exhibit 4.1 and Trotter and Needle, 2000b). Contextual assessment identifies the key conditions to be modified to reduce risk and enhance access to prevention and treatment programs. Contextual assessment data are used to develop an action plan of culturally appropriate interventions for the most vulnerable populations.

Risk and Health Consequences Assessment Module The Risk and Health Consequences Assessment Module identifies the types, extent, and nature of risks and the behavioral processes and psychosocial dynamics associated with risk taking. The risk behavior's broad implications for health, the behavior's social consequences, and its extent in the populations are primary foci. Assessment identifies the most vulnerable populations based on risk behaviors and identifies the factors that reduce risk. Risks are assessed at the level of individual behavior, communitywide norms and institutional processes, and the structural level of laws and policies affecting risk behavior.

Intervention Assessment Module Assessment of conditions affecting proposed interventions and their potential benefits builds on existing effective interventions. Interviews with the providers and vulnerable populations are key sources of data. The Intervention Assessment Module first considers existing interventions and their adequacy and effectiveness from the perspective of the major stakeholders. Existing interventions are assessed as to their targeting strategies, appropriateness and accessibility, and the sociocultural and structural factors inhibiting or facilitating their use. New interventions are developed based on gaps in coverage, lack of accessibility, and specific needs not currently met, particularly those of highly vulnerable populations. Proposed interventions consider environmental modifications; structural changes in programs and policies; and community changes in behaviors, attitudes, and knowledge to reduce risks. This information is summarized in a proposed action plan for incremental interventions based on existing programs and directed to changing behavior at individual, community, and structural levels. The approach is capable of being accomplished within the scope of local resources and through multiple integrated strategies addressing the spectrum of levels that affect risk and severity. Changes in the delivery of services focus on enhancing availability, accessibility, and relevance. Where necessary, political and policy changes, such as funding new programs or mandating free

BIOCULTURAL INTERACTIONS

Cultural Systems Effects on CVD

When we examine the multiple factors contributing to high levels of CVD in African Americans, it quickly becomes clear why a cultural systems model is necessary to consider all the factors affecting its manifestation. We can begin with the general ecological system, reflecting the poverty-level lifestyle that characterizes a disproportionate number of African Americans. Economic factors expose them to a variety of risk factors for CVD: poor neighborhoods, with rampant criminal elements and drug use, compounded by limited public health care facilities. These all constitute risk factors and contribute to increased stress, which exacerbates hypertension. Dangerous inner-city environments inhibit doing exercise (Bolton and Wilson, 2005), an important protective factor in CVD and stress reduction. Impoverishment affects dietary patterns, which are significant contributory factors in hypertension. Traditional preferences for salty and fatty foods, particularly pork and fried chicken, aggravate hypertension and contribute to CVD. The belief that their traditional foods are healthier than "white people food" can lead to neglect of medical advice regarding dietary changes (Schlomann and Schmitke, 2007). Treatment utilization is affected by family, community, and religious self-care practices, as well as the insufficient public education and community care facilities. Addressing all of these interacting factors contributing to high CVD rates among African Americans must begin with understanding their health culture and its effects on symptom recognition, treatment seeking, and compliance with care directives.

access to services for low-income groups, may be sought to address health problems more effectively.

CHAPTER SUMMARY

The effective provision of care requires an understanding of the effects of culture on health behavior and clinical relations. Effective cross-cultural adaptation requires an ability to understand individuals within the context of their cultural systems. This chapter has provided models for understanding cultural systems and performing community assessments. The RARE approach provides advantages in creating community involvement in health issues and assessments at the level of relevant cultural beliefs and behaviors. Beliefs provide the design for thought and behaviors, but ultimately it is what people actually do rather than merely think or believe that has the greatest implications for health. The next chapter addresses these health behaviors at the level of the family, community ethnomedical traditions, and professional health practices.

KEY TERMS

Anthropological medicine
Blended family
Care
Culture
Cultural systems models
Cure
Ecology
Extended family
Formative evaluations
Heal
Matrilocal family

Nuclear family
Outcome evaluations
Patrilineal extended family
Process evaluations
Protective factors
Psychosomatic disorders
RARE
Risk factors
Stakeholders
Triangulation

SELF-ASSESSMENTS

The Conceptual Framework for Cultural-Ecological System Health Assessments (Exhibit 4.1) and the RARE assessment modules provide models and foci for analyzing specific aspects of the social and cultural environments that affect health and disease.

Self-Assessment 4.1. Community Disease Assessment
Select a disease or illness that is important in your community and analyze factors that affect the incidence of that condition by applying these assessment frameworks.

Self-Assessment 4.2. Cultural-Ecological System Health Assessment
Use the framework in Exhibit 4.1 to describe the basis for the health conditions affecting your community or a region or ethnic community in your area.

Self-Assessment 4.3. Family Health Assessment
Are certain health conditions typical of your family historically? What are they? What does the family contribute to produce them, genetics, diet, environment, or some interaction among these?

What family titles do you consider to fall within membership of your "immediate family"?

Are these all biological relatives?

What form of family structure best characterizes your family?

Who would you want to be able to visit you if you were hospitalized? Would it include nonfamily members?

What are your expectations regarding a woman's behavior during pregnancy?

What are your expectations regarding her husband's behavior?

Would you apply different standards for people from different cultures?

How are these expectations based in your culture?

What role should the family play in interacting with health providers on behalf of their family members?

What are cultural views regarding the relationship of the menstrual cycle to fertility and disease?

What are your beliefs regarding sex and disease?

ADDITIONAL RESOURCES

Books

Michelle Issel. 2004. *Health program planning and evaluation: a practical, systematic approach for community health.* Sudbury, Mass.: Jones and Bartlett Publishers

Journals

David Richard Brown, Agueda Hernández, Gilbert Saint-Jean, Siân Evans, Ida Tafari, Luther G. Brewster, Michel J. Celestin, Carlos Gómez-Estefan, Fernando Regalado, Siri Akal, Barry Nierenberg, Elaine D. Kauschinger, Robert Schwartz, and J. Bryan Page. 2008. A participatory action research pilot study of urban health disparities using rapid assessment response and evaluation. *American Journal of Public Health* Vol 98, No. 1, pp. 28–38.

Chris Fitch, Gerry V. Stimson, Tim Rhodes and Vladimir Poznyak 2004. Rapid assessment: an international review of diffusion, practice and outcomes in the substance use field. *Social Science & Medicine* 59(9): 1819–1830.

R. H. Needle, R. T. Trotter II, M. Singer, C. Bates, J. B. Page, D. Metzger, and L. H. Marcelin. 2003. Rapid assessment of the HIV/AIDS crisis in racial and ethnic minority communities: an approach for timely community interventions. *American Journal of Public Health*, 93(6): 970–979.

G. A. Quintero, E. Lilliott, and C. Willging. 2007. Substance Abuse Treatment Provider Views of "Culture": Implications for behavioral health care in rural settings. *Qualitative Health Research* 17(9): 1256–1267.

Robert T. Trotter, II, Richard H. Needle, Eric Goosby, Christopher Bates and Merrill Singer. 2001. A methodological model for rapid assessment, response, and evaluation: the RARE program in public health. *Field Methods*, 13(2): 137–159.

CHAPTER

5

ETHNOMEDICAL SYSTEMS AND HEALTH CARE SECTORS

[T]he extent to which patients disclose their use of alternative therapies to physicians remains low. . . . The . . . "don't ask and don't tell" needs to be abandoned
—EISENBERG ET AL., 1998, P. 1575

LEARNING OBJECTIVES

- Describe the major sectors of health care resources—popular, folk, and professional
- Illustrate the popular-sector role as the first level of recourse to health resources through symptom recognition, pain significance, and decision making regarding the use of biomedicine
- Explore the roles of folk ethnomedical practices as a resource for addressing health maladies that may be alternatives or complements to biomedical treatment
- Examine the cultural basis for the appeal of alternative medicine in the United States
- Examine the cultural basis for the dominant professional sector, biomedicine

POPULAR, FOLK, AND PROFESSIONAL HEALTH CARE SECTORS

All cultures have ethnomedical systems: institutionalized practices for addressing health maladies. Westerners often consider biomedicine the only reliable health resource, but people around the world—and many in the United States—use other healing systems as well. Modern societies typically have **medical pluralism,** where within a single society competing ethnomedical traditions coexist and form distinct health subcultures with unique beliefs, practices, and organizations.

Kleinman (1980) illustrated this medical pluralism in showing that complex societies have three overlapping sectors or health care systems:

- The popular **(lay) sector** involving culturally based personal and familial beliefs and practices

- The **folk sector** involving cultural ethnomedical traditions and specialists

- The **professional sector** involving legally sanctioned professionals

The use of these sectors varies by immediate circumstances and as a hierarchy of resort or priorities. Generally, health concerns are initially addressed in the popular sector with self-assessment and self-help procedures in consultation with significant others. This may be followed by consultation with folk specialists or, if necessary and available, with biomedical or other professional services. Biomedical resources may be the first choice but are generally accessed through decision making at the family (popular) level. These sectors have implications for biomedicine because they are often used in conjunction with or as an alternative to biomedicine.

Popular (Lay) Sector. The popular sector, also referred to as *family care* in nursing, is the basis for most personal health care decisions. These cultural understandings derived from family socialization provide principal interpretations of health and generally pre-empt biomedical care, constituting a first line of resources. Family members and other interpersonal relations and social networks generally assist in assessing maladies and making decisions regarding treatment, including seeking biomedical care. The popular sector primarily involves what people, without recourse to specialists, believe and do about health care, including ignoring symptoms, and decide whether biomedical care is necessary or whether recourse may be made to the folk sector. Popular-sector health practices involve minor first-aid preventive measures such as lifestyle activities, hygiene, and vitamins and over-the-counter medicines. Informed sources on TV, the Internet, and numerous publications also advise popular health behavior. Knowledge of popular health beliefs and behavioral patterns gives health care providers the basis for appropriate inter-pretations of help-seeking behavior, symptom presentation and complaints, communica-tion about the body, and sick-role behavior and coping strategies. If health care providers are not aware of the cultural frameworks used by patients to conceptualize and communi-cate about their ailments, then **noncompliance,** patients' failure to comply with medical recommendations, is more likely. Case studies of African American health beliefs and Mexican American cultural factors affecting pregnancy and prenatal care illustrate the importance of the popular sector.

Folk Sector. The folk sector involves a variety of traditional cultural healing practices that are generally not part of an official or professional medical system. These include religious and spiritual healers, natural and physical healers (such as herbalists, midwives, and masseuses), and psychological healers (diviners, fortune-tellers). These ethnomedical systems have been called superstitions, charlatanry, quackery, and worse, and biomedicine has generally discounted their efficacy. But there is evidence that ethnomedical systems provide amelioration of suffering through curative social, psychological, and physiological processes. The appeal of this sector as both a complement and alternative to biomedicine is examined with specific examples from the U.S. subcultures such as Mexican *curanderismo,* African American religious healing, and Native American healing practices.

Other ethnomedical systems in the United States, often referred to as alternative medicine, are also of considerable economic importance, reflected in expenditures that exceed the out-of-pocket expenses for biomedical care (Eisenberg et al., 1993; Eisenberg, Davis, Ettner, Appel, Wilkey, Van Rompay, and Kessler, 1998). The extent of this alternative care indicates that health care providers need to understand this medical pluralism and how its utilization affects patient care. Other ethnomedical systems have implications for biomedicine because they may be employed as a complementary rather than an alternative approach. This simultaneous use of several health care sectors is illustrated in treatments for HIV/AIDS.

Professional Sector. The professional sector of medical care is generally dominated by biomedicine, although other professional healers are found both in the United States and cross-culturally, such as naturopathic physicians. The professional sector provides the official and legally sanctioned medical care services. In the United States, it includes biomedical practitioners, osteopathic physicians, pharmacists, chiropractors, auxiliary practitioners such as nurses and physical therapists, and competing and often marginalized professionals such as naturopaths, homeopaths, and acupuncturists. What constitutes the professional sector differs cross-culturally, reflecting the effects of culture and politics on health systems and practitioners.

The cultures of biomedicine are illustrated in cross-cultural variations in practice preferences and in differences between physicians and nurses. These cultural aspects of biomedicine affect clinical relations and can undermine patient compliance, requiring cross-cultural adaptation to be effective and competent in patient care.

The popular, folk, and professional sectors ideally represent the major differences in the principal health practices found in modern societies. There are differences cross-culturally in the practitioners found in each sector. The professional sector of one culture may function as a folk sector in another, such as Chinese medicine or acupuncture in China versus the United States. The distinction between sectors is not absolute: popular practices may overlap folk practices (such as herbal medicine use), and folk healers may adopt biomedical practices (such as stethoscopes). The relationships among practitioners and sectors may change as folk healers professionalize and collaborate with the biomedical sector or when professional healers adopt folk practices, such as acupuncture in biomedicine.

CASE STUDY

Alternative or Complementary Medicine?

The case of Lia Lee shows the pattern of the simultaneous utilization of multiple sectors of care: biomedical, popular, and folk practices. Lia Lee's parents did seek biomedical help for her powerful seizures, taking her to the emergency department during her more serious episodes. Physicians' services when their other children were ill in the refugee camps had proved useful. But they were not willing to give Lia all of the medications prescribed because of the numerous side effects. Instead, a variety of traditional remedies were also employed.

Hmong in the United States still use rituals, herbal medicines, soul recovery, coining and cupping, and various other ritual practices. Lia's mother had dozens of cans and buckets in which she grew medicinal plants used for treating a wide range of conditions: colds, stomach problems, postpartum conditions. Her mother gave her herbs from her garden and engaged in healing rituals designed to absorb the sickness into an egg. The Hmong also employed a practice known as cupping in which a small heated cup is applied to the skin, creating a suction that causes the skin to rise in a welt and "negative influences" to be extracted. Her family changed Lia's name so that the evil spirits could no longer find her, but the doctors undermined this by continuing to use Lia's name. A man's responsibilities as head of household include ritual offerings to ancestral spirits to maintain the health of the family. But many of the traditional ceremonies involve animal sacrifices that are prohibited in this country.

The failure of the biomedical approach to cure Lia and the limited effects from the traditional rituals led her parents to have several ceremonies carried out by shamans. The shamans also treated

The relationships among health care systems need to be analyzed according to structural superiority and functional strength. Structural superiority is concerned with the medical system's role in the national society and factors such as the power and wealth of its practitioners and their social prestige. The dimension of functional strength is concerned with the extent to which services are used and their distribution in a region. Biomedicine has achieved structural superiority in virtually all countries of the world, but the functional strength is highly varied across countries. Local medical systems often have greater functional strength, with many factors, including cultural relevance, contributing to their greater use. In most societies of the world, biomedicine dominates the political power structure, but this structural superiority is challenged by the functional strength of traditional healing systems.

This chapter examines some of the implications of these different sectors of care. Primary importance of the popular care sector involves the implications for the recognition of symptoms, care seeking, the significance of and response to pain, and the conceptualizations of the body and bodily processes that influence communication with providers. The considerations of folk healers illustrate why such practices are such an important feature of the American health care scene and why it is that alternative and complementary ethnomedical practices have such a strong appeal in the United States. This cultural perspective also helps reveal factors affecting the practice of biomedicine.

more mundane conditions such as colds and, ultimately, the final rites, drumming the ceremonious departure of the deceased person's soul. The shamans might also resolve medical conditions resistant to treatment by physicians. But the shaman was not the only source of traditional treatments. Thousands of dollars were spent to bring from Thailand sacred amulets filled with herbs. The parents brought in healers to help Lia with a coin-rubbing procedure. Christianized Hmong family groups may join together at the patient's hospital bedside to pray instead of calling the traditional shamanistic healers.

Lia's physicians, however, were seldom aware of the many treatments she received in her home and from community specialists. They didn't bother to ask. Despite their reliance on many traditional remedies, the Lees still tried to access the best biomedical resources available. In this regard, they were assisted by a social worker, Jeanine, who worked tirelessly as an advocate for Lia. She sought information for the family, procured needed medical equipment, arranged for transportation to special education centers, and ultimately created a system in which Lia's parents could effectively administer the needed medications. When Lia suffered a major debilitating seizure at the special education school, hospital tests confirmed that her parents had been giving her the required medications. Jeanine had successfully transferred the medical prescriptions and achieved compliance by Lia's parents. But the Lees now avoided biomedicine. To the Hmong, a healer's reputation is based on trust developed through past success and their respectful treatment of the family. The power of doctors to impose treatments contributes to Hmong tendencies to avoid doctors if possible or until conditions reach severity.

POPULAR-SECTOR HEALTH RESOURCES

When you feel ill, do you typically call the doctor first thing, or do you seek advice from a significant other or a friend? If you are like the vast majority of the world, you first rely on your personal network of resources for validation of your condition and information about how to treat it. Our decisions regarding the health care we seek begin with one's primary relations of family, neighbors, and friends and their knowledge of what a malady is and how to treat it. We are typically not left alone to decide whether to seek care. Family systems restrict and allocate access to care. This may be motivated by control issues within the family, economic resources, or concerns about the effects of illness disclosure on the family's reputation, as when families do not seek care for members with mental illness or leprosy because of the social stigma. The popular system is the nexus for health care; it is where symptoms are generally first noticed, their significance is evaluated, and initial treatment decisions are made. This may lead to a dismissal of symptoms as insignificant, the use of folk remedies, or the decision to seek biomedical services. The popular sector is the primary context for legitimization of the sick role and the context that supports or undermines clinical advice.

Thirty years ago, an estimated 70 to 90 percent of all treatment of health conditions took place in the popular sector (Kleinman, Eisenberg, and Good, 1978), and twenty

CULTURE AND HEALTH

Popular Health Practices Among African Americans

Snow (1993) did an ethnographic study of the ethnomedical practices popular among lower-class rural African Americans. Poverty and prejudice made the popular and folk health care sectors of considerable importance, particularly for lower-class African Americans and those of southern rural origin. These beliefs have less relevance for more educated and urban African Americans who, nonetheless, may still use traditional ethnomedical practices (see Baer, 1981a, 1982, 1984). African healing traditions underwent adaptations in America, where supernatural forces were an important conceptual defense because of the lack of access to societal resources and the dangerous nature of the outside world (Snow, 1983). Forced self-reliance instilled attitudes that one is better off trusting God as a source of healing. Regardless of treatment, faith in God is important because God can heal anything. Self-treatment is viewed as "giving God a chance to heal."

Self-treatments include over-the-counter patent medicines as well as dangerous substances such as turpentine and kerosene. Popular-sector approaches are holistic, involving body, mind, spirit, and other issues of social life. One must keep the body clean, well fed, and warm; failure to maintain a proper diet is considered a major cause of illness. Health is dependent on moderation and a balance of diet, exercise, work, cleanliness, rest, and the maintenance of one's personal and spiritual relationships. One must "eat right," "act right," and "do right," following the rules of God and society.

Coping mechanisms tend to be highly developed out of a need to deal with unemployment, single parenthood, poverty, and racism. Coping uses natural support systems and deliberate

---

years ago, self-medication was practiced by 67 to 80 percent of adult Americans every thirty-six hours (McGuire, 1988). The United States has become even more multicultural since these studies were published, so it is conceivable that these percentages are even higher today. Women are the main health decision makers for family members, particularly children. The popular sector also includes a wide range of resources beyond family: neighbors, self-help groups, churches, over-the-counter products in pharmacies, special foods and teas, patent medicines, diets, prayers, talismans, and ritual behaviors. A variety of people and activities provide recommendations for health problems, ranging from preachers to paramedical professionals and their family members, hairdressers, and people experienced in the care of a particular illness.

Popular-sector activities are important for public health education because self-care practices are core to health maintenance, preventive practices, and medical decision making. Activities affecting health are found in all aspects of life: environmental exposure, dress, activities, bathing, eating, social relations and conduct, and religious behavior. Cultural conceptions of what constitutes illness and appropriate responses, rather than biomedical disease beliefs, direct patients' interactions with providers. Mechanic's (1962) classic article, "The Concept of Illness Behavior," revealed that principal determinants affecting the inclination to seek medical care are social, cultural, and interpersonal factors.

avoidance of contact with institutions where powerlessness and discrimination have been experienced (Smith, 1995). Providers may be viewed as part of the prejudicial system. Accepting providers' advice requires that one make sense of the proposed treatments within the context of one's life, the ability to care for one's family, and maintaining a positive attitude. Biomedicine may be rejected because of previous prejudice, cultural pride, a lack of trust, and a fear that providers may "bring one down." Appointments may be neglected to avoid circumstances that create a negative emotional tone and interrupt tranquility. This may result in not finding out more about conditions if that would disrupt one's sense of well-being, causing worry and a loss of balance and control. Avoidance is central to coping by staying centered on the feeling of knowing what to do.

Smith (1995) found that coping with disease among healthy low-income southern rural African American families involves relationships with trusted individuals who help resolve uncertainty about how to manage life's circumstances. Being active and energized produces positive feelings and provides strength. Positive interactions with family and community, particularly female kin networks, contribute to a sense of control and self-sufficiency: the ability to survive on one's own, taking care of one's self and children. Worrying can make a person ill, so control of emotions was central to the maintenance of health. Prayer and meditation provided a way to reduce the effects of negative occurrences. Coping emphasized moral behavior, individual responsibility, God's help and blessing, right behavior, and helping neighbors by providing emotional and economic support and doing good deeds.

A greater frequency of health-seeking behaviors is associated with high levels of stress, particularly interpersonal difficulties. An overall inclination to seek medical care is significant in seeking care for any particular episode. People with a low inclination to seek medical advice are likely to ignore routine illnesses whereas people with a high inclination to seek medical care do so more readily. Economic factors affect seeking medical assistance for significant symptoms; a person's hardship in leaving work may impede seeking medical care. Those of higher economic status are more likely to seek medical care. Cultural factors may inhibit seeking medical care; those with greater social and cultural distance from physicians are less likely to seek services.

Culture and Symptoms

Zola (1966, 1973) pointed out that culture influences the recognition of symptoms as significant and requiring care, affecting health communication. Symptoms may be ignored in some populations because of their prevalence and relationship to the culture's value orientations. For example, the negative aspects of anorexia may be difficult for people to accept in a culture where "you can't be too rich or too thin." Similarly, symptoms that are considered to be of little danger are not as likely to lead people to seek medical care. Symptoms that are widespread and commonplace may be ignored. For instance, when lower back pain is customary, people who suffer may accept it as normal and not seek treatment. Even pathological conditions that are widespread may be considered normal. Ackerknecht (1943, reprinted 1971) pointed out that in areas of South America where parasitic skin disease is widespread, those not suffering from the skin disease were considered abnormal and ridiculed. The relationship between symptoms and cultural values also affects how they are treated. Hallucinations are considered a serious symptom in Western psychiatry but in other societies may be viewed as normal experiences. For instance, in Mexican culture, apparitions or visions may be interpreted as a spiritual communication and not considered to be abnormal or a sign of psychosis.

Zola (1966) analyzed differences in Italian Americans' and Irish Americans' symptom presentations and their perceptions of their health status and their conditions. Despite the lack of evidence for it, the Irish perceived themselves as being in poorer health. Nonetheless, the Irish were more likely to deny that they experienced pain from their illnesses. The Italians were likely to present far more symptoms and complain that the symptoms affected their daily lives to a greater degree than did the Irish. Zola analyzed these differences as illustrating a cultural fit between concerns with bodily conditions and value orientations. Italians' overstatement of their symptoms reflected an expressive quality and cultural dramatization of their conditions. The Irish style of ignoring complaints reflects a cultural use of defense mechanisms of denial. They minimized their symptoms, limited their implications, and generally denied physical problems. Zola suggests that the Irish failure to communicate complaints was part of a self-fulfilling prophecy that their lives were painful and difficult. Frequent locations for their symptoms—eyes, ears, and throat—were analyzed as symbolic reflections of their guilt regarding what they should not have seen, heard, or said.

Culture, Ethnicity, and Pain Responses

Cultural differences in the meaning of pain and responses to pain were popularized in the medical social sciences by the anthropologist Zborowski (1969). Zborowski compared those whom he called "old Americans" with Irish, Italian, and Jewish American men. The typical pain behavior of old Americans was stoic and controlled, not valuing the expression of pain or emotional reactions to it. The old American standard did not endorse crying or complaining. In contrast, Zborowski found that both Jewish and Italian men were likely to give vocal and expressive pain responses. Although the Italians were concerned with immediate relief of their pain, the Jewish men were also concerned about the implications of the pain. For them, pain relief was not enough. There was also a concern with what needed to be done to address the underlying causes of the pain. Like the old American pattern, Jewish men also tended to value an unemotional response to pain, preferring to withdraw socially rather than complain to others.

We generally think of pain as biological, but the experience of pain is shaped by social and cultural factors. Different ethnic groups not only report their pain in different ways, but models of pain suggest that cultural factors affect the physiological processes through which pain experiences are made conscious (Bates, 1987). Pain is not merely a sensation but an experience that has interpretive components based in emotional and social associations and their meanings, providing the significance of sensations. Bates and Edwards (1998) illustrate that the response to pain has learned components based in part in the cultural meanings attached to pain. The most consistent differences in the experience of pain intensity are a function of ethnic identity and locus of control, which they attribute to influences from ethnicity.

For more than half a century, social scientists have recognized that human experiences of pain sensations are affected by emotional and cognitive states (see Zola, 1966; Koopman, Eisenthal, and Stoeckle, 1984; Bates, 1987). Situational implications of pain were illustrated in a study of wounded soldiers; those who had highly painful wounds that were not life-threatening experienced little pain. These conditions were almost welcomed because they removed soldiers from life-threatening combat situations. Research by Bates, Rankin-Hill, Sanchez-Ayendez, and Mendez-Bryan (1995) comparing Anglo-American and Puerto Rican chronic pain sufferers found that a wide variety of factors affect pain experience independent of the biological conditions that produce pain. This is reflected in the dominant theory of pain proposed by Melzack and Wall (1983), known as the "spinal gate" or gate-control theory of pain. This theory is based in a recognition that the production of pain occurs in the interaction between the insulated fast nerve fibers and the uninsulated slow fibers. The relative activity in the fast and slow fibers contributes to the experience of pain. With extensive activity in the fast fibers, there is an inhibition or a closing of the pain gate. With little fast-fiber activity, even minor stimulation of the slow fibers produces pain.

Dramatic differences cross-culturally in pain tolerance suggest that this gating mechanism is influenced by psychological, social, and cultural factors (Bates, 1987). Cultural norms regarding pain expression and tolerance of stimuli also play a role in the experience of pain sensations, affecting the pain threshold and tolerance. A cultural approach is necessary for understanding how pain experiences are affected by environmental conditions, psychosocial characteristics, and economic and political dynamics. Culture affects the culturally appropriate way of reacting to and expressing one's feelings about pain (see the special feature "Biocultural Interactions: Ethnic American Pain Responses"). Intracultural variation (male versus female) also affects vocalizations of pain. Cultural expectations of appropriate gender behavior (a lack of manliness versus appropriate female expressiveness) affect individual responses and pain expression (see Kleinman, 1988b; Good and Good, 1981; Bates and Rankin-Hill, 1994; Bates et al., 1995; Koopman et al., 1984). If life is expected to involve suffering, then pain is more likely to be silently accepted.

The cultural expression of pain is affected by cultural interpretations of the significance of pain and the implications of the conditions that cause pain. Pain is expressed in both verbal and nonverbal communications, including specific sounds, terms, phrases, postures, gestures, and expressions. Distress is shared in a metaphoric language in which the symptoms express concerns about the relationships of the patient to others. This expression involves somatization, where somatic or bodily complaints reflect psychological dynamics and concerns. Pain expressions may reflect the social dimensions of suffering, the dynamics of guilt or shame, a protest against social expectations, or a social tool that obligates responses to the sufferer.

Providers need knowledge about ways culture affects individual expression of pain to appropriately interpret the significance of patients' complaints. Patients from cultures

BIOCULTURAL INTERACTIONS

Ethnic American Pain Responses

Anglo-Americans. Anglo-American chronic pain responses are often nonexpressive, as they live with pain but do not display pain behavior (Bates et al., 1995). An emphasis on individual responsibility for pain management reflects cultural values of autonomy and control of one's life. A dominant coping strategy is to isolate oneself and to be alone. Another strategy to cope with chronic pain involves staying active. The view of the physical body as the source of pain often makes treatment programs based on psychological, cognitive, or behavioral approaches ineffective and leads to an extensive reliance on surgical interventions to remove the cause of pain. Nonetheless, intracultural variation is also important, and some Anglo-Americans find that psychological approaches provide relief. The "old American" stoic response to pain no longer applies to many contemporary Americans, who may engage in a hedonistic use of pain killers. Euro-American providers may still have the expectation of a stoic endurance of pain rather than an open expression of suffering or indulgence in medication.

Hispanic Americans. Hispanic Americans tend to have a high degree of expressiveness of their pain and high-intensity experiences of that pain (Bates and Edwards, 1998), but general expression of pain may not always be given in clinical settings because it contradicts cultural values. The value placed on endurance in machismo inhibits men from an open expression of pain. Pain expression may be considered more appropriate for women, but there is a cultural value on silent suffering and endurance. Women in labor, however, may be vocal in their expression of pain. The arrival of the woman's husband often results in longer and louder cries, a communication to the husband of the suffering she is enduring on account of her pregnancy. Pain can play an important role in making Hispanics aware of the need to seek treatment. If there is an absence of

that encourage emotional expressiveness of pain may require less attention to their symptoms than patients from cultures where stoicism and lack of pain expression are expected. The cultural background may alert providers that they need to pay attention to patients who complain minimally but are experiencing serious pain and need to take pain medication. For example, failure to emphasize pain needs to be considered in the context of a cultural tendency toward repression and denial, whereas vocal and expressive complaints need to be put in the context of cultural emphasis on expressiveness. Understanding these cultural influences is essential to correctly interpreting the significance of a patient's complaints.

Differences between U.S. norms and those of other cultural groups affect practitioners' ability to accurately interpret pain expression by ethnic clients. Culturally competent medical management of pain requires that providers be aware of their own culturally mediated pain perceptions and those of their patients, requiring a detailed psychosocial and cultural history to determine variables affecting the chronic pain experience (Bates and Edwards, 1998). Without knowledge of their own cultural expectations regarding pain management, providers are more likely to be judgmental toward pain, good health may be presumed and treatment neglected. Pain expressions may also reflect somatization, with depression expressed in bodily symptoms.

African Americans. African American responses to pain have been characterized as highly varied, reflecting diverse influences on African American illness behavior and contextual or social influences on its expression. Silent suffering may reflect a lack of confidence in providers or the perception that they will not respond to the patient's needs. Conversely, empowerment and a sense that services will be provided to those who complain or demand them may lead to a far more vocal expression of pain. African Americans may also avoid pain medication because of the fear that they might become addicted.

Native Americans. Native American responses to pain are highly varied, reflecting the more than seven hundred Native American groups present in the United States. Kramer (1996) suggests that pain in Native Americans is often undertreated. This may be the result of pan-Native American emphases on passive endurance (Winkelman, 1998). The pain reports typical of this population may be indirect and general, expressed in reflections on how they feel uncomfortable, rather than direct complaints. Communication regarding pain may be indirectly through family members or friends, who are expected to relay this information to providers.

Chinese Americans. Responses to pain of Chinese Americans include the avoidance of medication either out of fear of addiction or because of acceptance of suffering. Chinese American patients may also decline offers of pain medication, relying on providers to determine their needs. Patients will not typically complain about their pain, requiring that providers be aware of nonverbal communication indicating pain, assess patients' likely experience of pain, and provide medications rather than wait for them to be requested.

patients who express pain in culturally different ways. This can negatively affect patient-provider relations and the care and treatment provided to patients. Awareness of the cultural basis of pain responses and experiences helps practitioners suspend their culturally based evaluative frameworks and understand the cultural dynamics of clients' expression of pain.

This awareness also helps providers respond appropriately to people from cultures in which the open expression of pain is not normative. If a culture emphasizes a stoic and silent suffering attitude toward pain, a provider cannot depend solely on clients' verbal statements regarding pain or their request for pain medication in assessing their needs but must look for nonverbal signs indicative of clients' need for pain medication.

A recognition of differences among ethnic or cultural groups in pain responses is not the same as stereotypes about pain responses within groups. Within cultures, there are also important differences in pain responses. But these differences are also culturally structured, with variations related to individual difference in locus of control, socioeconomic status, age, generation, consistency of ethnic heritage, and gender (Bates and Rankin-Hill, 1994).

Cultural Conceptions of the Body

Peoples' perceptions of the health of their body and its structures and functions reflect cultural, rather than biological, concepts of anatomy. The disjuncture of medical and popular conceptualizations of the body affects consultation, treatment, and compliance. Even when providers and clients share a common vocabulary, the meanings of words may differ considerably. For many, the "stomach" refers to the entire abdominal region between the rib cage and the pelvis, but to physicians, the stomach is a more limited area. Culturally derived perceptions of the body affect communication about symptoms and experiences. Cultural conceptions of bodily functions play an important role in hysterical pain, which generally does not correspond to neurological conditions but rather to cultural images of the body. Knowledge of cultural concepts of the body enables a better understanding of information relevant to diagnosis and patient education. Cultural conceptions of the body have important implications for health through

- Notions about normal bodily conditions and functions

- Desirable diet and environmental exposure

- The nature and meaning of bodily by-products (e.g., feces, urine, blood, mucus)

There are important health implications of ways we expose the body and what we do to it and put in and on it: sun exposure, oils, perfumes and other odorants, tattooing, implants, diets, clothing or protection, mutilation, liposuction, drugs, dietary practices, binding and flattening, circumcision, and clitorectomy.

Cultural conceptions of menstruation have important implications for health behaviors. Where viewed as a process by which the body rids itself of contaminants, even excessive menstruation can be seen as healthy and normal. Where bleeding is viewed as a loss of vital fluids, the lack of menstruation may not be viewed as problematic. Traditional African American beliefs that one could become pregnant when the uterus was "open" during menstruation contributed to unwanted pregnancies by encouraging the assumption that pregnancy would not occur during other periods of the menstrual cycle (Snow, 1993).

Cultural concepts about what is appropriate or dangerous for the body are important for biomedical practitioners in accommodating for effects of medical procedures, particularly invasive procedures like surgery, cranial intravenous insertions, irradiation, and chemotherapy. For example, a common procedure for inserting an intravenous IV drip into an infant is through blood vessels on the top of the head. This procedure may be particularly distressing to people from China and Southeast Asia, where the head is viewed as sacred and an aperture through which the spirit may exit the body. Cultural concepts regarding ideal body states produce differences in what is viewed as a health problem. In societies where obesity is a sign of social status and wealth, efforts to address it as a health problem may be ignored.

Alternative therapy models that postulate a number of energy, spiritual, or bioenergetic bodies that affect health expand biomedical concepts of the body (Cassidy, 1996). Most alternative healing approaches consider the physical body to be but one of several levels of the body on which healing may operate. Actions on spiritual, etheric, or mental levels of the body may be viewed as affecting the physical body. Homeopathic traditions consider the body to have three distinct aspects, including spirit or vital energies. Bioenergetic systems consider the body to include etheric and astral bodies operating on a spiritual plane as well as a mental body that interfaces with the spiritual body. Acupuncture systems also view the physical body as being complemented by a spiritual body that is affected by energetic manipulations.

Concepts of the body as having several levels are also found in the medical social sciences. Helman (2001) differentiates the individual body, which involves physical and psychological characteristics, from the social body, which involves ideas acquired through socialization. Both of these bodies are a metaphoric system for communication about the self and the world. Scheper-Hughes and Lock (1987) analyze the body as a socially constructed symbolic artifact, articulating a perspective on "three bodies":

- The individual body based in lived experience
- The social body, a natural symbol used to represent nature and society
- The body politic, reflecting how individual bodies are controlled by social processes

Biomedical approaches generally address only the biological body, failing to recognize the social and cultural expressions of the physical body or its psychological, spiritual, and mental dimensions. Your physician may attempt to address the physical trauma caused by an assault but not likely the collective social sense of vulnerability that women feel regarding the risk of assault. The interactions among these three bodies nonetheless have important implications for health; illness, sickness, and symptoms involve metaphoric communication about the relationship among the individual, social, and political bodies. For instance, when politics prohibits women's control over their reproductive processes, the individual bodies suffer from unregulated abortions.

CULTURE AND HEALTH

Hmong Concepts of Self in Souls

To the Hmong, one's well-being involves the condition of many souls, each of which has a different effect on behavior and life. There are a number of souls in each person, ranging from three to as many as thirty (Xiong, Numrich, Youngyuan Wu, Yang, and Plotnikoff, 2005). Of great significance to well-being is the possibility of the theft of one's personal soul by malevolent spirits, jealous ancestors, or evil ghosts sent to cause illness. Sickness and death may result from the loss of any one of the souls that provide vital essence and functions in human life. Cultural rituals are significant in maintaining the health of the soul, particularly when the challenges of life disrupt balance. Some of the souls are thought to be associated with specific organs and to be lost if surgery affects the organ.

CULTURE AND HEALTH

Mexican American Ethnomedical Traditions

Core aspects of traditional Mexican ethnomedical folk specialists involve the *curandero* (curer), *yerbalista* (herbalist), *sobador* (masseuse), *partera* (*midwife*), and *espiritualista* (spiritualist healer). These health care systems involve a synthesis of Indian and Spanish influences and sometimes biomedical traditions. Mexican Americans' traditional healing practices are in decline, but the beliefs may still play a conceptual role in shaping health behavior (Trotter and Chavira, 1997; and e.g., Chapter Two on illness concepts). Most are familiar with traditional treatment concepts, although they may not utilize them; some may even reject them as superstitions if they are highly acculturated. Only a small percentage of Mexican Americans still regularly use traditional practitioners because of their decline in the United States, but most of the populace has positive perceptions of curanderos and similar practices and is willing to use these ethnomedical resources for appropriate conditions (e.g., see Chavez, 1984).

The Curandero. Curanderos are folk healers who blend centuries of influences from European, Native American, Catholic, and international traditions. Curandero, meaning "one who cures," is a general term applied to virtually any Mexican-origin ethnomedical practitioner, including those listed below. These other Mexican practitioners may reject the term curandero, feeling the more specific term is more appropriate. Curanderos use charismatic power and rituals along with herbal treatments. They are primarily used for folk illnesses and appear effective for dealing with mental and emotional illness, resolving psychological and social problems, and strengthening social ties and relationships (Trotter and Chavira, 1997).

Self-Care and the Yerbalista. At the basis of Mexican American self-care are a variety of *remedios caseros,* "household remedies." These are largely herbal remedies but also include oils, ointments, natural substances, and patent medicines. The lay use of these substances is complemented by recommendations from professional herbalists known as yerbalistas. Chavez (1984) found that 70 percent of respondents had used herbs as medicines for treatments of gastrointestinal and cardiac problems, diabetes, respiratory illness, nerves, and psychological problems (see Kay, 1996). Medicinal plants are widely available in Hispanic communities in gardens, grocery

People's concepts of the body include internal differentiations in essences, emotions, and self-structures (soul, spirit, and other entities) that play a role in human understanding of their drives, emotions, behaviors, and needs. Chapter Six discusses this as part of an "indigenous psychology," cultural concepts of the person, and illustrated in Hmong concepts of souls.

FOLK SECTORS AND ETHNOMEDICINES

The folk or ethnomedical sector involves a variety of forms of cultural healing. Folk medicine traditions in the United States include midwives, spiritual healers, diviners, faith healers, herbalists, root doctors, and many others labeled as involved in magical, stores, and pharmacies and from folk healers. The widespread use of herbal medications and their pharmacologically active substances means providers need to know about their patients' use of these remedies so clients can be advised against the use of certain deleterious substances and guard against synergistic or conflicting effects with pharmaceuticals.

The Sobador. The sobador (or *huesero*) combines characteristics of a masseuse and a chiropractor. Anderson (1987) discovered beneficial as well as potentially dangerous effects from these practices and concluded that the sobador is effective in treating a range of conditions. The sobador treats musculoskeletal pain and stiffness and other conditions with massage, joint immobilization and manipulation, kneading, and tonic massages. A major treatment technique is "mobilization," small-amplitude repetitive movements applied rhythmically to the joints, extending the limb in its accustomed patterns but short of the normal full extension. Manipulation involves the sudden controlled thrust of a limb to the limit of its physical range, generally with a lot of force. This may include rotational manipulation of the neck, involving torquing the head to the limits of its range of movement.

La Partera. Important aspects of Mexican American ethnomedicine involve the practices of parteras, midwives, also known as *comadrona*. A partera may also be a curandera, sobadora, or yerbalista. The traditional practices of parteras are now augmented with aspects borrowed from biomedicine, including the use of sterile conditions, surgical gloves, and monitoring vital signs of mother and child. Parteras have remained important influences in border areas, but their overall use is minimal because of legal restrictions on their practice and Mexicans' needs to have births in the United States properly registered for citizenship purposes.

Espiritualistas and Espiritistas. The *espiritualista* and *espiritista* traditions reflect syncretic influences of European spiritualism and New World traditions. In Mexico, these traditions have integrated Catholicism and Native American influences (see Finkler, 1985a, 1985b). These practices involve mediumship, where a practitioner channels spirit entities for the treatment of physical, spiritual, and emotional illnesses. Espiritualista centers have a variety of activities, including regular healing sessions, training for mediums, and general services for the public.

religious, or superstitious practices. They also include the complementary or alternative medicine (CAM) traditions that involve folk practices and quasi-professionals aspiring for acceptance as professionals. The folk sector often incorporates both spiritual and secular influences in the same practice, with their practitioners emphasizing the power of faith and belief as central to mechanisms of their effectiveness and also claiming that their procedures are scientifically based (such as Christian Science). Folk practices overlap with popular religious practices such as prayer, where the intervention of deity is considered to be all that is necessary for cure. Today we find many religions that have a dimension focused on healing: Christian church groups emphasizing charismatic healing; Eastern mystical and philosophical traditions, including Islam and Buddhism; and New

Age healing practices and beliefs (meditation, crystals). New Age healing practices exemplify this combination of empirical (scientific) and spiritual approaches to health that typifies the folk sector.

A central aspect of ethnomedical practices worldwide involves a form of religious healing known as shamanistic healing (Winkelman, 1992, 2000). The basic functional aspects of shamanistic healing involve inducing an altered state of consciousness (ASC) that provides physical and psychological therapies (see Winkelman, 1991, 2000a, 2003a, 2004c, and Chapter Ten). Not all ethnomedical therapies involve shamanistic healing, but every society has practitioners who have instituted a human universal: community healing rituals involving the induction of ASC. All societies have rituals that are used for healing, combining the family or larger local residential groups together in ecstatic ASCs that provide healing. These healing rituals intend an interaction with what is considered the spirit world, a level of reality with powers to heal and kill. These rituals involve a variety of procedures to induce ASCs, including singing, drumming, and dancing and sometimes the use of drugs such as hallucinogens, alcohol, and tobacco. The theories of illness vary widely, but two aspects appear universally: illness can be caused by the intentions of evil humans and of spirits.

Societies worldwide also employ two other universal aspects of the folk sector: midwifery and herbalism. In all societies, women have developed local traditions for the management of pregnancy. These beliefs and practices provide an evolved response to the biology of birthing and the local cultural realities formed by the authoritative beliefs and practices regarding birthing. All societies have also developed traditions regarding the use of local plants as an essential aspect of health maintenance and disease treatment. These traditions are both widespread, where virtually everyone knows some plants, and professional, where common bodies of empirical knowledge developed through clinical experience are learned regarding plant use (e.g., Chinese medicine).

The folk sector generally does not form part of the society's dominant health sector politically or economically but may nonetheless constitute the most frequently utilized health resources. This functional strength reflects their role as long-standing cultural traditions that may diffuse to urban centers as populations relocate. These traditions provide important health services, many of which have well-established empirical outcomes (such as midwives, masseuses, herbalists) and psychological effects (spiritualists, healers, diviners). The contrast of folk practices with the professional sector reflects differences in professionalization and power. The folk-sector practitioners are generally nonprofessional, reflecting informal systems of training and apprenticeship, often within family lines. Access to roles of folk healers might also be through spontaneous ASCs, signs at birth, apprenticeship, and self-instruction. Some folk healers form indigenous organizations and have rules of professional conduct, engage in training, sharing of techniques, and formal recognition of successfully trained apprentices (see Green, 1996). Folk healers may professionalize as a consequence of interactions with biomedicine or state bureaucracies, seeking recognition from governments; this illustrates the fluid boundary between the folk and professional sectors. Furthermore, what may be a folk practice in one society may constitute professional practice in another, reflecting different relationships to the power structures of the particular society (Chinese medicine in mainland China versus the United States).

The roles of CAM procedures in contemporary health care are increasing. The growing body of data on the efficacy of CAM approaches is exemplified in the IOM's (2005) compilation, *Complementary and Alternative Medicine in the United States*. These CAM approaches are still strongly based in the universals of religious healing but have developed many professional dimensions as well. The centrality of religion is obvious, however, even in postmodern societies such as the United States (see Barnes and Sered, 2005). Despite general secularization trends, religious healing practices have persisted and even grown in popularity, exemplified in Csordas's (1994) study of Catholic charismatic healing. Despite the hegemony of biomedicine, it remains challenged by the recourse to religion for many aspects of health. The spiritual and religious approaches to healing are supported by the growth of the holistic health movement, which considers spiritual health among the many dimensions or levels of human health.

The healing traditions often referred to as complementary medicine and alternative medicine (naturopathy, acupuncture, chiropracty, herbalism, and homeopathy) fall in an ambiguous area between **folk healing** and professional medicine often referred to as holistic healing (e.g., see Trivieri, 2001). Although they reflect popular health beliefs and cultural traditions, they may also have specialized practitioners and professional organizations (such as discussed about midwives in Davis-Floyd's "Practitioner Profile" in Chapter Four). These wide-ranging CAM practices have important implications for biomedical providers because of the scope of their use. Studies by McGuire (1988) and Eisenberg and colleagues (1998) on the use of alternative and unconventional healing practices in the United States indicate their overlap with the use of professional sectors, reflecting the long history of these traditions in American culture.

Alternative Medicine Use in North America

Gevitz (1988) points out that contemporary American concerns with alternative medicine are deeply rooted in North American history and culture (also see Baer, 2001). Alternative approaches resulted from aspects of early American society: isolation from Europe, diverse healing traditions in a multicultural immigrant base, and independent and self-reliant tendencies. These fostered a reliance on local resources as cost-effective alternatives to expensive imported drugs. Native American herbal traditions were incorporated in an official nineteenth-century U.S. pharmacopoeia. Many alternative traditions today have roots in eighteenth-century herbalism, religious practices, and other healing traditions marginalized by biomedicine.

Social health movements have been prominent in this country for almost two centuries (Gevitz, 1988). These American folk medicine traditions reflect resistance to the medical establishment, emphasizing both a self-help individualistic approach and a concern with the toxic and political aspects of biomedicine. Biomedical precursors in the nineteenth century employed extreme methods such as bleeding, purging, sweating, and toxic substances in an approach referred to as "heroic medicine" that often killed patients (Baer, 2001). The attractiveness of alternative therapeutic approaches was reinforced by treatments that were often drastic, painful, and deleterious: blood letting, belladonna, strychnine, mercury, morphine, and cocaine.

These detrimental treatment effects empowered alternative approaches, including Thompsonianism, Grahamism, and Christian Science, health movements concerned with how individual behavior relates to health (see Baer, 2001; Gevitz, 1988). Prominent in the nineteenth century was Samuel Thompson, founder of the Thompsonian movement, a response to a public appeal for herbal medicine. He based his practice on commonly accepted procedures (emetics, warming substances, promoting digestion, and strengtheners), using remedies from Native American medicine. He also heavily marketed and made his practice available through publications, a society of practitioners, and a series of agents who represented the Thompsonian remedies.

Central to these health traditions were charismatic leaders with magnetic personalities and an astute understanding of mass psychology. They were revolutionaries and reformers and were often physicians rejected as heretics by their colleagues. These health movements were holistic approaches that emphasized the need to care for physical, emotional, and spiritual well-being, especially through diet. These nineteenth-century practices were often denounced by the professional society that was the forerunner of modern biomedicine, the AMA. The AMA achieved legislation requiring the licensing of doctors that led to dominance by biomedicine through prosecutions in the court system, driving healing movements from practice. Others retreated into the sanctuary of religion, which protected healing practices under constitutional religious rights.

Alternative treatment approaches appeal to American traditions of freedom of religion and rights to choice. These are reflected in religious connections that still exist within the health food and herbalistic practices. A focus on naturalism provides the emphasis for notions of balance and harmony that extend into cosmic and supernatural frames of reference. This approach sees energies as central to health and balance, a concept of "vitalism," a nonphysical vital force that permeates the universe and can be used for healing. Vitalism concepts are heavily influenced by Eastern traditions—yoga, meditation, and acupuncture—and scientific metaphors of energy. These energy concepts provide the basis for linking sacred and secular systems, a hierarchy of the universe where different levels or layers operate in different ways—harmoniously or in conflict—to create well-being or illness.

Unconventional Medicine in the United States

Eisenberg and coworkers (1993, 1998) assessed the national use of alternative medicine as "unconventional therapies": "medical practices that are not in conformity with the standards of the medical community . . . [and] not widely taught at U.S. medical schools or generally available at U.S. hospitals" (1993, p. 246). Unconventional therapies investigated included relaxation techniques, chiropracty, massage, imagery, spiritual healing, commercial weight loss programs, diets, herbal medicine, megavitamin therapy, self-help groups, energy healing, biofeedback, hypnosis, homeopathy, acupuncture, and folk remedies (summarized from table 2, Eisenberg et al., 1993). Prayer and exercise were also included in the original study, and the 1998 study added aromatherapy, naturopathy, and chelation therapy. The most frequently used therapies were massage, relaxation techniques, and chiropractic treatments. Unconventional treatments are used especially for chronic conditions such as back pain, renal failure, cancer, arthritis, AIDS, gastrointestinal problems, eating disorders, anxiety, headaches, and chronic pain.

CULTURE AND HEALTH

Peyote Religion as Community Healing

The **Native American Church** (NAC) is not a traditional healing practice but a syncretic religion that combines Christian elements with the use of peyote (*Lophophora diffusa* or *Lophophora williamsii*), hence its unofficial name as the "**peyote religion.**" The NAC has offered many benefits to Native Americans and their communities. Its moral code of devotion to family, abstention from alcohol, and obligations to the community help participants find the strength, motivation, and support to avoid alcohol and to accept personal responsibilities. The NAC has helped instill feelings of spirituality that played a fundamental role in traditional culture. The sense of oneness with the universe that these plants evoke has played an important role in recreating community identification that was undermined by forced acculturation to Euro-American culture. The psychotherapeutic effects of these plant medicines are widely established (see Winkelman, 1996a, 2001b; Winkelman and Roberts, 2007a; and the section "Total Drug Effects in the Social and Dynamics of Psychedelic Drugs" in Chapter Nine and "Biocultural Interactions: Physiological Bases of Hallucinogens' Therapeutic Effects" in Chapter Ten, which document their effects as "psychointegrators"). The positive effects of the peyote religion on psychological well-being and psychosocial adjustment are attested to in the accounts of Native Americans, the observations of physicians, and the reports of anthropologists. Aberle (1966) suggested that the use of peyote has many healing effects, including crises intervention; "miraculous cures"; release from guilt; providing guidance and purpose; and resolving marginalization, aimlessnesss, and helplessness.

People continue in the peyote religion for personal and social reasons. Revelations of personal significance from reflection on one's self, relationships, psychological problems, and conflicts provide the opportunity to resolve problems and create internal peace, harmony, and a feeling of purpose in life. Community relations provided by the NAC reinforce goals, commitments, and objectives formulated during the peyote ritual. The NAC provides a reference group that meets needs for approval and esteem, fosters adjustment between Native American values and those of the broader society, and guides a balance between collectivism and individualism. Peyotism offers status, countering prejudice and providing an affirmation of self-worth and validation of identity. Peyotism reinforces traditional values relating to spirituality and provides an alternative to the dominant society's values, emphasizing an ethical code of brotherly love, care of family, self-reliance, and avoidance of alcohol. Many substance abuse counselors in Indian country have avowed that the best way for Native Americans to achieve sobriety is through the NAC.

The use of unconventional therapies is found across different sociodemographic groups, with the highest levels reported for "non-Blacks," those aged twenty-five to forty-nine years, and those with higher education and income levels. The first study reported that 34 percent of respondents used an unconventional therapy within the past year. One-third of those saw a practitioner of those therapies; the other two-thirds employed an unconventional therapy without professional consultation. The 1997 study reported unconventional use rates ranging from 32 to 54 percent across different sociodemographic groups. The two studies by Eisenberg and coworkers suggest an increase in the use of unconventional therapies across that time period from 34 to 42 percent of the general population.

The first study reported that about 20 percent of patients seeing physicians for a medical condition also used an alternative therapy for the same problem; that increased to nearly a third of patients by 1997. The initial study found users of unconventional therapies also typically sought treatment for that condition from a physician (83 percent), but nearly three-fourths of these did not advise their physician of the concurrent use of alternative medicine. About half of the respondents reporting the use of unconventional therapies did so without professional supervision from either physicians or alternative healers. The unsupervised use of unconventional therapies suggests a potential risk for patients and indicates that physicians should ask their patients about their use.

Unconventional therapies are most likely used for "nonserious medical conditions, health promotion or disease prevention" (Eisenberg et al., 1993, p. 251). Backaches, headaches, insomnia, anxiety, and depression were more likely treated by unconventional therapy without medical consultation than vice versa. Only 4 percent used unconventional therapies for a "principal medical condition" without also consulting a physician. Eisenberg and coworkers' studies show the considerable role of **unconventional medicine** in the United States. They estimated the total use of unconventional therapies through extrapolation, suggesting 425 million visits per year for unconventional therapy, which exceeds the 388 million yearly visits to primary care physicians. Out-of-pocket costs for unconventional therapies were estimated at $34.4 billion annually in 1997, comparable to

CULTURE AND HEALTH

Ritual Healing in Suburban America

McGuire's (1988) study of alternative healing found the well-educated and economically comfortable middle and upper-middle class most often uses these practices. Alternative healing practices are part of a larger belief system that attracted adherents before their need for healing. Alternative healing practices provide meaning, describing what happens to the body, and imputing relationships with the wider society and issues of morality, community relations, and social status. Metaphors, symbols, and rituals evoke imagery, visualization, and positive expectations as a central part of the healing process, communicating ideas about the body and social relations. Many activities involve participants healing one another. Healing often works through empowering the individual to mobilize internal and external resources, such as the support of church groups or family networks. Many conditions treated—stress, loss of control, emotional and social disequilibrium, ambiguity, and helplessness—have psychosomatic implications. Alternative healing groups create a primary reference group that provides social and material support that strengthens people's ability to resist illness and disease.

PRACTITIONER PROFILE

Kaja Finkler

Kaja Finkler, Ph.D., is professor of anthropology at the University of North Carolina at Chapel Hill. Her major interests in medical anthropology have been comparative medical systems, including comparison between sacred and secular healing, the healing process, efficacy of healing systems, gender and health, reproductive technologies (especially as related to the new genetics), biomedicine, its beliefs and practices, and bioethics. The National Science Foundation and the Department of Health and Human Services supported her research in Mexico on sacred and secular healing processes and on studies of Western medical practices there. Finkler has been an invited and visiting scholar in Sweden, Germany, England, Australia, Israel, Buenos Aires, and Mexico.

During her thirty years as an anthropologist, Finkler's concern has been with issues in economically developing nations, especially with problems in medical anthropology. In more than eight years of fieldwork in Mexico and other parts of Latin America, she examined inter-related issues in medical anthropology, including the efficacy of healing systems, especially Spiritualist healing in Mexico and biomedicine; the anthropology of sickness; the cultural transformations of biomedical practice; and questions bearing on women's health, including domestic violence. She used ethnography, historical analyses, and analysis of the broader social systems to show how issues addressed in medical anthropology open a window to social, cultural, and historical processes.

Her research on Mexican Spiritualism and biomedicine led to publications such as *Spiritualist Healers in Mexico* (1985a) and *Physicians at Work, Patients in Pain* (1991). Further analysis of her Mexican data on differences in morbidity between men and women led to the book *Women in Pain* (1994b). Research in the United States focusing on concepts of genetic inheritance resulted in *Experiencing the New Genetics: Family and Kinship on the Medical Frontier* (2000).

out-of-pocket costs for all physician services. This view of "unconventional medicine" assessed only some of the many ethnomedical practices and used sampling procedures that eliminated groups (non-English speakers, people with poor health) likely to use alternative medicine.

Appeal of Alternative Medicine

Although biomedicine maintains a dominant economic and political role in American health care, folk and alternative professional traditions persist in part because of the appeal of these approaches. A dominant aspect of alternative medicine is the "holistic health paradigm" that emphasizes balance in the relationship between humans and the universe, providing a sense of meaning and connection often lacking today. Health and well-being are intimately intertwined with all aspects of life: the natural, social, spiritual, and cosmological. These healers provide a holistic treatment in a culturally relevant approach to an individual's concerns, operating within a shared worldview and value system. Important factors in the etiology of illness and mechanisms of cure are the patients' relationships to significant others, a holistic dynamic that reinforces its power and appeal. Understanding patients' personal and social situations enables these healers to treat illness, sickness, and personal conditions in ways not possible with biomedicine's focus on disease. Advantages of alternative over scientific medicine include

- Involvement of the family system and community in diagnosis and treatment

- Responsibilities of the family in both the sickness and healing processes

- Facilitation of the healing processes through meaningful explanations by the healer

- The closeness and informality of healing relationships

- The status of the healer in the community

- The healer's ability to influence behavior and to reinforce cultural values

- Culturally relevant explanations of immediate and ultimate causes of health problems

Factors contributing to the popular interest in alternative medicine include changing cultural and social conditions that have led to a reduction in people's perception of physicians' competence. Some people are attracted to alternative medicine because of negative experiences with physicians and dissatisfaction with the style of biomedical care. The highly technological orientation of biomedicine strikes many people as lacking the humanity and personalism they desire in medical relations. Whereas physicians prefer to rely on test results to determine a health problem, patients want to be treated as humans. Consequently, healing traditions that meet needs for affiliation and a relational style of care are more appealing. Biomedicine is also unable to deal with many conditions, making alternative therapies the only recourse for people with incurable diseases. Physicians' control style alienates patients who prefer an active role in healing decisions.

Many aspects of biomedicine are invasive and may even contribute to **iatrogenic** (medically caused) illness and mortality. Alternative therapies are often viewed as lacking the side effects and toxic consequences associated with biomedical practices. Alternative approaches also appeal to people who wish to take a more natural approach to their health, using natural products such as herbs and diet. Many people look for a holistic approach that addresses psychological, emotional, and spiritual aspects of the illness and healing processes and the individual's relationship to the broader ecological systems within which health is created.

Alternative healing practices often create a meaningful community and reaffirm spiritual beliefs. They generally enhance people's sense of involvement and responsibility for their healing, a collaborative relationship with the practitioner in healing. These approaches also have a focus on wellness, being concerned with the prevention and cure of disease through changing patients' lifestyle and healing by altering personal activities that contribute to imbalance. Self-healing is a basic principle underlying many healing practices that address disruptions in the body's balance and emphasize helping the body heal itself by restoring the body's natural balance. An appeal of CAM involves the limits of biomedicine. There are a wide variety of conditions for which biomedicine does not have effective treatment: colds, tiredness, diabetes, depression, cramps, allergies, aches, chronic pain, chronic fatigue syndrome, hives, arthritis, stress-related problems, Epstein-Barr virus, acne, anxiety attacks, allergies, back problems, pulled muscle, skin conditions, and until recently, fibromyalgia.

What alternative medicine places at the center of the healing process is not the disease but the person (Micozzi, 2001). Alternative approaches emphasize patients' experience of suffering rather than diagnostic categories. Emphasis on a person's experience reinforces patient participation with the healer, making the patient-healer relationship a significant aspect of the healing process. Alternative healing approaches are often eclectic and individualize treatment programs through the use of several traditions simultaneously, rather than just employing a single approach. A patient may use chiropractic treatments to align the physical body, herbs to strengthen certain organs of the body, and meditation to concentrate energy on maintaining healthy patterns in the body.

Evaluating Biomedicine and Alternative Medicine

Wardwell (1994) employed the term *quasi-practitioners* to refer to folk practitioners and characterized their therapies as "quackery," pretending to be scientific without a scientific basis for their claims. A dominant attitude of biomedicine toward alternative medicine is that whereas biomedicine is empirically established—based in science—the alternatives are not. University education and laboratory approaches to research serve as justifications for claims to a scientific basis for biomedicine. Nonetheless, many assessments question the extent to which biomedical practice is actually based in science. Cassidy (1996) reviews evidence indicating that only a small proportion of regularly utilized clinical procedures are scientifically established through double-blind clinical studies, in which a careful coding process means that neither physicians nor patients know if they are receiving a treatment or a **placebo** control (see Chapter Nine for discussion of placebos). By administering prospective treatments and a control substance in ways in which the physician and patient are both "blind" to whether there is a treatment or control, expectancy effects can be controlled for. Cassidy suggests that only 30 percent of biomedical practices are adequately tested with these gold standards of biomedicine; instead, much of medicine is guided by the traditions of clinical observation and experience, the kinds of verification used in folk medicine. Cassidy references the U.S. Congress's Office of Technology Assessment report that found that less than 20 percent of common medical practices were established as effective in double-blind clinical studies.

In many cases, biomedical approaches find it impractical or unethical to use the ideal standards of investigation. To deny patients in a control group some conventionally accepted treatment to establish the effectiveness of treatment in another group would raise ethical dilemmas, particularly if the treatment was potentially lifesaving. Other procedures raise serious questions about how to implement effective scientific controls. For instance, in the case of coronary artery bypass surgery, questions have been raised about the effectiveness of the surgical procedure as opposed to the broader lifestyle changes that occur along with life-changing surgery. The ability to carry out a double-blind clinical study of coronary artery bypass surgery would require surgically opening patients' chests without actually doing the bypass. Such dramatic interventions in a patient's chest and the associated changes in overall lifestyle recommended as adjuncts to coronary bypass (diet and exercise) also constitute forms of treatment and undermine effective control and comparison.

Difficulties with double-blind controls are even greater in alternative medicine where the patient's cooperation with the treatment protocol is essential. To reject alternative medicine for not adhering to the biomedical ideal of double-blind studies, which biomedicine itself seldom achieves, is a double standard and inappropriate for understanding alternative medicine and its effects. Clinical judgment, patient satisfaction, and an enhanced ability to maintain desired lifestyle activities are emerging as more appropriate criteria for assessing the effectiveness of alternative medicine as well as the quality of biomedical services.

Applying biomedical criteria to the evaluation of other ethnomedical systems is inappropriate. Holistic principles of individualized health care are in conflict with biomedical practices of evaluation: comparison of two identical groups, one with and one without a treatment. The scientific approach of testing for the effects of a single agent, using the same treatment for everyone with a specific diagnosis in a double-blind clinical trial with random assignment to groups, is not consistent with holistic approaches of individualized treatments adapted to specific characteristics of the person (McKee, 1988). Holistic views of the maintenance of health within a system of relationships are inconsistent with the determination of a single causal factor in treatment. Holistic approaches use the perspectives of synergy across a number of simultaneous treatment modalities, making it impossible to effectively evaluate in a double-blind protocol. Furthermore, assessing treatment outcomes cannot depend on a single biological measure because of the many effects of holistic treatments on a patient's life.

The health problems caused by the ideology of the biomedical focus on symptoms, following the allopathic ("against symptoms") approach, are seen in the consequences of the symptomatic treatment of CVD. In biomedicine, drugs are prescribed to reduce the symptoms associated with disease. For example, CVD and mortality are associated with higher levels of cholesterol, so medications are given to reduce the cholesterol levels. The assumption is that the cholesterol is a cause of CVD and that by lowering it, one reduces disease. By showing that certain drugs effectively reduce cholesterol levels, drug companies received FDA approval for that drug to be used to treat heart disease. Whether the drugs actually improve heart disease outcomes has been called into question by long-term follow-up studies of patients who were found to actually have higher rates of heart disease than untreated groups. The medication may effectively repress symptoms (cholesterol levels), but that does not mean that it prevents or cures heart disease.

A comparison of biomedical and alternative treatments is problematic because the very different conceptual systems and diagnostic categories prevent logical comparisons (Patel, 1987). Why would a spiritual healer want to treat cholesterol levels? How could a physician treat possession when the concept is not in his or her system? Comparisons within a single tradition using before-and-after measures of a patient's condition confound treatment with the natural improvement of conditions over time. Comparability of the efficacy of treatments requires assessments of patients' satisfaction with outcomes

BIOCULTURAL INTERACTIONS

Hypercholesterolemia as a Medically Constructed Malady

The disease of "high cholesterol level"—"hypercholesterolemia"—is created, defined, detected, and treated by biomedicine. High cholesterol levels do not produce illness; indeed, they may be associated with elevated mood. High cholesterol is defined as a disease based on the concentrations detected by laboratory tests. There is nothing natural about "normal" (or reference) levels; they are set by biomedical standards and lowered under pressure of pharmaceutical companies to diagnose more patients as having "high cholesterol" and therefore in need of treatment. Public health messages have come to reinforce the pharmaceutical industry's efforts to get people to take statin drugs to reduce their cholesterol levels. Patients, including children, are routinely screened and then convinced by their physicians to take drugs to treat a condition for which they have neither symptoms nor suffering. Statin drugs used to treat hypercholesterolemia reduce cholesterol levels by inhibiting an enzyme involved in cholesterol production. Statins also inhibit cholesterol metabolism products such as coenzyme Q10, which plays a key role in cellular activities. Q10 deficiencies weaken the muscles, including the heart, and produce a number of other adverse effects including neuropathy, dizziness, cognitive impairment, inflammation, muscle pain, and increased depression. The short-term successes of statins in lowering cholesterol levels and rates of heart attacks are countered by long-term effects that interfere with many useful functions of cholesterol in the body. This appears to actually lead to an increase in congestive heart failure, the condition statins are supposed to cure! (see Fallon and Enig, 2007).

and their overall health, particularly functional ability and desired life conditions. Evaluations of holistic treatment outcomes require assessments within systems of what they treat best and assessments of the enhancement of biomedical treatment outcomes when combined with complementary treatments (Patel, 1987).

Complementary or Alternative Medicine?

Some ethnomedical practices provide an *alternative,* something used instead of biomedical resources. But the actual pattern of simultaneous use of multiple sectors indicates that a more appropriate term in most cases is *complementary.* The same practice, such as massage, can be complementary or alternative, depending on whether it is used in conjunction with or apart from biomedical practice. Eisenberg's findings on unconventional therapies suggest that complementary is the more likely approach, with treatment used as an adjunct to conventional biomedical therapies rather than as an alternative. For example, Finkler (1985a) reported that patients' use of spiritual healers generally followed biomedical care and focused on problems not resolved in consultation with physicians. Because the differences between alternative and complementary therapies involve how they are used in relationship to biomedicine, the combined term CAM has come into vogue.

CULTURE AND HEALTH

Alternative and Complementary Therapies for HIV

The use of CAM among HIV-infected patients is extremely high. Furin (1997) found that 69 percent of a nonrepresentative sample of gay West Hollywood men infected with HIV used CAM; 92 percent also relied on biomedicine, illustrating that these therapies are complementary rather than alternative. Reasons for the use of CAM include the lack of an effective biomedical treatment and the political, social, and psychological dynamics of AIDS and CAM therapies. Furin suggests that AIDS activism is an important factor influencing gay men to use CAM in an effort to take control of their own treatment, lives, and disease. The social and political dynamics of CAM and HIV are also illustrated in a study of Canadian patients (Pawluch, Cain, and Gillett, 2000). They used CAM as a health maintenance therapy and coping strategy; a means for personal growth and maximizing the quality of life; a resistance to biomedicine; and procedures for mitigating the adverse effects of biomedical treatments, especially drugs.

The use of CAM was part of a health maintenance strategy to help ensure long-term survival. The patients' holistic perspectives viewed AIDS as a chronic condition rather than a quickly terminal illness. Their HIV diagnosis was no longer viewed as a death sentence; rather, CAM was part of an attitude of accepting responsibility for their health and a belief that they were capable of healing themselves. Their use of CAM focused not only on maintaining physical health but also on addressing spiritual, emotional, and psychological needs. They perceived these therapies as contributing to a sense of well-being, enabling the body's natural healing capacities to function. Lifestyle activities, enjoyable events, spirituality, and anything that facilitated natural recuperative processes and enhanced immune system functioning were seen as useful.

The view of CAM as complementary is emphasized in research-funding patterns established by the NIH's Center for Complementary and Alternative Medicine. The research protocols have generally been those that fit with the classic double-blind clinical trial approaches. For instance, instead of addressing the holistic lifestyle changes used in some ethnomedical approaches to cancer, single aspects such as dietary change may be investigated. This policy of emphasizing complementary rather than alternative treatment approaches is illustrated in the integrative medicine that combines aspects of CAM with mainstream biomedical approaches. Hess (1999) points out that the official biomedical position that rejects any notion of an alternative to biomedical approaches is an explicit endorsement of complementary approaches. Such policies often characterize the CAM approaches as palliative rather primary treatment modalities, further reducing their status and possibilities for funding. Given that few studies of the stronger "alternative-only" treatments are being funded, we are unlikely to see scientific studies that accurately assess the potential of these ethnomedical approaches because such studies would undermine power and resources controlled by biomedicine.

Other CAM users were less focused on addressing HIV and AIDS but, rather, with personal fulfillment, satisfaction with life, and broader philosophical and metaphysical issues. AIDS was even seen as a gift providing a transformative experience that helped them focus on the more important issues of life. AIDS enabled them to learn about compassion and address concerns about meaning and really important issues of life.

A few HIV-infected patients used CAM as alternatives to biomedicine, rejecting drug treatments. CAM was a political issue, a resistance against the biomedical system. CAM provided psychological resistance to negative expectations conveyed by biomedicine. Side effects and toxic consequences of biomedical treatments encouraged the use of alternatives without debilitating effects. More HIV-infected patients used CAM with biomedicine to address negative side effects of medication and as a strategy for addressing HIV and medication. CAM assisted in coping with the stress connected with HIV infection, helping to stabilize life, deal with anxieties and uncertainties, and reduce depression. This helped in maintaining lifestyle and personal relationships and meeting day-to-day obligations. CAM therapies could help people forget about the seriousness of their health and focus on enjoyable experiences such as massage, meditation, and music.

CAM is used by HIV-positive patients for a variety of reasons. These range from physical therapies to address HIV and their compromised immune system through a range of psychological therapies for dealing with stress and secondary effects of medication and treatments. They provide a sense of control, enhance optimism about their conditions, and facilitate resistance to the prejudicial attitudes of the dominant culture toward the high-risk HIV-infected groups (gays and ethnic minorities).

Important issues regarding consumer rights and choices are involved in whether biomedicine and society endorse a weak integration of CAM embodied in the concept of integrative medicine or a stronger integration of CAM implied by the term alternative. The existing division of resources in society allows these ethnomedical traditions only to supplement rather than provide alternatives to biomedical treatments. The stronger integration approach that would provide insurance and clinical support for alternative treatments has both benefits and drawbacks. Patients would have more choices, but they would run the risk of placing their health—and perhaps their lives—at the mercy of treatments with unknown efficacy.

The public's rights also invoke an obligation of the official bodies of medicine to protect consumers, with the burgeoning CAM phenomenon potentially producing a crisis for public health. The prevalence of these practices obligates public health professionals to investigate their use and effects, particularly their potential deleterious consequences, but generally without adequate knowledge of what is dangerous or what is effective. Administrative law provisions give public health officials unprecedented power to close ethnomedical facilities and ban practices that they view as being dangerous to the public

APPLICATIONS

Integrating Folk Healers and Biomedicine

Biomedicine often opposes the folk sector, but more recent developments have incorporated the folk sector into primary care of national health services. Some Asian countries (India, China, North and South Korea, Vietnam) already have incorporated nonbiomedical traditions into their national health plans. Economic barriers to access to biomedicine and pharmaceuticals reinforce the need to use locally available resources, an approach given official impetus by the WHO plan to encourage scientific evaluations of traditional treatments to ascertain which diseases can be effectively treated by traditional methods. This recognition of the efficacy of ethnomedical practices was embodied in the WHO plan of "Health for All by the Year 2000," established in the early 1980s to encourage scientific evaluations of traditional treatments to ascertain which diseases can be effectively treated by traditional methods. This was extended in the WHO's "First Global Strategy on Traditional and Alternative Medicine," launched in May 2002 (Northridge and Mack, 2002). This approach provides a framework for policymakers to use in evaluating the efficacy of these practices to ensure their safety and make them accessible and sustainable. These efforts require collaboration between ethnomedical and biomedical systems and mediation between the systems and their personnel. Anthropologists often play roles as mediators and project directors to help integrate the groups.

There also are roles for folk healers and CAM in modern societies where biomedicine is dominant (e.g., see *American Journal of Public Health* 92[10], 2002). The community mental health movement spearheaded the emphasis within biomedicine to recognize the importance of indigenous cultural practices in health care. A common role in the United States has been education of health care professionals about the cultural beliefs and the practices of populations served. This may be extended to using the traditional healers as consultants or to refer patients to them for specialized cultural treatments. Koss (1980) shows that joint training programs have led to joint referrals and collaborations in the development of treatment programs.

Knowledge of traditional practices can facilitate the work of biomedical practitioners. Folk systems influence patients' perceptions of etiology, severity of symptoms, natural course of illness, and communities. The ability to communicate with patients within their belief system enhances trust and rapport, the therapist's authority, and symbolic resources for influencing patients. Symbolically interpreting patients' behavior and symptoms permits assessment of psychocultural problems and the use of folk support systems to alleviate distress and control unacceptable behavior. Understanding cultural beliefs enables a therapist to use these powerful symbols and their effects on psychology, social relations, and emotions to enhance case management.

There is an emerging awareness of the significant role of CAM in the public health of modern societies. CAM is widely used in all parts of the world, but in many areas (particularly modern societies) it constitutes a largely underutilized resource base. Ignoring CAM is detrimental to public health, not only because of issues of potential debilitating effects but also because of the potential usefulness of such practices for communities. With appropriate knowledge of these traditional ethnomedical resources, public health practitioners can be more effective educators and promoters of the use of them.

A full engagement with CAM by biomedical practitioners will likely await further formal clinical evidence of its efficacy. But many sources of information can provide indications of efficacy, including (Winkelman, 1989)

- Long-standing traditional use patterns that provide "clinical" evidence
- Established similar applications in diverse parts of the world
- Congruence between the pathophysiology of diseases treated and the biochemical and pharmacological properties of the agents used

The WHO Traditional Medicine Strategy to generate research germane to establishing the efficacy of traditional medicine provides opportunities for anthropological input. This WHO plan focuses on addressing four principal areas to maximize the effectiveness of CAM:

- National health policy and regulatory oversight
- Access and affordability, including cooperation by biomedicine
- Determination of rational use, including training of biomedical practitioners
- Assessments of safety, efficacy, and quality

Anthropologists and cultural perspectives are directly relevant to the policy, access, and rational use concerns, particularly because most of these activities currently occur outside of the purview of biomedicine and official health systems. All of these issues must be addressed within the social, cultural, and economic contexts of practice. Addressing issues of appropriate national health policy for incorporating CAM requires engaging community and political organizations. Political action is essential to achieving legitimacy for CAM practitioners, as illustrated in the struggle of midwives to achieve recognition and protection under law (see Chapter Four). Policy directives must combine concerns with traditional use and sustainability with evidence of efficacy and the ability to integrate the CAM approaches within the context of biomedical and public health services. Such policy developments are social science rather than biomedical activities, requiring community assessments to determine what is available and being used as well as affordability and the sustainability of traditional use patterns.

Rational use requires education, a function that increasingly involves anthropologists and other cultural brokers within the context of medical training programs. Rational use also includes an assessment of relative efficacy and costs of CAM and biomedical approaches to produce an optimal balance. For instance, chronic conditions for which costly biomedical approaches have little ameliorative effect might be better served by CAM approaches, even if they, too, have limited effectiveness.

Anthropologists can also contribute to establishing the efficacy of traditional treatment practices (e.g., see Winkelman, 1986b, 1989, 1996a). Although the findings of double-blind clinical trials are often considered to be the criteria necessary for accepting CAM, there are clearly other forms of evidence regarding efficacy. Anthropologists have particular skills in assessing efficacy through ethnographic, observational, survey, and cohort studies traditionally used in public health epidemiological approaches. Cross-cultural comparative approaches are important to identify common treatment practices found around the world and in establishing efficacy, feasibility, and cost-effectiveness. Clinical assessments also require prior ethnographic investigations to clarify the approaches of traditional treatments that should be incorporated into formal studies.

interest. Balancing cultural and consumer rights with public responsibility requires considerable skill and knowledge, capabilities that are generally beyond the skills imparted in medical training but consistent with the cultural broker roles of anthropologists. As indigenous CAM providers are incorporated into public institutions, such as the integration of Native American healers into Indian Health Service units, there are issues of cultural sensitivity and appropriateness. The institutional culture of biomedicine in the United States has been hostile to these treatment traditions, making institutional cultural change a key to effectively providing CAM in an integrative medicine approach.

Because biomedicine is primarily concerned with biological well-being, other treatment approaches can address the emotional, interpersonal, and spiritual aspects of health not addressed by it. WHO (1992) has emphasized the vital role of traditional healing practices in providing contemporary health care, recognizing spiritual aspects of health and the necessity of having competent people to address these health care needs. The interaction of the spiritual aspects with community, psychology, emotions, and self-concepts reveals that spiritual approaches to health care are holistic: recognizing that mind and body, the spirit and the physical, are not separate but interact in producing health.

Cultural Expropriation and Indigenous Property Rights

As science turns its attention to alternative therapies, the social dominance of biomedicine and its leading role in the scientific study of healing have created a possibility for biomedicine to usurp significant aspects of traditional ethnomedical practices. As the empirical bases for the effectiveness of ethnomedical practices are understood (such as acupuncture), the practices may be incorporated into biomedical practice, but the traditional practitioners of these healing arts are not allowed entrée into the biomedical system and its privileged position. Even if these traditional healers do achieve professionalization through organizational development, they are typically auxiliaries or assistants in systems controlled by biomedical practitioners. What typically results is technical absorption (the adoption of alternative medical techniques by biomedicine) and organizational or administrative absorption (the control of alternative medical practices by biomedicine). This co-option of CAM by biomedicine is documented by Faldon (2005) and Baer (2004). This co-option reflects the power of biomedicine to do so and its profiting by responding to the increasing popular demand for these health services. In alliance with corporate elite sectors of society, biomedicine has managed to take over these modalities even though the training may be superficial (e.g., a few weekend courses in acupuncture versus six or eight years of study). Biomedicine's control of state regulatory and licensing boards and procedures may then often outlaw the independent practice of the modality by alternative healers. An even greater concern has emerged as traditional medicines are recognized as effective and efforts are made by pharmaceutical firms and other multinational corporations to seize rights to these plants or their extracts and compounds through patents. International law now protects the rights of customary knowledge holders, requiring cooperative agreements with these traditional communities. Acquiring the necessary informed consent and sharing of derived benefits from commercialization require deciding who constitutes the community and what are their norms regarding use and compensation. Such activities require cultural mediators and representatives to broker the gap between the global and local systems.

PROFESSIONAL HEALERS

The professional sector primarily involves the official and legally sanctioned health care services; it is dominated by biomedicine in most societies but includes other types of professionals as well. Professional medicine in the United States includes biomedical or allopathic physicians (M.D.s, "medical doctors"), Doctors of Osteopathy (D.O.s), Doctors of Chiropractic (D.C.s), Naturophic Doctors (N.D.s), and practitioners who function under the orders of these physicians, such as physician assistants, pharmacists, nurses, and physical therapists. Although we tend to think of biomedicine as the only "doctors," there are strong D.O., D.C., and N.D. traditions in the United States. In other societies, other health care systems have professional status, such as Chinese medicine in many parts of Asia and the Ayurvedic medicine traditions of India.

Cultures of Biomedicine

Biomedicine is referred to by a number of terms, including medicine, allopathic medicine, orthodox medicine, scientific medicine, capitalist medicine, and cosmopolitan medicine. In the United States, practitioners receive a university education, M.D. degrees, and licenses to practice from state boards, applying guidelines from the dominant professional association, the AMA. Biomedicine includes a variety of ancillary professionals who work largely or exclusively under the direction of physicians, such as nurses, respiratory therapists, laboratory technicians, and pharmacists. In addition, there are professionals that Wardwell (1992) calls "limited medical practitioners," who treat a specific part of the body (dentists, optometrists, physical therapists, etc.) or operate within certain boundaries defined by biomedicine (such as physicians' assistants and psychologists).

The power of biomedicine and its status as the exclusive legitimate medicine is of recent origin in the United States, a result of political actions taken by professional medical organizations in the late nineteenth and early twentieth centuries to exclude other forms of medical practice (see Hahn and Gaines, 1985; Starr, 1982). Informal and formal connections with court systems, legislatures, and official regulatory bodies (often created by and staffed with physicians) controlled and marginalized other healing practitioners such as chiropracty, homeopathy, naturopathy, herbalism, and midwifery, often making them illegal.

Osteopathic physicians (D.O.s) constitute a medical practice that managed to maintain autonomy of biomedicine, even operating in clinics and hospitals in a manner similar to that of physicians. Chiropractic was largely excluded from the arena of health care. Physicians were denied the opportunity to refer patients to chiropractors under threat of losing their license. The AMA's insistence that physicians could not make referrals to chiropractors, and their efforts to drive chiropractors out of business as a profession, was the basis for a criminal conspiracy lawsuit. The chiropractors won the lawsuit against the AMA and other biomedical organizations. The AMA's loss resulted in court orders to change its official rules to eliminate the formal exclusion of chiropractors. The success of chiropractors shifted them from a marginal profession, but they are still considered alternative and "unorthodox" medical practitioners (Eisenberg et al., 1993).

The political and economic dominance of biomedicine enables it to affect virtually all institutions of American culture. Biomedicine exercises controls from contraceptive access and preconception regulation of birth through the issuance of death certificates. This begins with prescriptions and advice regarding contraceptive practices, provision of prenatal care, managing the birthing processes, providing legally mandated neonatal treatments, and issuing birth certificates. Biomedicine's control continues with required immunizations and screening tests for schools and sports, provision of premarriage screening tests (blood type and Rh factor and AIDS tests), and validation of workers' compensation. Physicians are one of the most powerful and influential groups in the United States. Physicians' greater authority and control of resources in hospitals, public health agencies, and national politics dramatically counter the numerical inferiority of physicians compared with nurses. The power of physicians in American society has decreased in recent years, a reaction of the public to the increasing cost of medical services, and the changing infrastructure of health care provision created HMOs. HMOs have brought managers into the medical decision processes. Physicians and biomedicine, nonetheless, remain the dominant influences within the health sector. This power grows as physicians increasingly seek elective and appointive positions that determine the nature of health care policies and practices.

The biomedical practices have been presumed to be consistent, reflecting the view that they are based in objective scientific practice. The culture of physicians and biomedicine is not homogeneous. Among physicians there is a well-recognized stratification system in the prestige of various specialties. Surgery and internal medicine have ranked high on physician prestige scales, whereas psychiatry, pediatrics, general practice, and community medicine are viewed as inferior. Different principles of organization and types of care are found across cultures, between urban-rural settings, public-private services, and HMO-private physician practices.

The cultural aspects of biomedical practice are apparent in cross-national studies that find that cultural factors play an important role in different diagnosis and treatment decisions made by biomedical practitioners. Payer's book, *Medicine and Culture* (1996), examines variation in biomedical practices among European countries and the United States. Payer shows that even with the same condition, medical treatments differ considerably. Variations include the tendency to perform coronary artery bypass surgery, to use certain drugs, and to diagnose certain conditions. The aggressive American value system leads to more diagnostic testing, prescribing of drugs, and surgery. U.S. women are more likely to have cesarean sections, radical mastectomies, and routine hysterectomies at an earlier age. This reflects the value of aggressive intervention within the American medical system. The French concern with bodily aesthetics leads physicians to treat breast cancer through radiotherapy rather than surgery. German physicians diagnose cardiac conditions not recognized in American medicine but reflective of popular German health beliefs.

The internationalization of biomedicine and biotechnologies has influenced a homogenization of clinical practices around the world, but extreme cross-cultural variations in clinical practice remain (Good, Good, Brodwin, and Kleinman, 1992). What it means to be a good doctor and the standards for clinical practice and patient care are variable. For example, in the United States, laboratory tests are a basic standard of practice, but physicians practicing in many parts of the world do not have access to such technological assistance in making diagnoses. The practice of biomedicine is culturally and socially situated and shaped by local social expectations about the behaviors of physicians. The clinical narratives—physicians' explanations of diagnoses and treatments—are framed by local beliefs and expectations and local access to technologies and resources.

Nursing, Biomedicine, and Anthropology

Leininger (1976) analyzes the differences in the health cultures of nurses and physicians within the broader context of biomedicine in the United States. The profession of nursing has a particular position in the social systems of medicine. Nursing is the largest U.S. health professional group and traditionally was predominantly staffed by middle-class, European American women; the ethnic nurse population has grown considerably in recent years. Nurses outnumber physicians by about ten to one, but their power is miniscule in comparison. Nurses have been viewed as assistants to doctors. They nonetheless maintain some autonomous professional practice, beliefs, and responsibilities. Nursing remains distinct functionally and culturally, with its own specialized language, knowledge, and practices.

Leininger points to the production and maintenance of these cultural traditions through ceremonies recognizing historical founders (Florence Nightingale) and pledges and initiations at special ceremonies to confer full professional legitimacy. The old subcultural norms of nursing emphasize a compliant, deferent, and passive role of nurses with respect to doctors. This other-directed and service role was part of both patient care and the subservience of nurses to doctors. Nurses' activities, decisions, and actions were generally subject to review by physicians, and nursing activities were subjected to written and verbal orders from physicians. The dominance of nurses by physicians was accepted, reflecting broader patterns of sex discrimination of the culture. "It was truly amazing to find individuals manifest themes of behavior as being obviously compliant, deferent, and passive. Some [nurses] viewed [physicians] as 'mini' Gods because of their authority, and power, and control over so many people in the environment" (Leininger, 1976, p. 256).

The days of nurses being subservient assistants to physicians are largely gone; contemporary norms emphasize far greater autonomy for nurses. New subcultural norms were produced by increased education and professionalism of nurses in universities and broader cultural movements that have given women increased rights. Traditional aspects of nursing culture in the provision of direct care to patients have served as a basis for extensions of the nursing role into health maintenance and preventive care. Their role as assistants to physicians has become further defined and specialized as psychosocial agents. Nurses provide therapeutic services through interviewing skills, capabilities at group and individual interaction, managing relations between physicians and patients, and helping patients and patients' families cope with the effects of disease on other aspects of life.

CULTURE AND HEALTH

Cultural Aspects of U.S. Biomedicine

The norms of U.S. biomedicine are based on value orientations of middle-class European Americans. These are manifested in virtually all aspects of medical activities: concepts of illness and sickness behavior, criteria of normal weight and height, diet and body form, psychological and social normalcy, and communication styles and patterns. The resolution of cross-cultural conflicts in medical consultation requires adaptation to these cultural influences.

Ideology

Biomedical culture is manifested in its **ideology** or beliefs regarding the nature of diseases and the belief that mind and body are separate; this has been referred to as *dualism*. Biomedical ideology presumes that the body is more real. Mind has been viewed as secondary, and mental problems have been addressed through the manipulation of biology, using pharmaceutical agents to treat mental disease rather than examining how personal or social conditions produce those mental problems. The mind-body dualism of medicine produces biases and blinders, including an inability to explain placebo responses (see Chapter Nine).

Culture, Diet, and Weight

Cultural factors play a role in the criteria of appropriate body size. Cultural factors strongly influence perceptions of obesity. In previous eras, fatness was generally viewed positively as evidence of wealth and well-being. The shift in this century to views of thinness as evidence of well-being have become widely accepted because of the diffusion of Western cultural designs and preferences. Technology and marketing have also shifted the U.S. diet to decreases in fiber and increases in protein, conditions that exacerbate some health problems. Cultural differences in preferred body shapes and sizes provide alternative models of normalcy, beauty, and preferred shape and size. These, in turn, affect how patients view their health problems and desired conditions. It also affects how health providers and institutions respond to those culturally defined as having abnormalities. Although U.S. insurance companies charge an "overweight" premium for those exceeding "normal" size, cross-cultural studies do not support the contention of an association of body mass or fat with coronary artery disease, the widely presumed consequences. Biomedicine's normal body weight and height criteria are based on Euro-American norms, not cross-culturally determined criteria.

Communication

Communication in medical consultation is physician-dominated, largely from physician to patient. Effective participation in the dialogue depends on adopting the Euro-American approaches: assertiveness, independence, questioning, and demanding. Physicians generally view the important "information" coming from patients as involving the results of the lab tests rather than patients' verbal disclosures. The directness of American physicians in their communication is often seen as insensitive, conveying an authoritarian attitude designed to preempt patient challenges and concerns. Nurses, who interpret and explain for patients the information provided by physicians, often facilitate physician-patient communication. A cultural gap is often still present when physicians and patients share language and cultural background. The direct and frank communication reflects not only cultural expectations but also legal obligations for disclosure (Good, 1994). Communication with American physicians is framed in the context of broader cultural expectations about patients' "rights," including being fully informed and making their own decisions about treatment options. This contrasts with other societies' expectations of a paternalistic and protective approach.

Symbolism: The White Coat

One aspect of medical communication is embodied in the symbols associated with the practice of biomedicine: for example, the doctor's white coat (Blumhagen, 1979). The symbolic meanings associated with white affect perceptions of the image of physicians and reinforce their role in society. The purity of white conveys a significant aspect of physicians' ideal image. White had a functional role in indicating sterility in the context of early surgery; contemporary physicians have adopted white as a symbol of cleanliness. A second source of the white coat was from the laboratory (the lab coat), providing a symbol for scientific medicine. Cultural meanings of white imply life and innocence (as in the bridal gown), contrasted with black as a symbol of death and mourning. White's symbolization of justice, purity, cleanliness, and godliness facilitated physicians' transgressing cultural norms regarding the body and privacy, engaging in bodily examinations, particularly examinations of healthy people and pelvic examinations of women. This image of purity also facilitated physicians' entry into private places (bedrooms of the sick) and eliciting personal information that violated social norms.

Biomedical Values: Independence Versus Community Health

A central barrier to the effective provision of community health resources is a biomedical worldview, which adopts core American values without recognizing their cultural nature (Lefley, 1984). A central aspect of the deinstitutionalization approach for psychiatric patients is to help them achieve a social condition that reflects American values. This is represented in the idea of self-reliance and independent, solitary living. The therapeutic emphasis on an autonomous and independent lifestyle and reducing ties of dependency on others reflects core American values, increasing the anxiety that produces dysfunction in psychiatric patients. The anxiety of being alone and apart from dependency relationships is a socially induced illness resulting from cultural conditions that conflict with the psychobiological dependency needs of humans. The cultural emphasis on independence is at variance with human needs for support systems, and the emphasis on such independent approaches exacerbates feelings of low self-esteem.

Anthropological and cultural perspectives have contributed to the shift in nursing practice from the biomedical paradigm to a psychosocial framework (e.g., see Holden and Littlewood, 1991, Dougherty and Tripp-Reimer, 1985; Leininger, 1970). Rather than medicine's concern with disease and pathophysiology, nursing focuses on humans' responses to health problems, including perceived and actual consequences. Human health responses are more than the specific aspects of disease; they encompass being concerned with diverse areas such as self-care needs; pain experiences of disease and treatment effects; and changes in life processes, development, and stages (Dougherty and Tripp-Reimer, 1985). Nursing is concerned with peoples' views of their conditions and their social and personal needs. Nursing uses both disease and illness models, mediating between client perceptions and the biomedical orientation in nurturing patients' total well-being. Nursing has a long history of a focus on cultural issues to address clients' situations, incorporating cultural models into education and care long before medical school curriculums and physicians' training emphasized the need for cultural sensitivity. Social science curriculums were established in basic nursing education in the 1930s, and the concept of transcultural nursing was recognized almost half a century ago.

The theoretical formulations used in transcultural nursing reflect contributions of anthropological theory. Crucial elements in the domain of nursing theories—human nature, environment, concepts of health, and nursing care—have all incorporated anthropological perspectives (Dougherty and Tripp-Reimer, 1985). These include an understanding of human cultural and intercultural dynamics (e.g., ethnocentrism); cultural influences on well-being and on client behaviors, represented in cultural assessment modules; the recognition of the importance of illness as opposed to disease; and the role of nurses as cultural mediators and cultural brokers, facilitating the interface between client and physician cultures. Anthropological contributions to transcultural nursing include information on the way in which cultural belief systems affect health and risk behaviors, health care utilization patterns, and responses to providers. Anthropology has contributed both the culturally specific emic perspectives and the cross-cultural etic perspectives illustrating the universals of health care beliefs and practices.

The transcultural approach in nursing is closely allied with anthropological emphases on normal cultural patterns of behaviors, beliefs, and values and adapting nursing practice to accommodate cultural norms. Nursing broadly adopted anthropology's participant observation methodology in hospital and home care environments. The concept of the cultural environment has been a primary focus of community health nursing's emphasis on the broader environments—physical, social, cultural, and community—that impact health. Nursing has shared the anthropological identification with advocacy on behalf of the disadvantaged, brokering and facilitating relations of the poor and culturally isolated with institutional resources (Dougherty and Tripp-Reimer, 1985). Cross-cultural nursing courses teach culturally appropriate approaches to assessment and intervention, providing caring behaviors that conform to patients' cultural expectations. Knowledge of the cultural factors affecting patients' recognition of symptoms, beliefs regarding illness, and values regarding care can be used to support clinical interventions and enhance preventive health behaviors.

BIOCULTURAL INTERACTIONS

Body Image and Symptom Recognition as Contributing Factors in CVD

Various cultural health patterns and behaviors in the African American community increase the likelihood of CVD. The African American community has ideal body images that contribute directly to the prevalence of obesity and CVD. A large body is a culturally desirable feature, and a "big woman" is seen as attractive; there is a preference for a body that looks like it has "meat on its bones." This preference for a fatter body is a reflection of health beliefs that one is better off a little fat so that one can sustain periods of little food or have reserve resistance in case of disease. Women's body preferences are reinforced by African American men who consider women to be more attractive when they are what biomedicine would consider overweight (Bolton and Wilson, 2005). Biomedical norms regarding obesity are overshadowed by cultural beliefs regarding what is normal and preferable.

African Americans may also have misconceptions regarding significant symptoms of impending heart attacks, not considering headaches or a pounding heartbeat as possibly a warning (Schlomann and Schmitke, 2007). In general, the treatment of CVD is affected by a prevalent cultural belief that medications need to be taken only when pain or other significant symptoms are present. CVD is referred to as the "silent killer" because of its generally being without notable symptoms in personal experience. Disease may be present, but the experience of illness is absent. Consequently, African Americans may stop taking prescribed medications because they have no pain or symptoms. Repeatedly reminding an African American patient to continue to take antihypertensive medication despite the absence of symptoms is important because high blood pressure is generally symptomless.

CHAPTER SUMMARY

Health care providers need to understand their patients' illness beliefs and treatment resources in the ethnomedical sector that they use. These resources are of considerable importance because they are the primary source of health care and mediate the interaction with biomedicine. Assessing a patient's use of self and ethnomedical treatments is important because they tend to be used simultaneously with biomedical care, potentially compounding pharmacological consequences of medications. Physicians need to understand patients' models because they provide the basis for symptom presentation and communication with biomedical personnel. Cultural beliefs affect how symptoms are perceived and communicated. Health-seeking behaviors derive from many social, interpersonal, and situational factors, including knowledge, access to resources, motivations, and self-efficacy. Understanding and effectively treating patients' maladies depend on an understanding of their overall health management. This requires an informed inquiry into patients' self-care and complementary healing practices. This approach facilitates addressing all aspects of health and the inclusion of cultural resources and social support networks in treatment of integrating indigenous healing approaches to complement biomedical services. The roles of these ethnomedical traditions in health are addressed in the next chapter on transcultural psychiatry and indigenous psychologies.

KEY TERMS

Alternative medicine
CAM
Complementary medicine
Double-blind clinical study
Etiology
Folk sector
Lay sector

Medical pluralism
Noncompliance
Placebo
Popular (lay) sector
Professional sector
Unconventional therapies

SELF-ASSESSMENT 5.1. POPULAR BELIEFS AND PRACTICES

What are some of the steps that you personally take to avoid disease, illness, and other threats to health and well-being?

What kinds of health conditions would you personally treat for yourself or others without biomedical consultation?

For what kinds of conditions would you seek help only from a physician or other biomedical health practitioner?

What are some of the therapeutic activities or remedies that you personally take to address disease, illness, sickness, or other threats to health and well-being?

Are there other remedies that your parents or grandparents used?

Are there other home remedies that you have seen used?

People in all cultures have some home remedies that they apply to illnesses they experience. Do you or your parents or grandparents use their own remedies for any of the following conditions? What are they?

Indigestion	Cough	Sunburn
Vomiting	Flu	Sore muscles
Diarrhea	Fever	Cuts or bruises
Colds	Sore throat	
Congestion	Earache	

How do you obtain your medical services? Do you have a prepaid health plan (e.g., an HMO)? How does that affect your willingness to seek out health services?

Have you experienced health conditions that could not be cured by biomedical practices?

For what kinds of conditions would you seek help from alternative or complementary systems?

SELF-ASSESSMENT 5.2. INTERVIEW: FOREIGN HEALTH BELIEFS AND PRACTICES

Interview a person from an immigrant cultural group regarding their health beliefs and practices.

Where were you born? Your parents?

How long have you lived in the United States?

What are some of the illnesses that you would treat yourself or by members of your family or community rather than going to a doctor?

What are some of the causes of illness found in the beliefs of your culture?

What are some of the treatments provided by people other than physicians?

What were the treatments for?

What was provided in the treatment?

What was the outcome?

SELF-ASSESSMENT 5.3. FOLK HEALERS AND UNORTHODOX MEDICINE

Are there nonphysician healers that are part of your culture? What are they called, and what do they do?

Have you or members of your family ever been treated by one of these healers?

What are some of the treatments provided by these healers?

What are the explanations offered for these healing processes? How are they believed to work?

Have you (or a family member) ever used a religious healer? What was treated?

What treatment procedures were used?

What was the outcome?

Have you ever used any of the unorthodox medical practices described by Eisenberg and colleagues? Which ones? For what conditions? What was the outcome?

SELF-ASSESSMENT 5.4. EXPERIENCING BIOMEDICINE

Have you ever been a patient (or visitor) in a hospital?

Were there requirements or social practices that you found to be unusual? What were they?

Were there hospital rules that you found unpleasant?

Were there services or forms of care that you felt were lacking?

Was your family adequately accommodated and comfortable while they visited you in the hospital?

How do you feel about your hospital experiences in terms of the social relations? Were there things you wish would have been different?

Do you feel that you have been discriminated against by health care providers? How? Why?

When you see your doctor, do you feel that the doctor understands your needs? Are there communication problems? If so, why?

Are there communication or relationship problems in interaction with your physician? What kinds of problems? Why?

Have you ever experienced conflict in receiving the treatment that you felt you needed from physicians or biomedical practitioners? What caused the conflict? Was it resolved? How?

What role does the nurse play in mediating your relationship with the physician?

Have you ever had a condition that could not be effectively treated by biomedicine? What was it? How did you address the resolution of that health condition?

ADDITIONAL RESOURCES

Books

Abel, E. K. 2000. *Hearts of wisdom: American women caring for kin, 1850–1940*. Cambridge, Mass.: Harvard University Press.

Bailey, E. J. 2000. *Medical anthropology and African-American health*. Westport, Conn.: Bergin & Garvey.

Bonder, B. R., L. Martin, and A. Miracle. 2002. *Culture in clinical care*. Thorofare, N.J.: SLACK.

Clarke, A. E., and V. L. Olesen, eds. 1999. *Revisioning women, health, and healing: Feminist, cultural, and technoscience perspectives*. New York and London: Routledge.

Das, V., A. Kleinman, M. Lock, M. Ramphele, and P. Reynolds, eds. 2001. *Remaking a world: Violence, social suffering, and recovery*. Berkeley: University of California Press.

Davies, W. 2001. *Healing ways: Navajo health care in the twentieth century*. Albuquerque: University of New Mexico Press.

Finkler, K. 2001. *Physicians at work, patients in pain* (2nd ed.). Durham, N.C.: Carolina Academic Press.

Fraser, G. J. 1998. *African American midwifery in the South: Dialogues of birth, race, and memory*. Cambridge, Mass.: Harvard University Press.

Hahn, R. A., ed. 1999. *Anthropology in public health*. New York: Oxford University Press.

Hsu, E. 1999. *The transmission of Chinese medicine*. Cambridge, U.K.: Cambridge University Press.

Huff, R. M., and M. V. Kline. 1999. *Promoting health in multicultural populations: A handbook for practitioners*. Thousand Oaks, Calif.: Sage.

Kelner, M., B. Wellman, B. Pescosolido, and M. Saks, eds. 2000. *Complementary and alternative medicine: Challenge and change*. Amsterdam: Harwood Academic.

Ma, G. X. 1999. *The culture of health: Asian communities in the United States*. Westport, Conn.: Bergin & Garvey.

Sager, S. M. 2001. *Restored harmony: An evidence based approach for integrated traditional Chinese medicine into complementary cancer care*. Hamilton, Ontario: Dreaming Dragonfly Communications.

Journals

Alternative Therapies in Health and Medicine.
Journal of Alternative and Complementary Medicine.

Agency

National Center for Complementary and Alternative Medicine.

CHAPTER

6

TRANSCULTURAL PSYCHIATRY AND INDIGENOUS PSYCHOLOGY

*[T]he sociocultural environment becomes physically structured in . . .
neural structures in the brain [that] are altered in adaptations to
emotional stress and trauma, . . . experience, and cultural learning*

—CASTILLO, 1997A, P. 268

LEARNING OBJECTIVES

■ Illustrate cultural issues in diagnostic categories used in psychiatry and in determining normalcy, deviance, and mental illness

■ Introduce the use of cultural frameworks for the clinical assessment of pathology

■ Use biocultural frameworks to illustrate interactions of individual psychological
capacities with indigenous cultural psychologies in the development of the self

■ Examine possession to illustrate cultural concepts of self and normal personality
functioning

■ Provide biocultural and psychocultural models for examining the cultural bases
of personality, self, ethnicity, and illness

■ Examine ethnomedical syndromes cross-culturally to illustrate the interactions
of biology and culture and their roles in indigenous psychologies

CULTURE AND PERSONALITY

Your characteristics as a person, what you feel and think about yourself and others, are made possible by interactions of your biological capacities with the developmental influences from your cultural and social environments. Anthropology's perspectives help to reveal the relationships between an individual and his or her culture in producing "normal" personality, behaviors, and illness. This cultural perspective on normalcy expands the perspectives of psychiatry and psychology in understanding and treating mental health maladies.

Anthropology's "culture and personality" traditions (see Bourguignon, 1976a, 1976b; Bock, 1988) contributed to the development of cross-cultural investigations of the nature of human psychology and mental illness. This involved an investigation of the relationship between two levels of analysis: personality, the innate qualities and developed characteristics of individuals, and culture, the collective patterns of groups. A key concern was the relationships between the two: in particular, how does culture—the collective patterns—get imposed on individuals' personality development?

In attempting to answer these questions, anthropologists' interactions with Western psychiatry and psychology produced interdisciplinary research areas called transcultural psychiatry, cross-cultural psychiatry, ethnopsychiatry, culture and personality, and psychological anthropology. These involve cross-cultural studies on

- The interaction of culture and biology in producing universals of human psychology and illness

- Differences and similarities in psychology and mental illness in different groups

- Cultural effects on psychological states and predispositions to specific mental illness

- Ways in which mental illnesses are viewed and treated in different cultures

The sociocultural causation of psychological disturbance was made apparent by cross-cultural differences in psychiatric phenomena. Other cultures' conceptions of illness have contributed to the understanding of how culture affects health and the recognition of other well-developed indigenous psychological systems and treatment processes. Cross-cultural approaches illustrate the influences of culture on **personality** and other biological capacities for social and personal life. The differences between Western psychiatric conceptions of a person and those found in other cultures illustrate a need for an **indigenous psychology,** a culture-based view of the nature of personal psychology, identity, and illness. Expressive culture such as songs and myths embody an indigenous psychology, representing cultural concepts of persons and their internal structures and motivations.

Anthropology provides frameworks for describing how culture mediates and influences biological development and psychology, using socialization and symbols to teach us how to behave as members of society. Cultural effects on psychology and ethnic identity can be described in reference to universal features of social life: gender, attachment, emotions, self-concept, **status** (positions) and roles, developmental stages, and concepts of the person (personality). Cultural influences on life-cycle development have implications for clinical assessment. Psychological and medical anthropology address core questions about ethnicity, how culture relates to our personal and social identity, and the interactions among physiology, culture, and social contexts in producing disorders.

Although the biomedical perspectives presume a universally valid system for classifying mental illness based on symptoms, there are cross-cultural differences in the meaning of behaviors and their personal implications. This cultural nature of normalcy is illustrated in the phenomenon of possession, where what is seen as reflecting a psychiatric condition may be viewed as a normal cultural behavior in other cultures. These spiritual manifestations of self and others can play a role in cultural therapies and managing emotions and social relations among kin and community. Culture also plays a role in the shaping of psychological distress, manifested in ethnomedical syndromes known as "folk illness"

CASE STUDY

Hmong Conceptions of Well-Being

Hmong traditional beliefs consider a cause of illness to involve the spirits, who can steal one's soul, enter into one's unconsciousness, or frighten a person. One belief is that spirits may have sexual intercourse with people, causing them to be infertile. When physicians characterize an episode of possession as "being crazy," it embarrasses the Hmong because the physicians are ignorant of or denigrating traditional beliefs about the spirits that control them. Physicians label such beliefs as psychotic instead of recognizing them as cultural beliefs no more unusual than a barren Catholic woman praying to the Virgin Mary to help her get pregnant.

Accurately diagnosing the maladies of Hmong patients is a challenge. Psychiatric concepts of depression, schizophrenia, and other conditions have no equivalent in the Hmong language, even though psychological disorders are widespread among the Hmong in the United States. Physicians' questions regarding the nature of pain—deep, dull, sharp, radiating, or on a scale of 1 to 10—reflect cultural metaphors that are not useful in interviewing patients who merely report that they hurt. Consequently, their many emotional problems from war trauma and dislocation are manifested in bodily symptoms of somatization that doctors cannot distinguish from their discussion of organic problems. For example, the liver is a central organ in Hmong thought and somatization. It is thought to be central to emotional states, personal character (Xiong et al., 2005), and expression related to concerns about emotional distress. Somatization foci for the emotional life include the expression that one has a "broken liver" instead of the American "broken heart."

Fundamentally different concepts of bodily processes are seen in the doctor's diagnosis of epilepsy and the Hmong view of the seizures as a condition involving the spirits and potentially a blessing that may bestow special powers. Lia Lee's physicians did not seek her parents' view of her symptoms; consequently, they could not understand the parents' perceptions of her situation as a spiritual condition and their resistance to medical interventions. For the Hmong, a prediction of a dire disease outcome could be interpreted as a curse; the doctors' statements that Lia Lee would die were seen as evil curses rather than objective assessments.

and culture-bound syndromes such as possession, witchcraft, evil eye, and mental health conditions generally not recognized in Western psychiatry. Understanding these maladies in relation to the indigenous psychology reveals the culture-specific conceptions of personhood, self, and others.

This chapter helps you better understand both the nature of your self and that of others, providing models and perspectives that reveal relationships between individual characteristics and cultural beliefs that facilitate culturally sensitive health care. Other areas of interactions between culture and psychology are also considered in the effects of religion, rituals, and beliefs on physiological responses (Chapter Nine) and shamanistic healing practices and their use of altered states of consciousness as therapeutic tools (Chapter Ten).

CULTURAL CONCEPTS OF NORMALCY AND ABNORMALCY

Have you ever wondered what it means to be normal? What is "normal" is related to one's personal and cultural circumstances, including

- Cultural definitions of what is acceptable behavior and tolerable deviation

- Behaviors appropriate for different roles (e.g., priest versus church member)

- Behaviors appropriate for different contexts (e.g., school versus church)

- Influences on the significance of symptoms (e.g., when is a "late" menstrual period a concern?)

All cultures distinguish normal and abnormal behavior, but the specific criteria differ. Normalcy is what people of a particular group consider the ideal or preferred forms of behavior. One culture's concept of normal, even valued and esteemed, behavior may be seen as deviance from another culture's perspective. For example, some cultures' beliefs that illness is caused by witches, ghosts, and possession are viewed in other cultures as delusions and symptoms of psychiatric disorders. Western cultures' valuing of self-sufficiency is seen as deviant from many cultures' perspectives. Basic emotions such as aggression may be shunned and punished or used as a system for allocating prestige and esteem.

Cultural determination of what is normal or abnormal is illustrated in the following behaviors, which are normal in some cultural settings:

- Seeing spirits (hallucinations) of one's deceased parents or children

- Living with your parents as an unmarried adult

- Beating up your sister's boyfriend

- Drinking cow blood and smearing your body with dung

- Burning down your mother's house after she dies

All cultures recognize common symptoms of mental disturbance: for instance, when a person engages in behaviors that significantly depart from cultural norms, are erratic and unreasonable, do not make sense, or involve antisocial actions. But what may appear as unreasonable, delusional, or antisocial from one person's perspective may be a ritually structured acceptable behavior within another person's culture. An outsider may mistakenly view religious figures as psychotic and delusional when their behavior is seen as normal within their own cultures. Cultures distinguish ritual leaders from insane individuals. What constitutes deviant versus religious behavior is determined by cultural norms. Even if biomedical perspectives consider a condition to be an organic pathology, it may not be dysfunctional from the point of view of the culture. For example, temporal lobe seizures (epilepsy) manifested as possession may provide social benefits by facilitating ASCs (Winkelman, 2000a).

Labeling Theory of Deviance

Cultural perspectives are key to the dominant approach to deviance, the social labeling approach that views deviant behavior as the outcome of cultural and social conditions that "produce" deviance by determining what is normal and what is unacceptable. Culture and context, rather than biology, define most of what is deviant. Is it normal to kill yourself? Biologically it does not make sense, but many cultures induce such behaviors as self-sacrifice as well as leading its members to commit suicide because of failure, despondency, or mental illness. Although both involve effects leading to one's death, they are also culturally viewed as distinct.

Cultural norms also direct people to respond to deviant behavior in specific ways, including labeling of specific behaviors as abnormal and producing social responses that create further problems for those defined as deviant. These secondary consequences of labeling include expectations about the sick role and how others should treat a sick person. Even with biological diseases, social responses create additional biological consequences, as described in leprosy (see Chapter Two). The consequences of social responses are seen in the case of homosexuality. Men who have homosexual tendencies and are exposed to negative social labeling of homosexuality often react by internalizing society's negativity. This can produce guilt and shame and undermine self-esteem even before the individual actually engages in homosexual behavior. These responses are not universal; in some cultures, homosexual behavior is part of the normal development of all men, as described in Herdt's (1987) report on New Guinea culture.

Deviance reflects reactions to normative cultural values and expectations. Socialization processes communicate ideal values and norms and provide rewards and punishments to motivate people to adhere to those normative expectations. Those who do not adhere are deviants and are generally treated in ways to motivate them and others to conform to the expectations. Deviance can reflect intracultural diversity within the group (e.g., minorities), alternative cultural values (e.g., individualism versus conformity), an exaggeration of normative expectations (e.g., excessive materialism), or a protest against ideal expectations (e.g., hippie communalism). Deviance can reflect

- The loner who defies conventions

- Those who do not achieve the highest ideals

- Individuals who are unable to achieve normative expectations

- Social structuring of failure, such as labeling minorities as "mentally retarded"

Concepts of normal are cultural and situational (context specific) and related to particular roles (e.g., what is appropriate for men versus women). Beliefs considered signs of disturbed thinking in Western cultures (such as believing that witches are eating your liver or that your neighbor has used sorcery against you) are not signs of disturbed thought in cultures where they are normal beliefs. Even when a behavior is atypical or undesirable, whether or not it is evidence of an abnormality, can depend on situational expectations. Cultures recognize contexts in which departures from normalcy are expected (such as extreme grief, murderous revenge, or licentious sexuality) and permitted for short periods. Behavior is also evaluated as to the motivations of the individual for engaging in the behavior, such as religious inspiration, provocation, or confusing a person for a dangerous mythological being.

The relationships of cultural evaluations to the definition of deviance are seen in the different cultural views of possession, which vary from serious delusion to a normal cause of illness or to a source of divine inspiration. Possession is often seen as pathological or deviant, but where cultures have a positive view of possession, it may not have detrimental consequences.

Implications of Cultural Relativism for Concepts of Normal A major controversy between anthropology and psychiatry regarding mental illness involves the concept of cultural relativism and its implications. At the core of the controversy are questions about the biological universality versus cultural uniqueness of human experiences, including mental illness. Biomedicine and psychiatry have emphasized the universality of mental illness. Anthropology's emphasis on cultural relativism has different implications. Cultural relativism has weaker and stronger forms (Prince, Okpaku, and Merkel, 1998). The weak form holds that what is normal is culturally defined and can be understood only in the cultural context. The stronger form indicates that what is experienced in each culture is so unique that it is impossible to make valid cross-cultural comparisons. Whether one adheres to the weaker or stronger form of cultural relativism, the question of what is normal versus what is abnormal can be appropriately determined only in the context of a person's cultural expectations, beliefs, and situation. What is viewed as pathological aggression from one group's perspective might be considered righteous indignation and divine punishment in another. What constitutes a serious pathological disorder in one culture may be a reasonable adaptation in another. Symptoms must be evaluated in social and cultural contexts, as illustrated in the following section. Aspects of your own cultural concepts of normalcy may be assessed with the self-assessment exercise at the end of the chapter.

Culture and Personality Disorders

Because personality is created within a cultural system, it is necessary to assess behavior as normal or abnormal with reference to that context. The assessment of the cultural identity and background of clients and the cultural schemas for behavior in their culture enables the determination of whether they exhibit a personality disorder or a normative pattern. Behaviors that are characteristic of symptoms of a diagnostic category should not be considered as evidence of the existence of a mental illness if they are normal behaviors in a client's culture (Castillo, 1997a, 1997b, 1997c; Kleinman, 1980).

Castillo illustrates that some personality disorders recognized in the DSM-IV are normative patterns of behavior in particular cultures. Assumptions about a normal person in the DSM-IV are based on modern educated working or middle-class people. People socialized in premodern traditional societies may have religious beliefs or other behaviors that are viewed as symptoms of neurosis or psychosis in modern societies. Because dominant personality disorders emphasize behavior that is normal or typical in specific societies, it is vital that clinicians assess cultural identity dynamics to determine what a normal personality is for someone of that cultural background. This includes the individual's immediate psychosocial environment (family and community) and religious, spiritual, or ritual behaviors normative in his or her culture.

The failure to assess cultural expectations for behavior results in the ethnocentric imposition of a diagnostician's cultural concepts on a patient. The lack of consideration of cultural influences on symptom formation and expression can lead to errors in diagnosis and assessment. Paniagua (2005) provides basic guidelines for addressing the potential role of culture in psychopathologies:

- Self-assessment by providers to determine their own cultural biases

- Consultation with family members to determine if conditions are recognized as culture-bound syndromes or have particular cultural significance

- Asking questions using culturally sensitive and appropriate styles

Cultural factors can be assessed with the "Outline for Cultural Formulation and Glossary of Culture-Bound Syndromes" provided in Appendix 1 of the DSM-IV (American Psychiatric Association, 2000). This outline for cultural formulation is designed to supplement considerations of a client's ethnic identity and cultural background undertaken during the basic diagnostic process. The DSM-IV outline (p. 843) (also see Castillo, 1997a; Paniagua, 2005) stimulates inquiry into the following:

- The client's cultural identity, background, and use of cultural schemas, including involvement with the cultural group traditions and language and intracultural variation to avoid stereotyping

- Explanatory models (e.g., illness) for the client's conditions, including cultural influences on the expression of symptoms, cultural significance of the condition, and care preferences

- The client's level of functioning within the cultural-psychosocial environment. This requires an assessment of culturally relevant social stressors and social support, including emotional support, information, and material assistance from kin, religious groups, and the local community and the cultural views of and community responses to the patient's condition

- Cultural effects on client-physician relationships and communication, including differences in expected diagnosis and treatment and how the clinician's biases affect the encounter

- Overall cultural assessment of the significance of cultural variables in diagnosis and clinical reality, providing the basis for a negotiated solution in which the client's system (including family) and clinician agree about the course of care

BIOCULTURAL INTERACTIONS

Cultural Factors in Major Psychopathologies*

Adjustment disorders. The cultural background, acculturation, and family context need to be considered to determine whether the behavior is appropriate or excessive.

Anxiety disorders. Anxiety and panic disorders need to be assessed in relationship to cultural beliefs. If cultural beliefs in witches, sorcerers, and evil spirits are normative, these complaints need to be assessed in relation to what is normal within the community of reference for the client to determine if fear reactions are excessive. Phobias should be diagnosed only if the reactions are not in accordance with community beliefs and norms.

Avoidant and dependent behaviors. The cultural expectations regarding appropriate forms of avoidance, especially avoidance between people of specific status and relations (e.g., interclass, male-female, father-daughter-in-law avoidances) should be considered in making diagnoses.

Conduct disorders and antisocial personality. This diagnosis should not be applied to individuals living in areas of high crime, violence, and extreme impoverishment when the behaviors are in response to those conditions and adaptive for survival.

Delusional disorders. Content of potential delusions should be considered in relationship to religious and ethnomedical systems and the values and norms of the culture.

Depressive disorders. Diagnosis of depressive disorders needs to consider cultural expectations regarding demeanor and the normative manner of expression of depression (e.g., somatization).

Dissociative disorders. Attribution of dissociative disorders should generally not be made to clients in cultures where behaviors such as trance and possession are normative.

Learning disorders and mental retardation. The attribution of cognitive impairments should take into consideration the relationship of the cultural assumptions and biases of the

The failure to assess the cultural and social context of an individual can lead to many diagnostic errors, which are listed in the special feature "Biocultural Applications: Cultural Factors in Major Psychopathologies." The need for cultural assessments of normalcy is not just a clinical issue but a legal one as well. The fair treatment of people under law requires consideration of concepts of "reasonable behavior" and "state of mind" that are understood by a person from the perspectives of his or her cultural context. The application of these cultural concepts in assessing guilt or innocence in the cultural defense in criminal law provides roles for anthropologists as applied health advocates in their roles as expert witnesses (Winkelman, 1996b; also see the special feature "Applications: Cultural Defense as Advocacy in the Courtroom" in Chapter Three).

PERSONALITY AND SELF IN INDIGENOUS PSYCHOLOGY

An understanding of the dynamic relationships among biology, psychology, culture, and society is fundamental to explaining what is normal and abnormal as well as cultural illness and healing processes. Culture and biology interact through socialization testing instruments to the cultural background of the individual. These considerations should include language competence, familiarity with test material, and knowledge of social reasoning patterns and associations tapped by testing instruments.

Obsessive-compulsive disorders (OCD). Repetitive behaviors that are normative within the culture (e.g., religious rituals and customary behaviors or sayings) should not be the basis for OCD diagnosis.

Paranoid disorders. In making this diagnosis, considerations similar to those for delusional disorders are important (e.g., beliefs in aggressive spirits and witches, cultural expectations that their actions are frequent). Social norms regarding defensive behaviors, suspicions of others, fraud, deceit, and other aggressive behaviors need to be taken into consideration in determining the normative or abnormal nature of behavior.

Schizoid and schizotypal personality disorders. Cultural norms regarding social detachment and emotional expression and the expectations for people in specific positions (e.g., monks, law enforcement officials) need to be considered in assessment.

Schizophrenia and psychotic disorders. Behaviors and beliefs need to be assessed from the perspective of the client's culture. Behaviors such as spirit communication, hearing voices, and hallucinations that are experienced in culturally normative ways are not a basis for diagnosis.

Substance-related disorders. Diagnoses of substance abuse-related disorders need to consider cultural norms regarding substance use. Where cultures accept substances as normative and clients use them in normative ways, substance abuse disorders should not be diagnosed.

———————————

*Adapted from Paniaqua (2005).

experiences that elicit and shape biological development. This provides for the regularity of interactions among members of culture and their patterns of deviance and mental illness.

The regularity and predictability of behavior among people of a group derive from the effects of culture in patterning humans' biological capacities. Some aspects of social development and relations appear universally because of their necessity for human social life: for instance, awareness of self and others, gender distinctions, and the use of language. All humans require several models of themselves and others, a theory of mind that infers others' thoughts and intentions. This includes an indigenous psychology, a concept of normal personality and capacities, the internal motivations and mechanisms that explain what humans do and why. These overall conceptions of the internal capacities of humans are necessary for understanding others' intentions and achieving our goals as social beings. To achieve this, humans and other animals also develop concepts of self, identities related to internal differentiations in positions in society. These socially structured aspects of individual identity derive from a social position (status) within a network of different kinds of relationships (such as different positions on a team).

PRACTITIONER PROFILE

Richard J. Castillo

Richard J. Castillo, Ph.D., is professor of psychology at the University of Hawaii-West Oahu and clinical professor of psychiatry at the University of Hawaii School of Medicine. His interests are in how cultural factors affect the structure, etiology, and treatment of mental illness. His research and publications develop a holistic paradigm for the study of mental illness that integrates known neurobiological, psychological, social, and cultural factors. He was a DSM-IV Task Force Adviser on cross-cultural issues and on schizophrenia and other psychotic disorders. He serves as a cultural consultant on clinical cases for the Department of Psychiatry, University of Hawaii School of Medicine and the Hawaii State Hospital. He provides cultural sensitivity training for clinicians throughout Hawaii, nationally, and internationally.

Castillo chose to study medical anthropology because of Arthur Kleinman, who introduced him to the psychiatric concept of depersonalization, which is similar to the meditative experience of an observing self and a participating self. This experience is sought by Hindu yogis, but in Western psychiatry depersonalization is considered a symptom of mental illness. Because of many years of practicing yoga and meditation, this became the focus of his research. This led to articles published in the journal *Psychiatry* (1990) and in *Anthropology of Consciousness* (1991), in which he described nonpathological dissociation voluntarily sought through meditation practice.

Castillo made an important contribution that affected diagnostic criteria of dissociative disorders throughout the DSM-IV through published articles on cultural considerations for trance and possession disorders (1992a) and dissociative disorders (1992b). His work has also addressed the relationships among culture, dissociation, and the brain (see 1994a, 1994b, 1999). In addition, he has published two textbooks covering the cultural factors influencing mental illness: *Culture and Mental Illness: A Client-Centered Approach* (1997a) and *Meanings of Madness* (1998).

Concepts of personality and self embody representations of generic human qualities and capabilities as well as culturally specific notions regarding human capabilities and their sources, conceptions central to the notion of what is normal. They provide frameworks for understanding cultural and individual differences and similarities across cultures.

Personality and Indigenous Psychology

Personality involves the overall organization and dynamics of psychological processes that provide stability to behavior. Personality encompasses symbolic, mental, emotional, behavioral, and social capacities of a person as well as dispositions, drives, and memory. Understanding a person's personality and the *cultural* concepts of the nature of the internal organization and dynamics of the person allows us to make inferences about the meaning of that person's behavior.

All cultures have a personality theory: conceptions of the capacities and experiences of persons and models regarding how individual persons conduct themselves. These models often postulate souls, spirits, ancestors, lustful spirits, and possessing entities to explain behavior. Because such characterizations are not normally represented in Western psychological models, the concept of indigenous psychologies—cultural frameworks for understanding the bases of human nature and behavior—has been developed (see Heelas, 1981).

Indigenous psychologies meet human needs for concepts regarding what it is to be human (Heelas, 1981). They are necessary for understanding human beings to fulfill interrelated personal and social functions and to conceptualize aspects of the inner self, our emotions, motives and drives, personal will, sense of agency, and the soul. Indigenous psychologies provide a system of meaning to link an individual with the sociocultural order, sustaining the models of self that facilitate social relationships and enable the smooth operation of coordinated social life (Heelas, 1981; Lock, 1981a, 1981b). Indigenous conceptions of the nature of humans that are used in organizing collective social life employ supernatural concepts of identity, self, behavior, emotions, and agency.

Expressive Culture as Indigenous Psychology Indigenous psychologies are embedded in expressive culture: religion, mythology, folklore, music, and other aspects of culture that represent humans' appropriate social behavior, expected emotional reactions, and behavioral ideals. Expressive culture guides socialization and the development of personality through the models, ideals, and scenarios for behavior:

- Providing role models, exemplified in heroes and gods

- Expressing feelings and communicating culturally important meanings

- Formulating and expressing social sentiment

- Fulfilling psychological and social needs for understanding and identity

- Expressing ideal social behavior and social structure

Expressive culture's ideational and emotional content reveals personality dynamics, societal values, culturally important emotions, and the normative behavior of people. Expressive cultural material such as myths also manifests unconscious psychocultural dynamics, providing insight into the motivations driving cultural patterns. These sources of indigenous psychology express group sentiments and psychosocial dynamics, illustrating moral and ethical problems and exemplifying ideal responses.

Religion as Indigenous Psychology Religion is an important aspect of indigenous psychology, providing conceptualizations of models of the person and behavior through the values and meanings emphasized. Religious systems provide symbolic depictions of the ideal person and how to manage societal forces and interpersonal conflicts. Religions illustrate psychocultural dynamics and identity in ideals for individual behavior, rules for social behavior, and a cosmology: explanation about the origin and nature of the world, including humans. Religion provides a social identity in a "sacred self" (Pandian, 1997) that represents intrapsychic dynamics. Religious beliefs provide ultimate values and

CULTURE AND HEALTH

Indigenous Psychology and Self in Catholic Charismatic Healing

Csordas (1994) characterizes Catholic charismatic healing as engaging self-processes and emotions that are central themes of North American culture related to personal control and intimacy. Spiritual experiences provide release from the cultural emphasis on control in which believers surrender to deity and emotional needs for intimacy are met in personal relationships with Jesus. Charismatic healing processes affect personal identity through ritual practices that link the self, body, and the social world with the personal unconscious. Accepting the power of Jesus in one's life leads to a transformation of the self through relationships in which Jesus constitutes an "ideal other" for the creation of a positive sacred self.

Divinities play a role as internalized others that provide new self-models and facilitate the resolution of developmental blockages, fixations at earlier stages of self or emotional development. Csordas characterizes divine images as internal models that structure the development of a more mature self and relationships. A predominant theme in charismatic healing is related to the lack of intimacy or failure in intimacy, often stemming from childhood or marital relations. The divine embrace with Jesus substitutes for absent or lost parental or spousal intimacy, providing an enduring relation of interpersonal intimacy. The charismatic Catholic's personal relationship to Jesus

justifications, determining many attitudes and values, and organizing familial, economic, and political activities. Religions focus on conceptions of the inner self, emotions, consciousness, will, memories, and intentionality or agency, all exemplifying concepts of human nature. Understanding religious concepts in relationship to culture, psychological structures, and personal identity reveals their roles as indigenous psychology. Religious rituals can function as developmental guidelines derived from the influences of supernatural beliefs and entities as cultural models of the ideal person.

Self: Status and Roles

"Self" refers to a number of social aspects of identity (Spiro, 1993). Self is a socially referenced aspect of a person's identity based on relationships with others and their views of the person. Self is a consequence of the socialization of biological potentials for self-awareness through the development of personal and social identities in relationships with others. Self involves a social organism's representation of the organism, programmed by the expectations of the culture that provides information for both the organism and for others. Self includes many dimensions of identity, including social and personal perceptions of the individual as well as the desired self-qualities and identity in one's social presentation to others. Self is also experienced as one's internal locus of initiative and control, involving internalizations of the culture's conceptions of personality in general.

involving experiences of power, spiritual gifts, and inspiration produces a new sense of self through an intimate engagement with aspects of a primordial "real self." The divine entity provides protection and power that facilitates the patient in his or her confrontation with traumatic memories.

Csordas analyzes the charismatic movement's concern with demonology in relationship to its implications for the nature of the self. These evil beings are conceptualized as persons and intelligent entities whose qualities are represented in their names reflecting sins and negative emotions: greed, lust, anger, bitterness, and jealousy. These characteristics reveal negative attributes of the person. Demonic spirits are seen as attaching to the patient, bonding undesirable behaviors and emotions that must be severed to heal the patient. This freedom from bondage reflects cultural concerns with freedom and control. Demonic possession involves a loss of control that is compounded by the negative behaviors that the demonic entities produce in the person. These negative aspects are viewed as not-self, dissociated, and attributed to the demonic entity. Their effects on the person illustrate a crisis of control, a contested self, with the qualities of the demonic spirits reflecting cultural concerns about afflictions to the self. The nature of one's problem derived from the qualities of these demonic spirits may be exhibited indirectly in mannerism and mood of the patient, including facial and eye expression and bodily posture.

Self involves aspects of identity created by positions one holds in relationship to significant others, including

■ A sense of a status, a type of position within a social network

■ The associated **roles,** the responsibilities and behavioral expectations associated with that status or position

What is normal for a person is in part a function of one's position in various systems of status relationships (e.g., family, work, school, church, friends, clubs and associations). These socially ascribed status and roles may not, however, represent all personal identity. Social positions and roles provide models for behavior, but individuals may not completely adhere to those ideals. The person's private sense of self (self-representation) may differ from the social self presented for others. Socialization processes involve role negotiation, where people select their roles or try to change them.

Cultural ideals and norms regarding conceptions of status and the associated roles provide information about both common cultural psychology and intracultural psychological diversity. The specific status and the associated responsibilities defined within a culture illustrate primary ideal models for cultural identity. Cultural expectations for behavior of different statuses represent models of internal or intracultural variation in identity and psychocultural dynamics. Universal status positions and their role relationships (such as parent, child, spouse, sibling) are a basis for culture-specific roles (patterns of behavior, expectations, and identity) within categories of primary relations (i.e., culture-specific expectations of a father, son, husband, wife, brother, and sister). Cultural models of identity may be provided by the religious influences, exemplified in possession.

POSSESSION IN CLINICAL AND CROSS-CULTURAL PERSPECTIVES

Possession, the control of a person by spirits, takes many different forms and interpretations. Recall the scene of demonic possession in the movie, *The Exorcist,* where a small, frail girl acquires supernatural powers from the devil, along with a demonic appearance and an altered speaking voice. Although most possession episodes do not involve such extreme alterations of the person, the idea that a spirit takes over a person's body, will, and voice is common in cultures around the world. Possession involves experiences in which a person feels as though acted on by something experienced as an "other," controlling the person's subjective experience and behaviors.

The various possession phenomena indicate that cultural beliefs can play a central role in whether behavior is considered normal, a customary illness, a severe delusion, or valued conditions. Possession generally implies some ASC but may occur without it. Possession ASC—that is, manifested in dramatic changes in behavior and appearances, modes of speech, personality, consciousness, or awareness—is explained by a belief in a spirit or power that takes over and controls the person and his or her body and experiences (Bourguignon, 1976a, 1976b). The key issue is that although the culture views the person as being under the control of a spirit, biomedical views diagnose a mental illness.

Possession and Dissociative Disorders

Possession episodes are often characterized by symptoms taken as evidence of psychological disorders, such as "glazed eyes, psychomotor activity, change in facial expression and voice quality, and constricted attention, . . . sleep disturbances, depressed mood, psychosomatic ailments, anxiety and panic attacks" (Ward, 1989, p. 29). These associations have led to characterizations of possession as a **dissociative disorder,** where a split-off part of the personality temporarily controls the person. Dissociative reactions are considered to be adaptive, resulting in the creation of a separate identity and stream of consciousness that enables the person to continue to function by dissociating from the stress he or she experiences. Possession shifts responsibility from one's self by attributing the causes of one's actions and the sources of one's demands to spirits. Possession may permit the assumption of sick roles that can produce personal, emotional, social, and material benefits.

Dissociative disorders recognized in the DSM-IV include dissociative amnesia, dissociative fugue states, dissociative trance disorders, and dissociative identity disorders. Dissociative disorders typically involve a loss of consciousness or some loss of the integration of perception, motor function, memory, cognition, and personal identity (Castillo, 1997a). Dissociative disorders, like hysteria, involve sudden changes in memory, consciousness, identity, or motor behavior (Bourguignon, 1976a) as well as shivering, convulsions, physical complaints, and often periods of unconsciousness. There is not, however, a simple congruence between possession and hysteria because not all possessed individuals have hysterical characteristics.

Dissociative amnesia is characterized by the inability to recall extensive amounts of information. This memory loss cannot be explained as a function of ordinary forgetting and is usually the consequence of emotional trauma or stress. Dissociative amnesia is more frequently found in association with possession than other ASCs. However, when amnesia is associated with possession, it is amnesia for what happened during the possession ASC episode, not a general amnesia for what has happened in the immediate past (Winkelman, 1992a).

Dissociative fugue states involve the acquisition of a new identity or persona without awareness of a past identity and forgetting the new identity when the person returns to the previous one. The extended duration of the fugue state makes it an inappropriate diagnosis for possession because possession involves situations of a ritual specialist who returns to a normal social identity following the possession episode or a patient who has a temporary rather than a long-term change in identity.

Dissociative trance disorder is an additional DSM-IV diagnostic category involving a trance or a possession trance interpreted as the replacement of an ordinary personal identity by an entity. Castillo (1997a) considered this distinction necessary because of cultural differences in responses to dissociative disorders. Cultural differences in interpretation of the experiences produce different consequences for these dissociative experiences. In cultures where possession is accepted, dissociation can provide relief from distress. In modern cultures where such spirit possession is not normative, the dissociative experiences can increase distress. Castillo considers dissociative trance disorder to be an appropriate diagnosis only in conditions in which the possession trance is not part of the culture's religious practice or healing rituals and causes significant distress and social impairment, particularly in important areas such as occupational functioning (see DSM-IV, 1994, pp. 728–729).

Multiple Personality or Dissociative Identity Disorders

A diagnosis associated with possession is multiple personality disorder or its current term, dissociative identity disorder, where separate personalities develop dissociated from the ego. People in modern societies with dissociative identity disorder have symptoms similar to those of schizophrenia and are often misdiagnosed with schizophrenia (Castillo, 1997a). In premodern societies, the disorder is integrated into other syndromes, particularly possession by spirits.

Dissociative identity and multiple personality disorders involve two or more distinct personalities or identities with different periods of control over individual experiences and behavior. In this dissociative reaction, major aspects of the psyche, emotions, and behaviors acquire autonomy from the ego and control the individual's intentions and behavior. When the alternate personality is dominant, the ego is unconscious and subsequently amnesic, generally unaware of secondary identities, but secondary identities may be aware of one another and the primary identity.

Goodman (1988) explains why multiple personality disorder and possession are not role-playing, faking, acting, or self-hypnosis but instead psychological functions related to the neurophysiology of ASC. Although involving similar psychophysiological processes, these disorders differ considerably in the cultural perceptions of the phenomena. Dissociative identity disorder experiences are not interpreted in religious terms, and

BIOCULTURAL INTERACTIONS

Biological-Social Dynamics of Possession

The widespread manifestations of possession illustrate an underlying biological basis related to seizure phenomena. Possession has been associated with tremors and convulsions that indicate organic causes, which can be provoked by poor diet, trauma, stress, and disease (Winkelman, 1986b, 1992a). The conditions associated with possession—spontaneous illness and seizures, amnesia, tremors and convulsions, and compulsive motor behavior involving excessive, violent, and uncontrolled movements—indicate that behaviors and beliefs regarding possession may result from temporal lobe and epileptic syndromes. These may underlie the **possession trance** experiences of being controlled by something else: a spirit. Although possession concepts may be universal, their significance is associated with cultures of greater societal complexity (Bourguignon and Evascu, 1977). Possession experiences may be caused by social conditions, such as oppressive circumstances that destabilize consciousness, or by poor diet and mistreatment, which can provoke dissociation as a psychological defense. In formal cross-cultural studies of possession, both biological and social influences are involved as possession is significantly and independently predicted by both temporal lobe measures and political integration (Winkelman, 1986b, 1992a).

patients are generally ignorant of both the processes and occurrences (Krippner, 1987). Yet, most of the patients have an onset between the ages of sixteen and twenty-five years, the age range during which mediums and possession phenomena emerge cross-culturally (Winkelman, 1992a). Goodman suggests that behavioral similarities between possession and multiple personality disorder indicate that they are two different manifestations of the same human capacity. Major differences involve the ritual control exercised in possession cults, where cultural interpretations play an important role. Western cultures produce greater difficulties for a patient in treating the incidents as evidence of pathology, which compounds the patient's negative experiences and limits therapeutic success, in contrast to those cultures where the possession is accepted.

Possession as Normal Behavior

Possession may imply some illness or undesirable condition but may be a normative behavior that people emulate. The dominant psychiatric interpretations of possession as forms of mental illness fail to consider important positive cultural functions these conditions may have in healing, self-development, and personal expression. For instance, possession may be a professional qualification for healers, who acquire social prestige by being possessed by spirits. Positive cultural conceptions are illustrated in Goodman's definition of possession as a situation where a "supplicant asks a being of the other, the alternate reality, who possesses no physical body of its own, to descend into his/her body" (1988, p. 2). Asante (1984) describes possession as a transcendent state in African religions that involves enlightenment and a harmony with nature and the universe, one where the person possesses gods and goddesses and acquires their qualities.

A single culture or tradition may distinguish forms of possession, as described in Krippner's (1987) review of Brazilian spiritists' differentiations of five grades of possession:

- "Grade one possession" involves a person under the control of an alien spirit, feeling compelled to do certain behaviors but retaining a basic sense of self and identity, similar to the irrational behaviors associated with obsessive-compulsive neurosis

- "Grade two possession" involves past-life personalities or splits within the individual's psyche, such as hysterical personality syndrome and a negative alternate personality

- "Grade three possession" involves the control of a victim through practices of sorcery

- "Grade four possession" and "grade five possession" involve more complete forms of control of the individual by other spirits who inhabit their bodies and direct their behavior; these experiences may be deliberately sought in religious healing rituals

Possession involves a range of alterations of self and consciousness. Possession engages varying degrees of influence, different psychodynamic conditions, both dissociative pathology and normative social behavior where interpersonal communication with the spirit beings provides transformative influences on the self. Possession allows greater flexibility in relationships, the assumption of new statuses and roles, with negotiations mediated by the different "beings" presented by the possessed person. A meek grandmother becomes possessed by "the general" and commands the community to specific courses of action with the authority of a mythical figure.

Boddy (1994) characterizes possession as working on behalf of women and their families, using spirits to channel assistance in meeting responsibilities. Possession may provide a means of indirect communication by subordinate people who cannot challenge authority on their own but who do so through the possessing spirits. Possession is used to manage problems of everyday life, allowing spirits to change relations between spouses. Spirit communication contributes to health by using the threats of supernatural powers to modulate relationships with others and provide social support. Possession can evoke catharsis (release) of troublesome emotions, producing identity changes, altering power relations, and providing resources for managing stress.

Possession enables someone to be someone else, diversifying the self by incorporating the "other's" roles and associated behaviors to achieve specific goals. Possession provides processes for incorporating various others into personal development, reformulating and expanding identity and self-expression. Possession may even be incorporated into expressive modalities in drama, theater, and political activities where it functions as a mode of cultural resistance or accommodation to change through models provided for traditional identity.

Summary Possession has been attributed to a variety of psychiatric diagnoses, but whether a possession episode should even be subjected to psychiatric classification depends on the cultural interpretation. In cultures where possession is a valued and desired condition and entered voluntarily by an individual, there may be no justification for attributing a psychiatric diagnosis. Where possession occurs under specific social conditions and is viewed as illness, it may be considered pathological. Even where viewed as illness, possession may be a normative condition with positive psychodynamic functions.

BIOCULTURAL APPROACHES TO INDIGENOUS PSYCHOLOGY

Cultural acquisition and personality development derive from socialization, which develops universal psychobiological potentials into culturally specific psychodynamics. Universal psychobiological capacities for social identity are developed under cultural processes that instill collective patterns of culture, norms, and ideals into an individual's biological development. Humans' biological capacities for attachment, emotions, and behavior are formed in culturally specific ways.

Culture's Developmental Effects on Brain Plasticity

Castillo (1997a) outlines neurobiological effects of cultural adaptation, where cultural learning and memory formation induce developmental changes in the brain's neuronal microstructures. Culture gets wired into the brain through modifications in brain neuronal structures from learning cultural categories and responses. Cultural learning modifies the nervous system in producing long-term potentiation. This involves repetitive interactions with the environment through cultural schemas that result in the imprinting of the cultural patterns in brain microstructures and the formation of specific neural pathways to respond to cultural events (Castillo, 1997a).

This ability of learning to affect neuronal structures undermines traditional assumptions about the homogeneity of the human brain. Although all humans have the same brain macrostructures, the neurobiology of learning and memory imply the potential of culture to exert influences at the cellular, molecular, and neuronal levels as cultural schemas are internalized in the individual in the plastic neuronal structures of the brain. Learning, adaptation, environmental and emotional stress, and interpretations of these experiences evoke physiological responses; these have effects on the microstructure of the brain's neuronal system's dendrites, neurotransmitter receptors, and hormones. Culture becomes structured in neural networks through habitual interpretation, action, and thinking created by socialization (see the section in Chapter Nine, "Biosocialization").

The brain's neuronal formation through learning enables culture to have effects on causes, manifestations, and outcomes of mental disorders (Castillo, 1997a). Culture affects the formation of neural pathways through exposure of its members to stressful events as well as the resources provided for ameliorating stress. Some effects are a consequence of interpretive systems (meaning) and habitual patterns for responding to environmental stressors. Culture-specific schemas used in cognitive processing elicit emotion and cognition, stimulating the responses acquired in the development of the neural networks. The brain development acquired in response to cultural patterns can also induce maladaptive patterns of behavior and thinking, leading to mental illness through adaptations to emotional stress and trauma. Consequently, cultural factors can affect outcomes of mental illness using other cultural schemas—rituals—to elicit brain microstructures that can manage culturally induced mental illnesses.

Psychocultural Adaptations to Universal Biological Features

Basic areas of cultural influence on biosocial aspects of identity involve

- Biologically based needs, emotions, gender differentiation, and life-cycle development

- Psychocultural adaptations of self and personality to the indigenous psychology, the cultural models of a person

- Psychocultural adaptations to society, including ethnicity: individual identity in relationship to others

Universal biosocial features of human life, such as drives, emotions, gender, and developmental stages provide perspectives for examining cultural identity and personality.

Primary Needs and Drives The cultural significance and structuring of basic needs, motivations, and desires reveal cultural psychology. The socialization and development of primary needs (such as food, protection, procreation, affiliation) and their linkages to social values reveal psychocultural dynamics and priorities.

Emotions Cultural shaping of a person involves a selective expression of emotions. Emotions have both biological and cultural aspects (see Chapter Seven). Psychocultural dynamics are illustrated in the socialization of emotions and their culturally patterned manifestations. Emotions illustrate psychocultural dynamics because they are always shaped by culture. Culture influences what evokes emotions, their inhibition, and cultural ideals regarding their expression and significance. Normative and ideal cultural values associated with the expression of basic emotions illustrate cultural psychology. Cross-cultural perspectives illustrate cultural psychology in unique emotions and culturally typical emotional dysfunctions and illness.

Gender Roles Universal aspects of human psychocultural dynamics involve cultural differentiation of male and female roles, thus providing significant patterning of behavior and self-concepts. A culture's normative patterns for men versus women are fundamental aspects of psychocultural dynamics and cultural psychology.

Life Stages Development across the life cycle provides perspectives on psychocultural dynamics. Culturally patterned expressions managing universal features of human life—birth, adult transition, marriage, and death—illustrate enculturation of primary roles and emotional relationships. Culturally defined conceptions of life stages and changes in identity across stages reveal culturally specific aspects of the personality, social roles, and identity. Cultural adaptations to universal features of life-cycle development, and culture-specific stages and psychocultural dynamics, are relevant to appropriate health assessments and care (see the special feature "Applications: Culture in Human Development and Clinical Assessment").

APPLICATIONS

Culture in Human Development and Clinical Assessment

The notion that humans go through fixed universal phases of development, a feature of life span or developmental psychology, is generally presumed rather than demonstrated. For example, adolescence is generally considered to be a normal universal aspect of development, a consequence of puberty. This is despite evidence that adolescence is not present in all cultures but, rather, developed as a part of the historical social differentiation of the merchant class in Europe. Cultural differences in patterns of development are illustrated in the ethnographic materials from many cultures (e.g., see Munroe and Munroe, 1975).

An accurate assessment of health and developmental status requires a recognition of cultural influences on assessment and physical development. Criteria customarily used are based on norms for a middle-class U.S. population, whose average physical size is greater than that found for many other groups. If these standard norms are used, children from other ethnic groups, especially Asian, will be considered to be underdeveloped. Cultures differ in their ideals about appropriate care, socialization, behavior, and development. Cultural ideals may conflict with health care practices or law. Cultural influences on health change across the life cycle as new roles, expectations, and activities alter behavior and exposure to risks. Medical anthropology can help identify culturally mediated risk factors and developmental influences.

Age Reckoning

A misleading assessment of development may result from how people calculate the age of a child. Whereas Euro-American norms see the child as being zero years old at birth, others consider the child to be one year old at birth. Chinese traditions add another year to age at the Chinese New Year rather than the birth date. This can result in a child born at the end of the calendar year being considered two years old within months of birth by the Chinese system and mistakenly suggest an underdeveloped child.

Caregiving and Neglect

Cultural beliefs about appropriate caregivers vary considerably. Euro-American norms traditionally considered the mother to be the primary caregiver, but other cultures have considered grandmothers, aunts, or sisters to be the primary caregivers. Failure to appreciate cultural norms regarding caregiving has led Euro-American social service workers to consider a child abandoned or neglected when not under the primary care of the mother or nuclear family. This tragic cross-cultural misunderstanding has resulted in the forced removal and foster placement and adoption of Native American children.

Sleeping Practices

Sleeping relations with infants vary, ranging from cultures in which an infant is always in direct human contact to those in which newborns are isolated in their own room and bed. Most societies' norms for contact with infants are more intense than is typical in the United States. Many cultures have the mother or other caretaker constantly carrying the child on the chest or back, permitting immediate response to an infant's needs.

Infanticide and Neglect

Cultural preferences for male children affect infanticide and abortion. In cultures with strong preferences for male children, medical tests to determine sex may be used to make decisions to abort female fetuses. Similar preferences for male children are linked to female infanticide. However, not all "neglect" constitutes abuse; in some cultures, it is traditional to allow the mother to rest after birthing, "neglecting" her child who is cared for by other relatives. Neglect may also reflect realistic expectations about child survival and practices that allocate resources to ensure survival of healthier children (Scheper-Hughes, 1987, 1992).

Circumcision and Clitorectomy

Ideas about normal surgical alteration of genitals vary widely. American biomedical norms regarding male circumcision are based more in cultural tradition than empirical evidence. Cultural influences that guide providers' behaviors need to be countered with an understanding of other cultures' practices and preferences. Women who have had clitorectomy (female circumcision) and other genital procedures have special health care needs in terms of contact with male care providers and advice regarding sex, menstruation, pregnancy, and delivery.

Punishment and Abuse

Cross-cultural conflicts result from recent developments in the United States in which child abuse has been legally defined, and providers are mandated to report suspected cases of abuse. Cultural conceptions of appropriate punishment vary widely, placing health care providers in a position of needing to educate some clients about the law. Campaigns to discourage child abuse need to consider cultural differences in physical treatment and care. Understanding cultural practices provides a basis for appropriate health education and prevention of problems for the family. Cultures employ ethnomedical treatment practices with consequences that may be misunderstood as abuse. The Asian practice of "coining," where a hot coin is rubbed on the body, may produce welts and bruises. Failure to recognize the source of such marks and misreporting them as abuse can have catastrophic consequences. Cultural competence entails the ability to differentiate ethnomedical practices from abuse.

Puberty and Adolescence

Puberty and adolescence are closely related in America, which confuses biological and cultural stages of development. Puberty is a biological phenomenon of hormonally induced sexual development. Adolescence is a particular way in which the onset of sexual maturity is socially managed. Some cultures allow for marriage when puberty is reached, including constitutional laws that

Continued

authorize marriage at age fourteen years or younger (e.g., Mexico). Cultural differences create the potential for disastrous misunderstandings, where a man may be charged with sexual abuse of a minor for relationships with what his culture considers a legitimate mate. Social service agencies often consider these cultural dynamics in deciding the merits of maintaining a family relationship versus criminal prosecution.

Aging Processes

Both social expectations and biological processes affect aging and its debilitating consequences. Social class differences in morbidity and mortality illustrate social influences on aging. How the aged are treated and the respect and consideration they expect differ among cultures. Culturally sensitive health care requires the recognition of these expectations. Expectations for care of the aged are rooted in cultural beliefs. Understanding these expectations permits more effective care and enhanced patient satisfaction.

Death

Because death is a regular occurrence, biomedical personnel become accustomed, even callous, to death as part of the coping processes involved in uncertainty, powerlessness, and responsibility for the gravest of human issues. Medical attitudes of opposition to death as a sign of failure contrast with most cultures' acceptance of death. Life support systems create special problems in the care of a terminally ill person, especially where cultural norms dictate extreme dedication to one's parents. The termination of life support and do-not-resuscitate orders may be unacceptable or require culturally specific management. Knowledge of the appropriate death rituals and grieving procedures makes adaptation easier for health personnel and families. Knowledge of families' expectations in the hours following death enables staff to assist, plan, and adjust to accommodate patients' families in these difficult times.

These **psychocultural adaptations,** the development of psychobiological capacities in culturally specific ways, are illustrated in universal enculturation into

- Normative institutional goals, rules, status (social positions), and roles
- Situational norms for managing social and motivational pressures
- Behavioral patterns derived from personality dispositions and characteristics
- Satisfactions and frustrations of drives
- Behavioral disorders and deviant behavior (LeVine, 1974)

Ethnic Identity

The relationships of culture to psychology produce differences among ethnic groups. Ethnicity (individual identity as a member of a group) derives from individuals' relationships to the multiple influences of their own culture and the broader society. Ethnicity derives from interactions among psychology, culture, and society, that is, from how individuals develop their biologically based potentials for personal and social identity through relationships with their own culture and other social groups. Significant foci in representation of ethnicity include (Winkelman, 2001c)

- Beliefs regarding the inherent characteristics of people as social beings

- Concepts of persons and their inherent characteristics, an indigenous cultural psychology

- The self in contrast to models of identity provided by out-group others

- Formation of biological drives, capacities, and potentials in cultural patterns

Ethnic identity is multidimensional and implicit, an emerging knowledge about one's self created by influences operating outside of the self. Ethnic identity is affected by exposure to cultural and social learning experiences and historical and external factors. Awareness of ethnic identity is a developmental process, beginning with largely unconscious or taken-for-granted concepts, based on others' attributions, and potentially continuing through self-examinations leading to ethnic awareness or even the development of cultural competency and bicultural identities (see Winkelman, 2005, for discussion). Ethnicity is more than ascribed group membership but derives from relationships with others. This may produce an ethnic identity that varies across circumstances, with multiple selves expressed in different circumstances.

Ethnic groups are not homogeneous but have internal variability in characteristics of members of an ethnic group. This requires characterization of both normative cultural characteristics and the major patterns of internal variations in identity and behavior within the ethnic group membership. This occurs in differences such as generation; degree of acculturation; strength of identification; commitment to the ethnic group identity; peer group preference; interest, knowledge, and involvement in the culture; and minority status and experiences of prejudice, discrimination, and powerlessness (Phinney, 1996). Assessing these influences on individual psychology and well-being requires consideration of a number of dimensions of cultural psychology: influences from history and other groups; child-rearing environments and goals; behavioral ideals embodied in social statuses and roles; beliefs about human nature, an indigenous psychology; and cultural values and expressive ideologies and their effects on attitudes and behaviors. Frameworks for studying these diverse inputs to ethnicity are provided by conceptual models developed in psychological anthropology.

Psychocultural Model of Human Development

Anthropological approaches to personality and ethnicity view them as mediating between two main aspects of culture: the primary institutions of society (infrastructure and social structure) that provide formative experiences and the secondary institutions (ideological or superstructural beliefs: religion, folklore, mythology, cosmology, etc.) that manifest models for the personality processes and dynamics. Personality mediates between material experiences and expressions. Expressive culture (such as religion, myth, folklore, stories, song, drama, art, performance, literature, proverbs, poetry, music, ballads) project (or manifest) personality processes, cultural ideals, and normative patterns of behavior, constituting an expression of indigenous psychology.

The psychocultural model (Whiting and Whiting, 1975) provides a cultural-ecological systems approach for examining personality within the contexts of biological, environmental, social structural, and ideological influences. The psychocultural model emphasizes seven main influences: history, environment, the maintenance (cultural) system, child-rearing environment, innate needs, learned behaviors, and projective systems, including indigenous personalities reflected in myth and religion. LeVine's (1974) evolutionary model of population psychology emphasizes four cultural adaptations of individual personality: environmental, primary parental socialization, secondary socialization, and group adaptations to population norms. The psychocultural model, integrated with the evolutionary model of population psychology, provides a broad framework for examining the different components of cultural systems that affect cultural psychology and identity (Figure 6.1).

The diverse inputs into these models and the bases for variation across many aspects of the culture provide frameworks for assessing both intercultural (between cultures) differences and intracultural (within culture) variations (see Winkelman, 1998, 1999, 2001c, 2005, 2006a). Variations within the same culture may derive from differences in socialization experiences, environmental influences, family history and structures, economic opportunities, secondary socialization experiences (school, military, sports, religion, or prison), and immediate peer and adult models. Behavior and identity are produced within an integrated cultural system in which any aspect can impact socialization and development.

Environment Environment and its resources have many influences on development, not just physically but socially as well. Perspectives on environmental relationships are important for understanding how individuals may not have access to resources or may be affected by environments outside of their immediate setting (e.g., how the international drug trafficking and drug wars affect local communities without contact with the international level).

History Cultural history provides models for both parents and children in personality as well as relationships with other groups that play a role in the development of opportunities and identity. History includes cumulative cultural history and outside social influences that affect self and other conceptions and models for personal behavior.

Cultural System The cultural (or maintenance) system includes influences from the domestic economy of family, kinship structures, and community as well as infrastructure, resources, and the political economy. Patterns of work are considered particularly powerful influences on socialization experiences and value orientations imparted to children and have far broader influences on development and health, as detailed in Chapter Four.

History
Traditions and beliefs
Intergroup relations

Environment
Ecosystem relations and adaptations
Migrations and borrowings

Maintenance System/Cultural and Social System

Production
Subsistence and work patterns
Means of production
Division of labor

Domestic Economy
Family organization
Kinship patterns
Community organization

Reproduction
Population size
Fertility patterns

Political Economy
Political systems
Social structure and stratification
Law and social control

Child's Learning Environment
    Settings occupied
    Caretaker relations and teachers
    Tasks assigned
    Mother's work

Socialization of Biological Needs
Needs, drives and capacities
Emotions and attachment
Sex and family roles
Secondary social drives

Learned
Behavioral styles
Skills and abilities
Value priorities
Conflicts and defenses

Secondary Socialization
Stages of life-cycle development
Social roles
Initiation and adult transition
Mesosystems, exosystems, and macrosystem relations

Individual Adult
Material and social organization of behavior
Social roles
Population ideals and norms

Projective/Expressive Systems

    Religious beliefs and practices
    Art and recreation
    Deviance, crime, and suicide rates
    Indigenous psychology

    Ritual and ceremony
    Games and play
    Culture-Bound Syndromes

FIGURE 6.1. *Expanded Psychocultural Model*

Innate Potentials Cultures mold innate potentials in the formation of childhood personality. These involve physiological, psychological, and social functions, including bonding and personal attachment, eating, sex and reproduction, emotional relations and communication, self-representation and internalization of social others, and the direction of primary and secondary drives.

Child Rearing The child care environment and cultural customs that guide parents' interactions with children are in part adaptations to ecological pressures. Primary socialization involves parental behaviors, rewards, and punishments that shape children's behavior. These influences may be supplemented with secondary socialization influences—schools, military, peers, work, initiation—that produce a distinct self to adjust the individual to the normative expectations of adult personality, self-image, and social roles reflecting cultural ideals. Family influences are primary in the child's learning environment and transmission of cultural influences in the development of innate potentials. Although family is universal, its status, roles, and influences are variable, producing both cultural and individual influences on social roles, gender, personal identity, emotional expression, learning styles, and behavioral patterns.

Adult Personality and Projective Systems Adult personality and its characteristics and dynamics involve an indigenous psychology, a projective system expressed in religion, mythology, cosmology, ritual, art, drama, stories, proverbs, poetry, music, ballads, legends, and oral traditions. This expressive material represents cultural psychology and identity through displaying group ideals for behavior and models regarding the expression of emotions. Expressive culture reveals the cultural collective unconscious and psychocultural patterns. These representations of the cultural person provide indigenous psychologies. Theories of illness engage these beliefs about the self and the conditions and factors that affect it.

ETHNOMEDICAL THEORIES OF ILLNESS

How can we effectively conceptualize the differences among and similarities across cultures in their views of illness? Early approaches emphasized distinctions among scientific, folk, and primitive medicine:

■ Primitive medicine is based on magic and the supernatural world

■ Folk medicine is based on tradition, home remedies, and community healers

■ Scientific medicine is based on experiments and problem solving

These distinctions may have an intuitive appeal, but they are of limited usefulness because the categories share the characteristics that are supposed to distinguish them. Folk medicine also involves problem solving and includes magical methods. Magic is also based on tradition, takes problem-solving approaches, and includes empirical components such as plant phytochemicals, simple surgical procedures, massage, effects on emotions, and sanitary practices (avoidance of contamination). Biomedicine is based not only on scientific approaches but also involves clinical rituals and cultural traditions that are not always scientifically based, currently accepted, or actually useful for patients.

BIOCULTURAL INTERACTIONS

Susto: "Magical Fright"

Susto is an ethnomedical syndrome found in many Latin American societies and other parts of the world. The conceptualization of susto in Mexico and Latin America is that it involves the separation of an individual's spiritual aspect, or soul, from the physical body. Typically, it is believed that the individual's soul is driven away by a frightful experience that may happen directly to the victim or to a member of the victim's family. Weaker members of the family (women or children), rather than the individual who directly experienced the frightening occurrence, may be the victims of susto and soul loss.

Symptoms attributed to susto include generalized pains and fevers, listlessness ("low energy") and loss of strength and motivation, a depression or period of introversion, and weight and appetite loss (see Rubel, O'Nell, and Collado, 1985). Rubel and colleagues did an empirical study to test three major hypotheses regarding the cause of susto: physical disease conditions, psychiatric disorders, or social stress and social role performance. Their data, collected in the state of Oaxaca, Mexico, assessed organic conditions (physical health), psychoemotional conditions, and social relations, comparing patients diagnosed with susto (*asustados*) with a matched control group. Their primary hypotheses postulated that susto was the consequence of self-perceptions of personal inadequacies with respect to meeting social role expectations. They found significant positive associations of the social stress measure in those suffering susto. Their study also found a general association between susto and organic disease; however, no particular organic disease was implicated as being associated with susto. In general, the asustados had higher levels of sickness and organic disease than the matched control group. This higher level of organic dysfunction was clearly illustrated in a comparison of mortality in the control group. At a seven-year follow-up, none of the control group members had died, but about one-sixth of the asustado group had died, suggesting that this ethnomedical syndrome reflects more than just social failure.

However, the asustados did not show higher levels of psychoemotional illness or psychiatric impairment with respect to the controls, leading the authors to conclude that it was unwarranted to attribute susto to emotional pathology. Rather, it is a consequence of social role expectations and cultural understandings. The failure to meet social expectations and to fulfill critical aspects of social roles induces stress, which may account for both the occurrence of susto and the higher levels of nonspecific mortality due to organic diseases. Even though it is a psychological condition, it still has physical consequences. All maladies, illness as well as disease, are both biological and cultural, a necessary interaction.

All ethnomedicines rely on useful empirical knowledge for managing practical problems of illness and sickness. The predominant theories of illness found in cultures around the world have emphasized the importance of supernatural theories of illness. Magical and ritual healing activities have a variety of empirical, real, and adaptive effects.

BIOCULTURAL INTERACTIONS

Sleep Paralysis Syndrome

The Hmong experience an unusual incidence of what has been called "nightmare deaths" and sugar-coated with the term "sudden unexpected nocturnal death syndrome" (Bliatout, 1983). Death often occurs during sleep. The Hmong refugees in America experience nightmares of reliving horrific war scenes and being pursued by the dead. Some survivors report the sensation of a large spirit that sits on them, suffocating and squashing them to death. A sense of paralysis prevents them from resisting or calling out and leaves them exhausted and terrorized if they survive the experience. For the Hmong, sometimes such experiences have been interpreted as communication from the ancestors or warnings of impending disasters. Now, however, they are generally attributed to the consequence of their horrific experiences and trauma in Southeast Asia while fleeing attacks by communists.

Culture-Bound Syndromes

The term *folk illness* has been used to refer to many conditions not recognized in biomedicine, such as soul loss, bewitchment, and possession. Because of negative connotations of "folk," other terms have been introduced to refer to these maladies found in ethnomedical traditions around the world. **Culture-bound syndromes** refer to culturally recognized illnesses such as witchcraft or soul loss that are not included in biomedical or psychiatric diagnostic systems. Besides soul loss, these include "penis shrinkage" (in Chinese, *koro*), magical fright (in Spanish, *susto*), and "nightmare deaths." Culture-bound syndromes are conventionally understood as culturally specific systems of behavioral, psychological, cognitive, and emotional disorders that derive from the psychological, interpersonal, and social dynamics specific to a culture. Most conceptualizations of these syndromes have assumed that they are cultural illnesses without a biological basis. Yet, there are similarities, perhaps even universal manifestations, of some ethnomedical syndromes. Are these diverse illnesses derived from biology, from culture, or both?

Culture-bound syndromes are generally viewed in standard biomedical or psychiatric diagnostic schemes as not being real. This perspective has ethnocentric biases, reflecting cultural assumptions regarding what is real. Should only conditions with a biological cause be considered real? Even if not a physical disease, an illness may have consequences for mortality, as illustrated in Rubel's long-term study of susto (Rubel, O'Nell, and Collado, 1985).

The assumption that culture-bound syndromes are derived from a single set of cultural circumstances undermines any effort at scientific comparison and explanation. The classic notion of "culture bound" implies its presence in a single culture and, by extension, that the condition is a consequence of cultural and social causes, not biological factors. There are similarities in this syndrome in distinct regions of the world, implying that some have a biological basis (Simons and Hughes, 1985). Some ethnomedical syndromes

Some characteristic features of their nightmares are not unique to the Hmong, but parallel the "old hag" syndrome, a form of sleep paralysis reported in Newfoundland (Ness, 1985). This is an immobilizing dream in which one typically experiences an "old hag," a person or large animal, seated on one's chest while one struggles violently to free one's self. The individual normally leaves the paralyzed state and comes to full consciousness when touched or spoken to but feels exhausted. A well-recognized medical syndrome known as sleep paralysis exemplifies the physiological characteristics of being awake but unable to move, clarity of consciousness, and awareness of surroundings, often coupled with high levels of anxiety. This condition is recognized in the medical literature but not in psychiatrists' diagnostic categories (DSM). If it were more prevalent in our culture, it might become a clinical and diagnostic concern.

involve recognized biological conditions not yet formally categorized in the DSM, as illustrated in the cross-cultural manifestations of a sleep paralysis syndrome.

The parallels between the Hmong and Newfoundland cases illustrate why there are questions about the validity of the assumptions of culture-bound, implying unique cultural conditions that cannot be compared cross-culturally. Anthropologist Hahn (1995) has criticized the concept of a culture-bound syndrome as obscuring the interactive roles of culture and biology in illness, giving the false impression that some illnesses are culture-specific and independent of biology. This implication distracts from the multidisciplinary approaches necessary to understand the manifestations of illness in the interaction of one's physiology with mind, self-concept, and social relations.

An alternative to the term *culture-bound syndrome* is *culture-reactive syndrome* (Hughes, 1985). Rather than viewing these illnesses as specific and exclusive to a single culture, culture-reactive syndrome includes the possibility that a variety of cultures may produce similar psychological disorders. The concept of culture-reactive syndrome emphasizes that local cultural conditions or social relations predispose members of a population toward particular kinds of disorders. For instance, cultures that induce a lot of sexual anxiety produce the psychological generation of anxiety, illustrated in the genital retraction syndrome.

The perspective of a culture-reactive syndrome emphasizes the importance of considering the sociocultural factors disposing particular kinds of illness disorders. For instance, cultural factors in complex industrial societies may predispose our own culture-bound syndromes in conditions such as premenstrual syndrome, type A personality, agoraphobia (fear of leaving the house), obesity, anorexia nervosa, and road rage. The concept of "culture-reactive" nonetheless has problematic assumptions in implicitly suggesting that some ailments are not "cultural reactive." As discussed in Chapter Two, even physical diseases have cultural dynamics, a reaction to the cultural and social milieu, rather than

BIOCULTURAL INTERACTIONS

"Ghost Illness"

The interaction of physiology with cultural, psychological, and social influences is illustrated in the Comanche concept, "ghost illness" (Henderson and Adour, 1981). Ghost sickness, as the name implies, involves a belief that ghosts, often one's deceased relatives, can cause illness. Ghosts are thought to make their relatives sick to cause them to die and join them. Ghost illness is manifested by symptoms indicative of facial paralysis (Bell's palsy), such as drooping of the face, mouth, or eyelids on the affected side and facial contortions, impaired blinking, numbness, and tearing. Henderson and Adour's biocultural analysis reveals precipitating organic and psychosocial factors and an interaction between them that produces Comanche ghost sickness.

Biomedical research on facial paralysis has established a variety of organic factors. These include the disruption of nerve conduction caused by pressure on the canals housing the facial nerves, which can be caused by diabetes, infections, or physical trauma. A primary viral agent includes the herpesvirus, which may be dormant until stress results in its reactivation and disruption of nerve conduction. These viruses may provide a mechanism through which the widely recognized **psychogenic** ideology of ghost sickness operates.

Jones (1972) reviewed the psychosocial contributions to the manifestations of ghost sickness. The victims have often faced rejection in their efforts to reenter Comanche society, and their ghost sickness episodes reaffirm Comanche identity because it is a Comanche illness. Fright has also been implicated in the medical literature in precipitating facial paralysis. Vascular spasms can result from emotional trauma, placing pressure on facial nerves and disrupting nerve conduction. Cultural beliefs and expectations regarding contact with ghosts also contribute to the production of intensely frightening experiences that can trigger insult to the facial nerve through hormonal secretions. Ghost illness may be triggered by these and other contributing factors, including the emotional stress caused by marginalization, poor nutritional status due to low income, and lowered resistance to metabolic diseases or prior infection.

consequences derived only from biology. Hahn (1995) emphasizes that "all human conditions are *equally* biologic *and* cultural *and* social, cognitive, psychologic, *and* psychodynamic" (p. 59). Illnesses are determined 100 percent by biology and 100 percent by experiences produced in interaction with the environment. And as the incidences of ghost illness illustrate, the biological and the cultural are not separate and distinct influences when psychosomatic dynamics induce physiological responses to cultural beliefs.

Ethnomedical Syndromes Shortcomings of the terms folk illness, culture-bound syndromes, and culture-reactive syndromes illustrate the need for a more general term such as *ethnomedical syndrome*. Ethnomedical syndrome does not imply that a malady is

BIOCULTURAL INTERACTIONS

Genital Retraction Illness

Several ethnomedical syndromes in Southeast Asia and China involve genital retraction. Known in China as *koro*, it involves acute anxiety accompanied by the sensation of shrinkage of the penis. Genital retraction conditions are found in other parts of the world and are associated with a variety of medical conditions; it also occurs under conditions of panic without other major psychiatric disorders. It is not considered a disease or psychiatric illness in the Western medical literature, although there are reports of penile retraction, particularly by men under conditions of extreme threat to life experienced in combat. The lack of significance in Western cultures may reflect the lack of significant cultural concerns about this condition. The presence of the syndrome in cultures where it is not pathologized nor considered to be an illness illustrates that cultural beliefs are central to the acute anxiety associated with the condition. The interaction between cultural and personal implications, coupled with anxiety, can create a feedback loop in which the condition is exacerbated (continued penile decrease). Suggestion combined with hysterical panic reactions can create a cyclical pattern of manifestation of this syndrome.

The importance of psychocultural dynamics in koro is reflected in the epidemic occurrences of this illness in Chinese culture. These occurrences may not reflect physiological retraction but, rather, a panic reaction based on the fear of such retraction and its personal consequences. The relative lack of importance of this syndrome in some cultures, in comparison with its hysterical epidemic occurrence in others, illustrates cultural influences on a biologically based genital retraction syndrome. In some cultures, there is an extreme fear and anxiety associated with the belief in the illness, which is reinforced by others. This reinforcement creates a psychosocial dynamic lacking in cultures in which the physiological retraction occurs without social reinforcement. Other cultures have different ways of eliminating the fear using pharmaceutical substances to ensure erections.

unrelated to biology, and it may have similarities to biomedical syndromes when stripped of cultural features. Careful assessment of various ethnomedical syndromes blurs the distinction between conditions recognized in biomedicine and those recognized in other ethnomedical traditions. The conditions recognized by Western medicine can be labeled in a parallel way as *biomedical syndromes*. Ethnomedical syndromes are found in biomedicine as well; psychiatric concerns and diagnostic categories are not culture-free but also reflect cultural conceptions. Ethnomedical syndromes, like biomedical diseases, are manifested in a complex interplay among biological, social, and cultural factors with individual circumstances. Too much cultural specificity in a description (e.g., reference to specific myths that "explain" the illness) necessarily makes it appear culture-bound. Descriptions based on behavior rather than cultural interpretations make a syndrome more generalizable. The extent to which the surrounding context is included in the definition restricts ("culture binds") a defined syndrome. The term *syndromes* conveys the conception of a related group of symptoms that occur together, reflecting universals that may involve underlying biological processes.

Biobehavioral Perspective on Ethnomedical Syndromes

The culture-bound approach to ethnomedical syndromes emphasizes the importance of cultural meanings in determining the nature of these maladies. The similarities in ethnomedical syndromes in different cultures imply that they are not strictly *cultural* but share common biological underpinnings.

Taxon is an organizational framework for identifying underlying biological bases for similar ethnomedical syndromes (Simons and Hughes, 1985). The *taxon* is a biological concept that refers to groupings based on similarity in characteristics. Taxons reflect a *taxis* (plural, *taxes*), a biologically based reflex response (behaviors) of an organism to external stimuli. These stereotyped responses of a species, such as startle reflexes and defensive postures, reflect the genetic heritage that elicits and organizes stereotypical whole-body behavioral responses to significant events. All mammals show similar physiological and behavioral reactions to being startled by a loud noise, an adaptive defensive and orienting posture.

Biological bases for the similarities suggest the grouping of various ethnomedical syndromes based on common behavioral or descriptive data indicating a relationship to a known biological taxon. Simons and Hughes (1985) apply the concept of taxon to organize ethnomedical syndromes based on a sleep paralysis taxon (e.g., nightmare death), the genital retraction taxon (koro), the fright reaction taxon (susto), and the startle-matching taxon (e.g., *latah*). The special feature "Biocultural Interactions: *Latah* and the Startle Taxon" shows the tension between culture-specific interpretations of ethnomedical syndromes and the cross-cultural and universal perspectives based in underlying biological potentials.

There are biological, cultural, and psychodynamic influences on all ethnomedical syndromes. The biological substrate of human experience means that no events are completely culture-free nor completely culture-bound. This is reflected in Simons's perspective on the Malaysian latah as a cultural elaboration of the startle reflex, which is universal and biologically based, being found in other mammals as well. Cultures differ in the extent to which this biological reaction is elaborated in cultural activities or even shaped into a recognizable disease syndrome. Examining different ethnomedical syndromes for biologically based taxons does not reduce them to biology alone but seeks to explain the similarities cross-culturally in these conditions in how cultural conditions have effects on specific physiological structures. Simons (1985) emphasizes the importance of distinguishing between factors that provide the descriptive features, shape, or form of a syndrome and those that explain its prevalence in one area as opposed to another. The origins of the form or structure may be biological, but the differential distribution, and thus the proximate cause, must be explained by social and enculturation influences that elicit and shape these biological potentials.

Identifying social conditions that elicit these taxes requires a cross-cultural comparative approach to the social influences associated with specific conditions. Understanding

BIOCULTURAL INTERACTIONS

Latah **and the Startle Taxon**

A classic approach to culture-bound syndromes is illustrated in Kenny's (1978, 1985) work on the *latah* syndrome in Malaysia. The etymological origins of the term are not known, although it means something like "jumpy," "nervous," or" ticklish" (Simons, 1996). The Malaysian *latah* is the best known of what Simons characterizes as the "startle-matching syndrome." Latah is characterized by involuntary responses to sudden fright, an excessive startle. It is a response that may result in dissociation and compulsive behaviors, including the repetition of obscene words, disobedience to orders, and mimicking others' movements. For instance, a person who is startled by a loud sound might jump up and run around wildly, screaming obscenities, until calmed by others. Many other cultures have similar syndromes related to the startle taxon, leading Simons to consider the concept of latah to be cross-cultural.

Kenny, however, characterizes latah as culturally specific, related to broader meanings within Malay-Indonesian cultures, and reflecting marginality, in contrast with normative cultural expectations of order and self-control. Kenny considers latah to be a culture-specific exploitation of meanings related to identity. Although symptoms similar to latah are found in other cultures (the startle and fright reactions, mimicry, compulsive obedience, and unacceptable sexual verbalization), these elements are related in different ways in different cultural contexts. Kenny considers latah startle responses to result from social conditions rather than biological factors.

Although a hyperstartle response may be viewed as part of human nature, cultural patterns and social influences elicit these responses. The behaviors and their meanings come not from biology but from socially conditioned performances that are learned and exhibited in specific relations. To understand latah, we must examine the situation-dependent cultural meanings and the social performance of behavioral displays that originate in cultural learning and social expectations, rather than in reflex processes. Cultural meanings and situation-specific responses are the essence of the latah syndrome; the startle reflex provides no understanding of the cultural context that produces latah. Kenny's perspective reflects interpretive approaches where phenomena are understood strictly in terms of the local culture and their meaningful fit with other local meanings. This approach does not attempt general theories of behavior or social psychodynamics. Kenny's position is one in which the behaviors, practices, ideology, and values associated with latah fit only local circumstances found in Malaysia. In contrast, Simons sees the Malay-Indonesian latah as a specific example of a more general behavioral response sequence to environmental stimuli, a biologically based startle response that is elaborated in different ways in different cultures.

the culturally unique, socially structured, and biologically potentiated aspects of health maladies requires a multimethod perspective and approach to integrating many levels of observation and explanation (Browner, Ortiz de Montellano, and Rubel, 1988), including

- Indigenous theories of sickness, their emic descriptions of the condition, beliefs about causes, personal experiences, and understandings of the situation and treatment processes

- Use of comparative categories that relate cultural phenomena to universal structures

- Relationship of the condition to human anatomy and physiology to provide a standardized framework for comparison

These kinds of data are essential to relating ethnomedical syndromes of one group to similar syndromes found in other cultural groups. The characteristics of people in each culture who are more likely to be afflicted help to identify the contextual factors and social causes of the condition. Cross-cultural studies of theories of illness are part of this process of identifying the culture-specific causes of ethnomedical syndromes with cross-cultural research. The usefulness of combining indigenous theories with cross-cultural comparisons is illustrated in an examination of universal and cross-cultural theories of illness.

CROSS-CULTURAL ETHNOMEDICAL SYNDROMES

The efforts to understand the commonalities in the diverse ethnomedical systems of the world have produced systems that reflect the values and assumptions of Western thought. For instance, the separation of natural and supernatural theories is common, although many cultures do not make the natural-supernatural dichotomy characteristic of modern thought. Nonetheless, there are similarities across cultures that suggest the need to develop etic categories that represent the universal or cross-cultural commonalities in ethnomedical concepts of illness (see Erickson, 2008). Based on a cross-cultural study, anthropologist Murdock (1980) suggested some major types of theories of illness causation, both natural and supernatural (personalistic) forms. The supernatural categories were most numerous, including supernatural aggression and human magical aggression such as sorcery and witchcraft. There were other mystical forms of illness causation such as taboo violation and mystical retribution. Personalistic systems that attribute the cause of illness to human or supernatural agents that act against a person are found in most ethnomedical systems; they appear to constitute universal religious healing beliefs (Winkelman and Winkelman, 1991).

Natural Disease Causation

Naturalistic systems explain disease within an impersonal system, one of natural forces or conditions that are disturbed from their natural equilibrium. Although naturalistic beliefs are not prominent in most ethnomedical systems, they are universally recognized causes of maladies. Naturalistic systems include biomedicine, osteopathy, chiropractic and humoral medicine, Chinese medicine, Ayurvedic medicine of India, and many herbal traditions. Personalistic and naturalistic theories are analytically distinct but not mutually exclusive. Both may be present within a single disease: for instance, where sorcery (a personalistic cause) may dispose one to accidents (natural cause). Emotional causation of illness may fall into either category, evoked by supernatural (spirits, hexes) or interpersonal influences (threats, attacks, ridicule) that cause emotional responses.

Theories of natural causation ascribe maladies to the physiological consequences of something the victim experiences, such as traumatic experiences, infection, stress, organic deterioration, accident, and overt human aggression. Natural causation includes causes recognized by biomedicine (e.g., injury) as well as those not generally recognized by biomedicine (e.g., illness caused by cold temperatures, heat, wind, dryness, etc.). Although stress is considered to be a cause of illness in about half of the societies studied worldwide and overt human aggression as a universally recognized human impulse, Murdock (1980) reported that natural causes were rarely considered important in the overall explanation of illness.

This may reflect a failure to recognize the empirical, physical, psychosocial, and socioemotional aspects of ethnomedical practices. Green (1999a) points out that the natural causation theories are much more widespread than recognized (also see the special feature "Applications: Using Indigenous Contagion Theory in Public Health Education"). Another cross-cultural study (Winkelman and Winkelman, 1991) found that the shaman, often considered a spiritual healer, also uses physical remedies for diseases, accidents, and wounds based on assumptions of natural causation. These involve massage, washing and cleansing the body, using herbal remedies based on plant materials or other natural substances, and simple surgical incisions to remove foreign objects and abscesses.

Natural causation theories may also be embedded in supernatural systems of belief that reflect innate aspects of human psychology. Human nature is predisposed to a belief in spirits. This acceptance of the reality of spirits reflects a range of adaptive human tendencies, beginning with a "hyperactive agency-detection device." This concept reflects the notion that humans are hardwired to respond to the world as if there were purposeful unseen agents that are the underlying causes of the phenomena we experience. The human tendency to attribute illness to spirits derives from our ability to search for and detect unseen predators and to attribute to an unknown other our human mental, emotional, and social properties (Winkelman, 2004a).

Balance Both natural and supernatural models of maladies have concepts of balance among varying forces, such as dry and damp, hot and cold, air and fire, and many others. Although some of these contrasts are explicitly based in naturalistic frameworks, there are also many systems in which the contrasting principles of balance are not so clearly just material or physical, such as the Chinese medicine concept of yin and yang. A significant area of balance concepts of well-being that is found cross-culturally involves the notion that emotions, too, must be balanced for well-being and that excesses in emotions may cause illness.

Emotions Emotions are recognized as significant causes of maladies in most cultures, but emotional causes of health problems have not been significant in the biomedical view of disease causation. Emotional diseases have generally been recognized in biomedicine,

CULTURE AND HEALTH

Hot-Cold Theory in Mexican American Ethnomedicine

The hot-cold beliefs in Mexican American ethnomedicine are based on principles of classification that have little if anything to do with temperature. Foods are a primary area in which hot-and-cold concepts are applied, but the conceptual framework is also applied to colors and illness. Cold foods include fruits and vegetables whereas meats, spicy foods, and alcohol are considered to be hot. Similarly, red is generally considered to be hot whereas blue is a cold color. Conditions such as menstrual cramps and pneumonia are considered cold, but pregnancy, diabetes, and hypertension are considered hot. The classification of illness, medicines, and foods with respect to this system has a strong effect on patients' compliance with biomedical treatments.

The treatment of hot-cold diseases follows the principle of "neutralization" in which a condition is treated with a substance with opposite qualities. These principles can be employed by the health care provider to ensure compliance. If a health care provider prescribes a diet, treatment, or colored medication without taking into consideration the client's point of view with respect to their classification as having hot or cold effects, noncompliance may result. As an example, common colds are generally thought to be a "cold" disease that should be treated by hot remedies. However, the frequently recommended juices are seen as cold substances and therefore not appropriate for a cold disease. Rather than focusing on juices as a source of fluids, other liquids such as teas, soups, and the like can be given with the same (or better) medical effects and without conflict with the client's beliefs system.

The hot-cold theory, therefore, can be used by providers to reinforce adherence to the regular treatment regimen. For instance, if a client considers a disease and the remedy to be cold conditions or substances, compliance with the cold medical treatment might be achieved by providing the patient with an additional substance to counteract the cold properties of the medicine. These could be foods, activities, or other medications or placebos. However, because the hot-cold theory and its applications vary widely, the health care provider must determine the particular clients' beliefs and discuss how an appropriate balance might be achieved.

but they are seen more as the consequence of other causes rather than causes themselves. In many cultures, however, emotions may be seen as causes of illness. This includes a wide range of ethnomedical theories of illness found in Mexican and Mexican American cultures documented by Kay (1996). Besides susto, discussed earlier, these include *celos* (jealousy), *corage* (rage), *envidia* (envy), *tristesa* (sadness), *nervios* (nerves, anxiety), and others that have an explicit notion that emotions lie at the cause of emotional imbalance. Emotions are natural causes of illness, but these theories make assumptions about causes of maladies that are similar to personalistic theories: that a malady is the result of someone's or something's ill intentions.

Personalistic Theories of Supernatural Causation

The most prevalent and important theories of illness found cross-culturally in premodern societies involved theories of supernatural illness causation that involve personalistic assumption, meaning that some personal agent acted aggressively to cause the malady. These notions of personalistic cause, such as embodied in the concept of an evil witch or ghost causing illness, are based on assumptions not recognized by modern medical science as being valid. Although framed in supernatural terms regarding the powers of unusual humans or evil spirits, these theories may nonetheless represent important psychodynamic, social, and physical processes relevant to health. The most prevalent and important supernatural theories of illness are related to concepts of animism—the spirit world—where attacks or punishment from spirit entities are reflected in a universal theory of illness, what Murdock (1980) called "spirit aggression."

Animistic Causation Animistic causes of illness involve the actions of a supernatural entity such as a spirit or ghost; these universal beliefs involve the attribution that some unseen entity is the cause of our problems. Murdock (1980) considered two principal types of animistic causation: spirit aggression and soul loss. Spirit aggression is a universal belief that illness is caused by the aggressive action of spirits, an attack involving the spirits putting something into or doing something to a person's body. Spirit aggression also includes spirit possession (see above). Soul loss involves a person having an aspect of his or her self, the soul or spirit, leave during a dream or as a result of the soul being frightened or captured by a spirit or act of sorcery. This concept of soul loss as the absence of some vital essence of the person is examined in the context of shamanic practices in Chapter Ten.

Magical Causation Theories of magical causation involve the ascription of illness to actions of another person. This malicious human (sorcerer or witch) has negative effects on others' health from overt actions or inadvertent emotions, particularly envy or jealousy. A distinction between sorcery and witchcraft reflects important differences involving intentional and unintentional effects, respectively. Sorcery involves the impairment of health caused by the intentional aggressive use of magic, affected either by the individual's power or through assistance provided by a specialized sorcerer or spirits. Sorcery as a cause of illness is found in most societies of the world. The other societies generally have beliefs in witchcraft, an impairment of the health of persons, animals, or crops caused by involuntary actions of special types of humans with innate powers to cause harm (see Evans-Pritchard, 1937). Witchcraft is found predominantly in the circum-Mediterranean region, where it is nearly universal, but is rare in the rest of the world.

A similar belief involves the "evil eye" (see Maloney, 1976). In this belief, someone can inadvertently cause harm by looking at another's property or person. Evil eye power is frequently thought to emanate from the eyes (or mouth) of persons as a result of their envy. Murdock's cross-cultural research indicates that sorcery is strongly associated with preliterate societies whereas witchcraft is strongly associated with societies with patrilineal descent, substantial bride price, and social stratification. Evil eye beliefs are found in all major cultural regions of the world (Roberts, 1976) but are concentrated in the circum-Mediterranean region and mostly associated with complex societies. Murdock

BIOCULTURAL INTERACTIONS

Magical Malevolence as Causes of Illness in Mexican American Culture

Mexican ethnomedical beliefs involving a person causing illness to another through magical means—*mal ojo* ("evil eye"), *mal puesto, hechiceria,* and *embrujameinto* (witchcraft and sorcery)—are found in cultures around the world. These illness beliefs share a sociopsychological dimension in attributing the cause of an individual's illness to others with whom the person has strained social relations. Mal ojo occurs when someone who has "strong vision" looks on one with an evil eye. Strong stares of envy, a lot of attention, and looking at or praising (without touching) a child are thought to cause mal ojo. The consequences come from the emotional desire and may occur inadvertently through the power of envy. Mal ojo may be treated with "cleansing" with an egg, crossing the body, and saying prayers or removed if the person with strong vision touches the person they admired. *Mal puesto,* a sorcery or hex, has more severe implications, attributing illness to peoples' deliberate action, the intentional placing of a spell or curse on another. This may involve *hechiceria* and *brujeria* (sorcery), ritual acts carried out alone or with the help of a magical practitioner (*brujo, hechicero*).

Therapeutic approaches taken by Leininger (1973) with Mexican American witchcraft illness involve an initial interaction with the family of the victim, assessing their history and talking about extended social relations and past occurrences of witchcraft. This typically results in the expression of concerns that reveal unresolved problems within the extended family, resulting from accultura-tion conflict regarding sexual behavior, social roles, and mother-daughter relationships. The dynamics underlying witchcraft reflect conflicts within the extended family, with the witchcraft

(1980) suggests that sorcery is widely available in societies that have widespread access to supernatural power, where everyone can access supernatural power (e.g., see discussion of the guardian spirit complex in Chapter Ten).

Sorcery and witchcraft constitute complementary explanations of illness due to human malevolent magic. Sorcery is actually practiced whereas witchcraft is an attribution where the actual practices are likely absent. An earlier cross-cultural study (Winkelman, (1992a) found beliefs about specialized sorcerer or witch practitioners that were significantly correlated with political integration beyond the level of the local community. The social characteristics and psychodynamic attributes of illness attributed to sorcery and witchcraft reveal that they reflect social tensions, frustrations, and anxieties and function in social control (Middleton and Winter, 1963; Marwick, 1970). Walker (1970) illustrates how sorcery and witchcraft serve adjustive functions (explanatory, instructive, and ameliorative) and adaptive functions (social control, unification, and governance); they also have dysfunctional aspects in disrupting social relations (Finkler, 1985a). The psychosocial dynamics of witchcraft beliefs are illustrated in the special victims involving those who were accused of flagrant violations of traditional norms. The family is generally unaware of the displacement obvious in discussion of the witchcraft problem. As therapy resolves family conflicts, anger and displacement subside, as do witchcraft symptoms.

The out-group members accused of being witches often accept their designation but see their role as one of protecting their own family from the violations committed by the victim. Their denunciations of the witchcraft victim state the unacceptable behavior for their own families. In the context of diagnoses of witchcraft-induced illness, the projection of blame on extended family members enhances in-group cohesion within the immediate family.

Witchcraft beliefs play important roles in coping with problems generated by acculturative changes and expressing disapproval of new behavioral norms adopted by the younger generations. Expressive therapy allows a focus on social and family problems and assistance with acculturation changes, enabling the family to function as a viable cohesive social unit. In the process of therapy, the belief in witchcraft is not challenged nor is it interpreted as psychotic or delusional behavior. Rather, it is recognized as culturally normative and part of the intercultural adjustment process.

Cultural perspectives emphasize the actions causing the illness, whereas anthropological explanations tend to focus on intragroup or intergroup dynamics. Witchcraft accusations reflect group tensions and in-group and out-group attributions of blame and culpability. The causes of the attribution are found in many psychological and social interaction dynamics: tensions and stress, beliefs and practices, intergroup conflict, distrust, scapegoating, cultural and value conflict, and cultural change. Witchcraft accusations can displace the in group's responsibility for causing stress-induced emotional illness in one of its own members by blaming the cause of the sorcery or witchcraft on the out-group.

feature "Biocultural Interactions: Magical Malevolence as Causes of Illness in Mexican American Culture." In Chapter Nine, we discuss the psychophysical consequences of hex death and **nocebo effects**—or negative placebos.

Impersonal Supernatural Punishment Significant features of supernatural theories involve punishment for misbehavior, what Murdock (1980) called "mystical illnesses": the "automatic consequence of some act or experience of the victim mediated by putative impersonal causal relationships rather than by the intervention of a human or supernatural being" (p. 17). An impersonal supernatural *power,* rather than the deliberate actions of supernatural *beings,* is considered to be the cause. Four major categories of mystical causation considered by Murdock include

- *Mystical retribution,* the automatic consequences of violating taboos (forbidden acts) or moral injunctions; while perhaps mediated by supernatural beings, mystical retribution emphasizes automatic consequences (like touching an electrical wire) rather than supernatural judgment. The major categories of taboos are concerned with

CULTURE AND HEALTH

Contagious Magic as Adaptive Cognition

Anthropologist Frazer (1900) pointed to a universal law of magic, the "law of contagion" or "contact," wherein once there is a contact between objects, an influence is thought to remain even after the separation of the objects. Contagion is implied by beliefs regarding the transfer of some quality, essence, or effect from a source to a target, exemplified in pollution and contamination. Nemeroff and Rozin (2000) analyzed behaviors based on the law of contagion, where contact with an object is thought to transfer some of its qualities, a positive or negative charge. They point to principles embodied in the cognitive processes of contagious thought that have adaptive advantages.

Nemeroff and Rozin reviewed psychological research that illustrates the origins and functions of these aspects of magic, which are universal principles not only of primitive thought but also of modern thought. For example, laboratory studies show that the avoidance of objects that have been in physical contact with "contaminated" or "polluted" sources (e.g., AIDS patients) reflects contagion fears rather than any rational beliefs or empirical facts about transmission.

Why should we modern people behave in ways characteristic of the superstitions of primitive magic? These cognitive tendencies are a part of human adaptations that have survival value. Humans have adapted to avoiding contact with a variety of potentially harmful influences, including strangers, bodily excretions, decaying and dead objects, and other contaminated sources of potential harm. We are also disposed to seek out contact with positive objects—family and kin, holy figures, and powerful leaders—hoping that their influences will be extended to ourselves, enhancing our protection, well-being, and self-esteem. Contagious aversion appears to be reversed among close kin and with those with whom we have love bonds, illustrated in food sharing and sexual intimacy.

behaviors with respect to food, drink, sex prohibitions, etiquette, ritual, property, and verbal taboos. This reflects a moral dimension to the causation of illness, a belief that by transgressing the norms of society, one becomes ill.

- *Fate* is invoked to explain that an illness is determined by one's personal destiny, such as embodied in astrological systems.

- *Ominous sensations* include dreams, visions, or other sensations such as seeing certain animals or events that cause illness, including unusual people, sickness, or death.

- *Contagion* involves contact with a polluting object, including animals, substances, classes of persons, or bodily discharges, especially menstrual blood and corpses.

The concepts of contagion and associated avoidance behaviors reflect adaptive behaviors that also allow us to consider them as naturalistic theories of disease. Pollution ideas include the notion that rotten food, corpses, and objects associated with the dead are

Negative contagion fears are more developed than positive ones, probably reflecting the adaptive advantages of avoiding potentially contaminating objects. Contagion beliefs have adaptive value in the domain of food. Food avoidances based on contamination can help reduce microbial infections, and interpersonal avoidances may reduce the transmission of disease. The principles of contagion are well manifested in food aversions, where humans avoid food that has been in proximity to contaminated objects, motivated by powerful elicitations of the emotion of disgust.

Nemeroff and Rozin (2000) suggest that the concept of microbial contamination involves an empirically validated instance of contagion, exemplifying the magical belief that a negative influence can be transmitted by contact of a source with a recipient. They propose that the recognized mechanism of microbe-borne physical illness via the oral route (by mouth) is the original source of adaptation for beliefs regarding contagion. Contagion avoidance is linked to acts of cleanliness and hygiene that reduce the effects of germs on human health.

Magical thinking is natural and intuitive to human thought and in some cases literally true, mapping out the actual contingencies in the universe. Practical efforts to limit the effects of contagion are found in rituals that limit contact with the ill. The magical postulation of unseen forces can be seen as validated by modern scientific concepts of gravitational, magnetic, and electrical fields; invisible (to-the-eye) germs; DNA traces from our fingerprints; the effects of vaccinations; the mind-over-matter effects found in psychoneuroimmunology and placebo effects; and interpersonal influences on perception, emotions, and behavior. Such perspectives also apparently manifest a realization of microscopic pathogens, as illustrated in the discussion of Green's (1999a) work in "Applications: Using Indigenous Contagion Theory in Public Health Education."

dangerous; these can be considered as empirical beliefs about the transmission of disease. These principles appear to be deeply engrained in the human psyche, a part of our evolved psychology, as illustrated in the adaptive nature of the thought processes underlying contagious magic.

Summary There is a social psychology of supernatural illness beliefs. The specific social patterns found in the cross-cultural distribution of theories of illness illustrate the overall psychosocial dynamics of illness. All societies have beliefs about illness due to spirit aggression; most also have beliefs in magical causation (sorcery or witchcraft). In small-scale hunter-gatherer societies, three theories predominate: soul loss, spirit aggression, and sorcery. In complex societies, spirit aggression illness involves possessing spirits. As societies become more complex, theories of witchcraft and evil eyes (as opposed to sorcery) become more important. Naturalistic theories are found in all societies but become dominant only in a few modern societies.

APPLICATIONS

Using Indigenous Contagion Theory in Public Health Education

The incorporation of indigenous healers into public health programs is of vital importance because they provide the vast majority of medical services worldwide. Programs for the prevention of contagious disease typically fail to incorporate indigenous concepts regarding contamination; this is particularly significant because many involve avoidance of naturalistic infectious agents and polluting environments that biomedicine recognizes as sources of infection. Green (1999a) suggests that indigenous beliefs be used in public health programs for addressing contagious disease because they express ideas similar to germ theory. Health education programs that use the indigenous language and conceptual frameworks provide a culturally relevant platform that facilitates the adoption of preventive behaviors.

Green points out that concepts about diseases caused by small worms are widespread in Africa. These theories are overlooked because they do not fit with the stereotype that indigenous disease theories are animistic and supernatural, illustrated in Murdock's (1980) consideration of contagion beliefs as mystical causation and pollution as a supernatural belief. Validating the beliefs of indigenous systems enhances the ability to bridge traditional systems and health education.

Indigenous theories are in substantial agreement with biomedical models in interpreting some of Africa's most serious diseases in a naturalistic framework that Green calls "indigenous contagion theory." This theory assumes that diseases result from exposures, including a "folk germ theory" of naturalistic infection, pollution, environmental exposures, and taboo violation. Naturalistic infection theories reflect medically sound beliefs in considering diseases to be caused by the presence of tiny organisms, often worms or insects, and other entities invisible to the eye and emphasizing the avoidance of exposure to polluting, impure, and contaminating substances.

CHAPTER SUMMARY

This chapter shows that culture is a basic concern in psychology, psychiatry, and determinations of normalcy and the relevance of symptoms. These assumptions are part of the cultural formation of self and personality through the processes of socialization. Mental illness is a major area in which cultural perspectives contribute to an understanding of health maladies and illustrate the limitations of the biomedical perspectives as a universally valid system for diagnoses and classification. The manifestations of these cultural effects on personality and self are addressed through a biocultural framework that illustrates the basis for the interaction of culture and personality and the central importance of culture in understanding person, self, and identity. Anthropological models provide frameworks for describing cultural effects on universal biosocial substrates and cultural differences in psychology in terms of universal features of social life: self, status positions, roles, and concepts of the person (personality). Expressive culture provides materials for articulating an indigenous psychology theory whereas biosocial approaches provide frameworks for assessing cultural effects on human biological universals. These cultural influences on the normal formation

Naturalistic ideas are also emphasized in beliefs that certain environments cause illness, including excessive sun exposure and inhalation of air, dust, vapors, and fumes. Pollution beliefs involve the avoidance of contact with polluting substances: clothes, personal items, food, and other objects associated with a person with disease, as well as dirt, animals, and bodily discharges (menstrual blood, fetuses, pus). Indigenous contagion theory includes a belief that disease occurs as a consequence of illicit sexual intercourse.

Green (1999a) proposes that these indigenous contagion beliefs should play a central role in public health programs aimed at reducing the spread of AIDS. Indigenous healers are presented with perhaps most of the cases of STDs in Africa and treat many of these conditions. The treatments may not be adequate for curing AIDS, but the traditional beliefs may have an important role in prevention. Indigenous theories often attribute sexual illness to promiscuity and multiple sexual partners, and emphasize the importance of limiting sexual contact to marriage. Indigenous theories of STDs generally involve the belief that they are caused by microscopic or invisible animals or contact with bodily secretions; consequently, naturalistic infection and pollution are the dominant theories of the spread of STD, concurring with biomedical models. Prevention emphasizes appropriate moral restraint, cleanliness and hygiene, and taboo observances, particularly the avoidance of contact with reproductive fluids. Treatment practices involving traditional medicines, amulets, rituals, and purification may not be effective in curing STDs, but traditional beliefs regarding sexual relations are good prevention. Green proposes that health education campaigns use indigenous theories, language, concepts, and beliefs to make messages more meaningful, acceptable, and motivating to target populations.

of the person are illustrated in examinations of possession and other culture-bound syndromes that illustrate cultural variations in conceptions of personality and normal functioning. Analyses of these mental illnesses in relationship to cultural systems provide an understanding of their role as aspects of an indigenous psychology.

KEY TERMS

Altered state of consciousness (ASC)
Culture-bound syndromes
Dissociative disorder
DSM (Diagnostic and Statistical Manual of Mental Disorders)
Folk psychology
Indigenous psychology
Personality
Possession

Psychocultural adaptations
Roles
Self
Socialization
Somatization
Somatoform disorders
Status
Taxon

SELF-ASSESSMENT 6.1.   CULTURE AND PSYCHOLOGY

What do you view as the principal social positions ("status," such as mother, son, nurse, student, etc.) that define who you are?

What aspects of your cultural background motivate the ways in which you present your self-image and identity to others? What characteristics do you want others to note about you?

What aspects of your physical body affect your behavior? For example, do activities of any of your organ systems (heart, liver, gallbladder, or ovaries or testes) cause you to behave in certain ways?

What emotions do you think are basic to human nature? How does your culture evaluate those emotions? Which emotions do you feel form an essential part of your identity?

What personality characteristics do you think are innate to women? To men?

What personality characteristics does your culture instill in women? In men?

SELF-ASSESSMENT 6.2.   CULTURE AND NORMALCY

Assess each of the following behaviors and evaluate them as to their normalcy, from completely normal to highly deviant. What values determine your assessment?

A son burns down the house in which his mother died.

   Completely normal   Normal but unusual   Somewhat deviant   Highly deviant

A family kills their daughter because she lost her virginity before marriage.

   Completely normal   Normal but unusual   Somewhat deviant   Highly deviant

A family has a party to celebrate the birth of a child to their unmarried daughter.

   Completely normal   Normal but unusual   Somewhat deviant   Highly deviant

A person is condemned to death for providing a medicine (heroin) that makes people feel good.

   Completely normal   Normal but unusual   Somewhat deviant   Highly deviant

A woman wears black for the rest of her life following her husband's death.

   Completely normal   Normal but unusual   Somewhat deviant   Highly deviant

A woman drinks alcohol frequently after her divorce.

   Completely normal   Normal but unusual   Somewhat deviant   Highly deviant

A thirty-year-old unmarried man lives with his parents.

   Completely normal   Normal but unusual   Somewhat deviant   Highly deviant

A young woman stays up late night after night reading books.

   Completely normal   Normal but unusual   Somewhat deviant   Highly deviant

A young woman stays up late night after night going to bars and parties.

   Completely normal   Normal but unusual   Somewhat deviant   Highly deviant

A family hallucinates the presence of their son for months after his untimely death.

    Completely normal   Normal but unusual   Somewhat deviant   Highly deviant

A family consults with an oracle to decide whether to invest in buying a farm.

    Completely normal   Normal but unusual   Somewhat deviant   Highly deviant

A man behaves erratically and attributes his actions to the wishes of his deceased grandfather.

    Completely normal   Normal but unusual   Somewhat deviant   Highly deviant

Do you know of cultural groups in which these behaviors are considered to be completely normal?

Do you know of cultural groups in which these behaviors are considered to be highly deviant?

SELF-ASSESSMENT 6.3. CAUSES OF MALADIES

What do you think are all of the general classes or types of causes of maladies, including disease, illness, and sickness?

What role do you think emotions have in health and disease? Stress? Religion?

Are there any kinds of social interactions that affect your health, making you ill?

ADDITIONAL RESOURCES

Books

Chrisman, N. J., and T. Maretzki, eds. 1982. *Clinically applied anthropology: Anthropologists in health settings.* Boston: D. Reidel.

Seeley, K. M. 2000. *Cultural psychotherapy: Working with culture in the clinical encounter.* Northvale, N.J.: Aaronson.

Tseng, W.-S., and J. Streltzer. 2001. *Culture and psychotherapy: A guide to clinical practice.* Washington, D.C.: American Psychological Association.

Web Site

National Institute of Mental Health: http://www.nimh.nih.gov.

CHAPTER

7

MEDICAL-ECOLOGICAL APPROACHES TO HEALTH

*[M]edical anthropologist[s] . . . suggest strategies for both
clinicians and patients to make decisions about risk management
that are based on sound epidemiological principles*

—DUNN AND JANES, 1986, P. 27

LEARNING OBJECTIVES

■ Explain medical-ecological approaches to disease and provide examples of the interaction between biological potentials and cultural influences in disease

■ Illustrate biocultural dynamics in evolutionary adaptations to disease, nutrition, birthing, and healing responses

■ Present the triune brain model as a basis for understanding emotional disorders

■ Develop a biocultural perspective on the role of culture in emotions

■ Deconstruct racial categories as cultural concepts and explain the evolutionary adaptations underlying skin coloration

■ Introduce epidemiological approaches to the measurement of morbidity and mortality and illustrate the necessity of a cultural-epidemiological approach to address causes of disease

MEDICAL ECOLOGY AND DISEASE

Health is affected by many interactions with the environment. Medical ecology examines the relationships of health to physical, biological, and social environments, such as climatic conditions, plants and animals, and population dynamics. Medical-ecological approaches examine population health and disease as reflecting the group's biological, individual, and cultural adaptations. Ecological systems are conceptualized as having three major aspects—abiotic (physical), biotic (biological), and cultural—that interact with each other and the human population in the determination of disease. For instance, wet environments (abiotic) support malaria-carrying mosquitoes (biotic) whose opportunities to infect humans are increased by artificial lakes and crowded populations (cultural). Medical ecology focuses primarily on the health effects of abiotic and biotic environments and is the closest of the medical anthropology approaches to the perspectives of biomedicine.

Medical-ecological approaches use evolutionary perspectives to examine the relationship of humans' evolved genetic potentials to their health conditions. Human health and disease are produced in the interaction of human biology with environments through cultural activities that increase (or decrease) disease exposures. Some causes of disease are genetic, the outcome of human genetic variations that are harmful to their hosts, such as sickle cell anemia. Most diseases are not caused strictly by genes, however, but by interactions with factors in the environment. The different disease profiles associated with various ethnic groups are produced in a chain of causal and contributory linkages involving the interactions of agents such as germs or toxins with many factors:

- Physiological and genetic characteristics, including individual susceptibilities and resistances to disease

- Nutritional input and other protective resources

- Stress and resistance resources, including immunological status

- Social networks and support for combating disease

- Health beliefs and practices that affect health behaviors and the incidence and course of maladies

Cultural systems models help to identify the many aspects of life and society that can contribute to the incidence of disease in the confluence of physical, biological, and cultural environmental influences that create exposure to pathogens and susceptibility to their effects. Medical-ecological approaches investigate many environmental factors affecting health, including these principal foci (see Moore, Van Arsdale, Glittenberg, and Aldrich, 1980; McElroy and Townsend, 1996; Pope, 2000):

- Human behaviors directly related to adaptation and survival

- Reproduction and birthing practices

- Population dynamics

- Diet, nutrition, and foodways

- Functional brain organization and evolutionary psychology

- Psychobiological effects of stress

Traditional medical-ecological approaches (see Moran, 1979) have emphasized the importance of the effects of a hunter-gatherer lifestyle as part of our evolutionary heritage that influences our health today. Aspects of these hunter-gatherer influences include adaptations on health that are manifested in diet and birthing practices. Contemporary cultures often lack a balance with these ancient human biological adaptations and produce disease by departing from practices consistent with humans' evolved biology. The field of evolutionary medicine has emerged from the examination of the relationships of modern diseases to our acquired adaptations. This is exemplified in the consequences for modern obstetrics that have resulted from ignoring these evolved aspects of birthing in the modern birth practices of biomedicine.

The diseases of modern humans are also associated with cultural behaviors and social influences, as manifested in the ethnic differences in the primary causes of **morbidity** (sickness) and **mortality** (death). Anthropology is a core aspect of the integrative science of epidemiology, the study of the distribution of causes of death and disease. Epidemiology studies the conditions associated with a disease with methods for identifying the many social and cultural contributory factors that shape human health.

Although different disease profiles are associated with so-called races, biological differences between human populations play little role in explaining different rates of disease. Instead, medical-ecological approaches explain differences in disease rates of different racial categories as reflecting the effects of social and cultural factors, rather than of genetic uniqueness. Anthropology's biocultural approaches help explain the association of disease with racial categories, contextualizing these relationships in the context of individual and group patterns of acclimatization, the physiological adjustments made in the course of the socialization of biological development. Cultural approaches are keys to understanding the epidemiological findings, identifying the social and cultural behaviors producing exposures to diseases.

Medical ecology's biological approaches include a focus on the brain and the biological dynamics of health behaviors and the evolution of the human healing capacity. A **triune brain** model provides a view of the different functional systems of the brain, an interaction among behavior, emotional, social, and cognitive dimensions that provide frameworks for understanding the social production of emotional illness. Health involves aspects of human neuropsychology and evolutionary psychology, the roles of ancient brain structures in humans' interpersonal behaviors, emotions, and cognitive processes. Humans have evolved adaptations to the effects of disease; these include social responses to those with whom we have attachments and involve caring and altruistic behaviors that help others at one's own immediate cost. The evolutionary bases of human healing responses involve a ritualization of emotions and social relations that have deep evolutionary roots in the roles of ritual in primate social adaptation. This makes understanding emotions key to understanding healing responses.

Emotions provide key areas for understanding the interactions of biology and socialization in human behavior. Emotions are biocultural outcomes of the socialization of emotional potentials within the frameworks of culture and social relations; these relations

CASE STUDY

The Physical Burden of History

The Hmong experienced various war traumas: dislocations, hiding in the forest for years, witnessing massacres and suffering gunshot wounds, indoctrination in communist "re-education" camps, prolonged starvation, gang rape, the execution of family members, and refugee camps. They walked for weeks and hundreds of miles with little or no food, surviving on insects. Their centuries of adaptation as mountain people have made them susceptible to tropical diseases. To get accepted as immigrants to the United States, they had to pass a medical exam to ensure that they suffered no serious physical or mental illness. Fortunately for most, the exam was concluded in about ten seconds. But when they arrived in this country, their history of trauma came with them, producing serious physical and psychological conditions. Physicians seldom could fathom the history behind their complaints. That history—starvation, exposure to chemical weapons, tropical diseases, and numerous stressors—could have had effects on Lia Lee's mother in ways that ultimately contributed to Lia's epilepsy.

The cultural systems model illustrates the many possible causes of Lia's convulsions; medical-ecological and epidemiological approaches elaborate on the contributory factors that had effects on her health. What caused Lia's "big one," the final epileptic attack that left her in a permanent vegetative state? Where do the relevant factors begin and end? Understanding Hmong patients is not merely addressing what they are experiencing today in the consulting room but also recognizing the factors in their past that have produced their conditions. The presence of a Hmong child in rural Merced, California, was part of a long string of events that included the Hmong being recruited for a secret CIA war in Laos and Cambodia. Was Lia predisposed to convulsions from her mother's exposures to toxins in Laos and high levels of physical and emotional stress? Would she have received different treatment as a private patient rather than in the county system for the indigent? Was her progressive deterioration a consequence of the wrong medications, too much medication, or her parent's failure to appropriately administer the medicines? Was the major seizure a consequence of "septic shock," a bacterial infection missed by the physicians? Did infection result from the medications that compromised her immune system? How much is due to doctors missing the pulmonary infection for months or the most damaging infection acquired in the hospital? What role do we attribute to the county health institutions and their inadequate resources for translators that could have helped ascertain Lia's condition earlier? What contributory role to the final seizure was the family's decision to wait for an ambulance, which took an excessively long time compared with carrying her a few blocks to the hospital emergency department? And why was Lia, daughter of Hmong hill people from Laos, seeking services in a Merced country hospital? What role do we attribute to U.S. imperialism and the CIA's secret war in Laos to her trajectory toward a comatose condition? Did the war itself consume resources that could have otherwise been directed toward a better public health system with translators?

provide a context for appraising or assessing the significance of our physiological responses and their meanings. Although similarities with the emotions of other animals point to the biological bases of human emotional responses, cross-cultural differences in emotions point to their biocultural and biosocial dynamics, where specific cultural influences are imposed on biological capacities.

EVOLUTIONARY ADAPTATIONS AND HEALTH

Key concerns of the medical-ecological approach include **adaptations,** the physiological and behavioral adjustments made by an organism to an environment. **Natural selection** is the process by which genetic characteristics of a species are shaped as a consequence of adaptation. The genetic variation within species affects interactions with the environment. The influences of the environment drive the processes of natural selection. Members of a species with genetic characteristics that permit them to make more effective adaptations to the current environment are more likely to survive longer and produce more offspring. Genetically shaped features that vary among humans (such as height, strength, speed, or certain enzymes) and facilitate adaptations that enhance individuals' survival in their current circumstances will increase in frequency in subsequent generations. Consequently, adaptation and natural selection alter the **genotype,** the collective genetic codes of a species. For instance, animals like squirrels that are preyed on by coyotes are more likely to survive if they are fast and small enough to hide. This allows genetic characteristics that enhance speed and limit size to facilitate adaptation and, consequently, occur with greater frequency in subsequent generations of their species.

These perspectives have led to the development of a field of evolutionary medicine that addresses how our acquired characteristics contribute to disease (see Trevathan, Smith, and McKenna, 1999, 2008). The areas in which evolutionary adaptations affect health include such diverse areas as diet, obesity, stress, reproduction, menstruation, premenstrual syndrome, breast-feeding, sleep, addictions, back and spinal conditions, CVD, and mental illness. As evolutionary medicine progresses, it has discovered genes that contribute to the risk for many diseases.

Environment in Adaptation and Natural Selection

The environment includes many factors that affect natural selection and exert influences on genotypes and health. These include diseases, climatic conditions, food availability, other species (predators and hosts), and culture. The ecological niche, a population's specialized adaptation to an environment, both exposes the population to and protects it from disease. Factors such as diet, climate, family dynamics, social networks, community resources, and the generational structure of the population are involved in human adaptations to the ecology and, consequently, disease. Populations' adaptations to the environment establish equilibrium that is managed through fertility and death. Demography (the study of population dynamics) identifies how ecological influences structure health through population features such as density and pressure, age and sex profiles, fertility rates, fertility regulation practices, and migration patterns (Moore et al., 1980). For example, infectious diseases increase in dense populations with more person-to-person contact to spread disease.

BIOCULTURAL INTERACTIONS

Biocultural and Environmental Interactions in Malaria

The role of culture in disease and natural selection is exemplified in the relationships among malaria, sickle-cell anemia, and agriculture (Livingstone, 1958; Weisenfeld, 1967). Malaria has two hosts, mosquito and mammal. The malarial parasite is a protozoan (*Plasmodium falciparum*) that lives in mammals' red blood cells and destroys them through the consumption of cell resources and the release of waste products. The mosquito that bites an infected person takes the *P. falciparum* parasite into its own body, where the gametes develop; they later complete their life cycle on retransmission to a mammal that gets infected by a mosquito bite. Humans have evolved a passive resistance to malaria in a recessive condition of sickle cell anemia.

Sickle cell anemia was selected for in human evolution as an adaptation that provided a natural immunity to malaria because it interfered with the development of the malarial parasite in the human system. Hemoglobin S causes sickle cell anemia when it is **homozygous** (contributed by both parents), producing abnormal hemoglobin, which causes red blood cells to "sickle" (distort into a curved shape). Individuals with the homozygous sickle cell condition suffer severe anemia and seldom survive. Individuals with **heterozygous** hemoglobin S (contributed by only one parent), however, have immunity to malaria because this hemoglobin creates a short life for the red blood

Many environmental features affect disease (Kelsey, Whittemore, Evans, and Thompson, 1996):

- Physical and chemical: climate, environmental, and workplace contaminants

- Biological: other animals, food sources, habitats, and reservoirs

- Familial: housing, hygiene, age distribution, cultural or behavioral characteristics

- Occupational: work conditions, hazards, contaminants, and stresses

- Socioeconomic: nutrition, sanitation, and health resources

- Social environment: public health, day care and medical facilities, prevention programs

- Psychosocial: stress factors and support systems

- Intergroup interactions: travel, migration

Epidemic mortality is a major mechanism of natural selection, where diseases attack those with genetic weaknesses. Those with genetic immunity to diseases obtain selective advantages and reproduce at higher rates, leading to changes in the population genotype. This immunity to disease can have negative effects as well by lowering other adaptations, as illustrated in the relationship of malaria and sickle cell anemia.

The interaction between sickle cell anemia and malaria illustrates the need to examine human health in the context of interaction among acquired characteristics that resulted cell, which is insufficient for the parasite's reproductive cycle. The potential for a fatal genetic disease (anemia) is retained because it provides an advantage in resistance to malaria. Persistence of this genetic trait reflects lower reproductive rates of normal individuals in malaria-infested environments. Individuals with the sickle cell trait can resist malaria and, therefore, contribute disproportionately to reproduction. As a result, the gene pool in malarial regions was altered across generations in selection for the sickle cell trait.

Agriculture increased the need for ponds to store water, increased mosquito-breeding areas, and increased selection for genetic traits for sickle cell anemia. Concentrated settlement patterns and domestic animals such as cows enhanced opportunities for the transmission of malarial parasites between mammal and mosquito populations. The control of malaria involves human activities that affect the ability of mosquitoes to breed and transfer the parasite to humans. Eliminating standing pools of water that provide breeding grounds for mosquitoes is a primary means of prevention; applying chemicals that kill mosquitoes is another mechanism for reducing malarial cases. Other interventions involve changes in human habitation, work, and migration patterns to minimize contact with mosquito-breeding areas and other mammals that harbor the malarial parasite. Construction changes in housing and other barriers to mosquitoes (sleeping nets) help to reduce disease transmission.

from evolutionary processes of adaptation and natural selection with the current environment and resources.

GENETIC, INDIVIDUAL, AND CULTURAL ADAPTATIONS TO THE ENVIRONMENT

Human adaptations to environmental conditions affect health through

- Genetic characteristics of a population acquired through adaptation and natural selection
- Individual physiological adjustments called conditioning that occur during development
- Cultural behaviors that mediate exposure to risks and provide care

Evolutionary adaptations produced genetic characteristics that affect contemporary health (Trevathan et al., 1999, 2008) such as our acquired preference for high-calorie sweets that enable obesity but that contributed to survival when such foods were scarce. Although genetic features affect many aspects of our metabolism, whether a person becomes obese will primarily reflect individual physiological adjustments. These individual developments are, however, strongly influenced by contemporary cultural adaptations that provide fundamental determinants of a population's health status in the diet made available (Brown, Inhorn, and Smith, 1996). For instance, when international fast-food restaurant chains saturate inner-city markets with poor nutritional menus that cater to our genetic predispositions for sweet and fatty foods, people in these areas have little choice about diet. Health problems

BIOCULTURAL INTERACTIONS

Birthing in Evolutionary and Cross-Cultural Perspectives

Human birthing is often viewed as a physiological act, but it is also a social phenomenon shaped by culture, power dynamics, and local expectations. Since Jordan's classic *Birth in Four Cultures* in 1978, anthropological studies of the cultural context of birthing have made significant contributions to understanding human reproduction and delivery (see McClain, 1989; Browner and Sargent, 1996; Davis-Floyd and Sargent, 1997). Biocultural approaches reveal that interactions between human biology and culture produce the local circumstances of birth. Birth occurs not as a strictly biological response but one shaped by many social processes that reflect cultural values. Cross-cultural approaches reveal that arbitrary cultural beliefs and practices surround birth and provide a basis for transcultural perspectives to determine natural aspects of human birthing.

Although there may be little "natural" about birth because it occurs within a cultural context, cross-cultural perspectives indicate that many cultures have developed similar adjustments to accommodate the physiological aspects of the birth process. Throughout most of the premodern world, birthing occurred in a supportive setting facilitated by the experience of older women familiar with the process. Women did not deliver their babies alone but in the company of their mothers, grandmothers, and other experienced women. These ancient practices of social and emotional support are crucial for the well-being of the mother-infant dyad. Support for the empirical efficacy of traditional cultural birth practices also comes from evolutionary studies of human birth. Studies of birthing from primate and evolutionary perspectives contribute to an understanding of the importance of female support systems facilitating birth for mother and child (Trevathan et al., 1999; Trevathan, 1999). Women assist the birthing mother, providing physical, emotional, and social support during the delivery. Evolutionary and cross-cultural perspectives reveal the importance of supportive environments that facilitate the formation of mother-infant attachment processes.

Cross-cultural perspectives played a significant role in the resuscitation of midwifery in the United States, providing knowledge about options in the management of birth processes. This cross-cultural fertilization helped reestablish the legitimacy of traditional birth attendants and enlarged the scope of considerations in addressing maternal-child health. Cross-cultural differences in approaches to birth even by physicians reveal cultural aspects of biomedicine, contributing to the development of a critical perspective on the appropriateness of customary obstetric practices. The awareness of arbitrary cultural aspects of modern obstetrics has contributed to redirecting health modernization programs to include rather than replace traditional birth practices. Cultural perspectives help public health planners recognize traditional practices as important complements to biomedical approaches.

The "natural birthing" movement reflects the efforts of modern women to recapture these dynamics through incorporating influences from cultural traditions where the power of women over

often result from the disjuncture between the genetic characteristics and contemporary conditions affecting diet, reproduction, and resource allocation.

Our individual development involves tuning our physiological systems in response to input from the environment, which is shaped by cultural adaptations. Culture is the most prevalent form of adaptation in addressing threats to health because culture can make birth remained more intact. The successes of these cultural traditions indicate the inappropriateness of customary obstetric procedures of having women adopt the lithotomy position (on her back with legs extended upward in stirrups) and to undergo episiotomy (surgical opening of the vagina to facilitate passage of the fetus) (Trevathan et al., 1999). Women around the world sit, stand, or recline rather than lie on their backs, as emphasized in modern biomedical obstetrics. The conflict of modern obstetric practices with the evolved needs of pregnant women can be remedied by cross-culturally inspired perspectives. For instance, female birth companions that provide support and reassurance during delivery can likely reduce morbidity and mortality associated with birth, postpartum complications, and malpractice suits against obstetricians. Birthing chairs where women recline are better suited to women's evolved birthing capacity than are beds with stirrups to hang their feet above their heads!

Contemporary dissatisfaction with modern obstetrics is in part due to its failure to accommodate to this evolutionary heritage and its importance in facilitating positive birth experiences and postpartum physical and emotional health. Cultural approaches to childbirth question the presumed superiority of biomedical obstetrics and what constitutes authoritative knowledge in childbirth. Contemporary studies of midwifery (Davis-Floyd and Sargent, 1997) establish it as a reliable health resource with a role in the modern world. American midwives have engaged in formal education and professionalization in modernizing their practices, producing what Davis-Floyd refers to as the "postmodern midwife" who accommodates traditional practices to modern demands and circumstances. Anthropology has played a role in establishing the validity of midwifery and facilitating its political struggle for legitimacy and acceptance, as described in the "Practitioner Profile: Robbie Davis-Floyd" (see Chapter Four and http://www.midwiferytoday.com).

The anthropology of birth focuses on the political dimensions affecting the continued viability of traditional birth practices. For more than a century, biomedical organizations have used the power of the state to oppress and vilify midwifery, placing it in the context of witchcraft and charlatanry. National health programs in the underdeveloped world generally still neglect, marginalize, and even disparage indigenous midwifery. Traditional midwifery practices still constitute the most important maternal-infant health resource in many regions and are generally as effective as or better than biomedicine in routine deliveries. Biomedicine often contributes to undermining access to the basic health resources that women and infants need, neglecting midwifery's potential contributions and, instead, emphasizing high-tech biomedical approaches. Even when incorporated into national health education programs, midwives' knowledge is often marginalized in a focus on Western notions of hygiene instead of focusing on the expansion of midwifery as a basis for effective services. Anthropology's cross-cultural and evolutionary perspectives on midwifery may inspire changes in obstetric practice.

more rapid changes in responses than biological adaptations achieved through evolution. Humans are, nonetheless, left today with many characteristics acquired in our evolutionary history and processes of natural selection that produced features that are poorly adapted to today's ecology or cultural patterns. This is illustrated in the special feature "Biocultural Interactions: Birthing in Evolutionary and Cross-Cultural Perspectives."

BIOCULTURAL INTERACTIONS

Genetics and CVD

A reason for the increased incidence of CVD in African Americans is their higher incidence of hypertension, exacerbated by a greater tendency to retain salts. It has been hypothesized that this greater tendency was the result of genes that enhanced the retention of salt. These salt-conserving genetic tendencies made those who had them less likely to die from dehydration while chained in the holds of the slave ships transporting them across the Atlantic Ocean. This ability to retain salt also enabled them to retain cellular water, a trait that facilitated survival in the "sun-up-to-sun-down" field labor the enslaved Africans were forced to endure (Fackelmann, 1991). Today African Americans do not face these extreme risks of dehydration, and the excessive levels of salt (sodium) in the diet and body contribute to hypertension. Genetic influences on hypertension come from a gene that codes for a protein called angiotensinogen, which in interaction with rennin forms angiotensin. Angiotensin results in increased blood pressure by its constrictive action on the blood vessels and alteration of the sodium-water balance in the body. The genetically predisposed increase in angiotensinogen levels can have a cumulative effect, with its overproduction resulting in an increase in sodium concentrations, which cause expansion of the blood volume and a rise in blood pressure.

A medication targeted for African American hypertension raised some furor, suggesting to some that their problems with CVD were a consequence of some "Black gene" (see Russo, Melista, Cui, DeStefano, Bakris, Manolis, Gavras, and Baldwin, 2005). Although genetic features are associated with essential hypertension, they are not unique to a single ethnic or racial group. The functions of sodium channels in the epithelial layer of the kidney, which affect blood pressure, develop under the control of the NEDD4L gene located in chromosome 18q (Russo et al., 2005). Different mutations of this NEDD4L gene are hypothesized to be the cause of different blood pressure phenotypes. Russo and colleagues found that there was a significant association of several gene variants with hypertension across groups, including various "White" (U.S. and Greek) and African American individuals. Indeed, the chromosome 18q association with essential hypertension was originally discovered in a study in Iceland (Kristjansson, Manolescu, Kristinsson, Hardarson, Knudsen, Ingason, Thorleifsson, Frigge, et al., 2002). Although gene features that contribute to high blood pressure and CVD are more prevalent in African Americans than some groups, only a small percentage of African Americans have the gene. The limited role of these genetic features in CVD is reflected in the far greater levels of hypertension in the African American population. More than a third of African American men and women are estimated to have hypertension, and nearly half of their population is considered to have some form of CVD.

BIOCULTURAL INTERACTIONS

Prevalent Genetic Diseases Among Ashkenazi Jews

A significant health characteristic of the Ashkenazi Jews population is the large number of genetic diseases that occur in them (see Purnell and Paulanka, 2003). These genetic disorders are the effects of genes that are normally not manifested because they are recessive, but if contributed by both parents, the gene can result in fatal disorders. Tay-Sachs disease is one of the most deadly genetic diseases prevalent in the Jewish American population, causing central nervous system degeneration and leading to a loss of motor control, impairment of vision and hearing, severe developmental delays, and generally death in early childhood. In addition to the widely recognized Tay-Sachs disease, a number of other deadly genetic diseases manifest in an abnormally high rate in Ashkenazi Jews (Purnell and Paulanka, 2003). Most of these are carried by several percentage of the Jewish population but as recessive genes and, therefore, do not affect individuals' health. It is estimated, however, that as many as 25 percent of the worldwide Ashkenazi Jews carry recessive genes for one or more of these disorders:

- Gaucher's disease, the most common of these prevalent genetic diseases, is a defect in enzyme metabolism that results in weakened bones, easy bruising and nosebleeds, and reduced growth
- Bloom's syndrome results in a relatively short stature, sensitivity to facial skin lesions, heightened susceptibility to respiratory tract and gastrointestinal tract illnesses, and leukemia
- Canavan's disease is a degenerative brain disease that causes developmental delays, loss of reflexes, and early death in childhood
- Familial dysautonomia, or Riley-Day syndrome, causes damage to the peripheral and autonomic nervous system, undermines development, and generally results in death by early adulthood
- Fanconi's anemia results in low blood cell counts and causes bone marrow failure

The prevalence of these genetic diseases among Ashkenazi Jews is thought to involve two genetic mechanisms referred to as the *founder effect* and *genetic drift*. The founder effect reflects an ancient trait that has increased in prevalence across time because of inbreeding patterns in a small population and the birth of many children from a founder with a genetic defect. Although such defects were likely recessive for the founder, they increased in relative frequency as descendants interbred. The principle of genetic drift notes that the in-group marriage patterns of the Ashkenazi Jews lead to a concentration of a range of recessive genetic diseases within descendants because the recessive genes were not diluted by different gene pools from outside their culture.

Natural Selection and Adaptation in Disease and Health

Evolutionary perspectives of adaptation and natural selection underlie the field of evolutionary medicine (see Eaton, Shostak, and Konner, 1988; Trevathan et al., 1999), which examines disease in relation to genetic adaptations made over hundreds of millennia of evolution. Evolutionary medicine perspectives consider humans' ancient physiological adaptations to help explain contemporary health problems as acquired genetic diseases.

Other diseases are the consequence of a lack of congruence between the genetic endowments shaped by primate and hunter-gatherer adaptations and contemporary cultural conditions, lifestyles, and diets. Health problems resulting from the incompatibility of modern environments with humans' evolutionary heritage include sudden infant death syndrome, obesity, diabetes, CVD, colic, asthma, allergies, cancers, orthopedic problems, drug addiction, and menopause. These evolutionary effects are illustrated in anthropological studies of nutrition.

Nutrition in an Evolutionary and Cultural Perspective

Food is a physical and environmental influence on human health, but the substances consumed are largely a consequence of cultural preferences, not strictly biological needs. Biocultural approaches identify causes of contemporary nutritional diseases in the maladaptation of cultural practices to human biology. Mammalian evolution involved adaptations for lactation (breast-feeding); contemporary child-rearing practices are not typically in congruence with this evolutionary heritage. Using infant formulas has detrimental effects on infant and mother, blocking an appropriate accommodation to humans' evolutionary adaptations involved in breast-feeding such as hormonal influences on the mother's fat cells, mother-child bonding from the endogenous opioids involved in the letdown reflex in nursing, natural suppression of ovulation, and immune system enhancement. Abandonment of this biologically based pattern of nutrition has social and cultural roots in modern lifestyles: the availability of infant formulas, breakdown in family support systems, increases in stress, and changes in women's work patterns.

Food affects health and evolution, but cultural dynamics filter how the nutrition available in the environment exerts selective pressures on human populations. This is illustrated in cultural and regional differences in the ability to digest milk as an adult.

Nutritional Anthropology Nutritional anthropology (Johnston, 1987; Ulijaszek and Strickland, 1993; Quandt, 1996) is an area of medical anthropology that addresses the interaction of physical and cultural influences in human foodways—that is, how ecology, cultural traditions, and social factors influence what humans consume and its effects on health. Nutrition is a central focus in the assessment of the evolutionary consequences of the hunter-gatherer lifestyle on diet, metabolism, nutrition, and contemporary health problems. Selection under hunter-gatherer lifestyles influenced human genetics: it has been postulated that hunter-gatherers' irregular food supplies contributed to a "nutritional thriftiness" involving genetic factors that enhance a nutrient-efficient response to available foods (Quandt, 1996). Metabolic systems were selected for the ability to maximize the use of nutrients available in the food ingested. These adaptations for efficient metabolisms have produced health problems in modern societies, with the abundant availability of sugars, carbohydrates, and proteins.

BIOCULTURAL INTERACTIONS

Evolutionary Adaptations for Digesting Milk

Humans' mammalian capabilities for digesting lactose during infancy are generally lost by age six years in most populations. They become lactose intolerant—not capable of digesting lactose—because of insufficient activity of the enzyme lactase, which breaks down lactose into glucose. Lactose intolerance is common among Asian, Native American, and many African-origin groups. Cultures with high lactose tolerance in adulthood are primarily of Western and Northern European origin and some Northern African groups. Evolutionary adaptations explain differences in lactose tolerance, which is associated with cultures with a long history of using dairy animals and generally absent in people who have only recently adopted the herding of animals. The use of dairy milk for nutrition was a cultural adaptation that exercised selective influences on genetic characteristics of these populations. The exact mechanisms by which this genetic selection has occurred remain unknown. It is likely not a function of enhancing the availability of carbohydrates and protein and fat nutrients. Carbohydrates are normally plentiful in dairying cultures, and lactose-intolerant adults can still utilize protein and fat nutrition from milk. In some dairying societies with high rates of lactose intolerance, there are also mechanisms for reducing the lactose content of milk products (e.g., production of fermented milk products such as cheese and yogurt).

The medical-ecological orientation to the role of lactose in human adaptation has important contemporary applications. This knowledge provides the basis for countering the ethnocentric perception embodied in the marketing slogan, "Milk is for everybody." In some populations, many individuals are unable to digest cow's milk. Lactose intolerance has implications for foreign aid programs, where the use of powdered milk is inappropriate for nations with high levels of lactose-intolerant adults. Contemporary human foodways involving large amounts of sugars and fats are influenced by agribusiness, capitalist world system dynamics, and marketing, rather than human nutritional needs produced by evolutionary adaptations.

These mechanisms are proposed in the "thrifty-gene hypothesis" of Native American diabetes. The supposition is that thrifty hunter-gatherer genes are too efficient for the modern abundance of high-carbohydrate foods. This hypothesis of diabetes as a genetically determined disease is not borne out in research, as described in the special feature "Biocultural Interactions: Thrifty Genotype or Starved Phenotype?" which explicates the social, political, and dietary factors that have produced a diabetes epidemic among Native Americans.

Individual Physiological Adaptations

Individuals make adaptations to environmental conditions that affect the organism's **phenotype,** the physical appearance of an organism acquired in the adaptations of its genetic potentials to the environment. The individual's body makes a number of physiological adaptations during development to environmental influences such as climatic stressors,

BIOCULTURAL INTERACTIONS

Thrifty Genotype or Starved Phenotype?

Native American populations suffer from extremely high rates of type 2 diabetes (adult onset), with an incidence of 40 percent or more in the adult population (such as the Pima of Arizona; Bennett, LeCompte, Miller, and Rushforth, 1976). This tendency to obesity and high incidence of diabetes in these populations has led biomedical researchers to postulate a genetic predisposition in a "thrifty genotype" (Neel, 1999). This postulated gene is hypothesized to have enhanced survival under conditions in which the availability of nutritional glucose was severely limited. The reasoning is that these populations evolved efficient metabolic systems as a consequence of a long-term adaptation to feast-or-famine cycles. A quick release of insulin more efficiently converts available glucose into fat stores. When these physiologies shaped by selective pressures of Arctic-sub-Arctic hunter-gatherer food strategies were exposed to the high carbohydrate, protein, and fat diets of the modern world, their "superefficient" metabolisms were then a detriment because they produced excessive storage of fats (see Diamond, 2006). Extensions of Neel's original hypothesis have pointed to the adaptive benefits of insulin resistance (a diabetes precursor) in populations with high-protein and low-carbohydrate diets and its maladaptive consequences when consuming energy-rich high-carbohydrate diets.

Population and clinical studies (see Martin, Johnston, Han, and Benyshek, 2000; Benyshek, Martin, and Johnston, 2001; Benyshek, Johnston, and Martin, 2004; McDermott, 2006, for reviews and discussion) call this genetic hypothesis into question and propose an environmental and nutritional alternative to the thrifty genotype hypothesis. Studies show that low birth weight, reflective of malnourishment in utero, is a strong predictor of adult diabetes. Severe famine in utero leads to abnormal insulin and glucose metabolism in adulthood, especially for the obese. This suggests that diabetes is a consequence of developmental acclimatization.

Native American groups with an excessive prevalence of diabetes were exposed to periods of near-starvation during the later nineteenth and early twentieth centuries (Benyshek et al., 2001). This period of deprivation was followed by dramatic increases in all aspects of diet, particularly carbohydrates and fats. This was partly produced by the high fat and carbohydrate content of the government rations, inducing basic changes in diet that made fry bread a new "traditional food." Initial Native American cohorts diagnosed with diabetes were children of those generations exposed to severe nutritional deprivation. Laboratory and clinical findings show that hyperglycemic conditions during gestation produce insulin and glucose abnormalities in subsequent generations. The role of the gestational environment in fostering these abnormalities is illustrated by the far greater importance of maternal than paternal diabetes as a risk factor.

Laboratory studies with rats exposed to similar conditions (maternal nutritional deprivation in utero followed by high-fat diets) demonstrate that diabetes can be induced by gestational nutritional deprivation and dramatic increases in nutrient supply from pregnancy to postweaning periods. Deprivation in utero, followed by excessive food energy sources, leads to elevated insulin-to-glucose ratios, glucose concentrations, and insulin resistance in adulthood. Fetal malnutrition in the females shaped their own glucose and insulin metabolism, which shapes the metabolic adjustments of their offspring. These elevated levels of insulin resistance were not improved by placement on an adequate diet after weaning. Subsequent studies by Martin and colleagues indicate that the thrifty-phenotype rats (thin at birth due to nutritional deprivation) that have low-protein diets are insulin-deficient as adults, but that those fed high-fat diets produce too much insulin (hyperinsulinemia) and develop adult insulin resistance.

This research indicates that epidemic levels of Native American diabetes are not genetic but, rather, a consequence of fetal malnutrition that is transmitted intergenerationally through the intrauterine environment affected by the mother's metabolic system. Diabetes was unknown in aboriginal populations, emerging as a health problem in these populations scarcely more than fifty years ago. Native American diabetes may be understood as a consequence of the intergenerational transmission of disturbed insulin metabolism that began as protein and energy malnutrition during near-starvation in the early reservation period almost a century ago and was induced in subsequent generations from the high-energy diets that were subsequently available.

The implication of this model is that the Native American diabetes epidemic was produced by political and economic conditions, not genetic predispositions. Consequently, these populations are not doomed to a genetically determined susceptibility to diabetes but can reduce the incidence of diabetes through dietary manipulations, particularly during pregnancy. Glucose intolerance in the mother during pregnancy is a predisposing condition for later adult-onset diabetes in her offspring. Current high levels of carbohydrates in Native American diets reinforce these influences. Dietary change during gestation to reduce blood glucose levels is a possible intervention to interrupt the intergenerational transmission of susceptibility to diabetes.

Considerable difficulties impede achieving such changes in the current ideological, political, and economic environments that maintain the status quo, including the biomedical thrifty-genotype hypothesis. Additional challenges face this new thrifty-phenotype model that attributes the perpetuation of diabetes to the mother's gestational diet. Benyshek and coworkers (2001) emphasize the need to develop interventions that avoid blaming pregnant women and instead place their dietary behavior in the context of broader community influences and constraints. A community-level approach is consistent with the macrolevel political and economic forces that initiated the chain of events more than a century ago through famines. These political diseases produced through racist ideologies and their resultant social inequalities require political solutions that mend these intergenerational disruptions in foodways. The persistence of the genetic model involved in the largely discredited thrifty-gene hypothesis is a form of reductionism characteristic of biomedical thought that ignores the determining causal factors involved in the interactions between the lifeways of groups and the macrosocial factors of the broader society.

temperature, humidity, nutrients, microorganisms, and toxic substances. These leave effects on the body, such as how access to nutrients has determinant effects on height and weight. Imagine how different you might look if you had eaten only half the food you have consumed across your life—or twice as much. Those differences would reflect phenotypic variation made possible by your genetic characteristics.

McElroy and Townsend (1985) discuss three levels of physiological adaptation:

- Acclimation, a rapid, short-term adjustment to an environmental stressor

- Acclimatization, a pervasive but reversible response to exposure over a longer time

- Developmental (native) acclimatization, an irreversible adjustment to environmental stressors

Acclimation involves changes like feeling cold (or hot) when you first walk outside, but after a few days of similar temperatures, you may feel comfortable. Acclimatization will occur over longer periods of exposure, so that when you have spent two months of summer in the 110-degree (Fahrenheit) hot environment of Phoenix, a quick trip to San Diego where it is just 65 degrees might leave you feeling cold and shivering. However, in the winter, 65 degrees might feel like a hot day. Your temperature comfort zone undergoes regular shifts in acclimatization but establishes limits of flexibility early in life that involve developmental (native) acclimatization. For example, you could probably not do much physical work at 10,000 feet elevation or when it is minus 30 degrees Fahrenheit outside; this reflects your developmental acclimatization regarding lung capacity for low oxygen concentrations and temperature resistances that normally cannot be substantially changed once you are an adult.

Developmental acclimatization may affect not only individual metabolic development, for instance, where childhood obesity deposits fat cells for life. Acclimatization may also be passed from mother to embryo, as illustrated in the intergenerational transmission during gestation of disturbed metabolic effects that appear to underlie the diabetes epidemic in Native American groups.

Cultural Adaptations and Health

Culture and its resources for mediating stressors and accessing resources produce human health through mediating adaptations to the environment. Cultural practices with adaptive health functions include food selections, postpartum sexual taboos that affect breast-feeding and birth spacing, avoidance of the diseased and their confinement, and ethnomedical practices (such as plant medicines with antimicrobial or antiparasitic action). Human health is also adversely affected by human alteration of the physical environment, poor diet, drug use, sexual lifestyle and behaviors, and other dispositions that increase risks.

Health and disease result from a variety of adaptations (and maladaptations) at social, cultural, and personal levels. Humans today live in very different environments—physical and social—from those that shaped the human genetic makeup. Health problems result from a physiology adapted to hunter-gatherer lifestyles confronting conditions in contemporary societies that contribute to health problems (such as refined sugar contributing to obesity and diabetes, air pollution causing respiratory tract diseases, and concentrated drugs causing addictions). Modern technologies also facilitate contemporary adaptations (medicines, clothing, eyeglasses) and allow for the survival of people whose genetically produced conditions would have otherwise caused their early death.

Cultural behaviors also affect disease incidence by limiting exposure and disease consequences through ethnomedical traditions that provide therapeutic interventions. Behaviors are the most significant factors in controlling disease, even in modern populations, where increased longevity is primarily due to public health measures rather than medical care. Ethnomedical traditions are often considered to be *cultural* adaptations but may also reflect biological adaptations acquired through natural selection (see the section below, "Evolution of the Sickness-and-Healing Responses" and Chapter Ten on shamanic healing). Protective aspects of ethnomedical traditions may also occur through dietary adaptations to include plant species with protective or curative effects against prevalent diseases, as illustrated in the consumption of foods with antimalarial properties in areas with endemic malaria (see "Practitioner Profile: Nina Etkin").

PRACTITIONER PROFILE

Nina Etkin

Nina Etkin, Ph.D., is professor of anthropology at the University of Hawaii, where she is also a member of the graduate faculties of the Department of Tropical Medicine and Division of Public Health (Medical School), the Program on Population Studies, and the Social Science Research Institute. Her perspective on medical anthropology is biocultural: linking culture, physiology, and the substance and sign of medicines through fieldwork and laboratory studies to understand the dialectic of culture and nature in diverse ethnographic and ecologic settings. Her primary interests in medical anthropology center on the culture and physiologic actions of indigenous (primarily botanical) medicines, food, and health and infectious disease.

Etkin's research was on the biological dimensions of health and the evolution of population variability, epidemiology, and health through studies of sickle hemoglobin and malaria, blood groups and infectious diseases, and hypertension. Her interest in malaria led to a broad-based and long-term study of medicine, diet, and health in a Hausa village in northern Nigeria. This research integrated a medical ethnographic focus with plant chemistry and led to insights on the cultural construction of health and the physiologic implications of people's health-seeking actions.

Etkin did ethnomedical and ethnopharmacologic studies in rural eastern Indonesia, with a focus on plant use in diet, medicine, cosmetics, and craft production. The significance of this is that the use of pharmacologically active plants in multiple contexts results in increased exposure, thus a greater likelihood of preventive and therapeutic benefits. The methods that she applied to studies in Nigeria and Indonesia were modified and transposed to a study of Hmong perceptions of prenatal care in a community clinic in Minneapolis. She identified clients' dissatisfaction, mainly with the quality of communication with clinic staff, which resulted in a series of reforms that directly improved clients' clinic experiences.

Disease in Ecological Context

Human disease has three levels of causation:

■ The genetic characteristics acquired as a species and as individuals

■ The unique developmental influences on our biology from socialization and other environmental influences

■ The resources of our culture that provide both risks and protective factors

Exposure to diseases, and the body's biological responses to them, occurs within social and cultural frameworks. The approach of "disease ecology" (Brown et al., 1996) recognizes the central role of culture in mediating the interaction of human populations with the physical environment, particularly plant and animal species. Critical medical anthropology (see Chapter Eight) influenced the expansion of the disease ecology approach to include an emphasis on the "political ecology" (Goodman and Leatherman, 1998). This macrosociological perspective examines the implications of interactions between different groups, particularly classes and nations, that affect health and disease through impacting environmental conditions and access to resources.

The consequences of diseases, therefore, reflect cultural and biological interactions in the ecological setting through a host (person) who may or may not be susceptible to the disease. Variation in susceptibility reflects

■ Individual genetic variation in the species

■ Individual differences produced by nutrition, acclimation, and acclimatization

■ Cultural factors that provide exposures as well as protection and resources

This expanded disease ecology approach is concerned with how cultural systems affect human responses to pathogens at three major levels of disease causation (Brown et al., 1996):

■ Microbiology of the action of pathogens, such as intestinal parasites, on the human body

■ The cultural ecology of sociocultural influences, such as commercial waste-water systems that dump sewage into waterways, on individual risks

■ The political ecology of intergroup interactions that affect access to resources, such as whether a nation's financial priorities are directed toward clean-water systems or subsidies for major corporations and exemptions for polluters

An interdisciplinary approach is necessary to identify causes of diseases and the effects of social conditions on their incidence and distribution. Medical ecology uses epidemiological approaches that study the distribution of disease and death in populations and the associated conditions to determine the risk factors, exposures linked to increased **incidence** of a disease (such as cigarette smoking and lung cancer). Assessing how ecology relates to health problems requires many sources of information, including environmental, clinical, epidemiological, behavioral, social, and cultural data (McElroy and

Townsend, 1996). These interactive features are the foundation of cultural systems approaches used in many health sciences to understand the factors responsible for the manifestation and differential distribution of diseases. Disease occurs in the interaction among our genetic heritage and diseases, our individual genetic and developmental features, and the sociocultural systems within which we live. These systemic effects on health are illustrated in Table 2.1, which shows American ethnic groups' different mortality rates. These relationships between ethnicity and disease are studied by epidemiology.

EPIDEMIOLOGY OF DISEASE

Determining the conditions producing disease requires many different forms of information on the presence of maladies and the associated conditions. Epidemiology, as noted earlier, is the interdisciplinary study of the distribution of deaths, diseases, and other health problems. Epidemiology identifies the conditions associated with specific diseases to determine possible causes and contributing factors. This includes conditions in the physical, social, and cultural environments, including beliefs and behaviors such as drug use, diet, and lifestyle. The classic approaches of epidemiology assess relationships among an *agent* that can cause a disease, the *host* that can become diseased, and the *environment* they occupy. Causal agents exist in an environmental context that affects transmission. This environment includes vectors, other animal hosts in which the disease develops (such as mosquitoes in malarial transmission). The host interacts with an environment in ways that may facilitate or impede contact with the agent. The host's internal characteristics (strength, immunity, stress) and cultural resources affect the consequences of exposure to the agent. Thus, health and disease are the outcomes of complex interactions among cultural and physical systems (see Krieger, 1994, 1999).

Measuring Disease

To identify which of the many aspects of social and cultural systems and their environmental interaction are responsible for a disease, a variety of measures of population characteristics are assessed to determine the factors associated with higher rates of disease. Morbidity rates measure the percentage of a population suffering from specific diseases, injuries, or other disability; mortality rates measure the percentages of death in a population in general or that due to specific causes. Identifying the most frequent causes of morbidity and mortality in a population is vital for prioritizing health programs. Public health departments regularly collect data about disease trends. The U.S. National Death Index provides a computerized database of death information and certain characteristics of the deceased. Death certificates and birth records provide personal information for identifying risk factors, characteristics associated with the increased incidence of a malady. Major sources of morbidity data are from (Lilienfeld and Lilienfeld, 1980)

■ Communicable disease case registries

■ Mandatory reports from clinicians and laboratories to health departments and the CDC

■ Specific disease surveillance programs, such as for cancer and birth defects

- Public health programs (Medicare, Veterans' Administration) and hospital records
- School, industrial, insurance, and medical plan assessments of their clientele
- Biomedical research and population surveys

Measuring Disease as Rates Mortality and morbidity are measured as **rates,** which in this context is an assessment of the relative frequency with which a condition occurs in a population. Rates are based on the ratio of the number of diseased cases or fatalities compared with the total population at risk for a disease (the number of occurrences of death or disease due to a specific cause divided by the population size). For example, 450,000 deaths due to cancer in a population of 225 million (450,000/225,000,000) provides a cancer mortality rate of 0.2 percent, or 200 per 100,000. Mortality is generally reported as a yearly rate, the number of deaths in a given population or subgroup within a year, as shown in Table 2.1. Cancer mortality for the American population as a whole was 185.8 per 100,000 in 2004. This is the cancer mortality incidence for 2004, the number or rate of deaths during a specific period. It is a measure of the percentage of the population dying of cancer in 2004 (1.858 percent). Rates are often adjusted for age-specific assessments (e.g., the rate of coronary artery events among men aged forty to sixty-four years). Rates are used to compare groups and assess the association of specific diseases with particular conditions or exposures. For example, Table 2.1 shows that the rate of heart disease for African Americans is 280 per 100,000 whereas that for Hispanics is 158 per 100,000.

Disease Associations as Risks Risks are probability measures of the likelihood that a defined group of people has the occurrence of a disease (such as heart disease), given a particular condition or exposure (such as being a member of a specific group; e.g., an African American or cigarette smoker). Risk is computed by dividing the rate (probability) of a disease among the exposed group by the rate (probability) of disease among the unexposed group (or the general population). This ratio indicates the relatively greater risk the exposed group has for contracting a condition. Risk can be compared between groups. The risk of death due to heart disease for Blacks is almost twice that for Hispanics (280/158 = 1.77). Risk factors are conditions identified as significantly associated with an increased occurrence of a disease. Risk factors may not be causes of a disease but are associated with a disease because of their correlation with **confounding variables** that are not causes but are associated with direct or contributory causes. Confounding variables are conditions that are correlated with both risk factors (exposures) and their associated diseases (outcomes) but not because they cause the disease. For instance, there is an association between coffee drinking (a risk factor or marker) and low birth weight (a condition) because women who drink coffee are also more likely to smoke cigarettes (a confounding variable and cause of low birth weight). Coffee drinking does not cause low birth weight but is associated with low birth weight because coffee drinking is correlated with cigarette smoking, which causes low birth weight. Once the confounding variable—cigarette smoking—is controlled for statistically, the analyses then show no association between coffee drinking and low birth weight. Risk markers are then the

CULTURE AND HEALTH

Confounding in the Association of Smoking and Cervical Cancer

Confounding is illustrated in the correlation between cigarette smoking and cervical cancer. The traditional assumption is that the relationship is causal: cigarette smoking causes cervical cancer. But is this true? The relationship is based on a confounding variable—sexual activity—that spreads the virus causing cervical cancer (Papillomavirus) and is the confounding variable. The positive correlation between cigarette smoking and the number of sexual partners makes it difficult to assess the role of cigarette smoking in the causation of cervical cancer. By using controls with measures of the number of sexual partners, the relationship between smoking and cervical cancer decreases dramatically; with controls for Papillomavirus infection, the relationship decreases further. Studies of women with the papillomaviruses find that the traditional risk factors (cigarette smoking, age of first sexual activity, number of sexual partners) have no association with cervical cancer. The confounding in the relationship between cigarette smoking and cervical cancer involves extraneous differences between women who smoke cigarettes and those who don't; women who smoke cigarettes are, in general, more sexually active than nonsmokers and, therefore, have greater exposure to papillomaviruses. Sexual activity is a confounding variable for the relationship between cigarette smoking and cervical cancer.

associated risk factors that are without causal effects. Being Black rather than Hispanic has a risk ratio of 1.77 in terms of mortality from heart disease. Being Black does not cause heart disease, makes dying from it nearly twice as likely as if one were Hispanic contextualization of risks in cultural behaviors is necessary to explain the association (see the section "Cultural Systems Approaches in Epidemiology").

Identifying Causes of Disease

When you think of the flu, do you think of the body aches and fever, or do you think of the virus that has caused it? Most people think of the symptoms they experience, and diseases were traditionally classified in this way. However, as the underlying biological mechanisms were identified in specific microorganisms, etiological classifications based on underlying causes were developed. The identification of specific biological causes has not been possible for many major categories of disease, however. Consequently, they remain classified on the basis of their symptoms (such as cancers, musculoskeletal conditions, and psychiatric disorders) rather than on specification of their precise causes.

Even when biological causes are identified, they are generally not sufficient causes of diseases: factors that alone, in and of themselves, always cause a disease. Rather, diseases generally require other contributory factors. In the cases of some diseases (lung cancer), no single determinant is known. Tobacco smoking is believed to cause lung cancer, but many smokers do not develop lung cancer, and it does occur in some nonsmokers. Potential contributory factors to the actual occurrence of lung cancer include environmental conditions and host factors that influence both exposure and response. A range of conditions, including genetic, personal (emotions and stress), social (family and support groups), socioeconomic status, and occupation, have an influence on individual susceptibility to a disease, known as the "biologic spectrum," which ranges from no reaction or infection to death.

The occurrence of disease depends on contributions from a range of causes (Hahn, 1995). Causes of death are often viewed in terms of the immediate causes (such as heart attack, head trauma, HIV/AIDS, etc.), but these are generally not sufficient. For example, HIV infection may (or may not) occur as the consequence of behaviors that expose an individual to the virus. Becoming infected with HIV does not lead directly to AIDS, which requires other conditions that compromise the immune system (such as stress, poor nutrition, drug use).

The concept of cause has a number of different levels. Necessary causes are those that are required; there must be the presence of a certain infectious agent or condition for disease to occur. Necessary causes are seldom sufficient causes, those that alone invariably result in a condition. Sufficient causes seldom occur because contributing factors or cofactors are also necessary for the development of disease. **Determinants** are considered scientifically established causes with direct effects on the level of disease as the most proximal (nearest) causes. There are distal or remote causes, factors that initiated a malignant condition far removed from the disease outcomes (such as a mosquito bite leading to malarial infection). The more proximal or immediate causes (such as the plasmodial parasites' destruction of red blood cells) are generally biological changes that lead to pathological states. **Proximal causes** are often those medically treated (medicines for reducing blood pressure for those with heart disease), but the more **distal causes** (poor diet and lack of exercise) are those that need to be modified to prevent disease.

Epidemiology attempts to separate direct and indirect factors. **Direct contributing factors** affect the extent of a determinant (factors such as a mother's drug use and nutritional status that result in low birth weight and high neonatal mortality). **Indirect contributing factors** are less proximal to health outcomes but affect them by influencing directly contributing factors (such as how lack of access to food stamps indirectly contributes to infant mortality by compromising women's nutritional status).

A complex chain of events is generally responsible for a death. An immediate cause of death (e.g., heart attack) has antecedent conditions (sodium retention, arteriosclerosis, high blood pressure) that contribute to the outcome. Antecedent conditions may be traced back to an underlying cause that initiated the chain of events leading to the death (such as sodium retention or other genetic traits or diet that contributes to high blood pressure). If the cause of death was a car crash, head injury could be the immediate cause, vehicular accident could be identified as the antecedent cause, and if the driver was intoxicated, alcohol could be designated as the underlying cause. But what if drunken behavior was a response to spousal conflict, which arose from the loss of one's job? Where do underlying causes and contributory factors stop? Medicine tends to stop at the direct biological mechanisms; cultural perspectives may attribute primary causality to social factors, including the class system, economic factors, and the international capitalist system.

BIOCULTURAL INTERACTIONS

Factors in CVD

It is noteworthy that the symptoms of CVD—hypertension, high cholesterol levels, and arteriosclerosis—may be considered necessary causes in only a limited sense because a cardiac arrest can also be induced by physical (drug, electrical) and "emotional" shock. In that sense, hypertension and arteriosclerosis are contributing factors and are distal causes of CVD. More proximal causes are found in everyday life, such as diet, activity, and stress, particularly the consumption of high-sugar, -salt, and -fat foods that can have an immediate impact on hypertension. These influences can lead to obesity, which provides more direct contributing causes of CVD by placing a greater load on a person's entire system. Proximal indirect contributing factors include the physical environments of the inner city that increase risks by inhibiting good diet and exercise. Both deteriorated inner-city environments and the broader societal discrimination can function as contributing factors to hypertension, stress, and psychological discord. Indirect contributing factors would include economic and political factors that have inhibited a person's access to health care for addressing CVD. All of these together will not necessarily cause a heart attack; there are many people considered "walking heart attacks" who will eventually die of something else. Something must precipitate an episode in which situational factors exacerbate the problems faced by a stressed system, exemplified in the case study of Mr. Glover reported in Chapter Two.

Where does "cause" ultimately reside? Because the occurrence of a disease depends on a variety of circumstances, explaining the origins of a disease requires an ecological model to relate diverse causes, contributory factors, and resistance resources in a "web of causation" linking the interactions among many conditions (Mausner and Kramer, 1985). Epidemiology's methodological approaches attempt to distinguish correlated conditions from variables that are causes or contributing factors.

Cultural Systems Approaches in Epidemiology

Epidemiology faces problems because of an excessive adherence to a biological paradigm (McKinlay and Marceau, 2000); this illustrates the importance of cultural systems perspectives in epidemiology (see Janes, Stall, and Gifford, 1986; Trostle and Sommerfield, 1996). The biomedical approach exemplified in the risk factor perspective associated with ethnic groups and their genetic differences has limited ability to explain variation in disease across major diseases. Cultural approaches provide a corrective to the epidemiological and biomedical perspectives on individual characteristics and risks. Biomedical views that medical conditions are caused by the risk characteristics of the individual—such as their personal behaviors, ignorance, or faults—result in interventions designed to educate the individual. Instead, the focus should be on addressing the broader sociocultural dynamics that affect many individuals by placing entire groups at risk. For instance, is it more useful to educate mothers and children about the risks to health from playing in raw sewage running in open ditches in their neighborhood? Or is it more appropriate to change that risk condition by providing sewage disposal systems? A cultural systems perspective shifts the focus from individual risk factors to an understanding of the systems relationships that affect populations, a process of contextualizing risks.

The epidemiological approach linking diseases to symptoms needs additional information to explain the dynamic relationships among cultural factors that shape the group's risk for disease. Anthropological perspectives help in identifying the social settings within which risks occur. This is done by explaining the linkages across risk factors: for example, why smoking cigarettes is a risk marker for cervical cancer even if it is not a cause. The human-environment relations fundamental to disease causation are produced, mediated, and structured by cultural factors that link causes and contributory factors. Culture explains linkages among the necessary determinants, contributory factors, and other social conditions associated with a disease, addressing epidemiology's need to understand causal risk behaviors to modify them through prevention programs.

Public health programs require understanding of the contextual dynamics of disease transmission, how cultural effects on behavior are involved in a causal web that produces disease. Explaining the associations of risk factors with diseases, such as higher rates of CVD for African Americans, requires "biological plausibility," an explanation of how the interactions of direct and indirect causal effects with contributing factors occur in the presence of necessary conditions. Cultural approaches identify systemic cultural factors that produce risk behaviors and their association with disease. The plausible mechanisms for relating risk factors to disease occur in the social context within which members of society are differentially distributed with respect to those risk factors.

The role of culture in mediating human contact with pathogens makes cultural factors central to an epidemiological analysis of how culture affects mortality, as shown in Table 2.1. All five major U.S. ethnic groups have heart disease as the number one cause of death, but Blacks have rates nearly twice those of Hispanics. The second major cause of death in the United States as a whole is cancer (malignant neoplasms), but Asian and Pacific Islanders have nearly half the rate of mortality from cancers (186 per 100,000 versus 111 per 100,000, respectively). Cultural perspectives are necessary to explain how these risk markers (ethnicity) are related to mortality. Why do African Americans have nearly twice the death rates due to heart disease? Why is being a Native American associated with elevated risk levels of motor-vehicle fatalities (26 versus 15) and liver disease (23 versus 9)?

For a more complete understanding, these findings need to be contextualized within culture-specific lifestyles and behavioral dynamics. Cultural approaches help explain how risk factors are associated with increased mortality by providing an understanding of the social contexts and behaviors involved in creating elevated risks and disease outcomes. For example, the social context of much Native American alcohol consumption (off reservations, far from home, and at great distances from hospitals) increases the number of automobile accidents and the consequences of those injuries. African Americans' heart disease may reflect some genetic contributions to hypertension but also social factors affecting diet, access to health care, experiences of prejudice, and cultural conflict.

Cultural perspectives are key for both descriptive epidemiology in identifying factors that predict the distribution of diseases and in analytical approaches to determining the causes of disease. Cultural methods are essential for preliminary epidemiological research, providing qualitative data for the development of measurements appropriate to specific populations. Cultural differences are fundamental to concepts of population segments analyzed by epidemiologists (such as race or ethnicity, religious participation, and social class). Cultural approaches are essential to understanding the significance of epidemiological findings on relationships of racial categories to health. Ethnic differences in mortality rates and specific causes of disease might be seen as reflecting something about biological differences among groups. This idea of distinct genetic characteristics has been a longstanding assumption embodied in the concept of race and has been used often in medicine to understand cultural differences in disease rates. As the following discussion of race indicates, the assumption of genetic differences accounting for differences in disease rates does not have validity. Cultural perspectives are essential in understanding the interaction between biological and cultural effects in producing intergroup differences in health.

RACIAL AND ETHNIC CATEGORIES AND HEALTH

The classic perspectives on race implied that racial or ethnic differences in health risks might result from genetic differences among groups. Race has been used traditionally to represent what was presumed to be biologically different human groups, but anthropology and genetics have shown that these supposed groups are not based in biological differences. Nor are the different disease rates among so-called races determined exclusively, or even principally, by genetic differences among groups. Rather, these ethnic differences in health outcomes are the consequences of how culture and social relations, including the treatment of some humans by others, produce differences in diseases among ethnic groups.

Racial Categories as Cultural Concepts

The concept of race historically implied biologically distinct groups of humans, each with unique and exclusive biological traits that the group (race) presumably shared in common. When such classification schemas arose in the Western world, genetics was not known, and classifications were based on an easily notable difference: skin color. Skin color was the primary basis for historical racial classifications of the White, Black, Brown, Yellow, and Red races (Europeans, Africans, Malayans, Asians, and Native Americans, respectively). The concept of races began in the context of Western contact with other peoples during colonization. The race concept gained popularity as a justification of the exploitation and unequal treatment of groups defined as inferior races.

Although early anthropology contributed to the notion that there were biologically unique races, modern anthropology has rejected such notions as a consequence of systematic investigations into the relationship of biological features to racial classifications. As genetic sciences emerged, examinations were made of the distribution of not only the obvious features (e.g., skin, eye, and hair color) but also of less obvious features such as bone sizes and dimensions, tooth patterns, enzymes, blood types, serum proteins, hemoglobin, and nasal index.

The measurement of the distribution of these traits illustrates individual and group differences but also undermines the concept of biologically distinct races. The search for the biological basis for the racial categories led to a surprising finding: No genetic features uniquely separated one racial group from another. Moreover, as the actual genetic variation in the human species was studied, the differences resulted in the initial handful of races quickly exploding into dozens. Soon the idea of homogeneous populations with distinct genetic characteristics was abandoned in recognition that the so-called racial groups have considerable internal variation and share most genetic characteristics with other groups. There is more genetic variation within racial groups than between them.

This assumption of unique traits differentiating the racial groups is rejected by modern genetic research. Almost all human genetic material is shared in common, and no racial group has uniform and unique characteristics shared by no other races. Statistical differences between groups' genetic traits do not causally determine differences in behavior, psychology, or cultural achievement. Humans have among the narrowest genetic differences of all species, reflecting the recent origins of modern *Homo sapiens* and their considerable genetic homogeneity. Furthermore, members of the same racial group may have greater differences between them than they do with respect to members of other racial groups.

There are human genetic traits that can be traced in groups and lineages across millennia. There also are statistical differences in the frequency of genetic traits in different groups that make the group label useful in guiding health screening for specific diseases (such as sickle cell in African Americans and phenylketonuria among European Americans). Similarly, certain genetic diseases are present more frequently in Jewish populations (as described earlier in the special feature "Biocultural Interactions: Prevalent Genetic Diseases Among Ashkenazi Jews"), but the vast majority of Jewish people do not have these genetic traits. There are disease and biological differences between groups called racial or ethnic, but they are neither homogeneous within groups nor exclusive between groups. Africans are more likely to have sickle cell traits, but not all Africans do, and many non-Africans are also sickle cell carriers.

Population Biological Differences   There is genetic variation among humans and statistical differences in genetic features between groups, but these differences do not define distinct groups. The concept of the **cline** is an alternative to the concept of race for organizing information about human genetic variation. A cline is a variation in the frequency of a single genetic trait across a geographical area. For instance, the percentage of a population with the genetically coded enzyme lactase varies as a function of distance from the ancient centers of cattle domestication. Systematic analysis of single traits permits the determination of the relationship of the trait to ecological conditions, population movements, and other factors. Analyses of clines show that the concept of races is arbitrary because discrete geographical boundaries for genetic traits do not exist. The discordance of variation of more than one trait (e.g., blood type, lactase, sickle cell anemia) shows that the classification of people into races characterized by combinations of distinct genes is not possible. Instead, we generally find that different genetic features are nonconcordant, that variation in one feature such as height is not correlated with blood type, lactase, or other genetic variations. Human variation at the level of racial groups can be described only as different relative frequencies of genes, not their absolute presence or absence. And there is no exclusively "Black," "White," "Brown," or other racial group gene.

Brues (1977) suggested that we reconcile the traditional concept of race with the current scientific knowledge about biological variation by defining a race in terms of the frequency of hereditary traits, but not whether they are present or absent in individual members of a purported race and not found in other races. Trying to define racial groups on the basis of gene frequencies in populations is problematic. The inability of scientists to achieve a consensus as to which clusters or groupings of morphological and genetic data constitute a race is widely recognized. What specific genetic characteristics are to be considered relevant for this classification? There are no natural determinants of which genes should be used for the purposes of racial classification. Most patterns of biological variation (e.g., molar patterns, blood types) are not used to classify people into racial groups. Furthermore, any group defined on the basis of genes alone would include people who consider themselves to be of different races and would separate people who consider themselves to be of the same race.

The social and intercultural context is the primary determinant of the meaning and consequences of race and the potent effects of such labeling. Statistical differences in physical features are also found between specific ethnic groups that result from group influences on individual developmental acclimatization. For instance, poor diet, specific work, or recreational activities such as horseback riding leave telltale signs on the skeletal structure. These can be used in forensic science to assist in identifying people from skeletal remains ("Applications: Forensic Anthropology"). This use of racial concepts can also produce errors. Goodman (1997) points out that the use of racial profiles in forensic medicine has led to misidentifications and misdiagnoses, often conflating genetic traits with the consequences of lived experiences. Forensic research has often bowed to political pressure to provide "bureaucratic races" based on ideal types, ignoring methodological problems. The failure to control for the effects of environment, socialization, social class, resources, education, and other social factors confounds any presumed biological differences between races.

The use of the term "race," therefore, should be rejected because of the inaccuracy of its assumptions regarding the nature and basis of human differences. Rejection of the appropriateness of the term race is not to deny physical differences between *groups* in terms of the *frequency* of specific genetic traits in populations. However, these groups have internal differences so great that some members are more similar to the normative profiles of other races than those of their own self-identified race. For instance, many African Americans have more biological heritage from European or White ancestry than African ancestry but are still socially identified as Black. Similarly, people from India are often considered Black in the United States, although their racial classification is Caucasian and group genetic profiles are more similar to European populations than to African populations. Why cannot we simply classify people into races on such apparent characteristics as skin color? This requires an understanding of the nature and basis of skin color differences.

APPLICATIONS

Forensic Anthropology

Forensic anthropology is the application of methods of physical anthropology for the identification of unknown people and of the causes of their death through the examination of both soft tissue and skeletal remains. Forensic anthropologists may apply their skills to the study of ancient human remains, but many use their skills to address contemporary concerns, such as identifying victims of crimes, airplane crashes, mass deaths by burning, or mass burials. Forensic anthropologists apply their skills at the identification of behavioral effects on skeletal materials to assist in determining the cause of death. This knowledge also facilitates the identification of victims through knowledge of the effects of cultural activities and behavior on skeletal features, such as how motorcycle riding or horseback riding leaves specific effects on the development of the skeletal structure.

Forensic anthropology is based on human osteology (study of bones), skeletal biology, human variation, dental anthropology, and a variety of other specialized fields, including gross anatomy, comparative anatomy, human growth and development, nutrition, pathology, toxicology, entomology, taphonomy, odontology, laboratory and DNA analyses, and criminal psychology. Forensic anthropology also employs skills from archaeology and cultural and applied anthropology as well as a general understanding of criminal investigations and roles of expert witnesses in courtroom testimony.

This field involves an interdisciplinary collaboration with pathologists and homicide investigators in the identification of victims of homicides and finding clues to their killers. Forensic anthropologists may remove human remains and associated artifacts and subject them to laboratory assessments to help determine the elapsed time since death and the person's sex, age, cause of death, history of disease and trauma, and work and other habitual activities affecting the skeleton (such as motorcycle or horseback riding, carrying heavy objects above the head). Evidence of previous disease and injury is assessed. Facial bone structures help reconstruct the face to link remains

Skin Coloration as Ecological Adaptation

The genetic basis of skin color needs to be understood to appreciate why it does not provide a scientific basis for racial distinctions. A microscopically thin pigment-bearing layer of skin determines skin color. The same substance—a pigment called melanin—determines all colors of skin, hair, and eyes. Differences in skin color among humans reflect the operation of this single genetic factor in interaction with the environment, along with minor variations in color and tone from near-surface blood vessels and carotene in the diet. Natural selection has led to local populations with greater or lesser activation of this system, but all human skin color—white to black—uses this system.

Melanin granules are found in two forms, eumelanin, which produces brown and black shades of color, and pheomelanin, which is responsible for red hair. These forms of melanin are also found in many other mammals. The melanin granules are produced by melanocytes located in the deep (germinative) layer of the skin. The number of melanocytes is about the same for all different colors of skin, but the amount of melanin produced to missing persons' reports. Physical features that differ statistically across ethnic groups help narrow identification to specific ethnic groups. Once identification has been made and cause of death determined, the forensic anthropologist may be called on to testify in court.

Textbooks and manuals assist the forensic anthropologist in these processes (see Stewart, 1979; Galloway, Woltanski, and Grant, 1993; Haglund and Sorg, 1996; Rhine, 1998; Burns, 1999). Forensic anthropologists have a credentialing process through the American Board of Forensic Anthropology (see http://www.csuchico.edu/anth/ABFA) and a Physical Anthropology section within the American Academy of Forensic Sciences. Many forensic anthropologists are professors of physical anthropology in universities with forensic anthropology programs (such as Universitiy of North Carolina-Charlotte, University of Toronto, and University of Tennessee-Knoxville). Some forensic anthropologists work in public agencies, such as the federal (Grisbaum and Ubelaker, 2001), state, or county bureaus of investigation, medical coroners' and medical examiners' offices, and other federal agencies (U.S. Fish and Wildlife Service Law Enforcement).

Some forensic anthropologists work at the Central Identification Laboratory in Hawaii, identifying war casualties. They identify human remains from wars, particularly where genocide is an issue, such as in former Yugoslavia (Bosnia, Serbia) or in Guatemala, where government-sponsored death squads killed tens of thousands of Indians and peasants. Forensic anthropology is a tool in the struggle for human rights and punishment of those who commit genocide. Scientific documentation of the time, place, manner of death, and the presence of others provides crucial evidence for prosecution. Forensic anthropologists may also work on disasters such as explosions, bombings, and the flooding of cemeteries that displaces bodies. The 2001 disasters at the World Trade Center in New York brought forensic anthropologists into direct involvement in the recovery and identification of bodies.

and its distribution vary. Light-skinned persons produce melanin slowly, and dark-skinned individuals produce much more melanin and more rapidly. Individuals with darker skin also have their melanin granules more evenly dispersed to absorb light more effectively.

Thus, the differences between "Whites" and "Blacks," in those with light versus dark skin, is not with respect to the absence and presence of a genetic characteristic determining skin color. People with light skin and those with dark skin have the same pigment-producing cells, but they produce different amounts. Classifying people into races on the basis of the darkness of skin color is analogous to classifying people into races based on the thickness of their hair, their dental enamel, or subcutaneous fat deposits.

The differences in skin pigmentation reflect the mediation of bodily processes through the intensity of pigmentation: one provides for protection from the sun's ultraviolet radiation, the other for the production of vitamin D. Exposure to the sun's ultraviolet rays can cause serious burning of the skin. Exposure to the sun results in the stimulation of melanin production and its movement toward the surface of the skin, where it provides protection against the sun. Such protection reduces painful burns and skin cancer. People living near equatorial zones where ultraviolet irradiation is most intense have darker-pigmented skin as protection. Intense equatorial sunlight increases ultraviolet irradiation and the overproduction of vitamin D, which can cause calcium buildup in body tissues, kidney failure, and circulatory, joint, and other health problems.

The distribution of lighter-pigmented skin reflects a different but related process. The effects of ultraviolet irradiation on the cholesterol in the skin produce vitamin D. A bone disease called rickets can result from vitamin D insufficiency; when resulting in pelvic bone deformation, it causes great difficulty in childbirth and can lead to death of the mother and fetus. As populations moved out of Africa and into northern regions, the selective advantage of darker skin was replaced by the selective advantages of lighter skin. People living in the northernmost areas of the globe face a risk of vitamin D insufficiency because the limited sunlight both reduces ultraviolet irradiation and creates the demand for additional clothing that limits the skin's exposure to ultraviolet rays. Dark-colored skin with larger amounts of melanin would further reduce the amount of ultraviolet rays absorbed and vitamin D production. Therefore, light-colored skin is adaptive in these regions to ensure the sufficient production of vitamin D. Additional selective mechanisms for light skin in northern regions may result from a greater propensity for frostbite of dark-skinned individuals. More recent migrations have not resulted in changes in skin coloration because biological adaptations take place over long periods and because technology and culture (clothing, vitamins, etc.) are quicker adaptations to managing these interactions with the environment.

So why can't we effectively and scientifically use skin color for racial classification? There is nothing unique about skin pigmentation between groups. Some groups are lighter or darker on average, but there is no clear distinction. Furthermore, nature does not provide any natural cutoff points between shades of skin color. Skin color is not determined by genes alone but occurs as a consequence of developmental acclimatization experiences, including sun exposure that stimulates the body's protective responses and produces darker skin. Neither nature nor science tells us that skin color should be a principle for dividing groups, rather than other genetically influenced features such as hair thickness, blood type, eye color, and types of earwax.

Rejecting the Race Concept

What are called racial groups actually have their differences in culture—learned behavior and beliefs—and group identity formation called ethnicity. Race is a distracting term in interethnic relations because it implies that biological factors explain differences when the biological differences do not exist. Contrary to popular belief, races are not biological groups like species or subspecies but, rather, cultural constructs. Effectively addressing ethnic differences in disease requires considering causal cultural and social factors and not falsely presuming that the cause is in genetic differences between groups.

The use of race as a means of categorizing human beings can be seen as racism. The lack of a scientific basis for the concept of race and its historical use to justify discrimination reveal the racist basis of the belief in races. A belief in races contributes to racism because it imputes to people and groups inherent genetic characteristics and justifies social barriers, prejudices, and discriminatory treatments. Racial thinking is frequently used to reinforce differences, ignoring how economic or educational opportunities produce differences among groups. Abandoning the term race focuses attention on sociocultural causes of group differences, as manifested in the concept of **ethnicity,** the social identity of members of a recognized cultural group. This approach of abandoning race in favor of ethnicity is a formal proposal to the U.S. government by the American Anthropological Association. This group has recommended that the U.S. government phase out the use of the categories and term "race." This is based on the recognition that the concept of race lacks scientific justification and does not describe or explain human biological variation. The use of ethnic categories that reflect the cultural and social bases of groupings is a more appropriate approach.

Current governmental classifications make use of both racial and ethnic categories without any clear basis for differentiating between them. Research often makes use of these racial categories in studies of populations but without a clear justification for these distinctions. The term "ethnic" differs from the biologically based concept of race and directs attention to the social dynamics that define group differences and produce the social and cultural effects on health conditions associated with race.

TRIUNE BRAIN STRUCTURES AND FUNCTIONS

Interactions among physiological, behavioral, and mental levels of an organism in maintaining health are based in relationships among functional brain systems. MacLean (1990) proposes that the brain's principle functional systems involve a **triune brain,** as mentioned earlier: three anatomically distinct systems that provide behavioral, emotional, and cognitive functions:

■ The **reptilian brain** or R complex

■ The **paleomammalian brain** (limbic system)

■ The **neomammalian brain** (neocortical structures)

MacLean's model of three brain strata has limitations, but motor patterns, social and emotional dynamics, and advanced cognitive capabilities did emerge sequentially in evolution. These brain systems shared with other animals were elaborated in the human brain with new components, especially at the borders between systems. This triune brain model provides a framework for explicating the relationships of health to behavioral, emotional, and symbolic processes.

The *reptilian brain* (or R complex) regulates organic functions such as metabolism, digestion, and respiration and coordinates behaviors involved in reproduction and self-preservation. The reptilian brain provides programs for genetically based behaviors ("instincts") and survival activities, including territorial behavior, mating, hunting, power struggles, and social hierarchies. The traditional view of the R complex as a motor apparatus has been expanded in recognition of its more complex roles in the regulation of daily routines, behavioral (nonverbal) communication, social interaction, and ritual activities.

The *paleomammalian* (or *limbic*) *brain* emerged 100 million years ago in the primitive mammalian brain. This "emotional brain" mediates sex; eating and drinking; fighting or self-defense; emotions; social relations, bonding, and attachment; the sense of self; and feelings of certainty and conviction. The paleomammalian brain integrates emotions into behavior, particularly those responsible for self and species preservation. The paleomammalian brain expands the capacities of the reptilian brain in an increased array of emotional expressive states, including sociability and enhanced capacities for bonding through nursing and maternal care. The limbic system regulates interaction of internal organ and neurohormonal systems with external psychosocial systems through providing the basis for memory, personal identity, and social relations.

The *neomammalian brain* (telencephalon or neocortical structures) resulted from hominid encephalization, the growth of the frontal areas of the brain that led to the emergence of humans and provided the capacity for symbolic processes and language. The neomammalian brain underlies the uniquely human language skills (speech, reading, writing); analytical processes such as problem solving, complex learning, detailed memory, logic, and math; and the generation and preservation of information, including cultural transmission. Neomammalian structures improved sensory and motor functions, extended memory capacity, and reorganized older structures into more complex functional hierarchies. In humans, it provides the basis for self-reflective consciousness.

MacLean (1993) proposes that the reptilian, paleomammalian, and neomammalian brains provide the basis for different mental functions, which MacLean labels **protomentation,** emotiomentation, and ratiomentation. The reptilian brain uses protomentation in organizing the basic actions of the body. The paleomammalian brain provides emotional influences on thoughts and behavior through emotiomentation. Protomentation and emotiomentation both involve the expression of meanings and intentions through vocal, bodily, behavioral, and chemical systems. The neomammalian brain expands on these biologically based messages through the symbolic capacities of language, which elaborate on the meanings of basic behaviors and emotions by integrating them with higher-level information processing derived from culture.

Development of the neocortex provided new potentials, but the functions of the earlier evolutionary formations persisted. The modern human brain is based in the interconnected heritages of the instinctual responses of the reptilian brain, the autonomic emotional states of the paleomammalian brain, and the cognitive processes of the neomammalian brain. For instance, when you are at a zoo and a tiger approaches the edge of the cage, your hair may stand on end (reptilian brain reaction) and your heart pound with excitement (emotional brain), but your neomammalian "thinking" brain assures you that the zoo has taken adequate precautions for your security, allowing you to ignore the messages of danger from your "animal" brains while you marvel at the tiger. But these different brains may function relatively autonomously. For instance, have you ever driven toward school or work on the weekend when you actually intended to go to the mall to shop? Or have you been preoccupied by and dwelled on your emotional issues and personal relationships while you are supposed to be studying calculus? Our behavioral and emotional brains may still operate with a great autonomy from our modern brain structures and provide a basis for health problems.

Ancient Brains and Health

The interrelationships among these three functional brain systems are mediated both physiologically by hormonal systems and symbolically by systems of meaning that we associate with events. These interactions have many effects on health and illness: for instance, when our fears evoke stress hormones or when our religious beliefs provide relief and calm in the face of crises. Interactions among levels of the brain are not just through language but involve representational systems that use social, affective (emotional), and presymbolic (visual) information to assess significance for the organism's well-being. They mediate, evoke, and channel physiological processes, producing healing through effects on the autonomic nervous system. The relationship among the functions of different levels of the brain—innate drives and needs, emotional and social influences, and cultural representational systems—produce many kinds of health problems in anxiety and fears, conflicts, excessive emotionality, obsessions, compulsions, dissociations, and repression.

The brain's principal functions are to interpret the external and internal worlds of experience. Although language representations are salient aspects of this awareness, cognitive processes based in lower brain structures also have important effects. Left hemisphere language capacities provide the most complex representations of meaning, but subneocortical processes shape meaning. Neocortical activities use information provided by intuitive representations, affective associations, and decisions of the paleomammalian brain, which plays a crucial role in providing unity to experience and a sense of conviction to our beliefs (Ashbrok, 1993). These brain processes have been referred to as *subsymbolic*.

These protomentation and emotiomentation processes are central to healing processes and many culturally induced maladies. Protomentation provides the basis for mental processes underlying impulses and obsessions (MacLean, 1993). The reptilian and paleomammalian brains are fundamental to the nonverbal thought that underlies basic emotions and social interaction. The R complex plays a fundamental role in imitation and behavioral communication, coordinating the overall integration of the reactions of the organism. The R complex has "a mind of its own" (MacLean, 1990) and entrains social, behavioral, and physiological patterns that affect well-being. But it cannot effectively learn how to cope with new situations, nor does it have knowledge of the subjective self.

Paleomammalian Brain and Emotiomentation   Paleomammalian processes represented in intuitions and feelings are vital to higher cognitive functions and behaviors. Emotiomentation involves brain processes underlying affects (emotions) that influence behavior through subjective information manifested as feelings (MacLean, 1990). These influence self-preservation behaviors: procreation, emotions, nursing and maternal care, audiovocal contact, and play. The paleomammalian brain system also synthesizes internal and external data, combining what the reactions of our bodies tell us with what we interpret in the outside world. This integration is mediated by other paleomammalian brain processes involving personal memory, self-representation, and social context. Empathic caring emerged from the long-term dependence of infants on adults for survival, involving the development of attachment behaviors, smiles, kissing, caressing, and other intimate interactions. Attachments produce emotional security and identity with family, providing the basis for extension of such relations to nonkin and the religious realms. Emotions are psychological information and can provoke physiological changes when the organism is confronted with threats to the survival of self or those others with whom we have interpersonal attachments. Symbolic manipulations of paleomammalian brain processes have profound effects on the organism, transforming emotiomentation into physiological effects that are fundamental to cultural healing rituals.

Emotional Brain and Health The paleomammalian brain produces and uses information through expressions of the face, vocalizations, actions, and gestures that provide information about other minds and their motives and internal states. These behaviors involve projections of the paleomammalian brain into the neocortex and evoke similar experiences in other individuals, creating a common awareness. Emotions affect others' behaviors through the activity of their minds and the interpretations modeled. The paleomammalian brain mediates patterns of social signaling that promote a sense of community and provide for cooperation—physically, socially, and mentally—in ways that enhance human adaptation and survival. The basis of personal well-being is deeply intertwined with a sense of community, a social identity where empathy with other humans provides the basis for self and security. These interactions also provide the basis for a variety of health problems derived from relations among emotions, social interaction, and sense of self. The emotional functions of the brain have a role in the instinctual drives and are directly tied to psychopathology in the distortion of drives (such as hunger and sex). The paleomammalian brain's activities are affected by cultural healing practices, including manipulations of emotions, sense of self, attachments, and social relations, providing mechanisms for achieving therapeutic results (Winkelman, 1992a, 2000a, 200b, 2002b).

EVOLUTION OF THE SICKNESS-AND-HEALING RESPONSES

Evolutionary perspectives indicate that sickness ("behavioral expressions of disease and injury") and healing ("culturally meaningful social responses aimed at undoing or preventing the effects of disease and injury") have a unitary basis (Fábrega, 1997, p. ix). Fábrega suggests that humans have a sickness-and-healing response, part of an integrated social and biological adaptation involved in helping others. Our innate healing responses are derived from biological adaptations involving caring, altruism, and compassion for our offspring and relatives (also see Williams and Nesse, 1991). This healing response of the organism assists others directly and has broader effects in restabilizing the group, engaging natural recovery responses based in innate processes of self-healing. When an organism's systems are disturbed, they react adaptively, constructively, and protectively. For humans, this includes a psychosomatic mediation of physiological and hormonal changes, where beliefs, hopes, and rituals induce positive changes in physiological responses.

Humans' innate sickness and healing adaptations are part of an evolutionary trend in the hominid line that provided caregiving. The ancient roots of these behaviors are reflected in the ways in which chimpanzees respond to the ill, wounded, or dying. The protection, caressing, grooming, assistance, and food provisioning to the ill illustrate that humans' sickness-and-healing responses involve an expansion of abilities found in the hominoid lineage (humans and great apes). The much greater development of the human healing responses indicates that it was part of the adaptations involved in human evolution from common ancestors with hominoids. The origins of sickness-and-healing responses involve a biologically rooted sociality manifested in the care of infants and children. This dynamic is extended to helping relatives, an extension of the dynamics of parental investment. Sickness and healing adaptations are also part of self-care activities (protecting from injuries, maintaining temperature homeostasis by covering a sick person) and enhancing social harmony when sickness destabilizes relations.

Sickness-and-healing responses involve an emotional awareness of others, a primate tendency to respond to emotional displays of others with expressions of empathy and sympathy. Emotions that are natural healing elicitors are states of pain, suffering, and distress, which evoke responsive capacities of empathy, compassion, and altruism. Sickness-and-healing responses constitute an emotional communication based in the ability to take into consideration another organism's condition; this requires a theory of mind to make appropriate attributions of the condition of others, the inference that another suffers and needs assistance.

Evolutionary pressures selecting for sickness-and-healing abilities are also involved in selecting for social exchange, sharing, and reciprocity. Changes in social organization that occurred during the development of the *Homo* line included enhanced social bonds, family ties, and extension of kinship systems into social alliances and group organization (Fábrega, 1997). A common response to sickness is face-to-face interactions, particularly among family members, and group interactions in ceremonies. Fábrega suggests that the adaptations for sickness and healing generated many kinds of experiences, including the evolution of society and culture. Sickness-and-healing behaviors were necessarily linked to an awareness of death because the phenomenon it sought to treat—sickness—often ends in death. This link to death means that sickness-and-healing relations were necessarily extended to care of the deceased and ideas about spiritual domains, afterlife, and religion.

Shamanism as an Evolved Healing Response

In his examination of the evolutionary roots of religion, Hayden (2003) also reveals the emotional bases of the origins of human healing practices in a phenomenon called shamanism. Hayden argues that these behaviors emerged out of humans' unique innate emotional foundations, including those involving the functions of altered states of consciousness. The central role of ASCs in shamanic behaviors and healing practices worldwide suggests that the biological structures commonly associated with shamanic ASCs are the basis of religion; they also have important healing effects. ASCs activate the paleomammalian brain (see Chapter Ten), a key area of the brain for managing emotions and interpersonal relations. ASCs provided adaptive effects in producing a sense of connectedness with others. Hayden proposes that communal rituals involving these ecstatic states had the effect of strengthening alliances and permitting an expanded sense of community. Hayden suggests that ritually induced ASCs enabled early humans to overcome our natural tendency to engage in an in-group-versus-out-group mentality, fearing outsiders. Instead of rejecting outsiders from their own social group, ASC rituals facilitated experiences of deep bonds with others.

Hayden proposes that these shamanic ritual behaviors played a selective role in human adaptations during periods several million years ago when extremely inhospitable environments and resource scarcity exerted selective influences on human evolution. Early hominids better adapted to these hostile environments by using shamanic rituals to forge close emotional bonds with members of other groups. This facilitated survival by providing others who could be relied on for food resources and physical protection.

I have proposed that an expansion of earlier group rituals also found in chimpanzees were the bases for these shamanic adaptations (Winkelman, 2004b, 2008). Night-time group rituals in chimpanzees sometimes include drumming, group chorusing, and excited bipedal charging displays (dancing). These kinds of activities produce ASCs in humans that have the effect of strengthening emotional bonds among members of a group. Thus, ritual and healing have common origins in strengthening group bonds.

The evolution of human healing responses involved expansions of earlier ritual capacities of mammals and primates. Rituals have many adaptive functions in the animal world, constituting the most complex forms of communication and group organization and integration. Rituals have important protective functions, providing an enhanced awareness of danger through signals that share information in ways that unite the group in a common orientation to danger. Rituals also provide for a reduction of aggression and injury within the group, allowing signals provided by rituals to express dominance (and submission), thereby precluding the need to fight to establish it and preventing injuries. Rituals are also used in reconciliation among disputants and to provide assurance to subordinate animals, allowing a reduction of stress and fear. A central primate ritual of reconciliation and support involves grooming, where animals carefully examine one another's body to remove parasites and intruded objects (such as thorns) and to cleanse wounds. These activities have not only calming effects but also important hygienic functions, especially when done in areas of the body an animal cannot clean on its own (such as the back).

These aspects of physical care and ritual reassurance are the foundations of the evolved sickness-and-healing response of humans. Elsewhere I have also presented evidence that these evolutionary developments led to shamanism, a universal spiritual healing practice of hunter-gatherer societies (Winkelman, 1992a, 2000a, 2002a, 2004b, 2008; also see Chapter Ten). Shamanism developed as community ritual activities for manipulating biological responses (such as the relaxation response) as adaptations to the need for psychosocial, interpersonal, and emotional adjustment. These shamanic adjustments are based in the stimulation of ancient structures of the brain through many of the same ritual activities used by animals to coordinate and integrate their societies. Similarities in shamanic healing practices around the world reflect the operation of innate healing responses for community ritual healing. Cross-cultural features of shamanism are directly related to innate brain processes that are elicited through the induction of ASCs. That some of the activities that induce ASCs (such as drumming, chanting, and dancing) have analogous forms in chimpanzee rituals points to the deep evolutionary roots of shamanism and how shamanic healing utilizes a variety of ritual mechanisms to produce physiological, psychological, and social integration, particularly in the area of emotions. Humans, however, have far more elaborate rituals than other animals, particularly in the area of healing.

Foundations for Innate Healing Capacities

McClenon (2002) argues that the origins of religious healing and shamanism involve an inheritable quality manifested in hypnotic susceptibility and its interaction with suggestibility and placebo effects. A strong correlation exists between hypnotic susceptibility and dissociation, fantasy proneness and thin cognitive boundaries, all involving enhanced connections between unconscious and conscious aspects of the mind and a greater susceptibility to suggestibility. People who are highly susceptible to hypnosis are more likely to have anomalous experiences (such as seeing ghosts or having spiritual experiences), are more fantasy-prone, and often experience having a "calling" to provide healing services.

This hypnotic capacity, manifested in repetitive behaviors or stereotypy, has ancient roots in primate biology in mechanisms for reducing aggression and social stress and engaging the relaxation response. For humans, the repetitive behaviors associated with animals' hypnotic behaviors produce both an alteration of consciousness and a sense of intragroup cohesion experienced as "union" or "oneness," classic aspects of religious and mystical experiences. The hypnotic capacity has adaptive features in enhancing processes of innovation derived from access to the unconscious mind; consequently, it can provide survival advantages by facilitating the development of creative strategies. Hypnotizability involves focused attention, reduced external awareness, and a reduction of critical thought processes that facilitate a focus on internal images and an enhancement of beliefs and expectations. The thin cognitive boundaries characteristic of highly hypnotizable people give them greater access to the information in their personal unconscious and the communication of information to the conscious mind.

Hypnotizability and increased suggestibility are associated with placebo effects, where psychological expectations produce physiological reactions. Consequently, the hypnotic capacity provides a basis for miraculous cures that enhance survival. The survival impact of these healing practices exerted selective pressures for humans disposed to hypnotizability. McClenon (2002) contends that the origins of shamanic healing practices are found in the adaptations produced by hypnosis and placebo effects. The tendency to suggestibility, which is based in hypnotic capacities, contributed to a biological capacity for recovery from disease. Suggestibility enhances symbolically induced physiological changes, psychophysiological responses that facilitate healing. Shamanic practices appear successful in treating the same kinds of conditions for which hypnosis has been shown to have significant clinical effects: somatization; mild psychiatric disorders; simple gynecological conditions; gastrointestinal and respiratory tract disorders; self-limiting diseases; chronic pain, neurosis, and hysterical conditions; and interpersonal, psychosocial, and cultural problems (see McClenon, 2002, for review). These are also characterized as emotional disorders, making an understanding of emotions key to an appreciation of the nature of human healing.

EMOTIONS IN BIOCULTURAL PERSPECTIVE

Emotions involve interactions of biology and culture in the production and interpretation of experience. Emotions are central to the most enjoyable of human experiences, the worst of them, and most psychopathologies. Emotions involve

- Physiological functions, processes, and reactions

- Motivations and behaviors related to one's sense of well-being

- Interpersonal, social, and communicative processes involving cultural appraisals

Emotions involve cultural appraisals or assessments of circumstances, interpretations of significance that link physiological reactions and personal experiences with social context. Emotions involve reactions that orient individuals to circumstances of importance within the social niche based in personal and cultural appraisals (assessments) of their implications for the well-being of self and significant others.

The universality of some emotional expressions (Izard, 1980, 1991; Ekman, 1972, 1973, 1982, 1986, 2003) suggests a biological basis for emotions. On the other hand, considerable cross-cultural variation in emotions and their significance points to cultural foundations. These positions reflect a long-standing dichotomy within science, the nature-versus-nurture debate: the determination of behavior by biology versus socialization. Anthropology has been associated with the nurture or socialization position, with cross-cultural perspectives contributing to an understanding of emotions as culturally specific expressions of meaning. Anthropology also emphasizes a biocultural perspective that considers emotions to emerge from the interaction of innate capacities with socialization and cultural values. These very different conclusions are both true. There are biologically based emotional capacities that are part of the instinctual heritage of mammals, but they are elicited by culturally shaped triggers and manifested as socially appropriate responses. Human emotions emerge from interactions among biological capacities (nature), learning experiences (nurture), social and environmental circumstances (context), and the appraisals (attributions) that humans make of those experiences (meaning).

Human Emotions: Universal or Culturally Specific?

Cross-cultural research on the meanings of facial expressions (Ekman, 1972, 1986; Izard, 1971, 1980, 1991) illustrates universals of human emotions. Studies using photographs of emotional facial expressions of people from many different cultures indicate that some emotions are universally recognized: happiness, sadness, anger, fear, surprise, and disgust. Imitative expressions of these emotions by infants begin shortly after birth, reflecting the innate bases of these capacities. People cross-culturally make similar attributions of meaning to these basic emotional expressions: smiles generally mean happiness and frowns mean sadness. These findings show that basic emotional facial expressions are a nonverbal communication system involving hardwired programs. Neurological bases for basic emotions are further illustrated by similar dynamics in animals, which show rage, fear, panic, play, lust, and care (Panksepp, 1998). Panksepp (2000) outlines the neural systems supporting these behaviors, suggesting that they constitute neurobiologically grounded archetypal intentional systems and primary forms of consciousness.

These universal emotions are not expressed, evaluated, and experienced in identical manners in all cultures, however. Cross-cultural variation in the expression of basic emotions reflects cultural interpretations essential to eliciting any emotion. Cultural elaborations on basic emotions may intensify (exaggerate), minimize, modify, or mask their expression. Cultures have different interpretations of emotional expressions (Russell, 1994) and different evaluations of the appropriateness and response to basic emotions (e.g., how anger is viewed). Cultures may expect exaggerated emotional displays, a suppression of emotions to convey a neutral emotional state, or even masking one emotion with another (e.g., using a smile to conceal anger). Cultural norms and vocabulary affect the labeling and reporting of experiences to reflect cultural values.

The universalist approach to emotions contends that common physiological processes underlie basic emotional responses (Levenson, 1992; Scherer, 2000a). The nervous system and its adaptive responses underlie the physiological responses to similar emotion-inducing situations (Panksepp, 2000). For example, there are adaptive advantages, such as a widening of the eyes and visual field, associated with surprise, a response that helps to obtain more information. Although cultures differ in the emphasis placed on aspects of emotions, verbal reports of the physiological experiences associated with basic emotions show substantial similarities across cultures (Scherer, 1994). Evidence suggests that universal emotional expressions in facial, vocal, and bodily reactions are based in physiological adaptations affecting behavioral tendencies and communicative signaling (Scherer, 2000b).

Evolutionary and Physiological Perspectives

From a biological perspective, emotions are a part of our animal heritage that evolved because of their roles in adaptation and survival, providing automatic responses for handling crucial situations. Emotions provide information, revealing intents and motivations to others in ways that can facilitate social interaction and group bonding. Emotions are more elaborated in humans than in other animals and are central to human sociability, cognition, communication, and consciousness (Averill, 1996). Anger-induced violence, sexual behavior, attachment to offspring, guilt, jealousy, and envy are areas in which human emotions far exceed animals' responses.

Biological perspectives on emotions generally consider them to have bases in the sympathetic nervous system, which activates the fight-or-flight response that mobilizes our bodies for survival struggles through stress reactions, hormones, and neurotransmitters (Baum and Garofalo, 2000). Emotions involve not only this general arousal or activation of the organism but also linkages of information processing and behavioral responses across brain systems (Panksepp, 2000). Basic emotional states are associated with particular neurotransmitter and hormone profiles that contribute to the experience. Physiological pathways are not unique for each emotion, however. There are some systematic physiological patterns associated with specific emotional responses (such as activation of the amygdala in anger). Generally, however, different emotions are not characterized by physiological uniqueness because they all generally involve an increased activation and arousal of the body for response. What makes emotions differ has much to do with differences in cognitive appraisal, the assessment of the significance of the arousal and associated external events for the organism. This interaction complicates the question of whether the physiological reactions are causes of emotions or whether they are caused by subjective experiences. Do increases in heart rate and blood pressure make a person feel angry, or conversely, does feeling angry make one's heart rate and blood pressure increase? Probably both.

Despite cultural differences, there are, nonetheless, substantial similarities in how appraisal processes operate across cultures (Scherer, 2000b). The nature of an antecedent event results in a highly delimited range of responses. For example, there are strong similarities cross-culturally in appraisals of and emotional responses to threats to one's personal safety, the loss of loved ones, sexual opportunities, and the resolution of problems. These same studies, however, show cultural differences in the strength of responses and in the social and communicative aspects of the experiences. Particularly salient cultural differences are found in appraisals involving morality or justice (Scherer, 2000b). Contemporary views of emotions recognize culture as a necessary physiological aspect of the input to an individual's appraisal of situations that produce emotional responses. Cultures differ in their appraisal criteria and their guidelines for responses based in values, priorities, and meanings. For example, if you feel anger, should you "let it out" on the person who provoked it? Or should you blame yourself for letting your emotions get out of control? These differences lead some to consider culture rather than biology the essential defining criterion of emotions.

Constructionist Perspectives and Biocultural Correctives

These biological perspectives on emotions are challenged by the relativist approaches in anthropology, which tend to consider culture, rather than biology, to be the foundation for the genesis and expression of emotions. From this perspective, the biological substrate of emotions is no more relevant to their understanding than is the biological substrate of language for comprehending the meaning of utterances. Emotions are viewed as the consequence of cultural values, judgments, communications, and negotiations that are part of broader cultural systems of meaning. Constructionists view emotions as cognitive appraisals derived from interpersonal and social influences and cultural beliefs and values (Hinton, 1999a). Any emotional state is best understood in the context of culturally constructed interpretations and consequences.

The social constructionist approach challenges the biological basis for emotions with the argument that the emotional categories addressed in physiological approaches are actually based in a Western folk psychology. Biological perspectives on emotions as originating in the lower brain levels and provoking irrational experiences also reflect a cultural view of emotions as involuntary (Averill, 1996). The English-language concept of emotion has a historical foundation in interpretations based in perceptions of the subject's passivity; this assumption is still reflected in contemporary concepts of emotions as bodily changes that happen to us (e.g., "he made me angry"). This has shaped scientific conceptualizations of emotions. The view of emotions as biological primitives that happen to us is a cultural construction derived from the dissociation of certain processes from consciousness, a lack of awareness of our unconscious appraisal and response patterns that produce our emotional reactions.

Emotions are culturally directed acts that a person performs to restructure personal responsibility and alleviate feelings of anxiety, guilt, shame, or other intrapsychic or interpersonal processes. These emotional and expressive performances may not engage the ego or conscious processes but may reflect preconscious, subconscious, or unconscious processes. Culture plays a role in the creation of emotional conditions through defining the nature of the experiences humans have by virtue of biology, interpersonal attachment, and the sociopsychological dynamics that place them within an interpretive framework (Averill, 1996).

The social constructionist perspective is supported by culturally specific emotions that defy translation into linguistic equivalents in other languages. Translations may be made of aspects of emotional experience, but the complex meanings and contextual evaluations that evoke them cannot be adequately expressed in languages whose cultures lack the values and associations basic to elicitation and experience of the emotions (see Rosaldo, 1983). Extreme constructionist approaches view emotions as culturally specific interpretations and consider the physiological reaction as an irrelevant issue.

Hinton (1999a) points out that the extreme cultural constructionist approach to emotions constitutes a form of cultural reductionism that erroneously assumes that biological and cultural explanations are mutually exclusive. The antiphysiological bias of extreme cultural relativism ignores the necessary role of bodily processes in emotional experiences, of brain structures in emotional responses, and of emotional processes in human cognition. Cultural factors may produce emotions, but these cultural processes necessarily utilize our physiological capacities. Startle reactions, freeze responses, autonomic nervous system activation, and reflex responses are part of humans' biological heritage. Activation of these responses is based on personal and cultural appraisals, rather than the automatic adaptive species preservation functions from which they originated. Indeed, emotional responses may be maladaptive (see Chapter Nine).

Cultural Production of Emotions

A biocultural approach avoids extremes of biological reductionism and reductive constructivism. Physiological sensations are mediated by physical structures and processes but are also shaped by cultural and personal appraisals. The *conscious* cognitive appraisal processes have been emphasized, but significant aspects involve the paleomammalian brain's unconscious processes. Appraisals involve unconscious drives, attachments, desires, and the relations of self with important others. These processes tend to operate outside of explicit awareness, presenting to consciousness a decision. Emotional responses that occur through unconscious processes before and independent of conscious appraisal processes reject the fundamental assumptions of the constructivist approach.

The relationship between the biological potentials and cultural influences in emotions is a product of socialization processes that structure the developmental context and the self-related implications of emotions for identity. The cultural production of emotions occurs at many levels:

- Elicitation of physiological functions (threat responses, fear, anxiety, etc.) through significance

- Structuring of psychological self-system and its components

- Linguistic and conceptual designation of types of emotions and their causes and functions

- Cultural ascription of their associated meanings and appropriate personal responses

Learning plays a role in eliciting the brain structures that process emotional information, providing associations of contexts and evaluations. The biological processes involved in emotions are associated with the physical and social environment. These associations stimulate the development of the neural structures (synaptic connections) that mediate emotional experiences and, consequently, incorporate cultural assumptions into neural networks (see Castillo, 1997a; Chapters Six, Nine, and Ten of this book). Emotional potentials develop in an interaction of physiological and sociocultural factors. Attachments, threats to well-being, and the primary relations of self and others are part of the biological foundations of emotions that are managed by cultural systems where meaning elicits and mediates physiological reactions.

The relationships of emotions and physiology are produced through cultural mediation, where values and priorities instilled in socialization create patterns of socioemotional development that induce patterns of physiological reaction. Relations with others shape the learning of emotions and personal biological potentials. These relationships entrain psychological processes with physiological structures through both functional (intrinsic) conditions and symbolic (extrinsic) meanings (Averill, 1996). The engagement of physiological processes by cultural symbols is called **psychophysiological symbolism** (Averill, 1996), entrainment (Laughlin, McManus, and d'Aquili, 1992), or symbolophysiological processes. These processes associate emotional experiences and physiological processes through symbolic interpretations. These relationships among physiology, learning, and symbols play a central role in developing connections between paleomammalian brain processes and culturally based appraisals mediated by the frontal cortex. Learning incorporates cultural programming into the responses of the emotional (limbic) brain. This information or meaning is essential for the construction of emotions, advising us how to feel and respond to sensations and what criteria and significance to associate with the appraisal of circumstances and their implications.

Cultural justifications for feelings and normative expectations regarding appropriate responses are basic to the experience and management of any affect. Cultures vary widely in expectations regarding the expression of emotions. Cultures vary in the ideals they instill in their members with respect to introspection about feelings, sharing them, or seeking compensation for emotional wrongs. In some cultures, emotional talk for some experiences is taboo, and individuals suppress and attempt to modify emotions they feel. In others, emotions such as anger are elicited and developed to an extreme considered pathological in other cultures.

Culture manages emotional life by providing meanings for experiences and mediating the interactions with others that elicit emotional experiences and responses. Even emotions based in functional adaptations are engaged through social processes involving the attribution of meaning. Culture tells us *what* to feel with respect to even universal emotions. If normative expectations differ significantly from actual sentiments, repression may be the normative expectation. Or emotions may be transformed, as when the sorrow and grief of loss is transformed into rage and a burning anger for revenge. Meanings of emotions include cultural definitions of the self and expectations for asserting social identity through emotional expressions.

Emotions reflect cultural interpenetration of biological and mental processes (see Csordas, 1983, 1994), a linking of physiological processes and cognitive assessments. Emotions are a communication system in which the body's information is manifested for cognitive appraisal and in which cognitive assessments are returned as information that has physiological effects on the body. Emotions link the organism and social environment through physiological processes, behavioral activities, communicative interactions, and cognitive interpretations (Hinton, 1999a). If we encompass the notions of human drives and needs—protection, appetite, sex, security, affiliation, and bonding—within the broader domain of emotions, culture is the tool through which basic emotions are met.

An Anthropology of Emotions Understanding emotions is hampered by limited cross-cultural research for deconstructing the Western folk psychology that dominates even the physiological approaches. Emotions involve complex interactions within systems (Hinton, 1999a) that include

- Neurophysiological structures, processes, and reactions

- Motivational dynamics and attachments

- Precipitating environmental conditions and events

- Value orientations and cognitive appraisals

- Behavioral responses and communicational interactions

- Subjective and personal experiences

- Self-regulation responses

A cross-cultural examination of these factors helps reveal the genetic bases of emotions, the cultural effects on the development of emotional responses, and the limits to human emotional plasticity. Understanding emotions requires an analysis linking these different systems and their feedback in developmental processes that occur across time (Hinton, 1999b), a shaping of biological processes by the cultural environment during development. This interaction produces "local biologies" (see Lock, 1981a, 1981b) reflecting physiological plasticity and developmental indeterminacy in emotional potentials, structures, and processes that are constructed in the person environment interface and in response to the cues provided by others (Hinton, 1999b). Emotions are part of the cognitive evolution of the species, processes that promote personal and species survival through adaptations that are sensitive to the perceptions of other members of the species regarding ecological threats. Consequently, an understanding of emotions depends on cross-cultural data to document the variety of ways in which genetic potentials may be shaped over the course of development by cultural expectations: what others consider to be significant and adaptive and how this affects an individual's appraisal of situations. The profound ways culture influences emotional development is exemplified in culture-bound syndromes (see Chapter Six). The same emotional potential (such as anger) may be culturally elicited and shaped in dramatically different ways.

Emotions and Evolutionary Psychiatry The complex biocultural nature of human emotions, and their far greater complexity in humans than animals, indicates that human emotionality—and its pathologies—are products of human evolution. Understanding the interaction of biological and social factors in human evolution and in contemporary pathologies is the focus of the emerging interdisciplinary areas of evolutionary psychiatry. These approaches attempt to understand human mental illness as outcomes of the interaction between adaptive traits and human social and cultural dynamics. Many of human pathologies appear to have features that are adaptive in certain contexts or to limited extents. Paranoia, for example, can be seen as an extreme of an otherwise adaptive tendency toward vigilance. Obsessive-compulsive disorder may be part of human propensities for culture, repeating learned behaviors. Cleanliness associated with OCD is seen as an adaptive hygienic trait when displayed in moderate ways. Passiveness and aggressiveness may have adaptive contributions in some contexts, but certainly only to certain extremes. Whatever are the biological predispositions to human psychopathology, our genetic propensities are developed in healthy or pathological ways in interaction with the social context.

CHAPTER SUMMARY

In this chapter, we introduced medical ecology's biocultural approach that emphasizes the importance of evolutionary principles and ecological adaptations in understanding health and disease. Human evolution is reflected in disease, nutrition, birthing, and healing responses. Biocultural approaches are essential for understanding the interactions of genetics, environment, and culture in producing contemporary health. Biocultural interactions are manifested in emotions, where biological aspects are manifested in universal phenomena and culturally specific dynamics are reflected in cross-cultural differences. The necessity of cultural approaches to understanding determinants of health is illustrated in the role of behavior in the distribution of morbidity and mortality. Cultural approaches are essential for core aspects of epidemiology's efforts to determine the factors that play a causal role in the distributions, causes, and prevention of disease. Community health programs most dramatically affect health through collective approaches that address upstream macrolevel determinants. This depends on shifting attention from the biomedical focus on physiological processes to the broader social context affecting risks, the allocation of resources, and the development of needed programs. These approaches are illustrated in the critical medical anthropology traditions of the next chapter.

KEY TERMS

Adaptations

Cline

Confounding variables

Contributory factors

Determinant

Direct contributing factors

Distal causes

Ecology

Epidemiology

Genotype

Heterozygous

Homozygous

Incidence

Indirect contributing factors

Morbidity

Mortality

Natural selection

Necessary causes

Neomammalian brain

Paleomammalian brain

Phenotype

Prevalence

Proximal cause

Rates

Reptilian brain

Risk factors

Risk markers

Sufficient causes

Triune brain

SELF-ASSESSMENT 7.1. ECOLOGICAL ASSESSMENT OF DISEASE CAUSATION

Do genetically predisposed diseases run in your family? What are they?

Are there environmental or behavioral factors that influence the occurrence of these conditions?

What contagious diseases have you contracted? What were their causes? Contributing factors? Predisposing conditions?

Is your disease history typical for "your" group? Why or why not?

What risk factors do you have for those diseases?

What aspects of your behavior made you susceptible to those disease conditions?

Are there social conditions that exacerbate or reduce your risk for these diseases?

Are there social conditions that exacerbate or reduce the consequences of these diseases?

What are the environmental conditions in your community that contribute to disease? Which are necessary causes? Contributory causes? Immediate causes?

Pick a major disease affecting your community and use the cultural systems models of Chapter Four to analyze the potential contributory factors.

ADDITIONAL RESOURCES

Books

Bendelow, G., and S. J. Williams. 1997. *Emotions in social life: Critical themes and contemporary issues.* London: Routledge.

Counihan, C. M. 1999. *The anthropology of food and body: Gender, meaning, and power.* New York: Routledge.

Eisenstein, Z. 2001. *Manmade breast cancers.* Ithaca, N.Y.: Cornell University Press.

Farmer, P. 1999. *Infections and inequalities: The modern plagues.* Berkeley: University of California Press.

Inhorn, M. C., and P. J. Brown. 1997. *The anthropology of infectious disease: International health perspectives.* Amsterdam: Gordon & Breach.

Kin, F. 2000. *Social and behavioral aspects of malaria control: A study among the Murut of Sabah.* Phillips, Me.: Borneo Research Council.

Kroll-Smith, S., P. Brown, and V. J. Gunter, eds. 2000. *Illness and the environment: A reader in contested medicine.* New York: New York University Press.

Strickland, S., and P. Shetty. 1998. *Human biology and social inequality: 39th symposium volume of the Society for the Study of Human Biology.* Cambridge, U.K.: Cambridge University Press.

Tapper, M. 1999. *In the blood: Sickle cell anemia and the politics of race.* Philadelphia: University of Pennsylvania Press.

Web Site

Centers for Disease Control and Prevention: http://www.cdc.gov.

CHAPTER

8

POLITICAL ECONOMY AND CRITICAL MEDICAL ANTHROPOLOGY

[M]edical anthropology . . . [should] . . . set as a standard that our work be dedicated to comforting the afflicted while afflicting the comfortable

—SINGER, 1990, P. 185

LEARNING OBJECTIVES

- Introduce medical anthropology's political-economic approaches and critical medical anthropology's assessments of macrolevel impacts on health
- Show the effects of social class and economic conditions on health
- Demonstrate why social networks and social support are important in health and recovery
- Examine the micropolitics of medicine, how ideological and power relations are reproduced in doctor-patient relations and in treatment
- Illustrate how advocacy approaches can enhance health through fostering institutional change and organizational development
- Illustrate roles of community studies and cultural approaches in ensuring public health

POLITICAL ECONOMY APPROACHES TO HEALTH

The role of politics in health is apparent in many areas. Congress funds billions of dollars in health programs and research annually but has rejected legislative efforts to establish universal health care and prohibited Americans from taking advantage of cheaper pharmaceuticals available across the border in Canada and Mexico. The economics of health was obvious when American automobile manufacturer Chrysler was virtually given to foreign financial company Cerberus for the price of assuming Chrysler Corporation's obligation to pay the health costs for its prior retirees! The cost of health care in the United States exceeds 13 percent of the gross domestic product, the largest sector of the American economy. Who controls and benefits from this incredibly large sector of the economy? And why do Americans, who pay more than any other country for health care, not have the best health in the world?

These are the kinds of questions addressed in political-economic approaches to health exemplified in critical medical anthropology. These approaches assess the effects of social conditions on health. Economic resources are general mechanisms through which social conditions produce the distribution of diseases and health disparities. Economic institutions, business activities, and political decisions not only affect who gets diseases and access to health resources but also actively produce disease through creating contaminants and other risks. Social conditions produce disease through work exposures (pesticides and industrial pollutants), the location of factories (near poorer neighborhoods), exploitation of the underprivileged (low salaries, no health benefits), and political decisions about funding public health and medical care services. Social conditions also affect health through producing stress-related physiological dysfunctions that reduce resistance to disease. And conversely, social organizations and communities can combat risks through social networks, and support can enhance health and recovery.

Political and economic conditions also affect clinical interactions between providers and clients and the nature and quality of care. In clinical interactions, doctors typically express values that distract attention from the social causes of patients' problems. This may directly or indirectly blame patients for their condition instead of recognizing the origin of maladies in broader social conditions. For instance, biomedical approaches blame patients for problems, such as drinking, rather than recognizing their causes in social conditions (e.g., how structural unemployment contributes to alcoholism or Native American alcohol-related problems reflect the direct effects of federal regulations).

Critical medical anthropology emphasizes the need to identify how economic and political processes have effects on health and well-being through the production and allocation of health resources and services as well as other factors that affect risks and protective factors such as nutrition, housing, occupational risks, industrial pollutants, and other contaminants. Prevention requires that social influences on health be addressed as the ultimate causes of disease instead of focusing on the proximate causes found in microorganisms. For example, the health problems of lead-based paints or sewage seepage in the streets are not addressed by treating the effects of lead or bacteria but by taking political actions that prevent exposure to such conditions.

By being aware of the macrolevel social processes that affect well-being, providers and consumers can be empowered to use political processes to change societal conditions that have effects on health. Critical medical anthropology studies the effects of the economic, political, and ideological aspects of biomedicine on health to be able to understand how to address these societal effects. This knowledge is used in an activist approach to

- Acquire knowledge about the relations of resources and power to health

- Develop programs to change social conditions affecting health and the provision of services to address health problems

- Educate communities about the nature of medical-political relations

- Empower people to resist medical control of their health options

Mechanisms for addressing these institutional effects on health are provided by

- Public health education programs

- The development of public policy

- Advocacy on behalf of communities

- Programs to produce community empowerment

- Communities organized to act collectively to produce change

A central principle of critical medical anthropology's approach to improving health is community involvement in health planning and patient empowerment to resist biomedical control and **medicalization** of social distress. *Medicalization* is a process by which biomedicine has come to manage a wide range of life circumstances by classifying them as medical problems, even if they are not diseases in the conventional sense. For instance, is a drinking problem a disease to be treated by medicine? Or is alcoholism a socially induced condition? Should alcoholism be "treated" under medical supervision? Or should it be addressed through social work or community development programs? In the United States, alcoholism is medicalized and treated as a disease.

In advanced industrialized nations, this medicalization of life includes most of the phases of the life cycle, particularly for women (e.g., birth control, pregnancy, and childbirth). Pregnancy and childbirth are not illnesses, but in the course of the twentieth century, the midwives who traditionally managed birth in the United States were made "illegal" with legislation sought by the AMA and its representatives; consequently, the practices of birth became an almost exclusive purview of biomedicine for much of the past century. Medicalization extends to school entrance requirements for health exams; work qualifications for disability; the management of aging, menopause, and bereavement; and many other aspects of life that depend on medical certification, such as sports participation and mental health clearances.

Medicine intersects with virtually all aspects of life, encountering cultural differences and political struggles over what people consider appropriate, such as age of first sexual intercourse, education about and the use of birth control, a person's desired management of pregnancy, necessary inoculations and preventive behaviors, appropriate socialization and discipline, preferred food and nutrition, communication styles and negotiation approaches, and many other aspects of life.

CASE STUDY

The Political Power of Medicine

The political power of physicians directly confronted Lia Lee's parents. This began with home visits from public health nurses who tried to ensure the family's adoption of the recommended treatments. Their assessments characterized the parents as noncompliant and unable to effectively administer the medications to their child even with the help of colored labels and lines on the liquid bottles. Outdated medications were mute evidence of their failure to appropriately administer the medications necessary to prevent seizures and address bronchial infections. The side effects were a primary reason her parents resisted the pharmaceutical regimen. Lia Lee's emotionless facial expression after taking her medication convinced her parents that the drugs were harming her rather than helping her. Later one of her physicians concluded much the same.

The doctors came to conclude that they were not going to be able to get Lia's parents to administer the medication needed to effectively treat her. The resultant convulsions and periods of oxygen loss were apparently causing a developmental delay and portended permanent mental retardation. Her physician eventually wrote a letter to Child Protective Services (CPS) accusing the parents of failure to comply with the administration of required medicines for their child. Such failure, he argued, was both child abuse and child neglect because it could result in further seizures causing brain damage and possibly death.

The physician's recommendation that the child be placed temporarily in a foster home to assure proper medication was immediately granted by the court, which ordered that Lia Lee be removed from her parent's custody. Without advance notice, social workers arrived to remove her

To resist medicalization, critical medical anthropology calls for community organization and involvement in the public dimensions of health decisions. Community involvement is dependent on both organizational change in health institutions and the development of community coalitions that can participate in this planning process. Achieving this community participation requires health professionals with the cultural competence to foster institutional change in their organizations, stimulating them to facilitate the formation of community health coalitions. These community coalitions can have greater power to influence health behaviors of people and exert political influence to effect institutional changes, such as new programs for alcohol education or tougher drunk-driving sentences. Anthropologist-advocates are involved in the politics of health, making efforts to influence policymakers, bureaucrats, and government officials to change conditions that affect access to health resources. Cultural perspectives can be employed on behalf of individuals and communities when anthropologists give expert witness testimony, create community input through community coalitions, or provide policy analysis regarding needed programs.

Not all groups have equal access to resources for health. One of the principal foci of critical medical anthropology is the issue of health disparities: the adverse health consequences for the underprivileged, poor, and marginalized. Who speaks on their behalf? Medical anthropologists have often felt a moral obligation to speak out on behalf of these from her home and took her to an undisclosed location. Her parents did not see her or learn of her location for weeks. In a court hearing in the following days, Lia Lee's father Nao Kao was present. There is no record of an interpreter present, but the father is recorded as assenting to the foster placement, contrary to what he in fact desired. Lia had become government property and the rights of her parents superseded by the demands of biomedicine.

Lia's initial foster placement was in a home operated by Mennonite sisters. They strapped Lia Lee into a car seat to control her behavior. Later she was placed with a foster family that cared for six other children with special needs, but they spoke no Hmong, the only language Lia understood. The foster family soon decided, for the first time as foster parents, that a placement child—Lia—should be with her parents, but CPS did not agree. A visitation period back at home was arranged, however, as a test of whether she could be returned to the parents. A test done afterward indicated that they had not provided Lia with her medication, confirming the CPS conclusion that she should not be returned to her parents. In the foster home, Lia was forcibly medicated on the prescribed schedule, but her seizures increased rather than subsided.

In retrospect, her physician reflected that there might have been other options: arranging daily home nurse visits or seeking assistance from other members of the Hmong community to assure Lia's proper medication. The doctor's retrospective comments also revealed the political agenda behind his actions: teaching the Hmong community the lesson that they had to follow the rules laid down by doctors.

less fortunate communities and to directly confront the political power of biomedicine to intervene in people's lives.

CRITICAL MEDICAL ANTHROPOLOGY

This power of medicine to control our personal lives in such dramatic ways has driven the development of critical medical anthropology as an explicitly political opposition to the societal power of biomedicine and its associated industries. Singer (1989a, 1989b, 1990) criticized dominant trends in medical anthropology that focus on the biological and cultural aspects of health without examining the economic, political, and social causes of disease. He focused his criticism on medical ecology in particular. He rejected the medical-ecological presumption of providing a unifying framework for interdisciplinary approaches to health and disease. Singer noted that traditional medical-ecological views have often emphasized an environmental determinism, where physical conditions (such as bacteria) have natural and automatic consequences. Singer emphasized that we should instead recognize the environment as a limiting force that is profoundly shaped by cultural activities. For example, are bacterial contaminants in the community's drinking water best understood as a "natural condition" determined by the environment or as a "produced condition" that is the consequence of human activities? Medical-ecological assessments of population-environment interactions often fail to recognize that cultural factors (economic and political institutions) can be determinants of environmental conditions and adaptations.

Critical medical anthropology criticizes medical ecology's approach for emphasizing ecological balance and, by extension, a sense of order and balance in society. This model of ecological balance as equilibrium, a stable pattern, can reinforce an ideology of maintaining existing social relations. Viewing social classes as natural and inequalities and poverty as natural adaptations in effect blames the poor and diseased for their own predicament of a poor adaptation, or at least excuses it as a natural cause. This naturalization ignores political and economic factors that produce inequality and the associated diseases.

Critical medical anthropology criticizes medical ecology's characterizations of health as a function of the population's adaptation to the environment. The idea of adaptation suggests that cultural institutions and practices are adaptive when they may actually have negative consequences. Tobacco production is an economic adaptation, and cigarette smoking may be an individual's adaptation to stress, but both tobacco production and consumption have devastating consequences for the ecological system (soil fertility) and personal health (lung cancer). Medical-ecological concepts of adaptation and environment have not generally addressed the social relations that constitute a fundamental aspect of such adaptation and, consequently, neglect the social environment where determinant causal relationships are located. Why are people drinking bacteria-contaminated water? Is it because bacteria are part of the environment? Yes, but why are the bacteria at dangerous levels in the water supplies? Is it because companies dump their waste products into the waterways that serve as community water supplies? Or is it because governments do not

BIOCULTURAL INTERACTIONS

Pesticide Poisoning as the Production of Disease

Pesticide poisoning of agricultural workers is an example of how relations of power and control of economic resources and political agencies produce disease (see Singer and Baer, 2007). There is limited legislative control of pesticides in the United States and even less in other parts of the world where American-produced pesticides are distributed for use. Even in this country, agricultural workers and their families are at risk of disease because of exposure to pesticides that are responsible for cases of both poisoning and cancers. Workers are given the pesticides to distribute in the fields but without being provided with adequate protection. This exposure occurs directly in the fields and through airborne dispersion of the pesticides to adjoining workers' quarters provided for the farm workers by the agricultural employers. Farm workers also bring the pesticide home on their clothes and skin, exposing their children to the toxins. The lack of showers in employer-provided housing means that workers face prolonged exposure to these toxins and deposit them in the homes where their children live. To protect workers, changes in housing and the availability of running water and showers for cleansing them of their pesticide exposures are essential to reducing risks.

fund the construction of safe drinking water systems and sewage treatment plants? Whether from active pollution or exposure by neglect, diseases are produced by human activity.

Singer (1989b) points out that the analysis made by McElroy and Townsend (1985) of the exposure of workers to toxic substances neglects crucial considerations. What are the roles of the owners' motivation to extract profit rather than spend money to protect the workers from exposure to pesticides? This failure to address the behaviors of the owners whose deliberate actions place workers at risk contributes to the perspective that the exposure is natural instead of its social origin. Critical medical anthropology accuses medical ecology's approach of legitimizing inequalities and victim-blaming: attributing disease to the poor adaptations of economically and politically subordinated groups, rather than recognizing that their adaptations are affected by the activities of more powerful groups in society. Similarly, the conclusion that poor people's health problems are a result of their ignorance about nutrition and their failure to purchase nutritional foods distracts attention from the cause of their problem. What are the effects of class relations in the allocation of resources for acquiring food and nutritional education?

The concept of adaptation *to the environment* has often failed to consider how humans construct their own environments, transforming them to meet social and cultural objectives. The social structuring of the environment requires that we attend to the forces and actors making decisions that affect environmental conditions. Adaptations need to be assessed in the context of competing social groups and their relative resources in the struggle. The adaptive nature of social institutions must be viewed according to their ability to meet human needs, rather than viewing oppressed populations as suffering from their own poor adaptations to the social systems constructed by the more powerful classes of society.

Medical-ecological approaches have obscured the impact of political systems and historical processes and their contemporary consequences. Diseases of modernization and poverty must be understood as world systems' effects and relationships between classes, rather than environmental maladaptations per se. The focus on the environment distracts attention from social relations and their active and causal effects on the environment. When disease results from external political and economic relations, such as businesses that pollute environments or sell contaminated foods, calling the disease a consequence of maladaptation suggests responsibility on the part of the victims rather than the oppressors. Instead of disguising social relations as natural consequences, Singer proposes that medical anthropology investigate how classic medical-ecological assumptions of adaptation maintain the existing structures of environmental and social relations, reinforcing the power of capitalism and the materialist paradigms of science. By treating diseases and environments as natural, we ignore how the interests of the elite classes produce risk factors in the environment, such as when industrialists contaminate the environment in ways that directly impact the poor.

Critical medical anthropology also criticizes clinical medical anthropologists who work as cultural brokers to teach cultural awareness to health care providers. Cross-cultural training is seen as serving the interests of biomedicine rather than the needs of consumers or societal needs for the optimal distribution of health resources. Singer proposes instead a focus on understanding how health is produced by social structures, organizations, and conditions, particularly economic and political processes (Baer, Johnsen, and Singer, 1986; Singer and Baer, 1995; Baer, Singer and Susser, 1997).

Critical medical anthropology and similar political economy of health approaches use historical and cultural systems analyses to show how health is affected by

- The distribution of economic resources

- Social class and power relations between groups

- Racial classification, prejudice, and discrimination

- Sexual stratification: male-female differences in risk

- The global political economy and international pharmaceutical industries

Biomedicine as Capitalist Medicine

During the 1960s, anthropologists implementing public health programs in impoverished countries became aware of economic and political effects on health. Here they recognized that health disparities are increased by capitalist medicine and its effects on the ways in which governments allocate material and economic resources. Poor countries that build large centralized hospitals with high-tech coronary care centers to treat obesity among the rich do so at the expense of constructing primary community health care and public health programs that would provide benefits for the masses. This has led anthropologists to advocacy roles in an expression of their concern about the inappropriate exportation of Western biomedicine.

Universalizing biomedicine has favored America's international construction industries for hospitals and served the interests of the capitalist pharmaceutical companies. Biomedicine and pharmaceutical industries of Western societies have aggressively entered other societies, undermining traditional healing practices and influencing the allocation of health care resources. The internationalization of biomedicine has not focused on providing the greatest good for the most people through community-based prevention programs and basic care but, rather, through capital-intensive specialized services that maximize profit for health providers and the pharmaceutical industries. Poor countries adopt biomedical models because of the pressures imposed by Western governments, international health agencies, and capitalists' enterprises. International corporate influences include the construction of hospitals and specialized health facilities and medical equipment that reinforce the unequal distribution of resources.

Critical medical anthropology emphasizes that capitalism and biomedicine promote political outcomes that have direct consequences for the distribution of health resources (such as advocating against universal health care and socialized health programs or prohibiting the importation of cheaper medicines from Canada). These perspectives examine the health consequences of ownership of institutions, the effects of oppression of rights or the distribution of resources, and the consequences of work conditions such as exposure to toxic chemicals. Critical medical anthropology engages activist and advocacy approaches to empower communities with knowledge of how to gain control of resources and institutions that affect health.

The reconceptualizing of biomedicine as capitalist medicine recognizes the ways in which biomedicine and capitalist enterprises are interdependent. Anthropologists study how biomedicine's economic and political power and values reinforce the capitalist world system. This directs inquiry into biomedicine's power in the control of health resources and political decisions affecting health care. Biomedicine's control of key health resources and decision-making power include

- Reinforcing a capitalist system of health care where the poor are denied care

- The primacy of profit in health care decisions, limiting treatments or expensive drugs

- Laws and regulatory bodies that enable biomedicine to prohibit alternative healing practices

- Producing profits for pharmaceutical and medical equipment manufacturers while receiving favors from them

- Consuming enormous resources in publicly funded medical schools and hospitals

- Controlling programs of national governments and international health agencies

Critical medical anthropology shows the economic-political power of biomedicine in how it reinforces the class structure of society through

- The massive allocation of resources in medical research and treatment facilities and practices

- Biomedicine's roles in defining disease and acceptable treatments, including its massive collusion with the pharmaceutical industry in treating disease symptoms

- The receipt of massive amounts of public funds in medical treatments while thwarting socialized medicine

- Its regulatory roles in limiting alternative medicine practices

Biomedical influence and control in society are facilitated by physicians' upper middle- and upper-class status and their roles in the corporate structures that control health resources, including hospitals and medical schools. The recent era of managed care and HMOs has produced corporate entities with multibillion-dollar-a-year budgets that determine what care is provided, for whom, and at what cost. Biomedicine's political and economic influences determine the priorities for the allocation of resources for research and treatment, affecting the consequences of disease. These priorities are supported by a significant capitalist sector, the pharmaceutical industries, and their patented medicines.

The Pharmaceutical Industry and Disease Production

The internationalization of biomedicine is principally promoted by multinational pharmaceutical companies. The pharmaceutical companies promote biomedical ideologies in a variety of ways:

- They are the primary providers of continuing education, the required ongoing training of doctors

- They constitute some of the largest companies in the world, controlling an enormous economic base

■ They use their economic power to influence public preferences through marketing to potential patients ("Ask your doctor if the purple pill is right for you")

■ They provide many perks for physicians to induce them to prescribe their brand-name pills

The association of pharmaceuticals with progress has led people in modernizing societies to adopt them over traditional medicines. The abandonment of the use of traditional medical practices undermines indigenous economic sectors. This marginalization of traditional cultural knowledge can also mean a loss of indigenous medical traditions well adapted to local diseases and resources. Instead, local populations are enticed by costly foreign-supplied pharmaceuticals generally administered inappropriately and without biomedical guidance regarding dosage and durations of treatment, rendering them ineffective (Singer and Baer, 2007). The lack of similar regulatory control of pharmaceuticals in other countries makes the people who use them susceptible to a variety of misuses, such as the excessive and inappropriate self-prescription of antibiotics that contributes to the development of "superresistant" strains of germs.

The powerful pharmaceutical industry has been driven by profit motives rather than overall health agendas of public health and biomedicine. Pharmaceutical industry so-called education and marketing interactions with doctors encourage the off-label prescribing of drugs, using them for purposes other than those approved by the FDA. These unapproved uses may compromise health by replacing known effective treatments in the interest of increased profits. Doctors are led to make these unapproved prescriptions by the heavy influence of the pharmaceutical industry not only through its education programs but also from wining, dining, and lavish vacations at the educational facilities in prime vacation destinations around the world. To obtain more patients, drug companies have deliberately misrepresented data regarding the need to treat conditions. By lowering standards for the treatment of high cholesterol levels and targeting moderate-risk groups, the pharmaceutical industry has increased its patient market by encouraging the treatment of patients who did not actually require medication.

Former industry employees have denounced companies such as Pfizer for deliberately misleading doctors to make unapproved prescriptions to increase sales. The *Wall Street Journal* (Armstrong, 2007) reported a lawsuit in which Pfizer was accused of providing doctors with a deliberately misleading educational program as part of a marketing strategy to prescribe Lipitor as a treatment for high cholesterol levels for millions of patients who did not need it. Pfizer has previously paid millions of dollars in fines for unapproved off-label marketing of other drugs it sells (Neurontin). Pharmaceutical company Merck was involved in a long cover-up of the fatal side effects of its popular painkiller Vioxx, which is considered to have caused more than 100,000 fatalities. Because of its complicity in causing and covering up the increases in heart attacks and strokes caused by Vioxx, Merck was liable for almost $5 billion in consumer lawsuits. This pursuit of profit in the face of evidence of the fatal effects of Vioxx exemplifies the political and economic production of disease and death by profit motives rather than natural causes.

Similarly, tobacco companies produce more lung diseases by aggressively marketing tobacco and seeking to overturn laws and regulations regarding the promotion of smoking to the public, including minors. Singer and Baer (2007) suggest that the increased consumption of tobacco products will make it the leading cause of death in the developing world by 2020. One could say that the leading cause of death will be profits for tobacco producers and cigarette manufacturers. Alcohol effects on liver disease, motor-vehicle fatalities, mental illness, and other conditions constitute major causes of death that are produced by the promotions and enticements of the advertising industry.

Biomedical Science as Cultural and Political Activity

Critical medical anthropology challenges biomedical claims to scientific objectivity by revealing value-laden biases of biomedicine. It has challenged scientific ideology by placing medical research agendas, findings, and treatments in a sociopolitical context. It shows that biomedical assumptions about a value-free medicine are mistaken. This is illustrated by showing how cultural values affect

- The practice of medicine (individualism resulting in blaming the patient instead of recognizing the importance of social causes)

- The unequal distribution of health resources (capitalist medicine resulting in masses of uninsured)

- The quality of health care (which is undermined by the disdain providers often express about Medicare patients)

Biomedical practice is not strictly objective but influenced by politics and professional self-interests, such as the physician organizations engaging in lobbying against universal health care (socialized medicine). By illustrating the political nature of science and medicine, critical medical anthropology reinforces the necessity of addressing how political power affects health. The political power of medicine enables it to define poor health status as individual responsibility (genetic, personal, and moral) and deny the reality of social causes in inequality. It consequently emphasizes advocacy, adopting political agendas that address the needs of the underprivileged and disenfranchised. Critical medical anthropology proposes challenging the powerful and privileged to reduce their power to perpetrate class-determined disparities in health.

Critical medical anthropology challenges the biopsychosocial model of disease and systems approaches to cultures as *integrated* systems, arguing that these fail to address the conflicts and dysfunctions in institutional structures that affect health through inequality and discrimination. "A critical approach must define health as *access to and control over the basic material and non-material resources that sustain and promote life at a high level of satisfaction*" [emphasis in original] (Baer et al., 1986, p. 95). This requires identifying factors outside of biomedicine that affect health. Critical medical anthropology emphasizes a world systems perspective for understanding factors affecting health both within and outside the health care system. This includes addressing the relationship of broader societal ideological and political trends to medical care and how power and resources affect health across different levels. Anthropology uses a world systems perspective to analyze Western biomedicine and its primary collaborators and agents: multinational corporations, pharmaceutical firms, international health agencies,

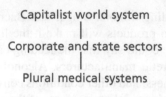

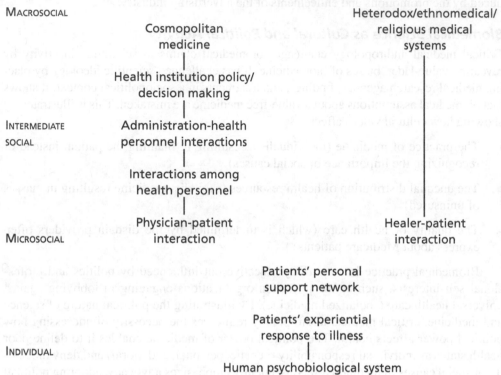

FIGURE 8.1. *Levels of Health Care Systems.*

Source: Adapted from Baer, Singer, and Johnsen, 1986

industrial firms, food suppliers, international agricultural businesses, and other chemical and technology suppliers (Baer et al., 1986). Examining access to health resources at different levels of the world system requires a complex set of interlocking models (see Figure 8.1).

SOCIAL CONDITIONS AS CAUSES OF DISEASE AND HEALTH

Social class is a condition recognized for its impacts on health, manifested in higher morbidity and mortality rates from most diseases for those of the lower social classes. Link and Phalen (1995) show global effects of social class on health in its significant association with all of the fourteen major causes of disease, ranging from higher infant mortality

PRACTITIONER PROFILE

Hans Baer

After teaching at George Peabody College for Teachers (Nashville), St. John's University (Queens, New York), the University of Southern Mississippi (Hattiesburg), and the University of Arkansas (Little Rock) and serving as a Fulbright Lecturer at Humboldt University in East Berlin and as a visiting professor in the anthropology departments at the University of California-Berkeley, Arizona State University (Tempe), and the Australian National University (Canberra), Hans Baer, Ph.D., now has a permanent position with a joint appointment in the Schools of Social and Environmental Enquiry and the Centre of Health and Society at the University of Melbourne.

Over the years, Baer developed an awareness of the political economy of health and a strong interest in osteopathic medicine. This led to a study of the sociopolitical status of osteopathy in Great Britain and an expanded study of chiropractic as well. He has also closely examined various aspects of chiropractic in North America and conducted ethnographic and archival research on American naturopathy.

In collaboration with Merrill Singer, Baer saw the need for the creation of a "critical medical anthropology" that would use the political economy of health as a broader framework for examining the settings within which medical anthropologists generally conduct their research. This led to sessions at annual meetings of the American Anthropological Association and other conferences that evolved into a special issue of *Social Science and Medicine* (1986). Subsequent work led to, among others, the books *Medical Anthropology and the World System* (1997) and *Introducing Medical Anthropology* (2007).

As a critical anthropologist, Baer is strongly committed to the merger of theory and social action. He has taken part in or organized peace and justice and Green Party political groups and conducted research on the political economy of nuclear regulation. Since immigrating to Australia, he has become involved in developing a critical anthropology of global warming.

rates to lower overall life expectancy as well as mental illness, coronary artery disease, respiratory tract conditions, and cancers. Class association with many different diseases establishes the general effects of social class on health. Specific characteristics of the lower-class lifestyle are associated with risk factors for poorer physical health (such as more undesirable life events: job loss, work problems, familial deaths, etc.). A lower incidence of intimate contacts and social networks and a greater prevalence of poor health practices among those of lower social classes increase their vulnerability to disease. What it is about class that constitutes an increased risk has been examined in terms of the specific class-associated aspects of *lifestyle* that increase risk. A poor individual's behavioral risks, such as occupations that produce exposures to toxic environments, do not appear to explain all of the association of lower social class with disease.

Individual foci are inadequate for explaining the persistent relations of class and disease. Social class itself, independent of specific effects on high-risk behaviors, has a causal role in producing disease. The effects of macrolevel social conditions on health are illustrated in the relationship between downturns in the national economy and the increases in the rates of specific health problems in subsequent years.

Most epidemiological research addresses individual-level variables, reflecting values of Western cultures and focusing on proximal (immediate) causes that implicate individually based risk factors rather than the distal causes found in social conditions. Is it individuals' problem if, because of poverty, they cannot adequately feed their children? Or is this a social problem affecting a whole class of people (the poor)? Link and Phalen (1995) argue that greater attention must be paid to the basic social conditions that affect access to resources such as nutrition, housing, and health care. These distal social causes, rather than individual proximal factors, are key to eliminating disease.

The limited relevance of biological factors in disease is illustrated by the widespread presence of infectious agents in individuals who do not succumb to those diseases. The poor, however, are more susceptible to virtually all classes of disease; this emphasizes the importance of determining the fundamental causes of disease in how groups of people are exposed to risk.

This determination involves **contextualization**, a determination of life circumstances and the economic and political forces that play a role in shaping individual exposure, providing information about the social and cultural factors that have the effects of placing groups of people at risk. Contextualization of individually based risk factors investigates why people are exposed to risk and under what conditions individual exposure to risk results in disease (Link and Phalen, 1995).

The role of social class as a fundamental cause of disease is exemplified by the fact that addressing the proximate mechanisms that link class to specific diseases does not eliminate the health effects of class. This is shown in the changing factors responsible for the association of social class and disease. Associations between social class and health noted in the nineteenth century largely derived from poor working conditions, housing, and sanitation associated with poor people. Public health practices that addressed infectious diseases led to a dramatic decline in the diseases associated with the lower classes. This decline did not eliminate the relationship between socioeconomic status and health. Rather, the intervening risk factors changed, leaving the relationship between social class and health intact. The elimination of risk factors associated with poor sanitation led to new risk factors (such as diet, exercise, and smoking) that mediate the class and health relationship.

The maintenance of the relationship between class and health despite changing risk factors reflects how socioeconomic status enables those more favorably situated to use their resources to either avoid risks or to deal with their consequences. Fundamental social class effects on disease persist; this reflects class influences on multiple risk factors and multiple disease outcomes. Addressing the proximate risk factors associated with individually based behaviors does not alter the fundamental mechanisms that link disease to social class.

This relationship makes programs based on changing individual risk behaviors inadequate because they fail to address the social conditions that are responsible for exposing people to risk factors. Link and Phalen (1995) suggest that policymakers should focus on fundamental causes that have the benefit of affecting many diseases rather than a single disease because these fundamental causes (such as poor nutrition) affect susceptibility to many different diseases. Focusing on high cholesterol levels in a patient does not eliminate the broader health effects of social conditions such as inequality in access to resources.

Economic Status as a Cause of Poor Health

Do you know someone who became ill after losing his job, or do you yourself feel less healthy in times of monetary hardships? These personal experiences can be seen in national trends, as revealed in the seminal studies by Brenner (1973). Brenner studied the relationship of unemployment and national economic downturns to increases in the incidences of cardiac disease, kidney failure, strokes, infant mortality, and mental illness. He found that economic recessions increase the amount of stress as a result of the intensified struggle for the necessities of life. Economically induced stress had psychophysiological consequences that resulted in increased mortality rates. Increased mortality from heart attacks usually follows the recession in two waves, one about three years after, the other at about five to seven years. The economically induced increases in infant mortality are much more immediate. Economic effects on increases in mental illness were hypothesized by Brenner to be consequences of provocation by economic factors in which stress from unemployment, economic problems, and the consequent dislocation from one's lifestyle causes mental problems.

CULTURE AND HEALTH

Alameda County, California, Longitudinal Study

Using data from the longitudinal Alameda County, California, study, Lynch, Kaplan, and Shema (1997) assessed the effects of economic hardship on measures of health functioning by examining measures of independent activities of daily living, activities of daily living, and clinical depression. These relationships were shown to be independent of age, sex, and adjustments for smoking, alcohol use, physical activity, and body mass index. Those with greater economic hardship are more likely to have difficulties with (independent) activities of daily living and higher levels of depression, establishing economic impacts on functional health status. The poorest group had a three-times-greater risk for disease, with the degree of economic hardship associated with measures of functional status and health. Illness at baseline was not a factor, and the significant relationships persist with controls for confounding from smoking, alcohol use, physical activity, and weight as well as adjustments for age and sex and control for prevalent diseases. The evidence does not suggest specificity of economic causes but, rather, a general impact of economic status on health. These general health impacts reflect social mechanisms that have effects on the distribution of and access to resources and, consequently, access to health services. The findings suggest that to enhance physical and psychological health of a populace, we need to remove economic hardship. Those most in need of medical intervention are the least likely to receive it. Government policies that create greater income inequality and a growing lower-income group detrimentally affect health, especially of children.

Individual Versus Social Interventions to Promote Health

Preventing disease and promoting health require a focus on specific factors in the social environment that increase exposure to risk agents or exacerbate contributing factors. Social networks are a crucial part of the human response to disease (see Chapter Nine), and the creation of social networks has been viewed as a means of ameliorating the health consequences of their absence. Principal ways suggested for modifications of social networks of individuals include (Berkman, 1984, 1985; Berkman and Kawachi, 2000; Kawachi and Berkman, 2003; Heaney and Israel, 2002)

- Promoting opportunities for individuals to enhance their existing social networks and establish contacts for new network linkages

- Improving individual opportunities for social contact through enhancing social skills

- Providing individual psychological treatment

- Using indigenous natural helpers

- Enhancing community networks for problem solving

These interventions that the authors suggest emphasize the development of *individual* social skills necessary to establish and maintain social contacts and relationships. A strategy of intervention includes convening the people available: kin, neighbors, friends, and other significant individuals. These individuals help a person by providing possible links to others outside the current direct network. Psychosocial interventions are designed to help individuals deal with psychological problems and the lack of personal skills that keep them from forming or maintaining relationships with others. More serious conditions may require community-based living centers to provide the support individuals need to develop social and personal skills.

The shortcoming of these approaches is that they view the relationship between social conditions and health problems as an *individual* problem, rather than recognizing the systemic social conditions that produce alienation and anomie and place entire communities at risk. The necessity of a more fundamental social change approach is illustrated by the findings that social conditions are fundamental causes of disease beyond the individual pathways through which they act in placing individuals at differential risk. The perspectives of critical medical anthropology emphasize the need for broad-scale social action to effectively change such fundamental causes. Failure to recognize general social conditions as global and fundamental causes of disease leads to the misdirection of public health efforts. The most prevalent causes of mortality are a direct consequence of drugs (tobacco and alcohol), poor diet, inactivity, firearms, and other social behaviors that are accepted as normative and can be effectively changed only by structural interventions. Optimizing public health requires that individual-level factors and systemic influences be addressed through a multilevel approach.

Social structural interventions address not only educational needs but also the lack of opportunities created by poverty, community disintegration, and segregation. This requires the creation of employment opportunities, community planning to create social connection and networks, and interventions that tie people into natural groups that can fill emotional and practical needs. In contrast to the individual-level interventions characteristic of social support and social network approaches, the critical medical anthropology perspectives recognize the need to change broad social conditions that affect health. Class interest, the control exercised by corporations, and the power of biomedicine are central concerns that can be addressed only through a radical transformation of the existing economic and political conditions. This transformation is manifested in the demand for universal health coverage and public health services. This requires a reversal of health expenditures from the predominant focus on biomedicine's treatment of disease conditions and, instead, directing resources to public health prevention of the social conditions that increase susceptibility to diseases.

BIOCULTURAL INTERACTIONS

Production of CVD in the African American Community

How does society produce CVD in African Americans? Many societal factors contribute to the production of CVD among African Americans, ranging from the economic effects on access to care to political decision making regarding public health education and community health funding. Preventive care is key in decreasing the number of cases and fatalities. Unfortunately, preventive care is often neglected by both physicians and public health programs. The incidence of CVD among African Americans also reflects medical production through treatment error. Some African Americans respond more strongly to certain pharmaceuticals, including the antihypertensive drugs that are frequently prescribed. For similar reasons, African Americans respond more strongly to caffeine, which has a recognized effect in raising the blood pressure. These effects on blood pressure place African Americans at greater risk in a society where caffeine consumption is highly promoted—perhaps even demanded for greater work productivity.

Economic factors also produce an increased incidence of CVD through the extensive exposure to advertising that promotes risk behaviors for CVD such as alcohol use, cigarette smoking, and fast-food consumption. Inner-city areas are plastered with billboards promoting cigarette smoking, and poor dietary habits are promoted by the deliberate saturation with fast-food outlets. Economic factors also affect CVD, as when decisions made by corporations affect the diet of African Americans. The mass marketing of unhealthy alternatives makes them readily available, often at a cost less than the ingredients for a healthy meal (e.g., the "99-cent menus"; Weathersbee, 2007). Community coalitions in the Los Angeles area are attempting to get local governments to limit the establishment of new fast-food outlets and provide incentives for the development of other kinds of food businesses. Such community-government coalitions may also be able to pressure supermarkets to locate new outlets in inner cities.

A local community-empowerment solution to the lack of good food is the development of community gardens. A community garden movement has begun among inner-city African Americans in Los Angeles in an effort to grow their own foods on the vacant lots that often dot the inner-city landscape. This form of community empowerment can have multiple effects on health through activity, community engagement, and healthier diets.

SOCIAL NETWORKS AND SUPPORT

Community development for health involves many mechanisms, including

■ The social distribution of resources and care

■ The psychological effects of social relations that are mediated in our psychosocial and emotional responses

■ Social effects on individual physiological responses, known as **sociosomatic** effects

The linkages of social relations to health were initially established by Berkman (1983), who found the effects of social networks and social support on morbidity and mortality (Berkman, 1984, 1985; Berkman and Kawachi, 2000; Kawachi and Berkman, 2003). The formal study of the relation of social support and networks to health was stimulated by the recognition that some people were protected from the effects of rapid social change through the mediation of "resistance resources," "psychosocial assets," and "social support" based in social and community ties. This led to Berkman's preliminary studies of the relations of social networks to health, based on data collected for other reasons. Although the initial studies lacked sophisticated measures of social networks, social support, morbidity, or mortality, her subsequent prospective studies have borne out these initial findings and refined them.

Explaining the effects of social relations on health requires distinguishing social networks and support and what they provide. **Social networks** are a person-centered web of social ties that link people and are assessed according to several aspects (Berkman, 1984):

■ Reciprocity in relationships, both giving to and receiving from others

■ Intensity of emotional closeness

■ The density of interaction among network members

■ Proximity, dispersion, and accessibility of members

■ The quality, frequency, intensity, durability, and strength of interactions

Social networks may or may not be supportive of health. One's social network may not be an asset but rather a drain on resources or involve negative interpersonal interactions that produce stress and illness. The quality and extent of the network relationships need to be assessed to determine their differential impact on health. *Social support* involves relations with others that provide a protective factor that can reduce the deleterious effects of stress through their availability and aid. Social support's structural aspects involve those with whom one has living arrangements, social activities, and interactions that meet basic needs. Social support refines the social network concept by determining what assistance is actually or potentially available from the network. Social support's functional dimensions are emotional, expressive, instrumental, material, financial, informational, and appraisal (which provides self-evaluation feedback) (Heaney and Israel, 2002).

Social Networks, Social Support, and Mortality

Berkman's early studies suggested that differential mortality risks are associated with a different extent of social networks or **social support,** the extent to which social networks provide physical, emotional, and other resources. Berkman reviewed studies indicating increased mortality associated with limited social support. Her Alameda study assessed social networks based on marital status, close contacts with relatives and friends, and participation in informal and formal groups, particularly churches. The relative risks were more than two times higher for people with limited social networks (men, 2.3; women, 2.8). Berkman (1984) reported that people with low levels of social connections had a higher risk of dying from not only CVD but also cancer and cerebrovascular conditions. These increased risks for those with limited social support were independent of their initial health status, including obesity and the use of preventive services; demographic, racial, and socioeconomic measures; and lifestyle features such as drug use (cigarette and alcohol consumption), physical activity, and life satisfaction.

BIOCULTURAL INTERACTIONS

CVD and Social Support

The Israeli Ischemic Heart Disease study found that psychosocial problems and lack of support from a man's spouse were important predictors of CVD (conceptualized as "coronary heart disease") (angina pectoris) (Berkman, 1981, 1984). The effects of anxiety are buffered by the support and love from a wife; men with high anxiety and without a wife's love and support had a risk factor of 1.8, almost twice the risk for CVD. The Tecumseh study indicated that a social support measure based on marital status, voluntary associations, public events, and other activities (classes and lectures) was associated with a significantly lower CVD risk for men (Berkman, 1981, 1984). The Durham, North Carolina, study reported significantly increased mortality risks associated with impaired social support (Berkman, 1981, 1984). Similar studies in California on the prevalence of CVD among Japanese Americans found social affiliation measures to be associated with a relative risk difference of about 2 (Joseph, 1980; Joseph and Syme, 1981). Comparisons of the CVD risk of Japanese men in Japan and the United States found that the most acculturated Japanese Americans had a CVD prevalence that was three to five times higher than that associated with the most "traditional" group (Marmot and Syme, 1976). These differences were not due to differences in the major coronary risk factors such as diet, cholesterol level, blood pressure, or cigarette smoking but, rather, with indicators of acculturation. Traditional norms emphasized collective in-group orientations focused on dependency needs and social relations that reduced tension. Social and cultural change, industrialization, and urbanization are associated with an increased incidence of CVD.

A principal hypothesis for explaining the observed associations is that the changes produce stress because the individual is unprepared to cope with the new environments. This makes the individual more susceptible to disease because the stressful situations compromise the immune system. Westernized lifestyles, industrialization, increased migration, and occupation mobility reduce the opportunities for the formation of enduring social ties, producing isolation and disconnectedness from others that reduce intimate contact and access to instrumental assistance.

Social Influences on Health

Research on the positive health effects of social ties indicates that they operate through many mechanisms (see Berkman, 1984, 1985; Heaney and Israel, 2002):

- Intimacy, companionship, social integration, and sense of belonging

- Opportunity for nurturant behavior and reassurance of social and personal worth

- Assistance with the provision of tangible resources

- Guidance and advice, particularly problem solving

- Access to new contacts and information

- Awareness of the availability of assistance

- Positive interpretations of circumstances contributing to perceived control

- Enhanced resources through community empowerment and competence

- Reduction of risk behaviors and enhancement of preventive health measures

Social support affects biological pathways through behavioral, psychological, and social responses. Social resources have effects on the physiological processes, especially increased heart rate and blood pressure, through their impact on stress-mediated responses in hormonal, neural, and immune systems (see the section, "Anatomical Basis of Stress" in Chapter Nine). Social relations provide the intimacy, nurturance, reassurance, and sense of belonging that can counteract the stress responses. Social networks can affect vulnerability to a range of psychosocial conditions through the coping resources provided through assurance of assistance. Social networks may inhibit an individual's stressful physiological responses associated with anger and depression by reinterpreting them or by changing behavioral or physiological responses that exacerbate the stress response. "Friends can cheer you up" reflects the popular recognition of the positive effects of social relations on mood. Social networks can facilitate coping through the emotional and cognitive strategies they share for managing stress. Good networks may enhance access to medical care or express concerns that lead to healthier decisions and behavior. The network may provide physical care as well as physical and economic resources and instrumental aid that enhance health. Social networks affect health through influences on the adoption of activities, including preventive medicine, compliance with treatments, and avoidance of high-risk conditions. Personal networks affect health maintenance behaviors and provide cues to preventive care, providing role models for appropriate behavior regarding health and risks.

The perception of the availability of support, rather than actual support behaviors, appears to be the factor most strongly linked to health outcomes. This suggests that culturally mediated perceptions affect health. The association of social networks with a reduction in a variety of diseases suggests that they affect overall resistance to disease. Different types of networks may be best suited for addressing specific circumstances or conditions (for instance, the intensity of relationships for affective support but the diffuseness of relationships for information).

The psychosocial relations with others can play an important mediating role in the subjective perceptions that affect responses to external conditions. Linkages of social networks to health derive in part from influences on personality factors, reflecting social competence relevant to the mobilization and maintenance of social support networks. Personality factors do not account for all of the relations and point to the need for ethnographic studies of social support networks and their relationship to health. Social integration and networks may enhance health by creating positive self-evaluations that, in turn, give a sense of mastery and purpose that prevent despair and anxiety and their detrimental physiological consequences. Social relations may also induce the release of endogenous opioids and their effects in enhancing the immune system responses (see Chapter Ten).

There are still many questions regarding the precise nature of the effects of social relations on health. Whether social support networks affect mortality through influences on exposure, recovery, or quality of care or through interaction with other risk factors has not been fully determined. Research is needed to establish the behavioral, social, cognitive, emotional, and physiological processes that create the linkages. This requires more sophisticated measures of different aspects of social networks and relations, a clarification of their various forms of support, and assessment of their influences on health.

MACROLEVEL SOCIAL EFFECTS ON CLINICAL HEALTH

The macrolevel approach of critical medical anthropology also assesses broader social influences on the microlevel physician-patient relationships (Waitzkin, 1979, 1991, 2001). These relationships are influenced by macrolevel political and economic contexts that structure the clinical encounter. Physicians are also agents of the ideology of the ruling classes. Key effects involve the control of access to treatments and the sick role (limiting access) and the medicalization of social distress, a form of social control that obscures socially produced conditions as individual responsibility.

Critical medical anthropology addresses how societal conditions affect the clinical encounter and patient care. Recognition of the role of power in the provision of care empowers an activist engagement with a community-oriented medicine designed to challenge the power relations of biomedicine by addressing the health inequalities produced by class relations and economic disparity.

Medicalization treats social problems as within the purview of medical treatment, such as when homosexuality, addiction, or delinquency are treated as medical problems. Assessing social conditions as diseases or pathogenic processes secludes a patient's condition from the political arena. Biomedicine constructs disease conditions and their treatment within a context where societal causes are ignored in favor of a focus on the individual. Medical control transforms social conditions into physical individualized and privatized circumstances.

Waitzkin (1991) shows that in face-to-face interactions in health care settings, providers maintain particular ideological relationships and social control over patients. Physicians define conditions in ways that make individuals responsible for their condition instead of recognizing a broader causation in the cultural-ecological system. For example, venereal disease might be blamed on immoral sexual relations or the lack of use of appropriate

APPLICATIONS

Changing the Micropolitics of Medicine

Have you ever left the doctor's office and felt unsatisfied with the communication between the two of you? Have you ever felt that the doctor misunderstood your concerns and explanations? Did you feel confused by or uncomfortable with the terms used by the clinician? Improvement in communication outcomes can be achieved through the creation of a collaborative, nonoppressive doctor-patient relationship. Patient education can encourage patients to question and challenge medical advice that serves as social control, empowering working-class patients to challenge the class dominance embodied in medical authority. Waitzkin (1979) suggests that it is necessary to clarify the verbal and behavioral mechanisms that are used in manipulation and social control of the physician-patient relationship to reverse the power relationships that are involved in the clinical realm of health care. Part of this involves ensuring that the communication from physicians to patients provides clear comprehensible messages.

Waitzkin (1991) proposes that it is also necessary to change the broader contexts affecting medical consultation to overcome the ideological and social control functions of biomedicine. Changes beyond the clinical context, a revolutionary restructuring of the broader society, are necessary to change the power dynamics of the medical encounter. Long-term strategies must address the entire health care system and the dynamics of power and finance that leave major portions of the U.S population without basic health care coverage or receiving it as disadvantaged Medicare and welfare recipients. Other needed social changes affecting health include altering the effects of work, unemployment, and class-based economic insecurity.

Viewing biomedicine as an ideological state apparatus that exercises social control provides people with a different understanding of medical consultation processes. These new perspectives help demystify the processes of medical control and reveal their political nature. This enables people to gain greater control over medical relations, as evidenced in the women's health movement and

protection, instead of attributing the exposure to the lack of community health resources for prevention, screening, and treatment. Waitzkin shows how physicians promote the dominant societal ideology of individual responsibility. Class relationships are reinforced in doctor-patient relations through the attribution of biological disease and individual responsibility for conditions that are basically caused by social factors (e.g., alcoholism, malnutrition, and infant neglect). The ideology of individual responsibility attributes the cause of such problems to the individual, obscuring the social and economic roots of these conditions. Biomedicine contributes to class control through the subtle manipulation of values, beliefs, and moral judgments that reinforce physicians' class interests.

Doctor-patient relations treat social problems in ways that reinforce social problems and keep people distressed. Physicians typically prescribe medications that help them adapt to those conditions (e.g., pain killers that allow patients to continue work activities that caused their problem or tranquilizers that enable patients to cope with distressing work conditions), instead of addressing patients' health concerns in the broader social contexts that create their suffering. The dynamics of doctor-patient communications alternative heath practices. Understanding the ways in which medicine exercises ideological and social control empowers resistance in the context of health care delivery. Rather than marginalizing patients' concerns stemming from social context, using ideological and social control messages, or providing a quick technical fix (such as medications), physicians should seek to understand the relationship between health problems and social conditions. By addressing the social contexts that produce personal problems, physicians can reduce further medicalization of social problems.

Medicine can address the social origins of illness, directing resources of community organizations, other professions such as social workers and public health, and political and bureaucratic functionaries to address social issues affecting health: from access to good food, safe streets, and playgrounds to programs that provide enriching social experiences. Facilitating patients' integration with community resources—groups, organizations, and institutions—is part of the solution. **Patient empowerment**—acquiring the ability to understand and affect the allocation of health resources—is a crucial issue. Empowerment includes understanding the broader social and political dynamics affecting health and the allocation of resources and the ability to take collective political action to ensure a just allocation of resources. Empowerment includes individual knowledge regarding the health system and how to use it effectively. For instance, individual empowerment involves knowing how to access public health facilities providing free immunizations; communal empowerment involves shared knowledge regarding how to organize and act to help ensure that local government agencies apply for federal funding for health concerns of the underprivileged. Individual knowledge is not sufficient; empowerment also requires increased community control over health institutions through democratic participation in governing health institutions and making political decisions that affect health resources. This is achieved by organizing local communities to participate in political processes that affect health.

encourages acquiescence to the difficult conditions of life. Physicians' lack of criticism of social context sends an ideological message of expectations of conformance. Medical advice and treatments encourage people to adjust without changing the social conditions that affect their lives.

Physicians promote ideology in encouraging adherence to social norms such as hard work and normative expectations of family and gender roles. In reinforcing adherence to gender roles, physicians provide medications that enable a woman to deal with the perceived burdens of housework and domestic commitments. Biomedicine exercises a critical role in the enforcement of industrial discipline, where excuse from work requires medical validation of the sick role. Physicians play a role in mediating patients' participation in economic production through medical excuses from work or the validation of workers' compensation. Adherence to normative expectations is manifested in encouraging people to return to work as soon as possible. Medication such as pain killers and tranquilizers help prevent dissent and control social discontent, enabling patients to continue in their work patterns, and reinforcing societal patterns of dominance, subordination, and exploitation.

Waitzkin (1979) analyzes medicine as an ideologic state apparatus, an institution that effectively instills particular ideologies through claims to be objective. This value-neutral stance and its esoteric nature place medical knowledge beyond the access of most of the population, forcing us to accept technocratic authority and social control. Physicians maintain dominance over patients by withholding information rather than allowing for a shared therapeutic decision. Through the use of inaccessible language and concepts, physicians foster patient submission, maintain stratification, and reproduce power differences between the classes. Patients feel personally responsible for their conditions, such as cardiovascular and respiratory tract conditions caused by inactivity, instead of focusing on the lack of public safety, night-time outdoor lighting, and parks that might make them feel more comfortable about exercising. When a man is encouraged to attend Alcoholics Anonymous for his drinking problems, the message is one of personal responsibility, rather than addressing the social contextual problems that motivate his excessive drinking.

Waitzkin (2001) suggests that these ideological and social control functions of physicians' behaviors are not deliberate but, rather, a result of uncritical efforts to assist their patients in their needs to cope. The inability of physicians to respond to the social context of patients' problems is in part a result of medical training that teaches them to treat the symptoms of social problems as technical problems to be remedied with medicine. There is also the imperative to interpret symptoms as personal problems, consistent with the broader societal ideologies and values of individual responsibility. This is illustrated in the biomedical approach to alcoholism.

Drinking Problems from a Critical Medical Anthropology Perspective

Alcoholism and other alcohol-related problems are generally treated by biomedicine as individual problems of genetic susceptibility or poor self-control. The individual is seen as being at fault, and the broader social conditions that contribute to alcohol-related problems are neglected (see Singer, 2008). The perspective of critical medical anthropology on alcoholism is illustrated in an article, "Why does Juan Garcia have a drinking problem?" (Singer, Valentin, Baer, and Jia, 1992). Rather than treating a case of alcoholism as an individual problem, Singer and colleagues assessed Puerto Rican drinking problems from historical, economic, and political perspectives. This macrolevel approach illustrates that heavy drinking of alcohol among Puerto Rican men is a function of social, economic, political, and historical forces. History reveals that alcohol consumption was part of daily activities of Spanish colonizers, and alcohol was used to pay plantation workers their salaries. Through this process, alcohol was incorporated into work, social life, and concepts of manhood in Puerto Rican society. Drinking was such an important expression of being a man that to refuse to drink was considered a sign of homosexuality. Drinking, however, was balanced with work.

The U.S. conquest of Puerto Rico changed the economic resource distribution. Whereas 91 percent of the farmers were the owners and occupants of land before, the consolidation of economic control through devaluation and credit freezes by U.S. interests produced forced sale of lands, leaving 80 percent of the population landless within a few decades. This resulted in the production of a seasonally employed rural workforce that experienced the alienated work relations of capitalism. Under these conditions, alcohol became viewed as a man's reward for labor, providing an external motivation for work that was not intrinsically rewarding. Alcohol became a cultural symbol of manhood, a privilege of economically self-sufficient men and a reward mechanism deeply embedded in Puerto Rican culture when industrialization produced massive unemployment and forced migration to the United States for economic survival. In the United States, drinking behaviors were expanded, but the marginalization and further unemployment of the Puerto Ricans transformed controlled social drinking into problem drinking.

This unemployment was a consequence of the transfer of industries from the United States to third-world countries where salaries were a fraction of U.S. labor costs. The widely established relationship of alcoholism with economic downturns, unemployment, and lack of control of one's life heavily impacted Puerto Rican men. Puerto Ricans have some of the highest unemployment rates of any U.S group. This unemployment denies manliness by thwarting self-sufficiency. The cultural emphasis on alcohol consumption as a symbol of manliness became an avenue of self-expression and escape. "Hard drinking replaced hard work, and alcohol, as a medium of cultural expression, was transformed from compensation for the sacrifices of achieving success into a salve for the tortures of failure" (Singer et al., 1992, p. 295).

Thus, the alcoholism problems of Juan Garcia are not the result of personal failure but of the general experiences in the United States of working-class Puerto Rican men. Various studies show that problem drinking among Puerto Ricans is associated with unemployment and a marginalized status. Confronted with an inability to succeed in life because of external structural circumstances in the economy, drinking became entertainment and a way to validate manliness with peers. Problem drinking is not an individual problem but a manifestation of a class problem produced by macrolevel circumstances. Similar dynamics are illustrated in cases of Native American alcoholism.

The "War on Drugs" Versus the Medical Marijuana Movement

You might presume that biomedicine and the FDA would determine, based on available evidence, the worthiness and availability of pharmacological treatments. This is not so. The U.S. government has created a political administrative hierarchy to control—even outright prohibit—the use of medicines based on political criteria. These political criteria are based on a perception of a substance having a "potential for abuse." The substances considered Schedule 1—such as marijuana, LSD, peyote, and psilocybin—are considered to be without medical applications despite considerable evidence of their therapeutic effectiveness for a range of contemporary diseases (Rätsch, 2001, 2005; Winkelman and Roberts, 2007a).

The use of politics to affect access to medicine is found in both the government's administrative and physical "War on Drugs" and in the community coalitions involved in the medical marijuana reform movements' efforts to change state legislation through the initiative process. The medical marijuana movement illustrates the crucial role of politics in determining access to health care resources and restrictions on health risks. Remember that Prohibition—the outlawing of alcohol use in the United States that was in force during the 1920s—required a constitutional amendment and ratification by the states. No such constitutional authority was given to the federal government to regulate marijuana. Federal regulatory control over drugs was not a power authorized by the original

BIOCULTURAL INTERACTIONS

Native American Alcoholism

Alcoholism is a substantial problem for Native Americans (May, 1994). Native American alcohol consumption rates are not higher than those of the general population, but there are higher rates of alcoholism and alcohol-related problems. This higher incidence of alcohol-related problems among Native Americans has been attributed to the social disintegration and breakdown that resulted from their domination and subjugation on reservations. Alcoholism became a rampant problem on many reservations as lifestyles were altered without meaningful replacement, and the enforced reservation restrictions increased tensions and frustrations. Problems with alcoholism became particularly acute among groups previously accustomed to the hunter-gatherer lifestyle and the freedom of movement it had entailed. Alcohol consumption has served not only as a means of reducing stress but, paradoxically, also as a means of asserting Native American identity. The Euro-American culture developed the stereotype of the Native American as an uncontrollable drunk, a perception strengthened by the increased alcohol use by Native Americans as a response to cultural and personal disintegration. Congressional action outlawed alcohol on reservations to protect them. These stereotypes reinforced for Native Americans the equating of drunkenness with "Indianness" and thereby served as a means of public assertion of Native American identity. For many Native Americans, drinking served as protests against Euro-American culture, especially during the prohibition movements outlawing alcohol in the early twentieth century.

Alcohol consumption among Native Americans is a means of establishing camaraderie; such use is particularly prevalent among young men. The population bulge of young Native Americans makes the incidences of alcohol consumption appear higher when not age adjusted. Most young male Native American drinking is not true alcoholism but instead the approximate normative patterns for other Americans. Their drinking behavior is an important part of life-cycle development: dealing with prohibited opportunities, peer group relations, and male solidarity (also see Kunitz, 2006).

Native Americans' drinking patterns and problems largely reflect the consequences of U.S. laws restricting alcohol possession on reservations. This forces alcohol consumption to be a public rather than a private affair. Because drinking is an off-reservation activity, it presents problems not encountered when people have the option of home consumption. Alcohol-related problems reflect consequences of the broader social systems. The federal governments' prohibition of alcohol on reservations results in off-reservation binge drinking, which presents additional problems when they are returning home on often poor two-lane highways filled with other drunks. The remoteness of reservations means access to ambulances and medical facilities for alcohol-related accidents can take hours, increasing mortality. Thus, for Native Americans, the problems of alcohol reflect macrolevel factors rather than strictly personal or cultural dynamics.

constitution or the approved amendments. Many have asserted that the federal government lacks the constitutional authority to regulate what we put into our bodies, including medicines and drugs.

So after Timothy Leary's successful Supreme Court challenge to the federal restrictions on marijuana, Congress enacted administrative control over marijuana and other political drugs such as LSD, psilocybin, and peyote by regulating them as medicines under public health provisions. No constitutional amendment was passed to regulate marijuana; instead, regulation was achieved by political maneuvering directed by the Richard Nixon White House staff. Legislation classifying these substances as medicines made them subject to regulatory control through the channels of the government's administrative law bureaucracy, rather than on the basis of the evidence regarding their medical effectiveness. The federal government has used this control to not only prohibit use but also to systematically block research into marijuana's therapeutic potential and to carry out a war against its citizens who assert what they view as their constitutional rights.

The federal government's administrative classification of marijuana and other ethnomedicines (e.g., psychedelics) as illegal drugs reflects an effort at ideological control over forms of consciousness permitted in society. Our society condones the production and distribution of drugs such as alcohol and nicotine that were at the foundation of American culture (see Winkelman, 2006a, Chapter Four), but other forms of drug-induced alterations of consciousness have been long criminalized in the West (Winkelman and Bletzer, 2005). The classification of medicines as substances with a potential for abuse is done in political terms and through political processes, rather than in terms of medically defined criteria regarding harm. Clearly, tobacco and alcohol have an enormous potential for abuse and are contributory factors in the major causes of mortality for Americans. Tobacco and alcohol are not classified as substances with a potential for abuse, however, and their use is not prohibited by the federal government. The right to kill ourselves with these drugs is part of our individual liberties guaranteed under the constitution!

The classification of a substance was formally awarded by Congress to the Attorney General of the United States, who delegated the power to the head of the Drug Enforcement Agency (DEA). Boire (2007) points out that this is a position traditionally held by law enforcement officials and people with legal backgrounds, not people with medical backgrounds. DEA appointees generally lack medical backgrounds and, instead, are political appointees and vocal proponents of the drug war that helps politicians look "tough on drugs." Consequently, despite specific requirements set out by federal law for scheduling a substance, the DEA administrator has acted against many substances in blatant disregard of the available medical evidence. Federal restrictions reflect the government's ideological use of political power to oppress medical freedom for patients. This control opposes patients' rights to treat themselves with the best remedies available.

The use of marijuana as an effective remedy for a wide range of conditions is substantiated by many forms of evidence (Rätsch, 2005). In recent years, medical studies have found it most useful for stimulating appetite in patients who have lost the will to eat from cancer, radiation and chemotherapy treatment, and the AIDS-wasting syndrome. One might presume that medical knowledge would determine the availability and applications of marijuana as a treatment for these conditions. Instead, marijuana is precluded from medical use by a federal administrator's regulatory decision, a political act that classifies it as a Schedule I substance, meaning it is considered to be without medical use and considered more dangerous than cocaine and morphine, which have "approved" medical uses.

The political battles over the control of consciousness continue today across America. States across the country have passed ballot measures that allow for the medical use of marijuana for the treatment of medical conditions. The local state's authorizations have been repeatedly challenged by federal officials, who have harassed and prosecuted doctors and medical marijuana centers even when they are legal under state law. The lack of constitutional authority has not precluded the powers of the federal government from contradicting the will of the people and attacking patients who depend on these substances for their health. The federal government's regulatory activities and War on Drugs have come to constitute a major force in compromising civil liberties.

The federal efforts to maintain a criminalized status for medical marijuana use despite enabling state legislation deprive patients of the treatments they need. The actions of the federal regulatory agencies place questionable government prerogative over the rights of individuals to have access to the medicine they need for comfort, health, and even survival. The federal government has criminalized their health behaviors, even driving many to suicide over the despair faced when their health issues are compounded by the stresses and costs of legal defense and incarceration (see the Web site of the Drug Policy Foundation, http://www.dpf.org). Continued federal efforts to criminalize even informing people about the potential beneficial effects of marijuana in treating their diseases reflect an ideological policy taking precedence over good medical advice.

Changing the oppressive federal climate regarding medical marijuana use, as well as the therapeutic application of other ethnomedicines such as those called hallucinogens and psychedelics, requires a broad-based effort involving many existing groups and coalitions. Winkelman and Roberts (2007b) have provided an overview of the multiple levels of society at which we need to act to change the current political climate that regulates these substances. Political pressure on federal regulatory agencies remains a central approach for opening up experimental use of these substances. This pressure involves many forms of coalitional action, including general education, education of the media, activities in public health, and policy organizations. What remains key is applying the cumulative scientific, clinical, ethnographic, and cross-cultural evidence regarding the immense potentials of these substances to public policy development to facilitate professional, media, and popular pressure to effect administrative changes in federal regulation. In *Psychedelic Medicine,* Winkelman and Roberts (2007b) have laid the groundwork for this public health and harm reduction endeavor. Education, public policy development, and collective political action, rather than additional science, is necessary to change opportunities for the use of psychedelics in the treatment of some of the most ravaging social diseases of our times, such as the addictions to alcohol, tobacco, methamphetamines, and opiates and their synthetic derivatives. The generally acknowledged success rates of the conventional addiction treatment industry is not much different from the spontaneous remission rate. In contrast, the effectiveness of the use of psychedelics, particularly peyote, ibogaine, ayahuasca (caapi), LSD, and ketamine, appears impressive (see Winkelman and Roberts 2007a, Volume 2).

Physicians have a moral imperative to seek the applications of these more effective treatments for these devastating psychosocial diseases. The complex legal maneuvers in federal, state, and local venues to protect medical marijuana patients, physicians, and dispensaries have relied on a variety of community coalitions that are networked across the country. The Coalition for Medical Marijuana has united medical, legal, and public policy efforts across the United States. Combined educational and legal approaches have been emphasized by the Center for Cognitive Liberty and Ethics (CCLE) (http://www.cognitiveliberty.org) as well. The CCLE is a network of scholars who address issues in the intersection of law and policy issues as they pertain to cognitive freedoms to use psychedelic medicines and other drugs. Their educational and policy approach has addressed policies necessary to preserve the ethics of the freedom of thought regarding these substances. The

PRACTITIONER PROFILE

Craig Janes

Craig Janes, Ph.D., is associate dean in charge of education programs for the Faculty of Health Sciences at Simon Fraser University, Vancouver, British Columbia. His interests in medical anthropology are primarily in global health, social epidemiology, and the political economy of global health reform. He has applied these interests in Mongolia, Taiwan, the Tibet Autonomous Region, China, Samoa, and the United States.

Janes's work as an applied medical anthropologist lies in sociocultural epidemiology; the impact of global, neoliberal health reform on local health care systems, particularly in transitional economies; and research on the mechanisms by which social inequality influences health throughout the lifespan.

In 1986, Janes participated in a public health-oriented study of alcohol use among a blue-collar working population. The goal was to identify disorder-producing aspects of the environment that might be amenable to programs of preventive intervention. He and colleagues identified workplace factors that contributed to high alcohol use, including migration, certain kinds of social network structures, and patterns of union-management relationships.

Later Janes began work on primary health care policy in China, particularly as it is being transformed by China's adoption of World Bank-promulgated neoliberal health care reform. This entailed looking at the role of indigenous Tibetan medicine in the rapidly changing health care in China, particularly in the context of ethnic conflict and transnational concerns with Tibetan independence or autonomy. Tibetan medicine had been rapidly expanded concomitant with Deng Xiao-ping's rise to power and China's retreat from the social guarantees of the Maoist socialist revolution. China has radically reduced its spending on health care; yet, the country is facing an unparalleled epidemic of tobacco-related disease. China may be refocusing its health care system so that indigenous medicines will expand to meet the needs of the growing number of chronically ill and dying citizens but in a model of health care delivery that is increasingly market driven. Janes recently launched a similar study in Mongolia.

CCLE has emphasized the importance of social impact litigation as a process for broadly advancing the potential to exercise our cognitive liberties and has filed legal briefs on the topic of cognitive liberty in federal court. Central to their efforts is raising public awareness of the emerging issues of cognitive liberty through outreach and educational campaigns designed to provide people with the information necessary so that they can empower themselves to participate meaningfully in public discourse and affect relevant democratic processes. This has been achieved through community engagement and coalitions.

CHANGING HEALTH THROUGH PUBLIC POLICY AND COMMUNITY INVOLVEMENT

Medical anthropologists have played a variety of roles in addressing the need for institutional responses of the health care sectors to cultural diversity, sociogenic illness, and the need for new policies and programs to address the relationships between health and social systems. Some of medical anthropology's principal involvements in this area include community coalition development, advocacy, and policy development. Some medical anthropologists have advocated on behalf of ethnic communities and their needs for health programs, obtaining public funding of community health programs. Although advocacy for the underprivileged is a long-standing anthropological tradition, some suggest that it can undermine anthropologists' credibility and effectiveness in the public policy arena (Boone, 1991). Anthropologists may be able to have a greater impact and be more successful in an indirect advocacy role realized through the following means:

■ Training in intercultural skills

■ Service as bureaucrats and expert witnesses

■ Roles on review panels and commissions assessing health problems

■ Involvement in processes of allocating funding for health program development.

Anthropologists' work on health policy has addressed virtually the entire spectrum of health concerns. Primary areas in health policy include AIDS and STDs, drug abuse, reproductive and neonatal health, nutrition, mental health, and concerns of minority populations. Cultural perspectives are central to health policy and program development because of the need to address the cultural mediation of high-risk behaviors and to obtain the involvement of the community in planning appropriate health programs.

Community Health Development

The "Health for All" projects of WHO stimulated international agencies, national governments, and local public health departments to reorient to assure community participation and to address the inequalities in resources allocated for health (World Health Organization, 1992). Approaches to improving community health typically place interventions in the context of the cultural system perspectives to understand the dynamics of health of communities and their resources and risks. This shifts attention from individual behavior and biological dynamics to the broader physical, social, and cultural environments that shape both health and the services of health care institutions.

Achieving the objectives of community health participation has constituted a social movement because such involvement is viewed as crucial for the success of health interventions. There are three critical aspects of institutional cultural change in order to achieve community health involvement (Smithies and Webster, 1998):

■ Organizational changes to accommodate community perspectives

■ Institutional outreach to communities

■ Interfaces between communities and organizations to achieve a permanent partnership

The central issues in culturally competent community outreach involve anthropological approaches and intercultural skills and competencies, including (Smithies and Webster, 1998)

■ Knowledge of the local culture

■ Knowledge of community involvement theories

■ The ability to manage conflict and negotiate differences

■ Understanding of cultural communication patterns

■ Skills in intergroup and intragroup dynamics and public relations

■ Cultural and social awareness of different communities and their needs

■ Skills in community involvement techniques and team building

■ Abilities to influence change in organizational culture

■ The ability to create inclusive work and advocacy organizations

The multileveled interventions necessary to change health risks are dependent on health organizations' competence in eliciting, responding to, and supporting community involvement in health programs through the formation of community coalitions. Organizational self-assessments by health institutions of their infrastructure and organizational culture are important to determine their preparedness, staff, and outreach necessary to facilitate community involvement. The public health sector and community health providers need appropriate input to develop the organizational culture and personnel capacities necessary for effective collaborative relations with communities. Effectively implementing community health programs often depends on changing the organizational culture of health organizations to facilitate acceptance of consultation and shared decision making. The IOM recommends that a variety of health professionals be educated and trained in cultural competence to support the community health improvement process. Preservice and midcareer training should be provided in public health, medicine, nursing, health care administration, evaluation professions, counselors, and social services.

Fostering community involvement requires knowledge of the culture of both communities and organizations within the health care industry. Knowledge is needed of the culture, values, beliefs, and social behaviors of the different ethnic or significant underserved social groups in the community, particularly with respect to health behaviors. Addressing the social context, the contextualization of disease, requires an understanding of how social and cultural systems produce health risks and disease. Such knowledge is essential for the development of many aspects of community health programs:

- Culturally appropriate assessments of relevant health-risk behaviors
- The development of socially and culturally responsive health policy
- The creation of health promotion campaigns and health education programs
- Engagement with cultural processes for facilitating community participation and empowerment in health care

An effective provision of services is dependent on the ability to engage diverse groups in a participatory democracy in which they contribute to determining priority health issues and the development of interventions to address those problems. Community health programs need people with anthropological skills, such as

- A knowledge of local cultures
- Processes for instigating organizational change
- The ability to train others in cultural competence skills
- Strategies for community involvement and empowerment
- The competence to work sensitively with target communities and concerned constituencies

Advocacy for Health Improvement

A major aspect of community health improvement involves **advocacy,** action on behalf of communities to help ensure their access to needed resources and services. There are many different forms of advocacy in community health (Smithies and Webster, 1998). Effective advocacy requires a knowledge of community needs and interests and skills for effectively communicating those to other social groups, including health institutions and bureaucracies. Effective advocacy requires a knowledge of both institutional organizational politics and processes of community mobilization. Effective advocacy depends on the ability to create structures for interaction among community members to elicit their perspectives and establish consensus. Advocacy skills include

- The ability to understand people in cultural contexts
- A knowledge of how to communicate in culturally effective ways
- The ability to mediate between different views and resolve conflict
- The ability to negotiate synergistic solutions
- A knowledge of culturally effective ways of promoting services and educational programs

Advocacy to change health policy and the social environments and physical conditions that produce disease also requires a knowledge of political and bureaucratic systems. Altering conditions of the physical environment that produce health risks requires access to resources. The allocation of resources takes place in a political environment in which a knowledge of organizational behavior and alliance building is essential. Major health issues in which anthropological input can affect the responses of health institutions to health care needs are the organization, delivery, and costs of services (Boone, 1991). Cultural understandings of organizations, social structure, and communication are vital in developing quality, cost-effective, and appropriate health care. Practical concerns about costs must be balanced with sensitivity to patients' concerns about health needs. Cultural perspectives facilitate understanding those needs and the effects of disease and treatments on people's everyday lives. Cultural responsiveness in health care systems is crucial to patients' experience of the quality of care, producing greater satisfaction through cultural sensitivity. Costs and benefits have important cultural dimensions but need to be addressed within a context cognizant of cultural factors affecting patient perceptions. Cultural responsiveness can enhance the recovery process, reduce the length of hospital stays and need for follow-up, consequently contributing to cost containment. "[M]inorities' [notions] of . . . 'good health care' derive so often from fundamental religious values that they can scarcely fit into a cost/benefit analysis" (Boone, 1991, pp. 32, 37).

Public Policy and Coalition Development

Managing cultural differences and value-laden political issues is central in the development of public policy. Public policy is based on a multidisciplinary social science approach that addresses concerns of diverse constituencies, including government, the public, and health industries. Concepts of culture and social systems are used to analyze policy issues and alternatives on health issues, enabling anthropology to make substantial contributions to the development of culturally responsive public policy. Anthropology's approaches include values analysis, case study methods, historical and cultural systems approaches, and cultural change models (Boone, 1991).

Medical anthropology's cultural systems perspectives can facilitate the creation of more effective institutional responses to health care needs through

- The development of health policy and prevention programs

- Promoting the institutional development of culturally responsive care and services

- Managing the people and perspectives involved in the intersection of academic science, policy science, and health organizations that contribute to health policy development

- Providing an integration of the interests of health constituencies (bureaucrats, health providers, and cultural groups)

Needed capacities of health departments and community programs include staff with the skills to effectively participate in intergroup dynamics and synergistic relationships among diverse stakeholders to produce political impact. Mobilizing communities requires health care staff familiar with the community and their activities and capable of engaging

APPLICATIONS

Developing Community Involvement and Practitioner Cultural Competence

Chrisman's (2005, 2007) work in the Seattle Partners for Healthy Communities exemplifies the anthropological contributions to developing health capacity in communities and cultural competence through programs that address a community's perceived needs in ways consistent with its values, strengths, and resources. This requires incorporating local members and existing organizations into program conceptualization, development, and implementation. Programs that build from a community's perceived needs are more likely to get acceptance and long-term support from the community. This collaboration with community is mandated by the new approaches in public health that recognize that prevention programs must be accommodated to community perceptions and realities and developed in ways that are self-sustaining.

Public health programs developed by hospitals and physicians without engaging community commitment and involvement are unlikely to persist beyond the time during which the outside agency is involved. To give permanency to initiatives, such as local weight loss or cigarette cessation programs, community organizations must be incorporated from the initial stages. Community involvement helps ensure that meaningful interventions are developed. For instance, in addressing obesity, nutritional advice based on a white American meat-and-potatoes meal plan is not likely to make sense to most Hispanic households who need to modify traditional diet for health reasons.

Chrisman (2007) conceptualizes cultural competence as requiring a systems approach that provides training through establishing linkages across diverse institutions in seeking to implement the goals of organizational cultural competence by addressing these principal components: having missions and goals in the organization that value diversity, diversity hiring and training within the organization, and intensive interactions through coalitions between the health institutions and the community. Chrisman emphasizes that these community partnerships are essential for the transformation of organizational culture to achieve institutional cultural competence. Partnerships must be developed among educational institutions, hospitals and clinics, community and public health agencies, and other groups involved in planning for long-term care. Chrisman emphasizes the importance of community networks and coalitions in providing the relationships necessary for training nurses and doctors. The community coalitions provide placement opportunities for reinforcing the concepts regarding cultural diversity acquired in the classroom setting.

Chrisman integrates nursing students into the community-based coalitions, such as his CDC-funded REACH program that established a diabetes intervention project in the Seattle area. This coalition included a variety of stakeholders in addition to representatives from departments of the local nursing, medicine, and public policy schools: representatives from community clinics; members of African American, Hispanic American, Asian American, and Native American communities; local faith-based organizations; members of the American Diabetes Association; local agencies providing services for public health promotion and disease prevention, including the State Department of Health; representatives from pharmaceutical companies; and a local company that addressed quality assurance in health care delivery. The coalition was subsequently expanded through efforts to recruit members from a variety of other organizations, including political groups, the government, and media outlets (Chrisman 2007).

Because of the diverse linkages across groups in the community, the coalitions are able to represent the diversity that must be addressed in cultural competence training programs. These cultural differences also create tensions that are often worsened by the long-standing neglect of local communities by medical, nursing, and public health programs. Trained facilitators are important for mediating the differences among the diverse stakeholders in the community coalitions and, preferably, to train different stakeholder groups in advance to reduce cultural conflicts and misunderstandings. Antiracism training may be necessary for all members of coalitions, not just members of majority groups and health institutions. This training can benefit the latter in their work, reducing the frustrations in dealing with different cultures. This includes training not only for appropriate clinical interactions but also in the context of community coalitions: training in relational, communication, and managerial styles appropriate for the ethnic communities involved.

Such preparation can facilitate the formation of the community coalitions, creating the skill sets necessary for different groups to work together productively and for medical personnel to recognize the importance of accepting community's conceptualizations of their needs. For instance, if the program is designed to reduce the effects of diabetes, why would a community want a community center constructed instead of providing free screening services in existing clinics? Is this justifiable? Why shouldn't community health programs focus on providing services instead of community building activities? Anthropologists have key roles in making the community health needs and desired programs intelligible to the "foreign" medical and public health cultures. A community center might have direct relevance to diabetes care on many levels: a place to receive training in new cooking styles, places for diet support groups to meet, a location for safe exercise in what are dangerous neighborhoods, and a place for socializing and social networking in ways that enhance healthy behaviors. This, in part, is related to **community empowerment**. Chrisman defines empowerment as "the group's belief in its capability to succeed in future actions" (2005, p. 177). There are also immediate project goals that require the functioning of coalitions: acceptance of a biomedical or public health intervention that requires some acceptance by the community, a sense that the program is appropriate for them. Without coalition development and participation, projects are likely to follow the long history of failing to include community perspectives necessary to get their involvement and utilization of benefits from the programs. Community building in general may also have significant health benefits, illustrated in the effects of social support and social networks in health and recovery.

APPLICATIONS

Mothers Against Drunk Driving as a Community Health Coalition

The roles of community coalitions in successful changes in health and mortality are illustrated by Mothers Against Drunk Driving (MADD). MADD used coalitional building to combat the health problems caused by alcohol—particularly the automobile fatalities that occurred among under-aged drinkers. MADD's coalitions had nationwide success in enacting laws that put tougher penalties on drunk drivers and in obtaining more stringent enforcement of laws against driving while intoxicated.

The focus on underaged drinking as a key aspect of the alcohol problem exemplifies why it is important to have community efforts. The problem of underaged drinking begins in a context of both the neglect of adolescents' activities and tolerance of their drinking alcohol. The concept of alcohol as a rite of passage is deeply engrained in American culture, going back to America's colonial roots (Winkel-man, 2006a). This glorifying of alcohol condones abuse of self and others. The belief that alcohol is a test and sign of manhood needs to be countered at many levels. A different perspective needs to be seen in community models, political leaders, schools, churches, sports teams and other peer groups, and in families to have the ability to counter the effects of these cultural traditions regarding drinking. Getting a new message in the public sphere has been a key part of MADD's efforts to change a culture of drinking that tolerates abuses and contributes to one of the major causes of mortality in the United States: motor-vehicle accidents caused by someone under the influence of alcohol.

MADD was successful in combating this alcohol-induced epidemic by focusing on underaged drinking and driving under the influence (DUI) and by addressing change at many different levels, including public policy development, legislative enactments, governmental involvement (police, courts, social services), and community engagement in public and private sectors. Among the many coalition partners that MADD has developed are the various agents of the press, churches, community groups, schools, substance abuse rehabilitation programs, medical and nursing associations, public health officials, community health providers, and educators, legislators, judges, the police, business, civic groups, and many others. Civic groups such as the Lions and Kiwanis were recruited to major aspects of policy development, legislative campaign planning, and public influence campaigns with the legal system, from local cities and police enforcement through legislative initiatives for more stringent laws regarding intoxication levels and penalties for DUI. Making

community members and coalitions to produce changes at the collective level. It also requires the ability to link voluntary organizations across a wide range of areas in the creation of public policy and coalitions that can affect changes in community health behaviors that place people at risk and institute changes in broader societal institutions that reinforce healthier behaviors.

Coalition-Building Processes

Effective advocacy includes the engagement of community involvement in ways that ensure effective community participation in consultation for assessments of health needs vehicular manslaughter due to intoxication a serious crime took many forms of pressure to change what had been a tolerant judicial climate regarding these crimes.

To change the perceptions and behavior of adolescents, public health messages were targeted at youth in many contexts: sports, school, TV, and work. Peer support and reinforcement for antidrinking messages are supported by placing them in youth-dominated settings such as sports teams, YMCA and YWCA activities, and numerous boys' and girls' youth and scouting clubs. The creation of alternate social activities such as dances, concerts, and other events that are in alcohol-free venues provides positive opportunities for socializing and avoiding alcohol. Public health ads with an antialcohol message were placed in various venues in businesses where youth are often employed or congregate, such as theaters and amusement parks. Legislation was sought to keep proalcohol messages out of such venues. Pressure was put on the alcohol industry to put "responsible drinking" messages in their advertisements. Legislative efforts were made in many places to keep liquor establishments even farther from schools than already required by law.

Central to MADD's approach was changing not just cultural perceptions regarding alcohol use but the laws and enforcement regarding drinking, particularly drinking and driving. Changing laws was often necessary so that those guilty of negligent manslaughter would not get off with six months' jail time or a few years' probation. Grass-roots community organizing was the essence of the power of communities to effect change. Through person-to-person contacts, people are organized to make phone calls, send e-mail messages, attend hearings, and meet with public officials. It is the public manifestation of numbers of the community, supported by media and other groups, that has enabled MADD to force legislators to enact stiff DUI and underaged drinking legislation despite the "good ole boy" drinking habits of many legislators. The states' alcohol control boards were enlisted to seek out liquor outlets with persistent violations by doing undercover operations and "stings" to attack the supply side of the alcohol problem, sales to minors. Working with police, the judicial system, and legislatures and using the power of numbers to make public statements of strength, MADD again and again pressured judges to give full sentences rather than the customary slap on the wrist to those guilty of manslaughter while DUI. The media has contributed to this broad community effort through public service announcements, the coverage of MADD activities, and news of alcohol-related adolescent deaths to drive the MADD message home: alcohol can kill you, your friends, and your family.

and the creation of the institutional and community adaptations to improve health. The development of community coalitions requires professionals with cultural knowledge and interpersonal skills relevant to their stakeholders and the organizational capacity of health institutions to incorporate such collaboration. Community participation requires both formal and informal organizational change within existing health institutions to incorporate community interests (Smithies and Webster, 1998).

Fundamental to community involvement is the institutionalization of a community infrastructure or coalition-building capacity for responding to health problems. This means that community organizations are created that have the capacity to recognize health problems and engage institutional assistance in developing appropriate solutions to the problems. These organizations of diverse constituencies are involved in the identification and prioritization of problems and collaboration in the development and implementation of interventions. Community participation may depend on rewards and benefits allocated by health institutions to foster the creation of coalitions. The creation of successful and sustainable coalitions requires the commitment of paid public health employees involved in the organization of contact among diverse stakeholders.

Effective coalition building and modification of community health require an empowerment framework in which affected populations assume a greater involvement in understanding the factors involved in assuring their own health. Community involvement helps ensure that local health institutions are responsive to community needs and allocate resources for programs that have high priority for improving the community's overall quality of health. Benefits to communities as a whole resulting from community participation include a shift in resources toward the prevention of disease. The involvement of communities also enhances health through increasing confidence, skills, self-esteem, and empowerment.

Community coalitions contribute to community resources by increased levels of training and awareness. Effective community involvement ensures inclusion of traditionally excluded groups, enhancing the overall health of the community by reducing the risks to the isolated group(s). For instance, intravenous drug addicts (heroin) are not likely to be concerned about their overall health, and many have diseases such as HIV infection and hepatitis. These isolated groups constitute a pocket of infectious diseases that are not likely to be treated without an aggressive outreach campaign. Untreated, they pose a risk to the broader population through the spread of their diseases by casual sexual contacts as they support their habits through prostitution.

Organizations that participate in community health coalitions may obtain benefits through the development of organizational skills relevant to relationships with diverse stakeholders. Providers and agencies can also benefit from community health coalitions that not only strengthen their understanding of health problems but also help ensure a better distribution of resources for primary health problems. Effective community coalitions need to include more than representatives from health professions and governmental agencies. Effective planning for the prevention of disease requires the inclusion of a broader group of stakeholders, including those concerned with the environment occupational safety, special interest groups, broader community organizations, schools and other training institutions, and diverse sectors of the economy.

Those groups traditionally denied representation, or who are at greatest vulnerability of being denied access to services, need to be given special consideration. These hard-to-reach groups are often at higher risk for many health conditions. Effective coalitions require the inclusion of appropriate representatives, particularly those who can influence community attitudes and behaviors. Community coalitions should represent individual community members and their organization but also other stakeholder groups, including private and public health care providers, epidemiologists, health researchers, relevant employers, school representatives, and other public organizations. Because of the increased interdependence of public health and managed care organizations, there is also a vital role for the latter in community coalitions (see the Lasker Report, 1997).

Smithies and Webster (1998) point out that community health programs are often staffed by people with little or no experience in community development work and who lack knowledge of culturally appropriate approaches. Effective community health workers need skills in eliciting from communities their own priorities and building a sense of trust, ownership, and participation. Consequently, cultural brokers and other mediators need to be involved in the process, creating opportunities for medical anthropologists in community health assessment. Effective participation in community coalitions requires the ability to create equality and acceptance across the diverse sectors. The traditional dominance of medicine and public health in making community health decisions means that they may need to make the greatest changes in accustomed practices and organizational behavior.

Successful community coalitions depend on the ability of institutionalized health services to create a culture of participation that contributes to the long-term involvement of community organizations (Meleis, 1992). Health care institutions and government-funded public health services remain as major actors in the control of resources. Consequently, they need to take a leading role in the redistribution of organizational resources to support the enhancement of community organizations that is necessary for successful community participation in health planning. Although community participation should be incorporated into ongoing projects, the ideal is to have community participation beginning with the conceptualization stage of programs (see the section, "Rapid Assessment, Response, and Evaluation" in Chapter Four). Public health agencies may need to take central roles in the formation of community coalitions to obtain their involvement. This will include recruiting membership, providing information, and coordinating activities and meeting places. Because this community interaction invariably involves different cultural groups, there is a need for cultural competence in outreach and organization, in addition to providers and administrators. Cultural knowledge and mediation and organizational skills are essential for bringing together the diverse stakeholders, community groups, and coalitions, and integrating their perspectives into health plans.

CHAPTER SUMMARY

A socially responsible approach to community health and care for the underprivileged must address changes in the existing conditions and institutions affecting health. The approach of critical medical anthropology advocates assistance to groups who struggle to address pressing medical problems through challenging the biomedical establishment and capitalist medicine. Scheper-Hughes (1990) emphasizes that it must be an "anthropology of affliction," with an orientation to praxis that resists the hegemony of biomedicine. An advocacy approach is necessary to counter the existing imbalance of power. Changes need to be made in the availability of services, the nature of the clinical encounter, and the broader societal conditions affecting health. These include the distribution of knowledge and resources and the industrial "manufacture of disease" produced by contaminants and work conditions. A crucial aspect of the critical medical anthropology agenda involves the development of clinics to provide services for underserved ethnic minorities and lower social classes to increase their access to medical care.

Services need to be provided in a culturally appropriate manner. A key issue involves changing the relations between providers and their clients in ways that empower clients through an understanding of medical encounters and the ability to take an active role in making decisions regarding their care. Care must be proactive, providing outreach and prevention services and restructuring the nature of medical practice to ensure its access and relevance, particularly for those who need it the most.

These changes require an examination of the roles of world economic systems in producing the social origins of diseases and the ways in which health policy is formulated. An understanding of how the elite classes control the poor and their access to resources is crucial to understanding how public policy and material and human resources affect health care. Because biomedicine constitutes one of the major interfaces between the working class and the capitalist class, its ideological impact on both clinical practice and broader social policies and its role in reproducing social relations and stratification must be addressed and modified. The assurance of health requires a fundamental restructuring of the infrastructural and structural determinants of policy development, resource allocation, and health care provision.

KEY TERMS

Advocacy

Contextualization

Critical medical anthropology

Empowerment

Medicalization

Patient empowerment

Social networks

Social support

Sociomatic

SELF-ASSESSMENT 8.1. POLITICAL-ECONOMIC EFFECTS ON HEALTH

1. Use the "Conceptual Framework for Cultural System Health Assessments" (Exhibit 4.1) in Chapter Four to describe the economic and political factors affecting health conditions in your community and, in particular, different ethnic communities in your region.

2. Review local newspapers to identify health issues that are impacted by the local government or for which the local government has the potential to make important contributions to their resolution. What are the political and economic factors that affect these actions? How could they be changed?

ADDITIONAL RESOURCES

Books

Andrain, C. F. 1998. *Public health policies and social inequality.* London: Macmillan.

Court, J., and F. Smith. 1999. *Making a killing: HMOs and the threat to your health.* Forward by Ralph Nader. Monroe, Me.: Common Courage Press.

Kiefer, C. W. 2000. *Health work with the poor–A practical guide.* New Brunswick, N.J.: Rutgers University Press.

Kim, J. Y., A. Irwin, J. Millen, and J. Gershaman. 2000. *Dying for growth: Global inequality and the health of the poor.* Monroe, Me.: Common Courage Press.

Lay, M. M., L. J. Gurak, C. Gravon, and C. Myntii, eds. 2000. *Body talk: Rhetoric, technology, reproduction.* Madison: University of Wisconsin Press.

Singer, M., ed. 1998. *The political economy of AIDS.* Amityville, N.Y.: Baywood.

Whiteford, L. M., and L. Manderson, eds. 2000. *Global health policy, local realities: The fallacy of the level playing field.* Boulder, Colo.: Rienner.

Journals

Journal of Health and Social Behavior.
Social Science and Medicine.

CHAPTER

9

PSYCHOBIOLOGICAL DYNAMICS OF HEALTH

The placebo effect is . . . a clear case of symbolic and meaningful events . . . having an apparently direct effect on human biology. . . the "meaning response"

—MOERMAN, 2000, P. 56

LEARNING OBJECTIVES

- Review evidence of the ability of religion to affect health and the various mechanisms by which religion and ritual have therapeutic effects

- Illustrate the symbolic mediation of all healing and the bases for causal effects of symbols on health through biosocialization, the learned association of symbols, and physiological responses

- Describe the psychophysiology of stress and illustrate the symbolic and cultural mediation of stress responses

- Illustrate factors affecting the physiological responses to placebos and examine the meaning-based mediations of placebos

- Examine mechanisms underlying the immune system and psychoneuroimmuno-logical responses, particularly the roles of cultural meanings

- Introduce the concept of metaphoric healing as a mechanism for religious efficacy

CULTURAL HEALING

The cultural or symbolic approach in medical anthropology emphasizes the efficacy of ethnomedical systems, pointing to a wide range of evidence that they relieve maladies. This presumed effectiveness of ritual healing implies that religion somehow has the power to heal. Indeed, anthropologists have often concluded that religious healing is effective in ameliorating suffering.

Singer (1989a, 1989b) criticized this anthropological support of folk medicine, considering its persistence a compensatory practice designed to cope with the consequences of the failure of societies to provide adequate health care. Are we to be chastised for glorifying religious healing because it provides a diversion from the realities of inadequate public and clinical health services? Scheper-Hughes (1990) suggested another view: that both clinically applied and critical medical anthropology fail to address the challenge to biomedicine's materialist premises that is posed by ethnomedical traditions that consider spiritual practices fundamental to healing processes. How is it that a ritual can heal? Why do people feel better and report improvements following a religious healing ceremony? An implicit acceptance of other cultures' ethnomedical traditions by anthropologists as being efficacious may imply that their mechanisms of action can be incorporated in biomedicine's approaches. Or can they?

Scheper-Hughes suggested the need to understand other ethnomedical healing practices as involving mechanisms distinct from those emphasized by biomedicine: "[I]f medical anthropology does not begin to raise the possibility of other realities, other practices with respect to healing the mindful body, who can we expect to do so?" (Scheper-Hughes, 1990, pp. 193–194). Examining the bases for the legitimacy of these practices is justified on the grounds of cultural relativism and cultural sensitivity and through an understanding of their physiological effects. Ethnomedical practices not only provide a meaningful understanding of health conditions, they are also often effective through different mechanisms generally addressed by biomedicine.

Biomedicine has generally discounted the effectiveness of ethnomedical traditions, suggesting that at best they provide benefits through suggestibility: self-fulfilling expectations of improvement somehow trick people into feeling that they are better when, in fact, they are not. Some may discount the apparent improvements as placebo responses, but placebo effects are real; expectations, cultural symbols, and personal meanings can have profound effects on biological processes and responses. These placebo responses remain a challenge to traditional biomedical approaches, illustrating the ability of the mental level of symbols to affect the physical. Furthermore, among the most effective ways of eliciting placebo responses are through religious symbols and meanings. The universal role of religion in health practices points to its ability to elicit a range of healing responses and its special roles in human health. Religious healing also involves aspects found in all healing, what Kleinman (1973a) refers to as **symbolic healing,** involving the effects of meaning on physiological responses.

There are a variety of generic aspects of all healing encounters, religious and secular. These involve a patient's engagement in a system of symbolic and social relationships. These relationships are based on a general explanatory system (e.g., a mythic system, religious beliefs, biomedical materialism, or theories such as psychoanalysis) that defines the nature of maladies and possibilities of healing. Healing is abetted by a socially esteemed individual who has a variety of recognized powers that induce an expectation of resolving the problem. These healing interactions provide emotional and social support for patients, enhancing their sense of self-worth. A major aspect of all healing traditions includes the power of the interaction to elicit **endogenous healing responses** based on innate processes such as relaxation. These include patients' reactions of susceptibility to suggestion, positive expectation and hope, psychosomatic reactions, relaxation, emotional enhancement, placebo responses, and psychological reactions such as guilt, shame, dissociation, and catharsis (emotional release).

Religion has been a major mechanism through which these and other symbolic effects are channeled to enhance human health. Religion utilizes a number of mechanisms by which meaning affects physiological responses. Understanding these processes promoted a cognitive revolution in psychology that is replacing the behaviorist paradigms with a new paradigm (theoretical framework) based on the recognition of top-down causation. This involves processes in which higher mental levels affect lower-level physiological responses, such as when our fears produce physiological stress. These symbolic effects on physiological responses present anomalies for biomedicine's reductionist and materialist perspectives. They also present a basis for a new paradigm that explores the effects of mental phenomena on the physical world, especially our bodies. These mental effects on health are more broadly reflected in the effects of culture on biology and manifested in phenomena such as religious healing, stress reactions, voodoo death, placebo effects, and total drug responses.

Socialization processes provide many mechanisms by which ritual can affect health through the acquired associations of symbolic, psychological, and social processes with emotions and physiological responses. Associations of symbols and socially (ritually) induced experiences and emotions learned during socialization link symbolic and organic processes, enabling symbolic and ritual elicitation and manipulation of physiological responses and emotions. Socialization processes associate symbolic processes with the neurological development of the brain, providing mechanisms for symbolic healing processes.

Ritual is not meaningless behavior but behaviors that affect humans at physical, emotional, social, and cognitive levels. The universality of religious ritual healing reflects its powerful therapeutic effects. These effects reflect the impact of meaning and social support on individual responses to stress by providing a sense of certainty regarding well-being. Social networks and support play an important role in maintaining health and enhancing recovery through a variety of pathways. Studies of the relationship among culture, stress, and disease reveal the health effects of social relations and cultural beliefs and attitudes.

The bases for religious and other symbolic systems having effects on our bodies are part of the makeup of human nature. For example, our ungrounded fears—an erroneous symbol—can nonetheless provoke physiological reactions, such as in activation of the

CASE STUDY

Nightmare Deaths and Stress

The Hmong in America discovered that their dreams could kill them. During the early 1980s, the American public heard of "nightmare deaths" in which Hmong immigrants were dying in their sleep or shortly after awaking exhausted from gruesome nightmares. For a while, this "sudden-death syndrome" was the leading cause of mortality among young Hmong men in the United States.

Although dreams were sometimes interpreted traditionally as communications from ancestors, the Hmong in America experienced horrific war scenes and being pursued by dead enemies. Survivors of these dream attacks also reported large animals sitting on their chests or spirits lying on their bodies, crushing them breathless and suffocating them. They lay there feeling paralyzed but frantically struggling, screaming in terror, and tossing in their beds. After agonizing minutes, they awoke exhausted by the protracted struggle.

Some never awoke. Physicians attributed their deaths to the emotional distress of the dreams that triggered cardiac arrest, but a definitive cause was not established. Yet, clearly stress was central to these fatal responses, which were thought to be a delayed reaction to the trauma of war in Southeast Asia and the challenges of acculturation in the United States (Bliatout, 1983; Tobin and Friedman, 1983). Breathing difficulties are a consequence of the anxiety, paranoia, and depression that result from extreme stress. Unconscious suicide due to survivor guilt and loss of self-respect and control over life was thought to have contributed to the deaths.

The Hmong, however, viewed the deaths as stemming from their failure to perform their mourning rituals for their parents who died in the war. This omission left them vulnerable, without

fight-or-flight response. The stress-induced **general adaptation syndrome** (see below) illustrates how personal and cultural interpretations affect physiological processes. For instance, when you become frightened because you think there is a snake on the ground in front of you, but it turns out to be a vine, a mistaken symbolic interpretation—snake—provoked physiological responses of fear, shaking, and perhaps even fainting. The interaction of symbols with our physiological reactions provides a number of explanations for the efficacy associated with ritual and religious healing, as well as "voodoo death." There are powerful health consequences of cultural consonance: the degree to which individuals feel culturally compatible with the people they live around. Such contextual factors and interpersonal dynamics also affect stress and, consequently, disease.

Placebo and nocebo effects involve positive and negative responses of the nervous and immune systems to our expectations. Cross-cultural studies on the variation in placebo responses to drugs illustrate the power of cultural, social, and individual influences on the actions of biological agents, whose physiological properties are mediated, shaped, and even blocked by mental factors. The concept of the **total drug effect** illustrates the powerful cultural effects of expectations and social and contextual factors ancestor spirits to protect them from evil spirits. Their guilt about their failures to perform required rituals made them prone to interpreting their experiences as attacks by offended spirits.

The Hmong use rituals to maintain health or reestablish balance when disharmony results in illness. When Lia Lee was allowed to return home to her parents, they celebrated traditional rituals to improve her health with the expensive sacrifice of a cow and a shaman making the appropriate chants honoring the animal. The sacrifice was accompanied by visits by many people to the Lee household. After the sacrifice, these people ate the cow—its blood, intestines, internal organs, and virtually the entire animal—in a festive occasion.

These rituals did not, however, prevent Lia from deteriorating further and experiencing a life-threatening seizure. After numerous medical interventions, Lia lay on a hospital bed, apparently near death. Rejecting the physicians' predictions of her imminent death, her family rebelled, requesting that the intravenous lines be removed. The medical staff viewed this as their acceptance of their daughter's imminent death.

In fact, they requested the termination of medical procedures because they thought that these were the factors causing their daughter's decline. They took her home not to die but to receive traditional treatments. An herbal bath on a shower curtain in the living room showed immediate effect: Her sweating stopped, and she slept peacefully. Her 104-degree temperature dropped to normal, but she continued in a coma. The doctors attributed her longevity to the reduction of brain swelling; her parents attributed it to the herbal teas they used to bathe her. We might conclude that the loving family who held her in their arms was also responsible for her partial recovery.

(set and setting) on withdrawal, addiction, side effects, and other drug response characteristics.

Linkages among emotions, beliefs, attachments, and physiological responses are the foundation of the medical field of psychoneuroimmunology, where psychological expectations and social relations are recognized as having significant effects on health. The field of psychoneuroimmunology demands an understanding of how our social and cultural lives affect our self and its psychophysiological responses, especially immune system responses. Emotional and psychological reactions are principal ways in which meaning affects the nervous system. Meaning is what shapes our interpretations of threats to our sense of self and social attachments and affects health by eliciting physiological responses that reflect appraisal of our situation. These responses can be countered by the power of metaphoric models of religion that elicit our sense of self and emotions and provide significant others who can produce personal transformations at many levels: physiological, emotional, psychological, and social. These models may enable symbols to heal or to kill.

RELIGION, RITUAL, AND SYMBOLIC HEALING

Have you noticed that people often turn to religion in times of personal or familial illness or other forms of stress? Have you heard that people who attend religious services on a regular basis tend to be healthier? Religious healing is often discounted as involving self-deception or placebo effects. Traditional viewpoints of Western science and biomedicine have contended that religion cannot really affect your health. Religious traditions claim, however, to affect the physical body through prayer and "miraculous healing." As noted above, many generic effects of healing encounters can elicit endogenous healing processes of the body. What mechanisms of healing are provided by religion?

Medicine's Symbolic Reality

The experience of healing involves cultural meanings and responses, a symbolic reality, even when addressing disease with biomedicine. Imagine how different you would feel if you thought you had the flu but your doctor told you that you had a serious infection of intestinal worms! Or how much better you might feel if your doctor told you that what you thought was mononucleosis was just a nasty cold. That is the power of symbols to affect not only our perceptions and experiences but even our physiological realities. People experience psychological and physical diseases in the context of cultural meanings associated with those conditions, and the physiological aspects of these conditions and our bodies are affected by how we interpret the world. Remember the case study in Chapter Two in which "Mr. Glover's" stable condition in the emergency department changed to a cardiac arrest when incompetent residents failed to start his intravenous line? That failed effort did not cause the cardiac arrest; rather, it was Mr. Glover's annoyance at the incompetence of the staff, his personal reactions, that provoked the physical heart attack.

All healing practices are embedded in cultural systems that manage the experiences of maladies through the symbolic implications of conditions and therapeutic practices. Receiving a diagnosis when we seek care has physiological, psychological, and social effects that structure the personal experience of illness. Symbolic elements of healing may have profound effects even if the healer's interaction is brief and impersonal. Even if your doctor sees you for only a few busy minutes, if you feel her concern and confidence in her ability to effectively treat you, you are likely to leave feeling better. This is part of "cultural healing," an automatic consequence of a patient's entry into the healing system. This inspires confidence, allaying patients' concerns, and contributes to mobilization of their own defenses and confidence. Through labeling, defining, and classifying illness, the unknown is transformed into known events, producing psychophysiological effects.

Despite their importance to understanding the outcomes of clinical encounters, the health implications of symbols have been given only what Kleinman called "superficial and somewhat embarrassed attention" (1973a, p. 207) by biomedicine. This neglect reflects the fact that the importance of this "symbolic reality," the patients' interpretations, contradicts the traditional separation of the biological and the psychological. Symbols link cultural events and psychophysiological responses, providing a basis for symbolic healing. Kleinman (1973a) notes that all healing occurs within symbolic systems, manifested in cultural expectations, values, and beliefs that are associated with both affective and physiological responses.

What remained to be explained in this early statement of the symbolic model of healing was how sociocultural reality affects the body. How do news stories about a possible terrorist attack cause us to feel physically bad? Why can worrying about something that does not happen still make us sick?

The symbolic healing processes derive in part from how culture organizes our experience of reality. Explaining how symbols influence physiological responses, the causal relationship between sociocultural factors and physiological responses, provides new theoretical frameworks for explaining healing processes. The recognition that thoughts and interpersonal dynamics affect biological responses is a new perspective reflected in the recognition of the causal effects of subjective mental forces: *top-down causation.* These linkages are the result of the combination of socialization and biological development in a process of **biosocialization,** where socialization processes have permanent effects on biological development.

Biosocialization

The mechanisms of ritual healing are illustrated in perspectives of *biosocialization,* which explain how ritual manipulates the learned associations of symbols with physiological processes. Theories of religious healing need understandings of how biological mechanisms are affected by socialization. Symbols and physiological processes are linked together through **entrainment,** the habitual association of symbols with neural structures and networks (Laughlin et al., 1992). For example, if a white rabbit is repeatedly introduced to you during a fearful experience, such as a loud noise, the image of rabbit becomes associated (entrained) with the physiological structures evoked by loud noises. On subsequent occasions, presentation of the white rabbit can evoke the physiological processes associated with fear without the presence of a loud noise. Entrainment enables the image (symbol) of the rabbit to elicit physiological processes associated with the neural networks mediating fear responses. Through the processes of socialization and emotional manipulation, symbols may be able to elicit the neural structures associated with fear, anxiety, contentment, and other emotions.

Rituals and symbols can affect health because socialization associates them with physiological processes. Mental effects on physiological processes are inherent to human functioning because the meaning of situations elicits physiological responses. Our genes provide **neurognostic structures** and endogenous healing responses. Neurognostic structures are the initial structural and functional organization of neural networks for representing information, which provide the basis for behavior and mind. For example, you have a neural fear response, but the activation of that biological process will be shaped largely by cultural experiences. Learning configures these neurological bases, leading to the development of habitual patterns of interpretation and response to the environment and, consequently, creating neurological pathways. Developmental socialization entrains neurons into symbolically mediated networks. This involves linking the autonomic processes of the reptilian and paleomammalian brains (such as the fear response) with the symbolic structures of the neomammalian brain (cultural concepts about what we should be afraid of). Thus, the neurological or neurognostic potentials for fear responses are canalized in their development, so that they are evoked by what your culture has told you are sources of danger. Similarly, our endogenous healing processes are elicited by symbols that are associated with these natural responses.

These associations are produced through the neurobiological effects of cultural adaptation of individual learning and memory on the development of the brain's neuronal microstructures (Castillo, 1997a). Synaptic structure formation is plastic, or malleable, a response to learning created by repetitive and synchronous activation of nerve fiber systems. The formation of learning and memory associations involves a repetitive use of cultural schemas to interpret interactions with the environment. This results in cultural schemas being imprinted in the brain microstructures during the formation of neural pathways. Learning, adaptation, stress, and cultural interpretations of these experiences have effects on the formation of neural microstructures, dendrites, neurotransmitter receptors, and hormones. Socialization thus embeds cultural patterns of thinking in the formation of nervous system circuitry (Castillo, 1997a).

Socialization links neurons into networks through adaptation to the environment, one that is mediated by culture and language. Symbolic relationships between cognition and behavior "tune" the body—its muscles, organs, and nervous system—into specific response patterns. For example, how do you respond to hearing "The Star-Spangled Banner" or your own national anthem? It likely evokes emotions, attitudes, and physiological reactions.

The symbolic process is fundamental to the neural organization of experience, the development of models of the environment, and organisms' basic affective, behavioral, and cognitive responses. Symbols present in socialization processes that evoke particular physiological responses—for instance, symbols associated with rituals that induce relaxation—create associations that subsequently enable those symbols to evoke the same relaxation responses. These response patterns become habitualized, responding in programmed ways that operate outside of consciousness.

Religious healing processes operate on these association patterns in repressed or latent material functioning outside of consciousness in what are called automatized structures. This enables symbols in rituals to evoke unconscious biological and personal structures that have been linked with cultural symbols through socialization. For instance, if you were raised in a religious setting that provided important input into your personal development, you probably feel a sense of comfort when you enter your church. Just thinking about your religion can have calming effects. Symbols evoke healing processes by operating on these structures, transforming them outside of awareness. Symbolic healing processes may result from reduced ego control that allows for the emergence of unconscious aspects of the self, the transformation of emotions, or the integration of latent or suppressed capacities (Laughlin et al., 1992).

This **symbolic penetration,** the effects of a symbolically elicited neural system on other physical systems, allows cultural meanings to influence a range of biological processes, including autonomic and endocrine systems, brain structures, and emotions. For example, what happens if someone quietly tells you, "Don't move, there is a spider on your neck"? If believable, those symbols will likely "penetrate" your autonomic and hormonal systems, causing the release of neurochemicals associated with fear. Culture elicits biology, and it programs biology to respond to its symbols and evaluations.

Religious systems represent models of cognitive processes occurring in lower brain structures that are not normally accessible to consciousness. Integration of this previously unconscious material into the conscious network may result in profound changes in an individual's experience of self and world, including alteration of behavior, personality, self-understanding, and autonomic balance. Symbolic healing processes use metaphors embodied in myths and religious beliefs to bridge levels of the body and mind, crossing domains of meaning, and entraining neurocognitive structures through their associative linkages. These symbols evoke physiological processes entrained (associated) with basic emotions, attachments, needs of the self, and conditions that provide the comfort and security that address fears, anxieties, and other psychodynamic processes. Symbolic systems also direct ritual behaviors with adaptive consequences.

Ritual as Technical Activity

Ritual has traditionally been conceptualized as the behavioral aspect of religion, a repetitive action that has no basis for producing the intended effects. Like religious beliefs, religious behaviors have generally been considered to have no effects on the real world. In contrast to this traditional characterization of rituals as lacking observable consequences, they do have effects on health at personal, emotional, symbolic, interpersonal, social, and physiological levels. Rituals often incorporate plants that have physiological effects, such as those known as sacred medicines and psychointegrators (see the section "Nocebo Effects and Voodoo Death"). Ritual activities may induce prolonged wakefulness or isolation, profoundly affecting personal experience and producing emotional and psychological changes through activities, techniques, and agents for altering consciousness (see Chapter Ten). Ritual healing experiences often induce powerful altered states of consciousness that reflect the integrative emotional and nonverbal processes of the right hemisphere and produce euphoria. Powerful ecstatic **religious experiences** may involve a direct experience of a sacred or spiritual dimension of the universe that changes the nature of self and identity.

Cross-culturally, the most common recourse to ritual is for healing; these critical rituals typically manipulate cultural symbols and induce responses at psychological, social, and physiological levels. Healing rituals typically require the participation of significant others, sometimes the entire community. The healing systems often consider the cause of illness to come from relations within the group and use ritual interactions such as forgiveness to create significant interpersonal changes in the relations between the patient and others. Ritual practices generally provide relief for the entire local group by reestablishing harmonious social relations. Rituals may also control relationships between an ill person and others, mandating certain care and protection for the ill person or protecting the healthy from contact with the diseased.

Rituals also guide developmental socialization through expressing expectations for social behavior and self in myths. Cultural approaches to ritual emphasize their expressive and symbolic action as statements of the culture's basic values, especially humans' relationships to other humans, nature, and the supernatural. Rituals shape human emotions and drives, integrating them within cultural frameworks. Ritual's symbolic enactments order experience and behavior by publicly displaying models for behavior and identity, exemplified in the enactment of the behaviors of mythic figures of the culture. Ritual symbols also elicit physiological responses through their associations with emotionally charged beliefs, provoking alterations in the autonomic nervous system. Rituals can have effects on entire groups, eliciting a crowd response or group hysteria to the charismatic dynamics of a leader. These group dynamics of ritual can alter individual and collective identity.

The principal effects of ritual healing occur through social relations. Ritual healing practices can transform a person's life through enhancing the personal experience of self in relation to others. Rituals create social obligations that mobilize others to provide support, relief, comfort, and protection. They link people in powerful ways that meet attachment needs, enhancing personal well-being through a support system that provides material assistance and a sense of belonging and comfort. Rituals also heal through integrative social effects, reestablishing social cohesion by resolving conflicts, maintaining group continuity in the face of loss, and modifying behavior to create group harmony.

A significant feature of group integration is provided by transition rituals that address life-cycle transitions and the linkages between cultural and physiological conditions (such as birth, puberty, marriage, pregnancy, and death). This assists with adjustments to an individual's new status and its implications for social relations. Rituals for social transition affect health through the reduction of ambiguity and, consequently, uncertainty and stress. Rituals may reduce high-risk behaviors (poor diet, inactivity, troubled relationships, excessive grief, and so on) that may provoke further health problems.

Ritual healing is a dynamic function of the psyche that provides mechanisms for the maintenance of health (Valle and Prince, 1989). Ritual uses behavior to engage fundamental structures of thought involving prelinguistic symbolism, ancient forms of representation and communication shared with other animals (Winkelman, 2000a). Rituals address emotions through the formation of attitudes, a categorization along a good-or-bad evaluative dimension (Hill, 1997). They manipulate attitudes to control autonomic processes that operate independent of higher cognitive processing, producing emotional responses. Higher cognitive processes have little control over emotional reactions (LeDoux, 1995), but ritual processes and their grounding in lower brain structures (paleomammalian brain and R complex) have direct effects on emotions, based on previous socialization and attachments. Ritual can, consequently, resocialize the associations among emotional, cognitive, and behavioral processes. It can also serve as a mechanism for guiding behavior in practical ways, exemplified in biomedical rituals in the surgical theater.

Religion's Effects on Health

Although biomedicine has traditionally dismissed any presumption of efficacy of ritual and religious healing, epidemiological analyses have established that there is a scientific basis for attributing positive effects of religion on health. Hundreds of studies of the effect of religion on health have shown statistically significant relationships of religious participation with lower morbidity and mortality rates (Levin, 1994; also see Koenig et al., 1999; Koenig, 2004; Koenig, McCullough, and Larson, 2001; Levin, 2001). A particularly well-controlled double-blind study (Byrd, 1988) illustrating positive effects of prayer on recovery provoked dismissive editorials in many medical journals. The effects

APPLICATIONS

Biomedical Ritual

Ritual has been typically viewed as nonrational behavior and a sign of primitive thought processes, but it is found extensively in biomedical practices, where it has important functions. Anthropological analyses show that ritual plays central roles in managing people in social situations and is particularly relevant in dealing with problematic social transitions and resolving anomalies. In her analysis of rituals in surgical departments, Katz (1981, 1999) shows that ritual is integral to surgical procedures and serves a variety of technical functions in maintaining "purity" or sterility in surgical settings. Rituals in surgical rooms contribute to technical efficiency by delineating permitted behaviors and resolving ambiguous states of sterility. These clarifications facilitate autonomous action of the participants, directing their attention and behavior in ways that prevent contamination. Members of the operating team typically avoid objects that are potentially contaminated. In the operating rooms, the color green is used to designate sterile objects and areas. The maintenance of sterility is facilitated by colored sheets of paper that symbolically separate sterile and contaminated areas.

Ritual also helps establish appropriate behaviors in operating rooms by distinguishing them from ordinary circumstances. Ritual contributes to shaping the mental state of the participants and allows them to participate dispassionately in activities that normally evoke strong emotional reactions. Pus-filled abscesses and other bodily conditions that ordinarily evoke disgust and avoidance are treated dispassionately in operating rooms because rituals mentally and psychologically isolate that context, creating a discontinuity from ordinary experience.

Principal areas of the use of ritual within operating rooms include

- Demarcating the stages of surgical procedures
- Addressing the management of unanticipated and ambiguous events
- Indicating contexts in which danger is present because of ambiguous categories

Rituals are used when there is a potential for confusion and when boundaries or limits need to be established. They help establish these for the participants, making differences and boundaries salient and clear. Rituals are particularly important during periods of transition in the classification of objects from sterile to nonsterile. They exaggerate boundaries to clarify changes in the status of objects.

By clarifying the status of objects, ritual increases the autonomy of the participants. Because of ritually established sterile areas, a physician is able to move freely within them without concern about contamination. Scrub nurses in the surgical theater are empowered by rituals that allow them to think ahead and anticipate a surgeon's orders. Rituals establish the respective obligations of all participants and the predictability of their behavior, enabling them to coordinate their activities without direct communication. The anesthesia rituals that render patients unconscious also increase the autonomy of the staff, enabling them to ignore patients and their concerns and even joke about or ridicule the patients. The aspect of autonomy reflects a widely recognized characteristic of ritual: permitting people to engage in patterns of behavior that are otherwise prohibited.

of religion on health are difficult to accommodate to the biomedical paradigm, but the accumulation of data has led to a recognition that there is a phenomenon to be explained.

In its reluctance to accept the findings of these numerous studies showing an association of religion with enhanced health status, biomedicine often points to methodological flaws (Sloan, Bagiella, and Powell, 1999). A particularly important concern is the initial health status and functional capacity of people. Poor health could result in a lessened ability to participate in religious activities; that is, healthier people are able to go to church more often, resulting in a spurious association of health with religion. These kinds of criticisms have been addressed by controlling for the baseline health status of study participants and establishing causal sequencing to show that religious participation precedes the health effects (see Zuckerman, Kasl, and Ostfeld, 1984). Zuckerman and associates illustrated the lack of differences in the initial health status of religious and nonreligious participants. The impact of religiousness on all causes of mortality was assessed by comparing the mortality rates in high-religious and low-religious groups over the next two years. A significant difference in the death rates for the two groups (rate ratio approximately 0.5) indicates that those higher on religiousness had a death rate of about one-half of those who scored low on the religious scale.

Levin (1994) reviewed the increasingly sophisticated studies linking religiosity measures to a large number of health outcomes, making the relationship increasingly difficult to deny. There are lower levels of risks among those religions that are stricter and lower morbidity and mortality among people with higher levels of religiosity. These findings hold true for both health in general and for specific diseases. Levin notes that the validity of this association is substantiated by the literally hundreds of published studies and the positive findings for nearly all ethnic groups and different segments of the population. The volume and diversity of these studies rule out the possibility of a bias resulting from an even larger number of unpublished studies that did not find a significant association. Studies have established the relationship of religion and health, showing that it is valid, and providing reasons why religion may have a causal relationship to health (Levin, 1994).

Many factors need to be controlled for to understand the bases for these relationships of health and religion. These factors include not only the genetic particularities of some religious groups but also a variety of social variables, particularly socioeconomic status, education, age, health status, recognized risk behaviors such as smoking and alcohol consumption, and dietary, sexual, and social activities. Studies that fail to control for these potential causal factors do not undermine the argument that religious participation lowers mortality and morbidity but suggest that the effects of religion are due to its effects on other recognized lifestyle risk factors (e.g., sex, drugs, and violence). Differences in health outcomes between religious and nonreligious groups are plausible in light of current knowledge about the psychosocial dynamics of health, which suggest that the causal effects of religion on health may derive from various aspects of lifestyle. There is still a need, however, to establish exactly which of the many psychological and social mechanisms of religion's effects on humans are responsible for which disease reductions. Such findings might then be interpreted as illustrating that religion is a confounding variable for the health effects of behaviors such as sexual abstinence, marital fidelity, and reduced consumption of nicotine, alcohol, and other drugs.

The issue of considering religion as a confounding variable needs to be critically assessed, especially when those presumed "true causes" (such as lifestyle effects on sex and drug use) are considered the mechanisms through which religion tends to affect behaviors. Confounding is an association between a falsely presumed causal variable (religion, e.g., in the case of those who object to the findings) and an actual causal factor (e.g., something that explains the differences in mortality, such as assistance provided when people are injured). It is inappropriate to introduce a control for the relationship if that variable was part of the direct effects of religion, such as increased social support or lower levels of vices. Finding that the relationship between religion and health disappears with a certain control (such as the extent of tobacco and alcohol use) helps establish mechanisms through which religion exerts its effects on health.

Researchers have established a number of pathways and causal mechanisms for the religion and health associations (Byrd, 1988; Levin and Vanderpool, 1989; Levin, 1994; Koenig et al., 1999). Part of religion's protective effects is in reducing exposure to well-recognized risk factors such as poor diet, alcohol and tobacco use, and high-risk sexual activities, plus emphasizing certain forms of hygiene (Strawbridge, Cohen, Shema, and Kaplan, 1997). Religious attendance can also affect psychosocial pathways that have outcomes on health and mortality (Koenig et al., 1999). Religion has psychodynamic effects through beliefs and their consequences for peacefulness and self-confidence that can help reduce stress, anxiety, and conflict, creating emotionally tranquil states that may facilitate healing effects. Religions also provide a sense of belonging that may affect health. Larger social support systems of frequent attendees provide greater surveillance for health problems and a network that enables people to cope better with problems, reducing stress, depression, and self-destructive behaviors and providing needed resources. Religion's impact on health is multifactorial and involves a variety of social mechanisms recognized as increasing well-being.

Social mechanisms do not explain all of religion's effects on mortality because religion's effects on well-being do not appear to be mediated by these factors alone. The relationship between health practices and preventive behaviors constitutes only part of the causal pathway through which religion affects health. Strawbridge and colleagues' study (1997) used longitudinal data from an Alameda County, California, study that included a range of sociodemographic measures, mobility impairment, perceived health and depression, health practices and conditions, improvements in health practices, social contacts, connectedness, and the stability of marriage across periods from 1965 to 1994. This assessment of baseline health conditions and changes across time permitted control for the timing of influences and outcomes to strengthen causal arguments. These analyses first included a range of socioeconomic variables and next added initial health conditions, then social connections, and finally health practices. These controls enabled them to establish that those who were more religious had lower mortality rates independent of initial health. Furthermore, the measures of social connection had little effect on the significant differences in mortality of the religious and nonreligious groups. They also found that those who frequently attended religious services were significantly different from nonattendees on a variety of social measures, including higher rates of group membership and social contacts and the greater persistence of their marriages. Differences in mortality of the religious and nonreligious groups persisted despite controls for those differences. Assessment of the potential confounding role of health practices and social connections reveals that they act both as intervening variables and as causes of the relation between religion and mortality. The model of intervening variables received stronger support: those who frequently attended church were less likely to use drugs, more likely to reduce their smoking and drinking, tended to increase their social connections across time, and were more likely to remain married.

Similar findings are provided by a study (Koenig et al., 1999) assessing the effects of religious attendance in enhancing survival through a six-year follow-up study based in the Established Populations for Epidemiological Studies of the Elderly in North Carolina. Frequent attendees have lower mortality, larger social support networks and confidants, and less alcohol and tobacco consumption. Adjustment for demographic conditions, mental and physical health, social connections, and health behaviors reduced the risk differences between religious and nonreligious people, but they remained significant. Koenig and associates (1999) suggested that the differences in mortality, independent of the well-recognized confounding variables (social support, health practices, health conditions, and socioeconomic status), indicate the need for further studies on the specific biological, behavioral, or psychosocial mechanisms by which these differences are produced.

Levin (1994) points to the many valid studies that have controlled for the principal lifestyle factors, providing evidence for a causal effect by something more nebulous about religion's positive health effects. The multitude of conditions positively associated with religion suggests that there is some general effect of religion on health, rather than just specific changes in lifestyle and risk behaviors. Levin reports that regardless of how religion is conceptualized, it appears to have a salutary effect on health outcomes independent of the type of religion or type of disease. The health effects of religion likely involve both general and specific mechanisms and effects because religion has effects on a variety of morbidity and mortality measures. The evidence for a general effect of religion can be inferred from the general physical aspects related to managing stress responses (see below). Religion also provides various specific effects on behaviors that have additional specific effects on health, such as sexual restrictions that reduce the spread of STDs.

Further research needs to address different aspects and concepts of religiosity; the possibility of distinct health influences of religion versus spirituality; and the impacts of specific factors such as spiritual experiences, prayer, and faith in health outcomes. A major area to be addressed is how religious behavior, conceptualized as rituals, affects health. In contrast to the idea of ritual as meaningless action, there is substantial evidence that rituals have a variety of technical effects related to health. Furthermore, they are social activities that have many effects on members, including relationships that may be salutary for health (see Chapter Eight on social networks and social support in health). The basic question, however, may be how it is that beliefs—symbols regarding things that science considers not to exist—can have such powerful effects on our bodies. This is not a process unique to religious healing but is part of all healing encounters, including those of biomedicine. This interaction of the mind with the brain and body provides principal mechanisms that underlie the efficacy of ethnomedical healing traditions. These involve the roles of meaning in adaptation. Why is meaning so important?

Meaning as a Mechanism of Religious Healing

Religion clearly has had a role in promoting well-being worldwide and providing resources for dealing with stress, uncertainty, anxiety, and depression. The association of religion with healing has functional bases in meaning and belief and their numerous effects on individual psychology, social relations, and emotional responses. The many mechanisms by which religion affects health range from the fundamental values and rules it provides to its psychosocial effects of the group and psychophysiological effects of rituals on participants. Religion organizes economic, familial, and political activities and provides rules for social behavior and explanations about the natural and supernatural world. Religious beliefs provide ultimate values and justifications, motivating numerous aspects of behavior. These pervasive influences make religion a principal institution of culture and healing.

An empirical study of religious healing indicates that primary mechanisms involve psychological reactions that broaden coping abilities and enhance self-esteem (Valle and Prince, 1989). Religious coping is associated with more favorable outcomes in the face of negative events, suggesting that a framework based on benevolent principles is particularly important when demands exceed personal coping capacities (Spilka and McIntosh, 1997). Religion, myth, and spiritual beliefs are useful in managing stress and its psychophysiological dynamics; they provide a sense of control by specifying one's situation in relationships to known possibilities and focus attention on behaviors for coping and the alleviation of distress. Malinowski (1954) attributed the origins of religion to mechanisms for managing emotional life and its stress, anxieties, and frustrations. Illness raises concerns about why maladies have struck and what can be done to restore well-being. Religion provides explanations, a worldview that makes maladies meaningful in the context of cultural life and may heal (whole) the individual by relieving emotional conflicts and distress.

Meaning affects coping and, consequently, health through

- Providing a worldview that explains personal circumstances

- Harmonizing social relations and attachments

- (Re)conditioning and desensitizing to stressful events and their representations

- Providing dramatic enactments that express repressed emotions

- Promoting a positive attitude that induces immune system responses

- Eliciting expectancy or placebo responses and their physiological effects

The significance of meaning in healing has to do with meaning's fundamental roles in eliciting and managing human stress mechanisms. Symbolic meanings—right or wrong—can activate the stress mechanisms and their potentially devastating physiological consequences. Religious healing provides a unified psychosociophysiological response in which personal significance (meaningfulness) and social support manage stress by providing assurance that instills confidence and counteracts anxiety. To understand how religion, ritual, symbols, social processes, and communal activities have direct physiological effects on the body and health, we must understand the inputs into and effects on the autonomic nervous system (ANS). Religion and other symbols can alleviate stress and the dangerously high levels of pituitary-adrenal activity that occur during the resistance stage of the stress reaction. Through creating positive hope and expectations, countering anxiety, and changing emotional responses, religious beliefs can alter the balance in the ANS. Reducing stress and its physiological concomitants enhances the immune system and the body's capacity for recovery.

Religion and other symbols provide meaningful input in eliciting physiological systems of the body in a variety of ways. Above we discussed how the healing power of symbols is acquired through the processes of biosocialization (Laughlin et al., 1992), where culture shapes the development of the nervous system and embeds its influences in our neuron systems. Additional mechanisms of religious and symbolic healing are described in the symbolic elicitation of stress physiology and the general adaptation syndrome, the symbolic processes involved in placebo effects, the response of our immune systems to personal and social events, and the powers of metaphors in evoking symbolic healing.

STRESS RESPONSE

Do stress and illness seem to come in tandem for you? Have you ever caught a cold or flu after or during a stressful week, when you needed your health the most? Stress and anxiety both contribute to illness and provide mechanisms through which religion and ritual can enhance health. These mental effects on physical well-being are found in the spontaneous remission of disease: the rapid and inexplicable disappearance of documented medical conditions coincident with participation in religious healing activities. Similar effects are seen in hexes, some of which are followed by an individual's demise, even when under medical supervision (Cannon, 1942). Effects of mind, symbols, and meanings on physiological processes are not just extraordinary phenomena. Mental effects on biology are also involved in ordinary stress responses of the body.

Stress is a consequence of personal responses rather than objective circumstances. For example, are you stressed out about whether the local professional sports team will win this weekend? Maybe not, but some people are. What about needing an A on the next exam? Does that cause stress for you? Some people in your class do not care about the grade as long as they pass, so they do not experience as much stress.

Stress is produced by how a person perceives his or her ability to manage the situation and the person's cognitive and psychophysiological responses to that assessment. A dangerous situation, such as transporting a live rattlesnake in a jar on a city bus, might not be stressful if you feel you can manage it, but imagine how other passengers might feel! Even a safe situation, such as transporting a nonvenomous snake, might evoke extreme stress in someone with snake phobia. Stress involves cognitive, emotional, and physiological responses to perceived threats to one's well-being. Anything can be stressful, positive as well as negative events, when they have implications for well-being or self-concept or challenge central assumptions people make about the world. Stress results from one's perceived inability to effectively adapt to circumstances and the reaction of anxiety and fear experienced in response. A promotion and a raise might seem like great news, but they, too, can provoke stress reactions.

Much stress is socially induced by interpersonal interactions or cultural expectations and an individual's interpretation of situations. Consequently, the same situation does not affect all people uniformly because everyone differs in expectations, resources, and perceptions. Stress derives from the interaction of the assessed meaning of a situation and an individual's coping behaviors. Whereas the body can adapt to chronic physical stressors, it does not adapt to chronic emotional stress. Emotional stress is managed through defensive reactions and coping responses that mediate the effects of meaning— one's assessments—on physiological responses.

Anatomical Basis of Stress

Not all stress has negative effects on the body. The ANS relies on positive stress to function properly. An organism's response to stress is maintained by the complementary functions and balance between the two divisions[1] of the ANS: the sympathetic (or ergotropic) nervous system and the parasympathetic (or trophotropic) nervous system. Various factors affect the ANS balance between stimulation (activation of the sympathetic division) and relaxation (activation of the parasympathetic division). The sympathetic system provides adaptive responses to the external environment whereas the parasympathetic system maintains internal balance. Sympathetic activation provides the energy for muscles and mediates alertness, arousal, strength, and vitality. Parasympathetic activity is involved in storing sugar, fat, and protein, and it mediates rest, recuperation, and sleep. The tuning or balance between sympathetic and parasympathetic systems is affected by conditioning (learning), so that a balance between the two is embedded in our daily activities. The time of the day when our bodies begin their activation (sympathetic) and deactivation (parasympathetic) reflects our cultural influences and personal adaptation. For instance, do you easily wake up at 4:30 AM or fall asleep at 7:30 PM? Not likely, but some people do; you have habituated your body to a different waking and sleeping schedule.

The sympathetic system underlies the fight-or-flight response, providing a global activation of the body for response. Sympathetic system activation is associated with increased brain activation and brain-wave frequencies, skeletal musculature tension, and an external orientation to physical reality. Sympathetic activation is associated with both positive and negative emotions, largely dependent on the interpretation made of the situation. The parasympathetic system regulates the vegetative nervous system, ranging from cellular activity through digestive functions and sleep. It is responsible for synchronization of the cortical electrical patterns, relaxation, control of somatic functions, and the repair and development of the organism, especially during undisturbed sleep. Parasympathetic activation causes a slowing and synchronization of brain-wave frequencies, relaxation of the skeletal musculature, and an internal orientation to mental reality.

The complementary activation and balance provided by the sympathetic and parasympathetic systems provide for a hierarchic integration of the activities of the somatic, autonomic, and neural systems. The cyclical daily shift from wakefulness to sleep and back mirrors the cycles of sympathetic and parasympathetic dominance.

The sympathetic and parasympathetic divisions of the ANS are capable of activation by both top-down and bottom-up mechanisms. *Top-down* means that higher-level mental processes can activate lower-level bodily processes. Our thoughts can elicit responses of the body, such as when dwelling on an injustice can get you hopping mad and physiologically aroused. Similarly, praying and thinking good thoughts and expectations can calm an agitated person. Conversely, our ANS and mental responses can be driven from the bottom up, where stimulants that directly affect the body and lower levels of the nervous system have upward effects on the mind (such as when too many cups of espresso make a person talk so much everyone wishes they would shut up).

Sympathetic-parasympathetic balance is a central mechanism of stress responses and cultural healing. The organism attempts to maintain a balance in relation to physical and social environments while meeting internal needs. Disruptions require adjustments; failure can result in system breakdowns when resources are inadequate to reestablish balance.

General Adaptation Syndrome

The general reaction to all stressors was discovered by Selye (1956, 1976) in the 1930s. He labeled this generalized stress response the general adaptation syndrome. This syndrome was revealed in the three stages of physiological response to stress by laboratory animals:

■ Stress or alarm reaction of the body

■ Resistance with a new adaptation at an increased level of pituitary-adrenal activity

■ Eventually exhaustion leading to disease or death

For example, the stress reaction of the body includes an immediate increase in the heart rate that may sustain permanently higher levels of blood pressure and further stress a weak blood vessel in the brain, causing it to burst (a cerebral aneurysm or stroke) and resulting in disability or death. The physiological responses to stress begin with an increase in sympathetic ANS activity. A generally undifferentiated arousal of the sympathetic nervous system is basic to the elicitation of emotions and the physiological responses that prepare the organism for action. Prolonged activation exhausts the resources of the body, making it more susceptible to disease. This excessive activity within the sympathetic system contributes to pathological conditions by provoking increased cardiovascular function and disrupting the ANS balance. Prolonged hyperactivity of the sympathetic nervous system can cause damage to organs and lead to cardiac failure and death.

The general adaptation syndrome causes the pituitary-adrenal cortex to secrete hormones that stimulate the release of other hormones by the endocrine glands. This release of epinephrine and norepinephrine mobilizes fatty acids for use as energy, accelerates cardiac activity, and raises the blood pressure. Stress hormones elevate corticosteroid levels, provoking limbic system activity that triggers the release of adrenocorticotropic hormone (ACTH). Stress also affects pathogenesis by eliciting activity in the sympathoadrenomedullary and pituitary adrenocortical areas that secrete corticosteroids in response to stimulation by ACTH. Cortisol modulates stress responses, but its overproduction can damage organs. Epinephrine, norepinephrine, and cortisol have negative effects on the immune system, increasing susceptibility to infection. Glucocorticoids hinder lymphocytic action, causing immunosuppression. The disruption of cortisol regulation also contributes to depression and anxiety.

Sustained stress results in increased brain activity, particularly of the central nervous system noradrenergic neurons. Long-term stress results in exhaustion and a decline in noradrenergic activity if the stressor's demands are too severe. Synthesis can increase the available norepinephrine, but this can be maintained for only a limited time until the vesicles are depleted. Prolonged activation exhausts pituitary and adrenal defenses and other aspects of the endocrine system, leading to collapse. The response to stress is nonspecific, affecting the weakest aspect of the organism.

The elicitation of the stress responses by social situations and symbolic meanings leaves the body activated and mobilized. If a person is unable to respond—to deactivate the stress—ulcers, hypertension, cardiovascular problems, and migraine headaches can develop. These and other problems are a consequence of the self's inability to respond suitably to social, psychological, and emotional aspects of life. Fear of situations can produce the same physiological responses as actual situations, with symbolically threatening situations producing the same general adaptation syndrome that evolved to deal with threats to physical survival. For example, when walking alone late at night, you may interpret shadows from a bush as an assailant; this will provoke the same physiological reactions as the appearance of an actual assailant. Interpretations, interpersonal interactions, and social conditions that affect an individual's perception of well-being are addressed with the same systems used to deal with enemies (the fight-or-flight syndrome). The symbolic threats do not permit a physical struggle, however; consequently, we do not use up the neurochemicals generated for rapid action. The body is mobilized, stimulating the cardiac system to the point of exhaustion or releasing energy for defenses. Because these are not used and thus dissipated, they are deposited in arteries, causing arteriosclerosis. The management of these emotional effects is central to cultural healing through symbolic processes. Failure to manage such stressors can be fatal, as shown in Dressler's investigations covered in the special feature "Biocultural Interactions: Culture and Social Relations in Stress."

BIOCULTURAL INTERACTIONS

Cultural Ecology and Stress in African American CVD

African Americans face many stressors that contribute to hypertension and CVD. Living in disadvantaged neighborhoods has a direct impact on increasing the risk of CVD independent of standard socioeconomic control variables (occupation, economic resources, and education) (Douglas, 2002). Living in decaying inner-city neighborhoods exposes residents to chronic stress from fear of violence and the depressing effects of rampant poverty and urban decay. This kind of chronic stress can be fatal: "The stress of poverty or racism may evoke a hormonal 'fight or flight' response that boosts heart rate and blood pressure" (Fackelmann, 1991, p. 254). Not only inner-city environments but also successful suburban environments can provoke a deadly stress, the result of a lack of "cultural consonance."

BIOCULTURAL INTERACTIONS

Culture and Social Relations in Stress

Dressler has carried out a range of empirical studies that examine the relationships among culture, stress, and disease to show the health effects of cultural factors such as beliefs and attitudes. "[R]isks and resistance resources are embedded in contexts of different social relationships . . . [and] how specific historical circumstances have generated specific configurations of stress, adaptation and disease" (Dressler, 1996, p. 253). Contextual factors and interpersonal dynamics alter the relationship between stress and disease through cultural effects on adaptive factors. The biopsychosocial model has considered the psychosocial mediation of stress apart from cultural meanings, community context, and broader sociohistorical trends. Dressler's research reveals that personal and cultural significance are crucial to the mediation effects.

Stress involves both risk factors, which are stressors, and social resources and relations, which facilitate resistance to those factors. Stress involves the individual's adaptation to the physical and social environment to produce a homeostatic balance. Inadequate resources for adaptation can disrupt physiological and emotional balance. Resistance resources are central to responses to stress. These resources include personal coping skills, social support, and a sense of social solidarity and perceptions of mutual group support (Dressler, 1996, p. 260).

Dressler cautions against a view of stress that emphasizes the individual's perception of stressful events. This mentalistic emphasis on perceptions contributes to neglect of the effects of the social environment. Individual perceptions and beliefs modify the impact of stress, but social conditions produce stress independent of perceptions. Stress interactions need to be conceptualized within ecological, person-environment, and systems perspectives that address adaptation as the effects of culture on stress and resistance processes. The need to assess subjective perceptions and the cultural significance of stress is illustrated in the variation across social and cultural groups in the effects of life events on depression, reflecting the importance of social context for well-being.

Contextual impacts on stress are illustrated in Dressler's cross-cultural studies of lifestyle incongruity, "defined as the degree to which lifestyle exceeds occupational class" (Dressler, 1996, p. 259). In examining socioeconomic status (SES) and disease risk among African Americans, Dressler and associates found a relationship to what he called "cultural consonance in lifestyle" (Dressler, Bindon, and Neggers, 1998). Disease risks are related to the degree to which individuals' behavior adheres to cultural models, as determined by cultural consensus analysis. Cultural consonance in lifestyle has a stronger association with hypertension than do the conventional SES measures. They

PLACEBOS AND PLACEBO EFFECTS

The health implications of mental expectations that produce stress reactions have an opposite effect that is illustrated by placebo phenomena. With placebos, our expectations generally produce favorable responses for our organism, such as a relaxation response that counters stress. Although typically understood as having positive effects, placebos suggest that the inability to live in accordance with cultural lifestyle norms contributes to an increased risk for coronary heart disease. A study in Brazil (Dressler, Balieiro, and Dos Santos, 1998) found that culturally defined lifestyle congruence was negatively correlated with cardiac measures, depression, and stress, independent of SES. The explained variance associated with SES variables could be accounted for by cultural consonance measures, indicating that cultural consonance in lifestyle mediates the SES effects on health. The relationship of lifestyle incongruity to disease is a universal, a cross-cultural invariant that is independent of the perceptions that individuals have of economic status, stressful events, and economic stressors (Dressler, 1996).

Dressler's cross-cultural research (1994) illustrates that social support comes from the cultural system and varies across societies. Effects of stressors may be similar cross-culturally, but concepts of social support systems and support relationships are variable. The kind of social support that affects blood pressure can vary within the same culture, as Dressler, Mata, Chavez, Viteri, and Gallagher (1986) found in Mexico. Whereas men had lower arterial pressure with higher support on all social sources, for women it varied as a function of age, with younger and older women showing opposite effects from support from relatives and friends. They interpret these findings in reference to a woman's place within a community's social structure, indicating the need for culturally appropriate conceptualizations of social support. Dressler's assessments of stressful events, circumstances, and resources show that the effects of social class on health interact with these circumstances in producing health outcomes. Cross-national studies show the association of CVD with social class reverses during the process of social change. The relationship begins as a direct one in which CVD increases with social class, but the relationship ultimately reverses, with higher CVD in lower SES groups. Symbolic meanings and social patterns implicate culture in the definition of the nature of stress and support. Cultural resources for responding to stress and the patterns of coping they inculcate constitute part of the social dynamic producing disease and health.

The cultural dynamics of stress and stress management are illustrated in personal coping resources based in beliefs, attitudes, and strategies for addressing stressful circumstances through cognitive appraisal and restructuring. The ability to redefine stressful events is an important aspect of managing negative emotional reactions through an active problem-focused style. Dressler's cross-cultural research shows that an active coping style (versus a passive style) enhances health status. This helps explain why religion can have powerful impacts on health status, providing an active means of addressing problems.

have been considered to have negative effects as well, known as the nocebo or negative placebo. "The nocebo effect is the causation of sickness (or death) by expectations of sickness (or death) and by associated emotional states" (Hahn, 1997, p. 607); if the placebo is understood as "I will please," the nocebo can be seen as meaning "I will kill." Both placebos and nocebos reflect the ability of our mental life and symbols, beliefs, and expectations to have powerful effects on physiology. The potential magnitude of placebo effects is recognized in the biomedical practice of evaluating the effectiveness of new drugs and treatments using double-blind clinical trials where neither patients nor doctors know who gets the real treatment and who receives an inactive control.

Placebos Versus Nocebos

Placebos are typically defined as inert substances without pharmacological effects based in their biochemistry; their administration, nonetheless, causes improvements in a patient's experience of well-being and measurable physiological responses in the body. Placebo effects present anomalies for the biomedical paradigm by apparently producing physiological changes without a biochemical basis. They illustrate that subjective expectations have effects on physiological responses, an example of "mind over matter."

Hahn (1995) suggests that most physicians misunderstand placebos, discounting them as not having real effects. Shapiro and Shapiro (1997) reject the concept of placebos as *inert* substances, insisting that their effects are real and constitute a major pathway through which all healing traditions provide relief for patients. They define placebos as treatments used for ameliorative effects but that are ineffective for the condition treated. This misses the point that placebo effects may be real and cure conditions. Moerman defines "placebo effects as the desirable psychological and physiological effects of meaning in the treatment of illness" (2000, p. 52). The key construct in defining placebos is that the substance itself does not have a biochemical mechanism for producing a physiological effect. Rather, it is the patient's or physician's belief that is thought to be the factor eliciting the physiological response. Placebo effects are distinguished from placebo responses. Although placebo responses are the behavioral changes occurring as a consequence of taking a placebo, the placebo effect is the symbolic response, a "nonspecific psychological or psychophysiological therapeutic effect produced by a placebo" (Shapiro and Shapiro, 1997, p. 41). Placebo responses may have positive effects, no effects, side effects, or even negative effects (nocebo effects).

Nocebo Effects and Voodoo Death In a classic "hexing," the witch doctor declares that a person has done wrong and will die. This pronouncement may be accompanied by oral spells, rituals such as pointing bones or thorns at the person, and perhaps a ceremony in which a crude doll representing the intended victim is buried or burned. The community then watches as the person withers and dies in the ensuing days. As Cannon pointed out in his classic article "Voodoo Death" (1942), sometimes these unfortunate victims die under medical care but from no causes known to biomedicine.

This nocebo effect involves consequences of negative expectations. Nocebo effects have generic manifestations in negative expectations, pessimism, a range of disquieting symptoms, or even death. Hahn (1997) characterizes the nocebo effect as a side effect of human culture where negative emotional expectations produce consequences that are responsible for substantial pathologies worldwide. These have considerable significance for both clinical medicine and public health (Hahn, 1997). These health implications include evidence that belief in personal susceptibility to cardiac arrest is a risk factor for coronary death, even in patients without recognized cardiac symptoms. The occurrence of epidemic hysteria in schools and workplaces also illustrates these health implications. Public health officials have been called to the sites of "epidemics" in schools and workplaces, only to conclude that the rash of symptoms arose from the effects of suggestion and emotional contagion. Mental states are capable of causing pathological outcomes even in the absence of other risk factors for those conditions.

Nocebos are causal in the sense that they increase the likelihood of sickness or disease through negative expectations. These negative expectations may come from many sources (Hahn, 1997):

- One's personal-mental configurations

- The diagnostic categories of folk or medical classificatory systems

- Sociogenic mass hysteria

- Other influences based on the communication of expectations

Nocebo effects may be activated through a variety of mechanisms (Spiegel, 1997; Hahn, 1997). The illness classification systems of a culture provide expectations about what can occur, producing negative social messages that affect a patient's psychological state. Ethnomedical systems may have unintended nocebo effects, producing the outcomes that they institutionalize in their belief systems. For example, belief in the koro (penis-shrinking syndrome) can create an anxiety that can produce the phenomenon. The role of cultural conceptions in inducing experiences is well recognized in medical students, who often feel that they have symptoms of the diseases they are studying.

Physicians can produce nocebo effects in clinical interactions with patients: diagnoses assigned to patients produced poor outcomes when there was no objective evidence for the malady (Kasdan et al., 1999). Negative expectations may also exacerbate the consequences of disease, such as when a diagnosis of cancer leads to a more rapid demise of a patient than typically occurs when information about the diagnosis is withheld. This may be a manifestation of a general effect of pessimistic attitudes as a risk factor for disease outcomes. Negative perceptions undermine morale and contribute to an attitude of learned helplessness that views future events as uncontrollable. This perception has effects in undermining the immune system (Kasdan et al., 1999).

Epidemic hysterias may occur as a consequence of people observing or learning from others about symptoms and sickness. Although the symptoms may be associated with known sources or stimuli, they do not fit biomedical models of disease. Those who are likely to be susceptible to epidemic nocebo effects are people who are socially isolated, overworked, subjected to high levels of stress, incapable of complaining to supervisors, engaged in repetitive jobs, and female divorced sole breadwinners. Personal conditions and the social environment contribute to mass somatization. Broader social conditions are also implicated: lower social class, uncertainty, and stress (Hahn, 1997).

These culturally based illness systems provide scripts for the performance of roles that are acted out unconsciously. This is particularly likely if there are other victims with whom the individual identifies. These cultural scripts include the role of powerful individuals who can define the condition of a person, creating self-fulfilling expectations.

Social conditions also create particular stresses and burdens on individuals in specific social positions, increasing their susceptibility. These social effects may be fatal, as exemplified in voodoo death.

Voodoo Death as Nocebo Effect Throughout the world, we find the belief that magical actions can result in the death of victims. Medicine men, sorcerers, witches, and others with supernatural power are believed to be able to cause death through rituals or magical incantations. Cannon (1942) pointed to the reports of such deaths by "competent observers," including physicians. Cannon's explanations of the mechanisms of voodoo death involve the effects of extreme emotions of fear and terror on the ANS, particularly the sympathetic division. A person's emotional reactions elicit physiological responses and disrupt the balance within the ANS through hyperactivation of the sympathetic nervous system. The belief by the victim in the efficacy of voodoo produces extreme emotional excitation and the mobilization of the fight-or-flight response. These fear and rage responses result in excessive activity in the sympathicoadrenal system. High levels of persistent excessive sympathetic activity lead to exhaustion of the body's resources (see the section "General Adaptation Syndrome") and a fall in blood pressure similar to that associated with shock. Stimulation of the sympathetic nervous system constricts blood vessels supplying the vital organs, reducing circulation. These physical insults on the body are compounded by social withdrawal and restriction of food and water to the victims of hexes. These physical deprivations further exacerbate the shock to the ANS, and unless action is taken to reverse these physiological responses, the victim dies.

Because those who are hexed normally have committed social transgressions, social withdrawal from the victim reinforces the progress toward death. Those in the immediate social environment often accept and support the hexing. Relatives may reinforce despair and withdrawal and withhold food, water, and care. The family may begin mourning rituals, reinforcing a giving up. Lester (1972) suggested that voodoo death was part of a "giving up-given up" complex in which both the individual and the social group accept the individual's inevitable demise. This acceptance is part of a psychosocial process through which physiological responses are elicited. This giving-up response, modeled on animal behavior, socially reinforces the physiological responses of the individual. Laboratory studies suggest that shock can lead to a sense of hopelessness in which rats succumb rapidly to stressors and allow themselves to drown rather than continue to struggle. This giving-up syndrome is also implicated in human responses to others' death and their own precipitous mortality while grieving the loss of a spouse. Humans experience this giving-up complex as hopelessness, worthlessness, helplessness, and a lack of meaningful interpersonal relationships and personal gratification. The individual is left with a reduced desire to resist disease and an enhanced susceptibility to opportunistic pathological processes. This giving-up model of voodoo death suggests a mechanism distinct from Cannon's view that the effects result from overstimulation of the sympathetic nervous system. Instead, the giving-up model suggests that hopelessness leads to excessive parasympathetic responses and a shutdown of the ANS.

Garrity (1974) reviewed the literature on sudden death and concluded that more than one mechanism was involved in voodoo death. In addition to Cannon's model involving excited behavior and Lester's model involving giving up and withdrawal, he proposed a third mechanism involving acceptance. These individuals accept an impeding death with peace and calmness rather than with fear or hopelessness and apathy. These types of responses are attested to in studies that show increased mortality rates immediately following important days (birthdays or holidays), suggesting some degree of personal control over the timing of one's death.

Both the sympathetic and parasympathetic models of voodoo death may lead to rapid demise through effects on the cardiac system. Clinical evidence reviewed by Garrity suggests that cardiac arrest can be precipitated by either response, particularly for individuals with preexisting coronary artery disease. Garrity suggests that the underlying mechanisms involving death with acceptance may reflect a biofeedback in which a will to die can result in the modification and termination of vital functions.

The various approaches to voodoo death illustrate the interaction of beliefs and expectations with physiological mechanisms. Social responses are crucial, including the withdrawal of support and the acceptance of the victim's demise. Symbolic processes and meaning are central to the three mechanisms for voodoo death that Garrity posits: the elicitation of physiological responses; the effects of depression, apathy, and withdrawal; and the giving-up response. Cultural mechanisms can also reverse the psychophysiological response, as attested to in ethnographic accounts of the ability of healers to remove the hex and prevent death.

The reprinting of Cannon's article in the October 2002 issue of the *American Journal of Public Health* was accompanied by a commentary on his astute perception of these mechanisms before they had been directly confirmed by laboratory studies. Current knowledge of neurotransmitters and neuropeptides indicates that they are elicited by fear responses that shape the wiring of nerve cells for even more powerful future responses. Hormonal stress responses activated by the brain's fear centers in the hypothalamus and amygdala trigger further chemical reactions in the brain with detrimental consequences, including cardiac arrhythmias and cardiovascular collapse. The link in these responses is emotions, triggered by cultural beliefs.

History of the Placebo Effect

Placebos have a long history in Western medicine, generally employed as a pejorative denying the validity of other physicians' treatments and imputing fraud or quackery. Early concepts emphasized that placebos did not have any effect but were "medications given to please." Placebo effects came to be a central concern of biomedicine in the mid-twentieth century as methodological controls. This was stimulated by a recognition that new drugs typically started with high levels of success but declined in effectiveness over time. Many physicians thought that some frequently used medications were ineffective and that controlled evaluations were needed. Comparisons with inert substances were used to assess true drug effects, but these inert substances produced a treatment effect, undermining evaluations of drug effectiveness. The concept of the double-blind clinical trial addressed one aspect of the placebo effect, the enthusiasm and positive expectation conveyed by experimenters who believed in the effectiveness of their treatment procedures and conveyed this to patients. Clinical controls for placebo effects indicate that an average of one-third of patients receive relief from placebos, with placebo response rates varying from 1 to 100 percent. A comparable proportion of people responding to active medications may also be placebo responders. Despite the use of double-blind clinical trials to minimize expectation effects, the ability of patients, physicians, and researchers to correctly guess a patient's assignment to drug or nondrug (placebo) conditions undermines control procedures. Active substances have distinctive effects and taste, making identical matching placebos with indistinguishable physical or psychophysiological properties problematic, if not impossible. Consequently, the ideal principles of double-blind procedures have not been generally achieved.

What Placebos Affect

Placebos parallel many effects of pharmacologically active substances, including peak effects several hours after administration, a cumulative effect over time, a residual effect following the termination of administration, and side effects including "nausea, diarrhea, vomiting, palpitation, faintness, headache, increase in blood pressure and heart rate, and impairment of motor performance" (Benedetti and Amanzio, 1997, p. 114). The effects of placebos have been predominantly conceptualized as their ability to reduce pain but also reduce symptoms of a variety of conditions. These include so-called psychosomatic conditions (asthma, hay fever, coughing, ulcers), mental health problems (anxiety, depression, and schizophrenia), and physical conditions such as cardiovascular problems (hypertension and angina pectoris), multiple sclerosis, Parkinson's disease, and rheumatoid and degenerative arthritis (Benedetti and Amanzio, 1997; Helman, 1994). Placebos do not appear to be effective, however, for high blood pressure or psychiatric conditions such as OCD. Because placebos are a part of all treatments, not just medications, the concept has come to be applied to "any method of therapy" (Shapiro and Shapiro, 1997). Placebo effects are necessarily part of all treatment and medical encounters because the provision of care expresses support and concern that can minimize stress and anxiety.

Psychotherapy's intrinsic effectiveness, as opposed to placebo effects, is difficult to assess. This is because a control condition for placebo that does not constitute some form of treatment is difficult to conceptualize. The "no treatment" comparison itself requires some interactions that appear as treatments to carry out the comparative assessment. Consequently, even untreated controls improve across time in part due to the placebo response.

Placebos and Total Drug Effects

The concept of total drug effects, reflected in a cultural variation in the response to drugs, illustrates effects of cultural, social, and mental phenomena on physiological responses to drugs. Physiological effects of active substances are mediated, and even transformed, by individual, social, and cultural characteristics. This is well recognized in cross-national differences in alcohol consumption and alcoholism. Although the French have about twice the per capita consumption of alcohol as Americans, Americans' prevalence of alcoholism and alcohol-related problems is far greater. Obviously the effects of alcohol have to do with more than just the amounts consumed.

The effects of drugs and medications on human physiology, emotion, and behavior are not strictly due to their pharmacological properties. The total drug effect includes nonpharmacological factors that are responsible for variations in individual responses, including the placebo effect and other social, interpersonal, and personal factors. Helman (1994) makes the distinction between macrocontextual and microcontextual effects. Macrocontextual drug effects involve influences from the sociocultural system; these include social, political, economic, and moral factors and influences from family, other users, advertising, and sales processes. These are illustrated in the greater effectiveness of brand-name analgesics over unlabeled sources of the same drug (Moerman, 2000). The contribution of these factors to drug effects produces variation in patients' responses and reactions. Individual expectations are central to microcontextual effects. These effects from drugs' actions are reflected in set and setting influences, the expectations of the recipient and the context of his or her medication that contribute to the psychodynamic effects of the drug. These nonpharmacological factors include arbitrary drug attributes such as color and shape, the physical setting in which the drug is administered, and the prescriber's characteristics such as status and personality.

Another part of the total drug effect is the "treatment effect," the placebo-induced responses to entering into a treatment setting. Treatment effects are universal aspects of health care derived from patients' expectations that treatment processes involving a culturally sanctioned healer will improve their condition. These effects derive from previous experiences with the medical system, its worldview, the healer's role within it, and the emotional attachments the patient ascribes to the malady, treatment, and healing. Treatment effects are poorly understood because studies seldom address the "pragmatic empirical activities, technologies, rites, symbolic therapies, roles, and institutions . . . [and their] organization, interrelationship, and manipulation . . . within a total system" (Kleinman, 1973b, p. 61). The patient's reference group and expectations of friends and family contribute to effects from treatment procedures through beliefs in the efficacy of treatments.

Contextual effects are particularly noted for recreational drugs, where the setting contributes to the total drug effect. The effects of culture and social setting are also well noted in the effects of alcohol consumption and in the cultural and social dynamics associated with addiction and withdrawal. Contextual effects on psychedelic drugs are so extensive that some of their principal effects are a consequence of these extrapharmacological factors.

Total Drug Effects in the Social Dynamics of Psychedelics

Plants called hallucinogens and psychedelics have had important roles as sacred medicines in ancient and contemporary societies, evoking powerful spiritual, religious, social, and cognitive reactions. Cross-cultural perspectives on their use and effects illustrate the influence of social expectations on the interpretation of their effects. These social influences can be the major determinants of the drugs' effects.

From the earliest recorded civilizations and throughout pre-state societies of recent history, these plants were viewed as sources of the sacred, a contact with the spiritual world that provided healing. Their worldwide magicoreligious and therapeutic applications and spiritual interpretations (Furst, 1976; Schultes and Hofmann, 1979; Dobkin de Rios, 1984; Winkelman, 1996a) led to their postulation as progenitors of religion, as claimed by many groups (La Barre, 1972). Many religions view their practices as inspired by what some have called **entheogens**—"god-containing plants"—reflected in indigenous terms meaning "flesh of the gods," "voices of the gods," and "little saints." Schultes and Hofmann (1979) in *Plants of the Gods* describe the uses and beliefs surrounding these substances. The principal aspects of their use cross-culturally involve establishing personal relationships with a spiritual dimension of reality and reinforcing community relations through group rituals. The drug-induced experiences have effects on personality by placing the self in a special relationship with a mythical level of reality. The social rituals enhance social identity formation, group integration, and cohesion.

The effects of these drugs reported cross-culturally differ from perspectives developed in biomedicine. When the Western world rediscovered these substances in colonized societies, the plants were demonized, seen as evidence of consorting with the devil. Their practitioners were tortured to death by the Inquisition and religious authorities. Similar negative attitudes characterized the initial biomedical engagement with these substances.

Macrosocial Effects of Psychedelic Use The use of psychedelics or hallucinogens in religious healing systems is primarily associated with shamans, who use ASCs in healing and divination (Winkelman, 1990, 1992, 2000a). Cross-cultural research (Winkelman, 1991) indicates that political factors, as opposed to strictly cultural factors (beliefs), have effects on the differential use of hallucinogens. As societies increase in political integration and structural complexity, oppression leads to reductions in the use of and access to plant hallucinogens and other ASCs (also see Dobkin de Rios and Smith, 1977; Winkelman, 1996a). As societies evolve hierarchical religious structures, the use of hallucinogenic plants is usurped by the elite segments and eliminated from widespread use. Political integration leads to restrictions on the use of **psychointegrators** because of their effects on social relations and personal interpretations of the world. Psychointegrators are generally used in local contexts, where expectations and interpersonal relations play powerful roles in interpreting the experiences. The context-specific idiosyncratic interpretations could threaten hierarchical control of religious consciousness and central political authority. Key aspects of the traditional applications of hallucinogenic plants include inducing a profound visionary experience guided by traditional cultural values, beliefs, and goals. These community-based rituals reinforce a local traditional mythos and social order, as opposed to the ideological and political orders promulgated by state religions.

Psychedelics are also used by cultures to deal with the effects of social change, as illustrated in the Navajo adoption of the Native American Church (NAC; peyote religion) (discussed in Chapter Five) and the use of ayahuasca in the Amazon Basin. Andritzky (1989) discusses the widespread use in the Amazon Basin of ayahuasca in collective rituals. It assists in dealing with the problems of acculturation by mediating between the Euro-American and indigenous worlds and strengthening social cohesion and group identity. This symbolic synthesis of the traditional and new is through the emotionally charged images produced by the ayahuasca. These provide a method of symbolic confrontation and psychosocial adjustment. Aberle's (1966) work on the historical development of the peyote religion (NAC) illustrates that early Navajo adherents were predominantly those who experienced the greatest relative deprivation. Although antisocial and antiestablishment tendencies may be associated with peyote use in the broader American society, it is not so among Navajo and other groups participating in the NAC; this reflects both macrosocial and microsocial influences of the respective groups.

Microsocial Effects of Psychedelic Use Psychedelics have a variety of general and specific therapeutic effects (Winkelman and Roberts, 2007a; Winkelman and Andritzky, 1996; Ratsch, 2005), but these widespread therapeutic applications, which have also been noted cross-culturally, have not generally been apparent to biomedicine. Instead, the effects expected of psychedelics have reflected their own cultural expectations. LSD was initially used in Western medicine with the assumption that it produced psychosis, and clinical interactions (such as isolation of subjects and their observations through one-way windows) indicated that it could produce paranoia and psychotic reactions. Military applications as weapons in unsuspecting victims further confirmed that paranoia and delusion could result from uninformed administration.

However, in other settings, the experiences were different. The typical positive LSD experience—a "good trip"—changed the user's perception of ordinary reality. The sense of self underwent dramatic changes, with powerful experiences of mystical union and dissolution of self into a unity with the universe. These experiences led to a new medical paradigm, the psycholytic approach, which integrated a series of low doses of LSD in regular therapeutic sessions to alter the relationship between the conscious and unconscious. This facilitated psychoanalytic psychotherapy by weakening psychological defenses and heightening emotional responsiveness. These substances released unconscious material and promoted emotional release, enhancing and accelerating the therapeutic process. Profound personality changes were also found to be associated with LSD-induced mystical experiences, especially among people with these perspectives. This led to a new clinical paradigm, the psychedelic paradigm of LSD. Large doses were used to induce mystical experiences and insights to produce life changes and enhanced self-control. These different paradigms, in part, reflect effects derived from "set and setting" influences, the extrapharmacological factors derived from expectations and situational circumstances (Grob and Bravo, 1996).

Cultural Effects on Drug Dependence and Addiction

Drug dependence refers to the psychological need a user feels for a substance. Both psychological dependence and physical addiction are influenced by individual and cultural factors that contribute to the total drug effect. These needs can be a consequence of the desire to feel certain ways or to reduce symptoms of withdrawal. Addiction or physical dependence is also influenced by psychosocial and macrosocial factors. These cultural influences contribute to the determination of what is normal and acceptable behavior and how the use and effects are viewed, experienced, and treated. For example, in the United States, only relatively recently have alcohol, coffee, and tobacco been considered to be drugs.

BIOCULTURAL INTERACTIONS

Alcohol Effects and Culture

Alcohol use in any culture and its consequences are products of many sociocultural factors, rather than just the physiological effects of alcohol. These are mediated by many factors, including attitudes toward consumption, norms and values surrounding alcohol use, contexts and patterns of consumption, and expectations regarding those who consume it and their consequent behavior. Genetic variation greatly influences individual susceptibility to the effects of alcohol, but cultural patterns of use and their consequences reflect interactions among physical, psychological, and social aspects in the total drug effect. For instance, physical effects associated with chronic alcohol use (organ damage), can be accentuated or attenuated by cultural factors (such as diet, activity, and setting). Pharmacological consequences are mediated by concentration, dosage, and setting, which may dramatically exacerbate the effects (such as hard liquor versus beer or diluted wine). Health outcomes such as automobile fatalities are largely a consequence of consumption patterns (e.g., home or neighborhood consumption versus driving to bars).

What constitutes normal drinking (socially acceptable, whether daily or ritual) as well as drunkenness and the effects on health are to a great degree a function of cultural expectations and social effects. O'Connor (1978) (also see Heath, 2000) has investigated different cultural attitudes toward drinking. She conceptualized these as involving four major types: abstinent, ambivalent, permissive, and overpermissive:

> *Abstinent cultures*: Alcohol use is prohibited. These tend to have drinking and personal problems that are greater than those found in permissive cultures. The higher rates of alcoholism and problems are a consequence of the lack of social norms and supports for a normal drinking pattern.

In the case of both illegal and prescription drugs, symbolic and social meanings of drug use are important contributors to the overall effects. Symbolic effects of use are inferred from the continued use of tranquilizers over years, when their actual physiological action declines within weeks to months to levels at which they no longer have effects. Tranquilizers may help maintain certain kinds of lifestyle relationships and expectations: being self-controlled, sociable, patient, and able to perform normal role expectations at work or in the family. Although the physical properties of the drug are no longer effective, their continued use may reflect latent functions symbolizing the patient's condition or eliciting specific responses from friends and family. These effects are part of the macrosocial context of drug use derived from social relations. Physicians may contribute to this process by prescribing drugs for taking care of problems, rather than assisting patients in dealing with them directly through addressing the macrosocial conditions that produce stress.

The use of substances as aids in maintaining social roles and expectations and in improving social relations and one's own emotional state is referred to as "chemical

Ambivalent cultures: Have contradictory attitudes toward alcohol consumption. Some consider alcohol consumption a normal part of life whereas others encourage abstinence. The lack of a cultural consensus and accepted norms for the control of drinking behavior leave the individual in an ambivalent position that may contribute to alcoholic behavior.

Permissive cultures: Have norms, values, and customs that support drinking behavior and provide a context for its control. The culturally normative use of alcohol, especially in conjunction with meals, contributes to low levels of alcoholism. This is particularly true where norms do not condone drinking between meals or drunkenness.

Overpermissive cultures: Have norms, values, and customs that support moderate drinking behavior and attitudes that contribute to deviant patterns of drinking and the associated problems. In such cultures, drinking is often viewed as a sign of male virility, and the social acceptance of intoxication contributes to problem drinking. The generally lower levels of alcoholism in permissive and overpermissive cultures than in abstinent and ambivalent cultures reflect the control and acceptance of behavior, as opposed to its pathologization.

O'Connor's further studies show that the lowest incidence of alcoholism is associated with cultures in which there are

- Early life exposures to diluted alcohol within the context of food consumption
- Parental examples of moderate drinking
- Perceptions that alcohol use does not have moral implications nor does it serve as a sign of manhood
- A social agreement that abstinence is acceptable and drunkenness is not acceptable

coping." Drugs that are used as part of coping strategies—chemical comforters—include not only the physician-prescribed medications but also caffeine, tobacco, alcohol, and illicit drugs. Social factors affecting drug effects are particularly notable in subcultures associated with the use of "hard" illegal drugs: lifestyle consequences (poor diet, housing), vectors (exposure, common needle or bottle use), and the social response of others (such as police, employers, and family).

Ways that subcultural context contributes to addiction and withdrawal effects are indicated in a number of studies. Studies (Robins, Helzer, and Davis, 1975) of U.S. servicemen addicted to heroin in Vietnam found that most were able to leave the drug completely with little difficulty or withdrawal symptoms when they returned home. This reflects macrosocial context effects both in Vietnam (where it was easily available and a subculture supported its use) and the United States (where price, availability, required new contacts, and family and friends' disapproval inhibited use). Other effects include the reduced coping demands of home in comparison to those experienced under battlefield conditions. Global subcultural effects on addiction are illustrated in the widely acknowledged effects on drug use patterns caused by drug shortages, when heroin addicts would temporarily switch to methamphetamines (which had pharmacologically opposite effects) while maintaining the heroin subculture behaviors and lifestyle. The subcultures of addicts have powerful effects on addiction maintenance from nonpharmacological factors; consequently, there is an inability to end addiction without addressing the microsocial and macrosocial factors that influence individuals and their behaviors.

Theories of Placebo Mechanisms

The mechanisms by which placebos affect illness and disease remain uncertain because of a lack of systematic investigations (Shapiro and Shapiro, 1997). Nonetheless, a number of mechanisms of placebo effects have been implicated, including individual psychosocial response characteristics, elicitation of endogenous opioid and psychoneuroimmunological responses, conditioning, and meaning. It appears that the *meanings* of placebos are fundamental mechanisms through which they cause physiological responses.

Personal and Social Characteristics The characteristics associated with people most likely to have a placebo response involve "patient's preference for treatment with drugs and psychotherapy; patient's desire to leave the choice of treatment to the physician; drug expectations; patient's attitudes; physician's attitudes; anxiety and depression" (Shapiro and Shapiro, 1997, p. 220). Placebo responses are greater when patients have positive expectations regarding treatment. This includes the belief that their symptoms warrant clinical treatment and are treated with an appropriate drug. Placebo responses are also enhanced by a patient's attitude toward the physician as competent and attractive. Other nonspecific factors enhancing placebo outcomes include (Shapiro and Shapiro, 1997)

■   Patient perception of an efficient and comprehensive evaluation

■   Seeing patients punctually in a pleasant atmosphere and prestigious settings

■   Experienced staff using both psychodynamic and drug-oriented therapies

■   Staff interested in testing both drug and placebo effects

Placebo effects are associated with acquiescence but not with most personality variables. Placebo responders tend to have higher states of anxiety, suggesting that the reduction of anxiety is a mechanism through which placebos act (Benedetti and Amanzio, 1997). The attitude toward the physician, particularly confidence in his or her diagnosis and proposed treatments, is a significant factor in placebo responses. Because the vast majority of underlying causes of complaints involve emotional dynamics, releasing these concerns can enhance one's well-being. These effects reflect the general relief provided by placing one's concerns in a context in which they are intelligible and manageable, evoking the symbolic healing response. Part of the placebo effect is derived from patients' attitudes and beliefs; a positive belief seems necessary, and disbelief subverts placebo effects. Beliefs may produce even stronger effects than the specific drugs for which they are substituted (Shapiro and Shapiro, 1997) and may even produce effects opposite to the physiological actions of agents (see below).

Therapeutic Relationships Therapeutic relations are an essential component of placebo effects. Helman (1994) suggests that they may be based in "a reactivation of the feelings of basic trust adherent to the original mother-infant dyad" (p. 197) that provides a basis for a sense of security. Healers' characteristics producing placebo effects include culturally validated symbols of position such as status, age, appearance, and authority. These enhance a patient's confidence in the healing process. Placebo effects are created by the confidence healers convey through the style of relationship with patients and are augmented by congruence between healer and patient in understandings of the therapeutic approach and treatment processes.

Endogenous Opioids One area long recognized as possibly explaining the placebo effect involves endogenous opioids, the body's natural opiate substances (Benedetti and Amanzio, 1997). The role of the endogenous opioids in the placebo effect has been established through experiments in which chemical substances (naloxone) were administered that block the effects of endogenous opioids. Eliminating placebo effects with these blockers provides evidence that opioid mediation is involved in placebos. This is complemented by studies that enhance placebo responses through administering substances that counter the antiopioid action of other natural chemicals (cholecystokinin). Pain intensity also mediates placebo responses, with higher levels of pain eliciting stronger placebo responses. Placebo-mediated conditioned analgesia (pain relief) is directly tied to high-anxiety and fear situations. Stress can elicit opioid-mediated analgesic responses, even without the administration of placebos. The desire for pain relief is central to the placebo-mediated reduction in pain, which is elicited by the expectation that pain will be reduced by the specific treatment procedure or agent. Although endogenous opioids are elicited in some placebo responses, they do not account for all placebo effects. It also leaves open the question of the mechanisms by which expectations elicit endogenous opioid production or release. The endogenous opioids do more than reduce pain; they also play broader roles as messenger molecules in the body, particularly in the emotional centers of the brain. Thus, they constitute a communication system that operates on levels distinct from the cognitive paradigm dominant in psychology and reflect the operation of a "second brain" (see the section, "Psychoneuroimmunology").

Classic Conditioning Another basis for placebo responses is classic conditioning, the association of neutral stimuli with pharmacological responses. For instance, a previously neutral stimulus (such as a white pill) becomes conditioned by its pairing with an unconditioned stimulus (such as the effects of the pharmacological agents it contains) and its unconditioned response (such as pain relief). Repeated associations with a once-neutral stimulus (white pill) with the pharmacological effects of the pills can give the once-neutral stimuli the capability of eliciting the unconditioned response, pain relief. Or similarly, going to a doctor's office (neutral stimulus) becomes associated with a variety of unconditioned responses because of the subsequent reduction of suffering; consequently, just going to the doctor's office can elicit such physiological responses. This drug-mimicking response is found in animals administered inert substances in conditioned settings; once they have become accustomed to receiving medications in certain settings, being placed in the settings evokes therapeutic placebo responses. The therapeutic context is a conditioned stimulus that acquires effects because of its association with the unconditioned stimuli (active pharmaceuticals) that reduce pain. Benedetti and Amanzio (1997) illustrate the role of expectation in producing placebo responses in differential responses to drugs. Information given to subjects receiving epinephrine (a stimulant) had dramatic effects on the consequential experiences and symptoms; when told that the agent was a tranquilizer, their behaviors and experiences corresponded to depressive, not stimulant, effects. Similarly, substances such as emetics that produce vomiting may elicit the opposite of their pharmacological effects, both subjectively and physiologically, when patients are given opposite expectations: assurances that the substance will reduce nausea (Harrington, 1997).

The environment is a central aspect of the framework of expectations within which an individual's subjective experience is produced and acts on the body. It appears that placebo responses are not produced just by pairing of conditioned and unconditioned stimuli but, rather, by response expectancy and its self-confirming nature (Kirsch, 1997). Desire and expectation, like hope and faith, have roles in eliciting placebo responses. The conditioning and expectancy paradigms must include a cognitive component because of the central roles of meaning in placebo responses.

Information and Meaning as Placebo Mechanisms

Experimental procedures to distinguish classic conditioning from response-expectancy mediation of the placebo effect challenge the conditioning theory of placebo effects (Montgomery and Kirsch, 1997). This is the idea that conditioned stimuli (pills or treatments) associated with active ingredients are subsequently capable of evoking therapeutic effects because of their learned association with unconditioned responses. They propose that placebo phenomena be viewed from an information perspective where the response to a drug is an unconditioned stimulus. The association of drugs (or placebos) with these unconditioned effects provides the basis for response expectancy: pills produce changes, so when pills are taken, changes are expected and produced. Expectancies produce the physiological responses analogous to the ways in which our intentions elicit our voluntary behaviors. Response expectancies are based in our thoughts and feelings that produce responses in our bodies. One consequence of this is that placebo effects are resistant to extinction—they are not eliminated—and may actually increase over time. Extinction is prevented because placebo responses confirm the expectancy that generated them. This leads to the conclusion that the effects of conditioning on the response to placebos are completely mediated by expectancy, illustrated in the finding by Montgomery and Kirsch (1997) that verbal information can be used to alter expectancy and obstruct the effect of conditioning. Their results show that it is the interpretation that affects placebo responding. The basis of placebos is similar to the broader cognitive effects of treatment expectations. Treatments are unconditioned stimuli that mimic drug effects and confirm expectations.

Information is important in the generation and modification of placebo, nocebo, and drug responses (Flaten, Simonsen, and Olsen, 1999). Flaten and colleagues used a muscle relaxant (carisoprodol), together with a placebo, and information that indicated that the agent given was either a stimulant or a relaxant. The effects of both the drug and the placebo were in the direction suggested by the information provided, acting as a stimulant or a relaxant depending on the information provided. These effects were not only psychological but also physiological, as indicated in the differential absorption of the drug by the body. Subjects given a relaxant experienced increased tension when told they were receiving a stimulant. This group had lower drug absorption and higher tension than the placebo group receiving stimulant information. The authors suggest that the differences between expectations and experience produced increased tension, suggesting that both placebo and drug effects are mediated by subjective information.

Moerman (2000) illustrates cultural effects on placebo responses in his assessment of placebo and drug responses by ulcer patients. Whereas the causation of ulcers is commonly believed to involve stress and stomach acid, there is limited support for this. There was a recent belief that ulcers are caused by bacteria, but although most ulcer patients are infected, the infection rates are far higher than the ulcer rates, and most of those infected will not develop ulcers. Moerman assessed treatment by cimetidine for ulcers using seventy-two studies from twenty-eight countries. The placebo control groups in the study had placebo response rates ranging from 0 to 100 percent, and the effectiveness of the active drug was strongly correlated with the placebo rate. Moerman's (1983) cross-cultural assessment of the effectiveness of cimetidine versus placebos suggested that the trials indicating its effectiveness were a consequence of low placebo effects, which provided for a significant difference between treatment and controls. The nonsignificant studies found healing in an average of 58 percent of the placebo group, such high levels of success that the drug treatment was not significantly different.

These data raise important questions about the cause of considerable variation in placebo effects and how such large numbers of people could apparently be healed of ulcers with nothing ("ulcer healing was confirmed by endoscopic examination" [Moerman, 2000, p. 58]). Highly variable placebo effects for anxiety disorders and cross-cultural variation in response to placebos indicate that the response is a function of what treatments mean to people.

Moerman (2000) suggests that the effects of placebos are derived from a "meaning response," the attribution of meaning by patients. These attributions are influenced by a physician's enthusiasm, the interaction between provider and patient, and cultural influences (such as the colors and forms of the pills). Moerman suggests that there are three types of healing processes: "*autonomous ones* based on the immunological and homeostatic processes . . . *specific ones* based on the pharmacological or physical dimensions . . . and *meaningful ones,* based on knowledge and interaction" (Moerman, 2000, p. 56). Placebo's meaning effects are part of the general therapeutic effects derived from the process of attributing meaning to self and others that structures the experience of well-being. Meaning is inescapably part of all medical treatments, whether pharmacological, surgical, or interpersonal, involving meaningful symbolic acts that have effects on patients' physical condition.

The placebo effect can be considered physiological consequences of expectation mediated through the effects of hormones and neurotransmitters. But the specific ways meaning, belief, and interpersonal dynamics produce physiological responses remain to be specified. The meaning-based models of placebo action involve satisfying explanations, care and concern, and enhanced control (Brody, 2000). These aspects of meaning are individually variable and situated in individuals and their immediate sociocultural environment. Consequently, the study of placebo mechanisms requires investigation into the social and cultural conditions of meaningfulness.

Summary Understanding the nature of placebo effects has changed across time to recognize that they are a part of all medical treatments. Placebos may be far greater in surgical than in pharmaceutical treatment because there are no requirements for double-blind clinical studies in the assessment of the efficacy of surgical procedures (Shapiro and Shapiro, 1997). Shapiro and Shapiro suggest that the large-scale overuse of surgical interventions is likely in areas such as cardiac bypass surgery and other cardiac procedures, cesarean sections and hysterectomies, and transplants. Because of ethical issues, it may be difficult to carry out placebo and double-blind assessments of many surgical procedures. Although the placebo effect has often been viewed by biomedicine as something to be eliminated, the current understanding suggests that we should attempt to enhance placebo effectiveness. Placebo effects are an important aspect of the overall effectiveness of all treatments. Consequently, understanding placebo effects and how to elicit them is an important part of cultural contributions to biomedicine. Placebos' dramatic symbolic influences on bodily functions reflect personal and cultural processes, where beliefs and expectations have causal effects. Motivational, affective, and cognitive processes, particularly meaning, modulate placebo effects. The integration of the biological and cultural sciences is necessary for understanding the precise mechanisms through which meaning has effects on physiology and how to integrate those potentials into medicine. The general understanding we have of placebo mechanisms is that these mind-body communications involve expectations that have effects on the central nervous system, ANS, and peptides of the immune system, affecting the energetic and informational systems of the brain and body (Rossi, 2000). "Perhaps we should search for ways to enhance the placebo effect, which in turn may stimulate hope, optimism, and the motivation required to deal with a difficult world" (Shapiro and Shapiro, 1997, p. 236).

PSYCHONEUROIMMUNOLOGY

Psychoneuroimmunology emerged from the recognition of the ability of symbols, personal expectations, and social relations to have effects on immune system responses and health. Psychoneuroimmunology has investigated interactions among the central nervous system (CNS), endocrine system, and immune system (Lyon, 1993), particularly symbolic tuning between the nervous and immune systems (Varela, 1997). The interactions are not strictly material but involve the organism's adaptations through cognitive models, psychological states, and social relations. In the *Social and Cultural Lives of Immune Systems,* Wilce (2003) and other contributors help show how social life plays a fundamental role in the operation of our body's basic defenses.

The field of psychoneuroimmunology derived from findings that immune system processes are affected by organisms' responses in adaptation to the environment. The immune system and health and disease processes are affected by the interactions among psychosocial, emotional, and physiological processes and the ways in which thought, feeling, and behavior interact (Lyon, 1993). These interactions between an organism's biological and social levels are based in subjective emotional experiences and the sense of self. Immunological responses involve relationships between biological and social levels of being, an interaction of individual physiology and social psychology that is the context for effects at cellular levels (Lyon, 1993). Lyon suggests that this context involves human emotions, which are both biological and cognitive and produce both disease and healing. Interpersonal interactions and social experiences affect the immune system through emotions that are intervening influences between individually felt meanings and their somatic responses (Lyon, 1993).

The immune system operates as one of the most fundamental adaptations of the organism to the environment, a system that detects and responds in protective ways to pathogens: germs and other toxic threats from the environment. The immune system is one of the body's most complex systems, responding to the full array of pathogens that threaten the body, including microorganisms such as viruses and bacteria, fungi, allergens, and toxins (Hirsch, 2004). When these pathogens penetrate outer defenses in the skin, mucous membranes, and digestive systems, the immune system responds with the production of antibodies. Immune reactions are elicited by the detection of foreign proteins distinct from the organism's own. When a foreign antigen is detected, the body produces memory cells that are prepared to combat this pathogen if it reoccurs in the organism. The immune response is in specialized white blood cells called leukocytes, including lymphocytes (B and T cells), monocytes, and granulocytes (Hirsch). When a B lymphocyte is triggered by the recognition of an antigen, it stimulates the production of antibodies (immunoglobins) that have a wide range of specialized functions in combating entities that are foreign to the organism.

A systems perspective is necessary to understand how symbols bring about physiological changes in the body and how effects are communicated across domains of mind and body. Lyon (1993) proposes that these communicative functions of the immune system produce an "immunosemiotics" that involves "biological meaning" based in immune system cognitive functions of discrimination, inference, and memory that provide the basis for an "immunological self." The immune system can be conceptualized as a sensory system within which the white blood cells function as "messenger molecules" for communication among the CNS and immune and endocrine systems (Lyon, 1993). Peptides found in both the immune and neuroendocrine systems provide the basis for signaling the immune system in response to noncognitive stimuli such as viruses and bacteria. This immune system's sensory function enables it to relay information to the neuroendocrine system and initiate physiological changes. CNS responses to emotional stimuli change hormonal levels that affect the immune system as messenger molecules that act on the immune system indirectly through hormones and directly through neurotransmitters (Lyon, 1993).

Varela (1997) characterizes the immune system's structure and functions as a "second brain" that provides a self-regulating control of the body's responses to the environment. The immune system has organs distributed throughout the body (lymphocytes, B cells,

T cells of the thymus, the spleen, and the lymphatic system) that adapt through learning and memory. Through the interaction of mind and emotions with the nervous system, our psychological conditions influence health, as discussed above in the stress responses. This provides mechanisms for interaction between the CNS and the immune system. CNS response to stress causes the release of hormones (glucocorticoids) that interact with the lymphatic system through their surface receptors. This stimulates the immune system to release lymphocytes and immunotransmitters that act directly on neurons of the limbic system (paleomammalian brain), the center of emotions and self. Hirsch (2004) characterizes the brain-immune system communication underlying the immune system response as involving the sympathoadrenomedullary system and the hypothalamopituitary-adrenocortical system, both of which are paleomammalian brain regions aroused by the sympathetic nervous system's fight-or-flight response. This activation triggers the endocrine system of glands that release a wide range of chemical messengers. Hormone receptors are found throughout the immune system, organs, and the neurotransmitter systems. Their interaction across these different systems enables the hormones to play a vital role in communication across self, body, social context, emotions, meaning, and immune system responses.

Self

Lyon (2003) emphasizes that we must see the immune system as coterminous with the self, a system that has the function of distinguishing the "not-self" at the level of the cellular recognition of foreign entities. Wilce and Price (2003) note that the concept of the self is central to theories of psychoneuroimmunology because the most basic response made by the immune system is to the presence of an outside entity. Psychoneuroimmunological approaches have traditionally assumed that immunological processes work through a precultural level of the self involving the body and its emotions, a primordial aspect of personal identity that includes a sense of the body, its internal processes, and its emotional relations to family and significant others. The immunological self is not the rational, language-based thinking mind but, rather, a much deeper embodied self of behavior, habits, nonverbal communication, and social and emotional dynamics that are the foundation of our participation in society. This behavioral level is a semiotic (meaning) system shared with other animals in our embodiment and expression of meaning and intention through behavior. This body-based preverbal system is the basis for a metalanguage of communication within the organism and across its verbal, behavioral, neural, and immune systems (Wilce, 2003).

Body and Embodiment

The metaphors of the body found cross-culturally and throughout cognitive domains derive their structures from an innate basis, the necessary relationship of all knowing to the body. The body and its ability to act are necessarily the primary ground of experience and become the metaphoric ground for experiencing everything, including society. Wilce and Price (2003) use the term somatosocial, "body-social," to expand on the bases of the concept of sociosomatic, where social relations affect the interaction between mind and body. Somatosocial is a recognition that the body is before the conception of the social and a metaphoric basis from which we understand social relations. For example: He is the "head" of the group. She is the "heart" of the organization. He is the "brain" behind this. They are just "hired hands." He has our "back" on this one. We must "arm" ourselves. Who will "foot" the bill here? Does this project have "legs"? Can we count on you to keep an "eye" on things? He has a "nose" for this kind of problem. Can you "face" them? Do you have the "stomach" for this? Bodies are natural systems of meaning but also acquire their significance from local meanings and circumstances. The material bases of the symbolic and social world produce interaction patterns that have powerful effects on cultural concepts of the body. The presence of varying culturally induced concepts of the body within a person (such as the physical body, the phenomenological or experienced body, and political or economic bodies discussed in Chapter Five) implies embodiment, a process by which cultural beliefs, social relations, and political structures are imposed on our bodies during the development of bodily habits and personal subjective experiences of body and world. These are expressed naturally in behavior, an innate representational system of the body known as mimesis.

Mimesis

Mimesis is the core of human symbolic systems, with the body and its ability to act the most fundamental representational system and basis for metaphor. Mimesis is generally used to refer to imitation or modeling, a body-based cognitive process in which movement establishes relationships of meaning between humans and other objects, based on correspondences of the body to social processes. Mimesis, the body's ability to imitate and represent through action, is the common basis of both somatic and symbolic levels of reality. The level of representation of mimesis is manifested in our bodies as habits, the individual behavioral patterns produced by conditioning the lower centers of the brain into typical response patterns, an engagement of both bodily processes and associated psychological reactions. Habit also provides an emotional engagement, with a sense of control and security derived from the regularity or patterns of experience. These reflect conditioned effects derived from classic conditioning and associational learning and in which personal experiences and social conditions are symbolically and physically incorporated into the development of bodily responses. These and other learned meanings affect emotions, morale, mood, and experiences of depression and powerlessness. These bodily expressions of internal states are the most fundamental aspects of our relationships to the outside world. Body metaphors have the power to express meanings by their natural ability to mediate between the sensory domains of felt experience and the verbal domains of expression, employing analogical reasoning that uses the body as a common template for integrating felt experiences *and social reality*. Culture provides the social context in which the metaphors of our "bodyminds" are engaged by the social context that defines their meaning.

Social Context

Wilce (2003) points to the central role of social and cultural factors in immune systems, which reflects the intimate relations of our immunological system functions to our social relations and the symbolic expressions found in society. Social context is more fundamental than metaphoric systems in the emotional processes of the self that produce the integration of social life within bodily processes. Psychoneuroimmunology emerged from the recognition of the vital role of not only psychological aspects but also social processes and interactions in the functioning of the immune system. Our immune status is apparently affected even by our relative social status in society, making the hierarchy of social relations a part of the systemic effects on the health of individuals. Lyon (2003) proposes that the relationships of social life to the immune system are mediated through the habitual effects of conditioning on our behaviors, producing a mimetic enactment of personal and cultural patterns, which provide the basis for emotional contagion, the linkages between social life and bodily processes.

Kirmayer (2003) points out that anthropological research is essential to detailing the cultural dynamics of sociophysiological responses. These include ways in which a person's meaningful individual experiences have salient effects on physiological responses and the ways in which these events are socially distributed, contextually elicited, and impact the lives of individuals and cultures. Fundamental to metaphor theory of sociosomatic-psychosomatic interactions are the underlying emotional dispositions to act, in which cultural specifics shape the underlying biology of emotion. Lyon (2003) notes that the role of emotions as mediators between our experienced body and social relations allows them to represent the processes in the broader social structures that shape our social relations. The most relevant cultural metaphors of the body are those related to the management of our emotions.

Emotional Empathy and Contagion

Emotions are the representations of how the body subjectively experiences the self and the social world through interrelations in intimate social networks. Our emotional capacities involve self and physiological mechanisms for adjusting to the social environment. Through emotions, personal experiences are linked with social relations, the process through which individual psychophysiological dynamics and the social world are intimately interlinked. The symbolic processes and social relations play a fundamental role in eliciting emotions and in producing empathy through a contagion that transfers experiences from one body to another. Emotional contagion is based in unconscious imitative bodily processes that are derived from the dispositions produced by attachment, where the integration of body, emotions, and the social awareness of others first occurred. Emotional contagion is concerned with the co-occurrence of the same emotions among members of a group together in a setting. Across species, emotional contagion is based in imitative processes, including mimicry and other behaviors that place animals in attunement or synchrony. It is a multilevel phenomenon influenced by physiological, behavioral, and social aspects.

Elicitation of Psychoneuroimmunological Responses

Psychoneuroimmunological theories consider the meaning of events to play a role in the regulation of the immune system. Kirmayer (2003) notes that there are many forms of meaning, including those of cognitive, affective, behavioral, and social representation. These provide the bases for feedback loops between the psychosocial dynamics of life and the functioning of the immune system (Kirmayer, 2003; Lyon, 2003). Some contributions involve unconditioned effects, natural biological responses of the body such as grief from the loss of a family member, marital conflict, and a disruption of mother-child relations. Most have learned components, however, including conditioned effects from socializations and learned systems of meaning embodied in metaphors.

METAPHORIC PROCESSES IN SYMBOLIC HEALING

Kirmayer (2003) proposes that metaphor theory explains how learned behaviors, interpersonal relations, and communication dynamics are imposed on bodily experiences and physiological processes through socialization. These practices and experiences link (associate) the symbols of language with activities in the sensory and motor systems of the brain, thus making them capable of eliciting those same brain processes through the images evoked by metaphor. It is this power of metaphor that underlies the psychoneuroimmunological response.

Healers' activities and treatment processes reorganize patients' emotional conditions by providing interpretations of their situation in a world of known possibilities. Cultural healing processes manipulate a worldview that shapes the patients' experiences. Dow (1986) describes the universal aspects of symbolic healing as based in processes through which symbols affect the mind and, consequently, the body. For instance, if your patients told you that your visitor is a child-molester, could you give the person a warm hug? The label "child-molester" implies much that you likely despise; if you accept the accuracy of that label, it would so powerfully shape your attitudes and emotions that a warm hug would likely be impossible. Even if you doubted the truth, the labeling process may make you feel uncomfortable around the person. On the other hand, if you were told that the Pope was coming to visit you, it might so powerfully motivate you that you would get up from bed with considerable enthusiasm and energy, even if stricken with the flu.

Metaphoric healing involves processes in which the healer evokes for the patient a generally shared cultural belief, a mythic system that the healer uses as the context for interpreting a patient's condition. The attachment of a patient's emotions to mythic symbols transforms the patient through the association of the symbols with aspects of the patient's personality, self, and identity (such as souls, spirits, and morals). Healing is produced through remodeling the self within the structure of the mythic world, as illustrated in Christian charismatic healing.

Dow (1986) elaborates on the mechanisms of symbolic healing within a model of the hierarchy of living systems; for a similar example, see the diagram of the biopsychosocial model of the hierarchy of natural systems (Figure 1.1). Personality is part of a hierarchy of interrelated systems that extend from the atomic and physiological levels through the self and cultural systems. Our experiences are influenced by many factors "below" the personality (such as hormones and neurotransmitters) as well as those "above" or "beyond" the personality, such as interpersonal relations and national crises events. Agitation that we personally experience can be caused by factors at all of these levels: excessive epinephrine or medications within us or physical threats or bomb scares in the news.

CULTURE AND HEALTH

Metaphoric Processes in Catholic Charismatic Healing

In Catholic charismatic healing (Csordas, 1994), healing of the self has its basis in a conception of the person as involving body, mind, and spirit; this tripartite division of the person is manifested in Jesus, God the Father, and the Holy Spirit. Religious traditions (mythology and metaphors) are involved in characterizing these three aspects of the person and in healing the physical body and the emotional distress of memories. Charismatic healing processes affect personal identity through ritual practices that link the self, body, and the social world with the personal unconscious through the use of Christian images and metaphors and their associated meanings.

Charismatic healing processes use images of Jesus to evoke a transformation in one's orientation toward one's sense of self and relationships with others, particularly those who have caused emotional trauma. This transformation of the self first involves an elicitation of repressed memories considered to be the basis of a significant trauma to the self. During the healing ceremony, the patient experiences internal images that are considered to be a sign of divine presence. These images are also a form of information linking the patient's personal past, relationships with self and others, and interactions between mind and body. These images reveal the repressed emotional dynamics created by trauma; healing ritual allows for their safe retrieval from the subconscious in a supportive context.

Healing traumatized emotions requires that the victim forgive the perpetrator of the trauma. This is achieved through an imaginal reenactment of the trauma, recalling memories in the context of healing ceremonies in ways that allow the model of Jesus to intervene and heal the trauma. Charismatic practices heal emotional trauma by producing a personal growth toward maturity through forgiveness modeled on Jesus' unending love and forgiveness. Evoking these memories in the presence of healers and the models provided by Jesus helps to neutralize the negative emotions and memories. Trauma is overcome through the powerful heartfelt influences provided by the concept of Jesus' protecting love. Religious belief systems play a central role in modeling these self-processes of release and forgiveness. Accepting the power of Jesus in one's life leads to a transformation of the self through relationships in which Jesus constitutes an "ideal other," a set of ideal characteristics used as a model for the creation of a sacred self and identity, relief of trauma of the past, and protection for the future.

Although each level (physiology, body, personality, social relations) is a complete system, each is affected by the other levels (such as how our physical condition or how others treat us affects our psychological health). Many forms of communication, including the symbols found in myth and ritual, manipulate the personality of patients and affect the physiological levels of organisms. Personality shares unconscious thought processes of the body's physiological level, enabling psychological influences to have effects on the physical body. For example, when you think someone is following you and you are paranoid because you were recently mugged, those psychological beliefs and dispositions can elicit the stress response, even if the risks are not real. Belief trumps reality in the effects of psychology on physiology.

Dow (1986) suggests that symbolic healing is based on the human capacity for interpersonal communication, which derived from a prior capacity of humans to communicate with themselves through emotion. Through evolution, this intrapersonal biological communication mechanism was extended into symbolic systems and language. Consequently, symbols can reciprocally affect biological processes and produce a cure through symbolic effects on unconscious and somatic processes (Dow, 1986).

These emotional mechanisms are reinforced through processes of suggestion by others, emotional restructuring from interpersonal influences, and the dramatic aspects of therapeutic rituals. A link between self and body occurs through the emotions, and healing occurs through a patient's opportunity to relieve emotional tensions. Emotions are basic integrative functions, summarizing for higher levels of the organism the complex processes occurring at lower levels (Dow, 1986). Emotions can play this fundamental linking role because they acquire their meaning and the elicitation of physiological responses from personal, social, and cultural levels.

Kirmayer (1993) uses metaphor, the representation of one thing through something else, to explain the mechanisms of symbolic healing. Metaphors involve language, images, gestures, and actions to create meaning: "the active relationship of receiver to message of self to world worked within thought, feeling, imagination, and social transaction" (p. 162). Meaning is relational, involving feelings, sensations, behaviors, and cognitive transformations: "the use *of* something *by* someone *for* some end" (p. 162). Psychoanalytical approaches produce healing through revelation of unrecognized information about the unconscious self. In psychoanalysis, a patient's speech and symptoms reveal psychological dynamics of the unconscious. These dynamics may be healed by symbols that provide representations of distress and a balance among different aspects of the self. For example, by explaining a troubling dream (such as of a monster) as a symbolic representation of a real-life problem (such as your boss), one is able to understand the meaning of what was before only a distressing symptom. Structuralist approaches illustrate that healing occurs through meaning derived from an internal logic of the relationships in a total system, as exemplified in the analysis of myths that provide social and personal order. This is exemplified in the peace and tranquility that Christians experience when they turn their life over to Jesus, accepting that whatever happens to them is part of his plan.

Metaphors affect thoughts and feelings and produce experiences. If someone says, "You are a pig" or "You are an angel," the statements affect you, even though you are neither a pig nor an angel. Kirmayer (1993) suggests the need for a "biological psychology that grounds symbolic cognition in the body and in the exigencies of local power, relationships, and ecology" (p. 167). The effectiveness of ritual healing is not explained merely by the analogies produced between mythic materials and the sufferer's physical condition (such as the analogy between mythical processes and the woman's birth canal in Levi-Strauss's [1963] classic article, "The Effectiveness of Symbols"). Efficacy is derived from ways in which analogy and metaphorical processes produce psychophysiological effects. These metaphorical effects are shaped by expectations created by ritual, cultural traditions, and the associated feelings and images.

Kirmayer (1993) reviews Dow's (1986) universal aspects of symbolic healing as involving

■ Establishment of a generalized mythic world

■ Persuasion of the patient to particularize his or her problems within that mythic world

■ Attaching the patient's emotions to the mythic world symbols

■ Manipulation of those symbols for assisting emotional transactions

For instance, a charismatic healer *establishes* a general mythic world by using ritual and prayer to evoke the image of Jesus' healing heart; *persuades* the patient to identify with the image by committing to wanting to be healed; *attaches* the patient's emotions through evoking the image of Jesus and the patient's desire for his healing power; and *manipulates* the emotional dynamics of the patient by addressing his or her traumatic memories with the felt experience of the healing power of the love of Jesus.

Kirmayer (1993) suggests that "establish, persuade, attach, and manipulate" are processes that operate at physiological, psychological, and social levels. The metaphoric concept involved in thinking about one thing in terms of something else facilitates thinking by mapping the most obvious features of one domain onto another and then transferring qualities from the new domain back to the original one. If someone says, "He is such a pig," the existing conceptual framework of the disgusting qualities of pigs is easily transferred metaphorically to the person. Metaphor integrates *sensory, affective,* and *cognitive* concepts and shapes experience through this combined information. If you are a devout Christian, what does the phrase "the healing heart of Jesus" evoke in you when you contemplate this? A *sensory* image of Jesus or the "sacred heart"? An *affective* (emotional) sense of love and warmth in your chest? A belief (cognitive) in the infinite power of Jesus to heal? These are likely to all occur or not at all; if you are a Muslim, Jew, or atheist, none of the experiences are likely to be evoked. If non-Christian, you lack a belief in the metaphoric system that Christians depend on for their integrated experience and self-transformation.

Metaphor operates through three levels: "the mythic level of coherent narratives, the archetypal level of bodily-givens, and the metaphoric level of temporary constructions" (Kirmayer, 1993, p. 170). In charismatic healing, Christianity provides relevant narratives; our emotional capacities are an archetypal basis for the experience of love and forgiveness, and the images and processes of ritual temporarily construct our sense of self in relation to the archetypal capacities (forgiving love) that are evoked by the narrative accounts incorporated into ritual.

Metaphors have power in the symbolic realm and in the physical body and society. Metaphor uses representations linking the body and society, where the archetypes[2] of the body (the innate structures of the neural and motor systems) are manipulated by cultural myths and beliefs. Myths are generally powerful tools because they are based on archetypal images such as love and involve natural processes of the body that are linked to cultural meanings. This combination of archetype and cultural myths has powerful effects because it links biological processes and experiential meanings to the conventions of society (embodied in myths), making subjective experience appear as objective knowledge. For example, the ritual processes allow others (society) to confirm the powerful emotional experiences of love (an innate or archetypal capacity).

Kirmayer (1993) suggests that metaphor, myth, and archetype represent distinct levels of meaning: social, psychological, and bodily. Each constructs a worldview that contributes to meaning. The integration of those meanings through transactions among bodily, psychological, and social processes provides mechanisms for healing. Myth organizes and structures thought and behavior through its ability to evoke and reorder experiences. Kirmayer (1993) suggests that metaphors provide for healing by

■ Implicitly structuring conceptual domains through the logic of metaphoric implication

■ Evoking strong sensory-affective associations that transform abstract constructions

■ Bridging the archetypal and mythic levels of experience

Metaphors provide new images, ones with sensory and emotional qualities that extend the capacity for empathy. The healing efficacy of myths derives from their ability to unite disparate aspects of human experience, especially deep contradictions. Archaic myths still work today when they can be interpreted in ways that tap into patients' archetypal structures and unite the abstract and concrete, the sensory and affective, and thoughts and feelings, into the same image, producing meaning and understanding (Kirmayer, 1993).

Healing uses metaphors to evoke cultural myths and link them to bodily experiences. By using the religious belief, myth, or metaphor of the "healing heart of Jesus," Catholic charismatic healers evoke a system of well-understood ideals about Jesus that then become experientially available for application to one's self, heart, and emotions. Metaphor is a tool that can create meaning by linking bodily experiences with meanings in the domain of social life. Meanings of metaphors are experienced sensorially and corporeally. What does it mean to be a "Mother Teresa"? Would being sincerely called that make you feel good or bad? If that metaphor resonates with your previous experiences and cultural values, evoking meanings of service, sacrifice, and saintliness, then reflecting on her qualities will probably make you feel good and maybe inspire some act of kindness toward others. Metaphors have a way of "penetrating": entering into our bodies and influencing our experiences and behaviors.

CHAPTER SUMMARY

Religious healing elicits top-down causation, where cultural, symbolic, and mental phenomena affect human physiology. The principal mechanisms through which they operate involve meaning, including the effects of cultural congruence and social connectedness on one's sense of well-being and, consequently, homeostatic balance in the nervous system. These symbolic effects on health are manifested in the important roles of social networks and support in maintaining health and enhancing recovery. The relationship among culture, stress, and disease shows the health effects of cultural beliefs, attitudes, and consonance. These meaningful social responses to health concerns are central to cultural healing responses and the ways in which religion and ritual affect the brain, emotions, consciousness, and other bodily processes. Cultural healing occurs through the symbolic elicitation of learned associations that link symbolic and organic processes. This biosocialization involves symbolically mediated responses to the environment that link autonomic processes, symbols, and affects (emotions) and imprint cultural schemas on the microneurological organization of the brain.

Symbolic healing uses meaning and metaphoric processes to elicit endogenous healing responses. Ritual healing practices have effects at symbolic, psychological, social, and physiological levels and on cognitive and emotional responses. Religious healing practices are able to have effects on health through the physiological consequences of meaning, assurance, and social support. These effects intervene in stress reactions and the general adaptation syndrome. Emotional and psychosocial responses are principal ways that meaning stimulates and maintains homeostasis in the nervous system. A sense of self, social attachment, and bonding form part of the linkages among affect, beliefs, and physiological responses that are manifested in cultural healing and psychoneuroimmunological responses. These are elicited by natural metaphors that blend innate representational systems of the body with our cultural beliefs and metaphors.

KEY TERMS

Autonomic nervous system

Biosocialization

Double-blind clinical trials

Endogenous healing responses

Entrainment

General adaptation syndrome

Neurognostic structures

Nocebo effects

Parasympathetic nervous system

Placebos

Psychoneuroimmunology

Social networks

Social support

Symbolic healing

Symbolic penetration

Sympathetic nervous system

Total drug effect

SELF-ASSESSMENT 8.1. PSYCHODYNAMICS OF STRESS AND WELL-BEING

Have you ever been sick because of stress? How did stress cause your illness or disease?

Have you ever used religion to help you deal with illness? What effect did it have? How did this effect occur?

Do particular behaviors or rituals make you feel better? What are they? What effects do they have on you and why?

Are there particular metaphors that you use to express your states of well-being and sickness (e.g., "strong as a horse," "sick as a dog," or "feel like a million bucks")? What do the metaphors express about your internal emotional dynamics?

Have other people's behaviors had effects on your health and well-being? What happened? How did it affect you?

Have you ever felt as though someone "hexed" you? What were the effects on you? How did you deal with them?

What are your social support resources for maintaining health and combating disease? Who can you call on if you are sick? What are the resources that others could provide you if you were ill?

ADDITIONAL RESOURCES

Books

Dohrenwend, B. P. 1998. *Adversity, stress and psychopathology.* Oxford, U.K.: Oxford University Press.

Kunitz, S. J., and J. E. Levy. 2000. *Drinking, conduct disorder, and social change: Navajo experiences.* Oxford, U.K.: Oxford University Press.

Marmor, T. R. 2000. *The politics of Medicare.* 2nd ed. New York: Aldine de Gruyter.

Rice, P. L. 1998. *Health psychology.* Pacific Grove, Calif.: Brooks/Cole.

Stimson, G., D. C. Des Jarlais, and A. Ball, eds. 1998. *Drug injecting and HIV infection: Global dimensions and local responses.* London: UCL Press.

NOTES

1. These should be technically discussed as the ergotropic system and the trophotropic system. The anatomical basis of the ergotropic system includes the sympathetic division of the ANS, the posterior hypothalamus, and portions of the endocrine system, reticular activating system, limbic system, and frontal cortex. The trophotropic system includes the parasympathetic division of the ANS, the anterior hypothalamus, and portions of the endocrine system, reticular activating system, limbic system, and frontal cortex.

2. By archetype, Kirmayer (1993) means "the bodily-given—whether rooted in the nervous system or emergent in the form and exigencies of social life. Archetype stands for subjectively compelling images/experiences that seem to be presented to us before reflection or invention" (p. 171). "Attempts to ground thought in basic physical actions also imply an archetypal basis to thought in the structure of the motor system and bodily constraints" (p. 171). Archetypes arise from the interaction of given aspects of the body with a culturally patterned environment.

CHAPTER 10

THE SHAMANIC PARADIGM OF ETHNOMEDICINE

Shamanism represents adaptive potentials, an enhanced operation of consciousness derived from integrative brain functioning . . . [I]ts potentials and processes still have important implications for humans

—WINKELMAN, 2000A, P. XIII

LEARNING OBJECTIVES

- Explain shamanism and describe its characteristics derived from cross-cultural research
- Relate universals of shamanistic practices to brain structures and functions
- Describe adaptive effects of shamans' initiatory processes and healing activities
- Analyze shamanic healing practices by the psychophysiological dynamics of altered states of consciousness, social elicitation of endogenous opioid responses, and the integrating effects of ritual
- Explain the roles of spirit concepts as psychological structures representing self, others, and psyche
- Show the manifestations of shamanic potentials in contemporary religious experiences, psychotherapy, illness, and their applications in the treatment of addictions

386 Culture and Health

WHAT IS SHAMANISM?

The nature of the shaman and shamanic practices has been subjected to much debate. Some deny the legitimacy of the concept altogether and others apply it to such numerous phenomena as to make it useless for delimiting a specific phenomenon. Understanding the nature of hunter-gatherer **shamans** and the related **shamanistic healers** found universally has faced many challenges. This difficulty derives in part from the modern origin of the concept of the shaman coming from outside Western cultures and distortions in understanding produced by Western biases and perspectives of rationalism.

Shamanistic practices involving the use of ASCs for community healing rituals are found throughout history and prehistory, but the modern impact of shamanism on the Western world began in the seventeenth century in the context of the Enlightenment (Flaherty, 1992). The modern origin of the term "shaman" in the English language is from the Tungus of Siberia; similar cognate forms of the word are found widely in Eurasian languages across language families. The accounts of Russian expeditions into Siberia that contacted these cultures brought the activities of shamanism to the attention of Europe. Reports on shamanism focused on the sensational and outlandish, producing a view of the shaman as a madman and fraud who by deceit and guile controlled a simple-minded community. This "exotic other" and its dramatic ritual activities impacted Western cultures. Shamanism came to be seen as representing an irrational side of human nature, contrasting with the rationalism of the emerging scientific ethos of Europe.

Early nonprofessional ethnographic studies of cultures with shamanistic practices led to more complete descriptions of them by the twentieth century as they were linked to practices in other parts of the world by English translations of earlier sources (see Czaplicka, 1914). Combined with a growing body of professional ethnographic data (Benedict, 1923), this led to an emerging interest in what appeared as significant cross-cultural similarities in shamanic practices: they were found in foraging (hunter-gatherer) societies all around the world. Common features of shamanistic practices in cultures around the world contributed to a growing recognition of shamanism as a universal form of religion and ritual healing intrinsically tied to human nature. For example, the role of trance, ecstasy, or ASC, a special mode of consciousness providing access to the spirit world, was recognized as central to shamans' training and healing practices. These ASCs were recognized as having biological bases, being induced by rituals and plant medicines.

Although shamanism was alien to the orientations of Western cultures, by the early twentieth century, scholars began to relate shamanism to our own past in the literary and mythological phenomena of classic antiquity and themes in theology, mythology, and literature; eventually it impacted anthropology, the other social sciences, and more recently medicine. Today, shamanism is understood as a cross-cultural phenomenon and a natural biologically based paradigm for healing processes.[1]

Ethnomedical traditions around the world persist, with practices derived from the biopsychosocial basis that also produced shamanism. The nature of this primordial spiritual healing practice is revealed by cross-cultural research that identifies the strikingly similar characteristics of spiritual healing in practices reported for hunter-gatherer societies. These similarities have their foundations in the use of ASCs, which have psychological and physiological effects that have adaptive benefits.

The adaptive basis for the ritually induced ASC is the brain response that has integrative functions. ASCs involve brain-wave discharge patterns that synchronize information processing across the levels of the triune brain (see Chapter Seven), producing an integration of the behavioral and emotional dynamics of the lower brain into the frontal cortex. Shamanic universals reflect their foundations in neurological bases of knowledge; the experiences are produced through the ritual elicitation and integration of innate capacities of the brain for representing self, others, their intentions, and the natural world. Shamanistic rituals manipulate psychobiological structures of consciousness and self-representation derived from our ancient brain structures. Ritual involves adaptive processes that are part of the animal kingdom and integrative social rituals that are an ancient part of mammalian and primate genetics. Shamanic ritual engages these and other innate capacities, particularly the visual symbolic system of dreams that provides significant representations of self, others, and emotional life. Shamanic rituals stimulate the autonomic nervous system, the basic processes of consciousness, and the associated emotional and attachment mechanisms. The stimulation of these integrative brain processes provides healing effects through a variety of mechanisms: relaxation response, psychological integration of unconscious material into consciousness, and the stimulation of endogenous healing processes. A variety of endogenous healing mechanisms are associated with the stimulation of **serotonin neural pathways** and the release of endogenous opioids provoked by the effects of ritually induced ASCs and community bonding.

These neurologically based aspects of shamanism remain in humans and continue to be manifested in contemporary religious experiences and psychological crises. The presentation of shamanic features in spiritual and illness experiences even today attests to the continued relevance of shamanism for healing processes. The contemporary application of shamanism to health problems is found in the use of drumming circles and other shamanic practices for the treatment of addiction.

Ecstasy, Spirit World, and Community

The significance of shamanism was revealed by Eliade in his (1964) *Shamanism: Archaic Techniques of Ecstasy,* which revealed its cross-cultural patterns. Eliade summarized the core of shamanism as involving the use of "techniques of ecstasy" in interaction with the spirit world on behalf of the community. The shaman's ecstatic state, which today is characterized as an ASC, was typified in an experience of magical flight, when the shaman's soul is thought to leave his body and fly to the sky or descend into the lower world (Eliade, 1974). The shaman controlled spirits to accomplish many tasks:

■ Healing, where they assisted in the recovery of lost souls and protection against spirits and sorcerers

■ Divination, clairvoyance (clear seeing), and diagnosis, where their personal animal spirits traveled to obtain information

■ Obtaining food, with their communication directing hunting activities

CASE STUDY

Shamanic Treatment of Soul Loss

To the Hmong, soul loss is a condition that can be treated by ceremonies and might even be prevented by the spirit-strings the shamans carefully tie around an infant's wrist; unfortunately, nurses often cut off what they view as filthy objects. Some family members can perform a "soul calling" ceremony to get it to return, but soul loss normally requires a professional "soul caller" (*tus hu plig*) or the most powerful of the traditional healers, the *tus txiv neeb,* or shaman. One specialization of the Hmong shaman was known as a "fixer of hearts," mending the soul that is at the core of their concepts of illness. Its loss can lead to sickness, which can be addressed by the shaman who brings the lost soul back by offering the soul of a sacrificed animal as an exchange to appease the spirits that had afflicted her.

In a ritual involving the sacrifice of several chickens or a pig, the shaman links the soul of the patient and the sacrificed animal, a bonding that makes the animal's soul an acceptable substitute for Lia Lee's soul, appeasing the afflicting spirit. The ritual for Lia was carried out on plastic tarps covering the living room floor of the Lee's house, the family gathered closely around, with the cord tied to the pig's neck also wrapped around the family, connecting their souls. Lia and the pig were bound together with twine, their souls united in a spiritual marriage. The pig's soul, released by the sacrifice, would protect them. A second pig was also sacrificed for Lia in the hope that its soul would be substituted for her soul held by the spirits.

Then the spirits were called with rattles and a gong, and on their arrival, the pig was paid with paper money for his soul and given instructions. Seated on a bench and accompanied by assistants who chant and loudly beat gongs and drums, the shaman placed his consciousness in a winged horse that could fly off in search of the lost soul. The shaman, his head covered, entered into a trance driven by the sound of the gong and rattles that carried his soul to the spirit world. Chanting and dancing, he accosted the spirits, seeking to negotiate the release of Lia's soul in exchange for that of the pig. The pig's soul was commanded to remain with the spirits in agreement for the release of Lia's soul. To complete the pact, the pig's throat was slit, its blood splattering around the room, "washing" the money and the patient.

Although Lia's soul did not return, some rituals of calling the soul back do work. Ng (2003) recounts the situation of Pa, whose soul was frightened away when FBI agents came to arrest her grandson. She eventually became comatose and was unresponsive to rituals to call her soul back. She was hospitalized, but an extensive array of diagnostic tests revealed nothing. Desperate, her husband brought in another spirit doctor. This ceremony, using gongs and cymbals to call his spirit helpers, enabled the shaman to travel through a series of gates in the unseen spirit world. There he eventually found Pa's soul and negotiated with the spirits the rituals necessary to obtain her soul's return. She recovered within the thirty days agreed on, and her family provided the requisite ceremonies and sacrifices, which cost hundreds of dollars.

Shamans' soul flights involve visionary journeys where some personal aspect—a soul, spirit, or animal familiar—enters into the spirit world. This soul flight may be in the spirit body or in the transformed guise of animals or spirit allies. In soul flight, shamans feel their spiritual body separate from their physical body, a vehicle that allows them to fly to the spiritual world. Shamans may also engage in a **soul journey** for other forms of healing or for combating spiritual forces, acquiring needed information, helping others, determining the fate of separated family members, finding lost objects, acquiring information for hunting, and escorting souls to the land of the dead. The interactions in the spirit world typically involve dramatic struggles to recover a patient's soul, which has been lost due to neglect or fright or its theft by other shamans or spirits.

The shamanic cosmos is populated by spirit entities that affect all aspects of human life and nature. The spiritual includes the essence of natural forces, humans, and other animals, especially animal spirit helpers. Animals and their spirits controlled by the shamans are the vehicles through which shamans determine the causes of illness. Through transformation into animals and soul flight, the shaman engages the spirit world, ascending into the sky, moving through the earth, and descending into the lower world. A central shamanic feature is the *axis mundi,* the "world axis," a center of the world. The axis mundi is generally symbolized by a tree, post, or pillar that connects the shaman's three worlds: sky, earth, and lower world. The axis is a portal or path along which shamans, spirits, and gods travel.

The shamanic ritual was the social activity of greatest importance in hunter-gatherer societies. It was the context for the expression of the basic cosmological, spiritual, religious, intercommunity, and healing activities. Shamanic ritual structured the relationships of the individuals to their cosmos, providing a ritual that brought the local community into an experiential interaction with the spirit world and a confirmation of their worldview. In a nighttime ceremony attended by the entire local group, the shaman enacted struggles within the spirit world, summoning spirit allies while excitedly beating drums, singing, chanting, and dancing. The group's mythological accounts are recounted as the shaman travels to the various levels of the world and engages with the spiritual powers of nature, the planet, and the cosmos. The shaman collapses exhausted and, through soul flight, enters the spirit world to address health concerns of the community.

Eliade (1964) and others (Hultkrantz, 1978; Siikala, 1978; Halifax, 1979; Harner, 1990) have considered shamanic universals to include an ecstatic state of communication with the spirit world on behalf of the community. Other universals ascribed to the shaman include

- Being found in hunter-gatherer societies
- Selection for the position through a calling by the spirits
- A vision quest
- A death-and-rebirth experience
- Soul flight
- The ability to transform oneself into an animal such as a bird or a wolf
- The use of spirits as assistants to accomplish tasks
- The potential to be a sorcerer with negative powers to make people ill or die

Shamanism as a Cross-Cultural Phenomenon

The idea that shamanism is universal was accepted before being established by systematic research. Some, however, consider shamanism to be found only in Siberia (Siikala, 1978) whereas others consider any practitioner who voluntarily enters an ASC to be a shaman (Peters and Price-Williams, 1981). Systematic cross-cultural studies illustrate empirical features of shamanism.

A Cross-Cultural Study of Magicoreligious Practitioners A scientific cross-cultural study (Winkelman, 1985, 1986b, 1990, 1992a, 2000a; see Winkelman and White, 1987, for data and methods) established universals of shamanism. This was based by evaluating a wide range of characteristics of religious practitioners, including selection and training, ASC-induction characteristics, relationships to spirit entities and powers, professional activities, healing and divination practices, and sociopolitical powers. An assessment of characteristics of religious healing practitioners around the world revealed that shamans share substantial characteristics; whether in Africa, Asia, or the Americas, hunter-gatherer societies had the same kinds of healing practitioners, which I call shamans. These empirically derived shamans differ significantly from other types of religious practitioners found in other cultures in the regions of the world. I have labeled these other kinds of empirically derived healing practitioners as shaman-healers, healers, and mediums (see Winkelman, 1992a).

Cross-Cultural Characteristics of Shamans The empirically derived characteristics of shamans elicited from cross-cultural research closely conform to Eliade's (1974) and others' descriptions. In addition to hunter-gatherer societies, shamans are found in simple agricultural (horticultural) and pastoral societies that lack political hierarchies. These societies have their organization and leadership limited to the local residential community and are not controlled by the power of a chiefdom or state. In these socially simple communities, the shaman is a highly esteemed charismatic leader. Shamans initiate the most important collective ritual activities, organize communal hunts, and decide group movement. Shamans normally provide healing on behalf of a client but typically involve the entire local community (a band) in healing rituals, including divination for a diagnosis. Shamans are also believed capable of engaging in malevolent (negative) magical acts, attacking others with spirits, sorcery, or by stealing their soul. Shamans control spirits, particularly animal spirits. A feature of the shamans' initiation is a death and rebirth experienced as dismemberment and reconstruction of the initiate's body.

ASCs are the basis for shamans' training and professional services. The spirits select shamans through the outcomes of deliberate vision quests, involuntary visions, illness, or other signs. Shamanic ASCs are generally referred to as a flight or journey but do not involve possession in which a spirit takes over and dominates the individual. ASCs are induced through a great variety of procedures, including

■ Prolonged periods of extensive exercise such as dancing and drumming

■ Periods of prolonged fasting, water deprivation, and the use of emetics

■ Exposure to temperature extremes such as staying in cold places

- Ingestion of plant medicines called hallucinogens or other psychoactive drugs

- Austerities involving cutting the body or other means of inducing pain

- Periods of prolonged social isolation and sensory and sleep deprivation

Physical Healing Shamans are generally considered spiritual healers, but they also use remedies for natural illness causation (Winkelman and Winkelman, 1991), such as

- Rubbing or massaging the body

- Sucking on the body to extract an object considered the cause of illness

- Blowing on the patient's body or fanning it with objects

- Surgical incisions into the body to extract infections and foreign objects

- Washing and cleansing the body with water or other liquids

- Administering herbal remedies or other natural substances

Biological Bases of Shamanic Universals The cross-cultural distribution of the shaman with similar characteristics, activities, and beliefs has a biological basis. Similarities such as the ASC (ecstatic) experiences, spirit world, animal powers, visionary experiences, soul journey, death-and-rebirth experiences, and healing and divination activities reflect neurological structures (Winkelman, 2000a, 2000b, 2002c, 2004b, 2006b, 2006c, 2008). Shamanism found in hunter-gatherer societies around the world reflects similarities that come from two sources: the ecological and social adaptations of hunter-gatherers and the psychobiological nature of humans involving the structures and functions of ASCs. ASCs involve an integration of brain waves and areas. This integrative brain-wave pattern is produced by high-voltage, slow-frequency brain-wave activity originating in the limbic system-brain stem connections that drive synchronizing patterns into the frontal brain (Mandell, 1980; Winkelman, 1992a, 1996a, 1997, 2000a). These synchronous brain-wave discharges across the neuraxis (the nerve bundles linking the strata of the brain) integrate the levels of the triune brain and produce a synthesis of behavior, emotion, and thought.

Shamanistic Healers Besides the universal characteristics of shamans described above, shamanistic healers also share other characteristics (Winkelman and Winkelman, 1991):

- Interpretations of illness as being based in spirits and their effects

- The use of spirit entities as projective mechanisms in therapeutic processes

- Ritual manipulations for restoring individual psychodynamics and social relations

- The attribution of the causation of illness to the ritual actions of other humans

Other shamanistic healers generally do not have specific characteristics of shamans: soul flight, transformation into an animal, control of animal spirits, the death-and-rebirth experience, or assistance in hunting. Other shamanistic healers reflect an institutionalization of practices for altering consciousness and producing healing through integrative brain functioning.

Evolution of the Shaman Shamanistic healers developed from shamanic potentials over the course of sociocultural evolution (Winkelman, 1986a, 1990, 1991, 1992a). Other types of shamanistic healers emerged as human societies shifted from the nomadic band-level hunter-gatherers into agricultural societies and later those with a hierarchical political organization and class stratification. This evolution of the other shamanistic healers from shamanism is illustrated by my cross-cultural analyses that show the relationships of different types of shamanistic healers to subsistence and social conditions. Shamans were found throughout the world, mostly in societies with hunting, gathering, or fishing subsistence patterns; a few were also associated with pastoral societies and those with simple agriculture. The transformation of shamans' practices into characteristics of shaman-healers was largely a consequence of the effects of living in sedentary agricultural societies and the resultant effects on lifestyles. The large social groups led to the development of a new level of religious practitioner, the priest, who is involved in administration societies with a political hierarchy for group integration. These new societies minimized the importance of ASCs, exemplified in the new practitioners, healers, who used rituals, spells, and amulets for healing. Mediums are also found in these societies with political integration beyond the level of the local community as well as social classes or stratification; the mediums reflect the persistence of the biological bases underlying shamanism, the capacities for using ASCs for healing (see Winkelman, 1990).

THE INTEGRATIVE MODE OF CONSCIOUSNESS

Shamanistic practices reflect operations of brain structures that are revealed by the congruencies of universal shamanic practices and experiences with brain functions. These congruencies reflect an integrative mode of consciousness, a biologically based functional system. Scientific and mystical approaches concur in the recognition of four fundamental conditions, or modes, of consciousness:

- Waking consciousness, typified by fast (beta) brain waves

- Deep sleep, characterized by the slowest (delta) brain waves

- Rapid eye movement sleep (**REM** or dreaming), a mixed brain-wave pattern

- Transpersonal, mystical, or transcendental consciousness, characterized by slow brain-wave patterns in the alpha (six to eight cycles per second) and theta (three to six cycles per second) range.

The first three modes are noted in the primary patterns of variation in brain activity, behavior, and experiences of many animals. The last mode appears to be exclusive to humans; its physiological characteristics suggest that it be referred to as "integrative consciousness" (Winkelman, 2000a).

The modes of consciousness reflect basic functions:

- Waking: learning, adaptation, and survival needs

- Deep sleep: recuperative functions, regeneration, and growth

- Dreaming: memory integration and consolidation and psychosocial adaptation

- Integrative: psychological, social, and physiological integration

Different modes of consciousness involve the activation of different physiological, personal, and social information-processing functions. Modes of consciousness manifest some variation cross-culturally but have basic similarities everywhere, reflecting underlying biological processes. There is an involvement[2] of all brain areas in all modes of consciousness. There are, however, different patterns of activation of the different neurotransmitter systems (Hobson, 1992) and elicitation of different functional systems of the brain in different modes of consciousness (Winkelman, 2000a). For instance, although the waking mode of consciousness reflects activity in the frontal lobes, the integrative mode of consciousness has extensive activation of lower centers of the brain (paleomammalian structures) and structures involved in visual processing of information. Multiple mechanisms for accessing the integrative mode of consciousness and inducing ASCs attest to their innate functional nature (Winkelman, 2000a).

All cultures recognize the integrative mode of consciousness, but they differ in support for accessing it. Some cultures vilify ASCs, considering them to be the work of the devil or evil spirits, whereas others make inducing ASCs central to religious behaviors (Laughlin et al., 1992). Cultures differ in their "psychotechnologies," methods for altering consciousness to produce a "warp" in consciousness: a conscious transition between different modes of consciousness. Accessing the integrative mode of consciousness requires entraining neural functions that normally operate outside conscious awareness or intention. Shamanistic ritual is a primary way humans discovered to control operating structures of consciousness and stimulate integrative brain operations that produce healing.

ASCs in the Integrative Mode of Consciousness

Different types of ASCs frequently noted—soul flight, possession, and meditation—refer to different *states* of consciousness within the integrative mode of consciousness. These involve the activation of different aspects of the self and emotions (Winkelman, 1997, 2000b).

Shamanic ASC The shamanic ASC occurs in a dramatic ritual encounter within the spirit world. Procedures used to induce shamanic ASCs involve extreme activation of the sympathetic nervous system through singing, drumming, and dancing. This leads to exhaustion and collapse into dominance of the parasympathetic nervous system. This state is generally accompanied by the experience of intense visual activity involving the personal soul or spirit leaving the body and encountering spirit entities. Although appearing unconscious, the shaman remembers the visionary experience. The shaman's ASC may take the form of a visit from the spirit world, transformation into an animal, or entering into the spirit world. The soul journey or flight is an essential feature of shamanism, but not all of the shaman's ASCs involve soul flight.

Possession ASCs Possession ASCs emphasize auditory (versus visionary) experiences and a "takeover" by spirits that initially occurs spontaneously. Possession ASCs are associated with amnesia and convulsions, characteristics of temporal lobe seizures that suggest a physiological basis for possession ASCs involving paleomammalian brain structures, specifically, the amygdala in the hippocamposeptal region (Wright, 1989; Mandell, 1980). Possession ASCs involve dramatic changes in identity, personality, behavior, and emotional expressions believed to result from the influence of spirits (Goodman, 1988). Cross-cultural research (Bourguignon and Evascu, 1977; Winkelman, 1986a, 1992a) shows that possession ASCs are largely found in complex societies with agriculture, class stratification, and a political system with a jurisdictional hierarchy providing political integration of local communities into larger entities. Possession ASCs generally occur in women's cults among the lower classes, who face oppressive conditions that predispose them to seizures.

Meditative ASCs There are many forms of meditative ASCs, referred to as enlightenment, satori, transcendence, bliss, and many others. Meditative states generally involve an inward focus of attention, an isolation from the external world and emotional attachments in an effort to achieve emotional calm and nonattachment to desires. Some of the classic meditative states are associated with what are considered universal mystical experiences, such as what is referred to as "cosmic unity" and "void." In cosmic unity, the person feels connected with the entire universe across time. In void experiences, there appears to be absolutely nothing at all that can be perceived or stated about the universe: nothingness. Meditative ASCs are often induced through sleep deprivation, chanting, fasting, dietary restrictions, and sensory deprivation. Meditative ASCs emphasize self-control, concentration, low arousal, emotional detachment, loss of sense of self, and content-less experience (see Winkelman, 1997).

A Physiological Model

Physiological similarities underlie ASCs induced through many procedures,[3] including

- Hallucinogens and other plant medicines

- Dancing and other forms of physical exertion and fatigue

- Auditory stimuli, including drumming, rattles, chanting, and singing

- Sensory stimulation involving austerities, such as physical stress and temperature extremes

- Sensory isolation and deprivation

- Food and water deprivation, emotional manipulations, and social isolation

ASCs' effects on the brain involve overstimulation of the sympathetic nervous system, leading to activation of the parasympathetic system and a state of extreme relaxation. Extremes of parasympathetic dominance normally occur only during sleep or coma. This typifies the shamanic soul journey, but instead of unconsciousness, self-awareness and memory persist.

ASCs involve the reduction in inhibition of the limbic area, increasing synchronous slow-frequency brain waves (especially theta). Limbic brain circuits integrate information from lower brain structures, bringing preconscious or unconscious emotions and memory into conscious awareness.

Enhanced relationships between cognitive and emotional processes and the integration of information from different functional systems of the brain are produced by ASCs. This is exemplified in the shamanic practices of coactivation of dream and waking modes. Hypnotizability also reflects these integrative brain processes of limbic-frontal integration associated with enhanced theta wave production (McClenon, 1997). The ability of highly hypnotizable people to focus on internal imagery reflects a fundamental characteristic of shamanism. Highly hypnotizable persons have great cognitive flexibility, an ability to shift awareness and cognitive strategies, become deeply engrossed in imagination, and engage in holistic information processing reflecting integration of brain systems.

Rhythmic auditory stimulation is a universal feature of shamanistic ASC induction that produces coordinated alpha and theta brain-wave patterns. Music can also reduce anxiety, increase relaxation, and facilitate the integration of unconscious information into consciousness. Music's effects reflect information processing in the right hemisphere and subcortical areas of the brain, accessing expressive capabilities that existed before spoken language (Oubré, 1997). Chanting involves an ancient audiovocal communication system that creates group solidarity by providing information about emotional states of members of the group. These expressive capacities are epitomized in the ability of songs to evoke emotions (Newham, 1994). The shamanic use of song also affects humans through symbolic meanings, linking emotions, prior experiences, and unconscious psychodynamics and producing emotional reprogramming through expression of cultural themes and motivations.

Shamanic ASC induction generally begins with food restrictions and water deprivation. Fasting induces a hypoglycemic state (low blood sugar levels) that stimulates the hypothalamus and hippocamposeptal areas, emotional control centers of the limbic system; their activation produces theta wave discharges and increases overall brain-wave synchronization. Food reductions contribute to the induction of ASCs. Shamanic practices activate the sympathetic nervous system through painful stimuli (burns, extreme cold, pain, injury, and toxic substances), leading to exhaustion and a parasympathetic dominant response. Shamanistic activities stimulate the release of endogenous opioids, the body's natural opiates, through procedures such as painful stimuli; extensive dancing and other exhaustive rhythmic physical activities (clapping); temperature extremes; emotional manipulations, especially fear and the elicitation of positive expectations; and nighttime activities when the levels of endogenous opioids are naturally highest (see Winkelman, 1997, 2000a, for reviews). The release of endogenous opioids stimulates synchronized slow-wave brain discharges. Rituals that enhance social cohesion also elicit endogenous opiates (see the section below, "Opioid Release and Emotional Healing through Community Bonding").

Shamans may use psychoactive plants to induce ASCs (Harner, 1973; Dobkin de Rios, 1984; Furst, 1976; Schultes and Hofmann, 1979; Winkelman and Andritzky, 1996; also see the special feature "Biocultural Interactions: Physiological Bases of Hallucinogens' Therapeutic Effects"). Their effects include the parasympathetic response, slow brain-wave patterns, and intense dreamlike visual imagery. These substances have a long history of use as therapeutic agents and for inducing mystical experiences. Indigenous terms for these substances often translate as "sacred plants" or "plants of the gods" (Schultes

Physiological Bases of Hallucinogens' Therapeutic Effects

Shamanistic practices sometimes incorporate plants called hallucinogens, psychedelics, or entheo-gens in training and treatment practices (Harner, 1973; Schultes and Hofmann, 1979; Dobkin de Rios, 1984; Winkelman, 1996a, 2007b). Cross-cultural uses of these substances include (Winkelman, 1996a)

- Establishing contact with the supernatural
- Healing, including death-and-rebirth experiences that provoke personal transformation
- Developing personal relationships with animal and spiritual powers and mythical reality
- Diagnosing disease and divining needed information
- Creating social solidarity and reinforcing community relations

LSD, mescaline, psilocybin, and many other hallucinogens have virtually identical clinical effects. These and the cross-cultural similarities in experiences induced by diverse substances illustrate common biological mechanisms from effects on the serotonergic neurotransmitter system (Aghajanian, 1994; Mandell, 1985). The serotonergic system mediates primary effects of these substances by reducing habitual repressions of limbic brain structures, stimulating integrative brain processes by producing synchronous slow-wave brain discharges and visions.

These substances are called "psychointegrators," reflecting their effects on both neurotransmitter processes and personal experiences (Winkelman, 1996a, 2001a, 2007a). Psychointegrators stimulate emotions and "mind, soul, and spirit," inducing an integrative experience. This integration by serotonergic stimulation of limbic system-brain stem connections enhances linkages of the ancient brains and frontal cortex. Psychointegrators stimulate memories and emotional dynamics, integrating them into consciousness. This enhances healing through the recovery of repressed memories, integrating emotional concerns with rational processes, and resolving personal conflicts.

Important variations in psychointegrator-induced experiences are influenced by individual attitude, motivation, mood, and personality factors and the characteristics of the physical and social context of use (Bravo and Grob, 1989; Yensen, 1996). Shamanistic healers ritually manipulate these personal and situational factors, integrating knowledge of the client's situation in mythological systems to shape the patient's emotions and psychology. Psychointegrators' powerful mental (set) and social (setting) effects are illustrated in the different psychotherapeutic traditions that emerged in the clinical study of LSD (see the section in Chapter Nine, "Total Drug Effects in the Social Dynamics of Psychedelic Drugs"; Yensen, 1985, 1996; Bravo and Grob, 1989), reflecting the extreme neurobiological and emotional flexibility created by psychointegrators.

Psychointegrators' therapeutic effects derive from enhanced access to traumas and conflicts underlying personal problems. Psychointegrators stimulate traumatic memories and lead to a dissolution of self, releasing egocentric fixations and enhancing access to the unconscious (see Grof, 1975, 1980, 1992; Grof and Grof, 1989). Psychointegrators reduce habituation, the lack of response to habitual stimuli, altering relations between the conscious and unconscious and producing changes in self-perception. High dosages of psychointegrators force a focus on internal images, bringing memories into consciousness, and integrating insights from preconscious levels. Stimulation of the limbic self and attachment processes facilitates management of developmental or crises-induced needs for the integration of conscious and unconscious processes.

Contemporary Applications of Psychointegrators

The current legal classification of psychointegrators as Schedule I drugs without therapeutic applications ignores clinical and cross-cultural studies that illustrate their therapeutic effectiveness. The adverse consequences reported (Burgess, O'Donohoe, and Gill, 2000; Parrott, Sisk, and Turner, 2000) involve a pattern of frequent use rather than the occasional use in traditional therapies; most reputed claims of harm from psychointegrators are unfounded, although their use should be avoided in people with specific risk profiles (Frecska, 2007). Many reports that hallucinogens cause organic damage are unfortunately lacking controls for the confounding effects of psychiatric illness and polydrug abuse (Halpern and Pope, 1999). Nonetheless, there are clear contraindications for the use of some psychointegrators (monoamine oxidase inhibitors) with serotonin reuptake inhibitors (Callaway and Grob, 1998).

Traditional patterns of use provide guidelines for therapeutic applications (see Metzner, 1998; Leary, 1997). Traditional use involved administration in periodic sessions, often involving the entire community and within a spiritual worldview. Typical traditional patterns of use involve the management of developmental change (initiation) (Dobkin de Rios, 1984), health crises, or the need to orient to changes in psychosocial relations (Andritzky, 1989).

Contemporary applications typically combine psycholytic and psychedelic approaches, first using large doses to induce transformative experiences, followed by low doses for processing psychodynamic material (Passie, 1997). The psycholytic approach uses these substances to reduce fear, inhibitions, and repressions and to promote therapeutic alliances. These substances ease memory blocks and promote catharsis (emotional release), accelerating the course of therapy. They are especially effective with chronically withdrawn patients with repressed conflicts, stimulating the dissolution of psychological defenses and heightening emotional responsiveness. The ability to relive early memories and to retain them for subsequent sessions facilitates psychotherapy. The ability to weaken defense structures makes psychointegrators useful in patients with rigid defenses, severe character neuroses, depressive and mood disorders, anxiety, and OCDs and for placing fears and emotional traumas in a more realistic perspective (see Delgado and Moreno, 1998; Greer and Tolbert, 1998).

The psychedelic model indicates that inducing mystical experiences results in profound personality changes and enhances therapeutic progress. Mystical experiences provide a sense of interconnectedness, unity, and meaningfulness, promoting a resolution of personal conflicts, and providing awareness of a sense of a higher self. These experiences give a sense of self-control and promote life changes. Psychointegrators enhance self-healing through purging negative affect and promoting psychological integration. They have also been used in ethnomedical treatments of substance dependence (Jilek, 1994; Heggenhougen, 1997).

Psychointegrators were used in many cultures as therapies and in meeting innate human drives to seek ASCs (Siegel, 1990). The innate basis suggests that there are consequences for societies that attempt to repress these substances. Ignoring and prohibiting these substances has not led to their disappearance, as illustrated in the current societal rediscovery of these practices in the use of the recreational drug Ecstasy (also known as MDMA) and at raves. The need to address these issues with an informed approach derived from cross-cultural ethnomedical uses is emphasized by their continued use.

and Hofmann, 1979). Ethnographic, clinical, and laboratory studies[4] illustrate evidence of the therapeutic effectiveness of these agents for the treatment of a wide variety of psychological and physical conditions. Support for claims of therapeutic effectiveness are also found in laboratory evaluations, clinical studies, and other forms of data on LSD and many other psychedelics (see Winkelman and Roberts, 2007a, 2007b; Passie, 1997). I have detailed the biochemical basis of the effects on perceptual, cognitive, and emotional experiences elsewhere (1996a, 2001a, 2007a), and they are discussed in Chapter Nine (in the section "Total Drug Effects in the Social Dynamics of Psychedelic Drugs") and below.

Dreams and Shamanic Consciousness

Shamanic practices integrate the dreaming and waking modes of consciousness[5] (Winkelman, 2000a; Peters, 1989). Nighttime ritual activities deliberately blend dreaming and waking modes, with ritual activities before sleep, reducing barriers to the awareness of dream experiences. This practice reflects physiological effects of dreams that facilitate induction of the integrative mode of consciousness. Sleep induces parasympathetic dominance and other characteristics typical of ASCs, including vivid imagistic experiences and changes in sense of self. Dream patterns are similar to those of hallucinogens, evoking visual imagery and slow brain waves (Mandell, 1980). Dreams involve a presentational or visual mode of symbolic information (Hunt, 1995). They involve the closest contact of the ego with the unconscious (Laughlin et al., 1992) and reflect an "unconscious personality" and its emotional needs (Winson, 1985).

Evolutionary perspectives on dreams and their functions illustrate the role of dream processes in integrative consciousness. Most mammals dream (Graham, 1990), reflecting brain functions that emerged about 140 million years ago as a mammalian adaptation to integrating learning through "off-line processing"; this is achieved by using the frontal cortex as an association area for consolidating memories during REM sleep (Winson, 1985, 1990). Dreams involve an ancient neural information system, limbic structures (hippocampus and amygdala), that are core processing areas for the assessment of emotional associations, transferring experience from short-term to long-term memory, and the formation of strategies (Graham, 1990; Winson, 1985). Dream (or REM) sleep is an activated state of hyperorientation. REM sleep is like a paralyzed hallucinatory state, with sensory structures functioning with internal input but with inhibition of the muscle system, allowing for intentional behavior without bodily movement. Dream sleep involves intense lower-brain processes that suggest the active rehearsal of behavior patterns.

REM sleep engages presentational symbolic capabilities (Hunt, 1995), a system of information processing based in visual images. Dream characteristics of imagery, emotion, and visual symbols are cognitive processes of this presentational modality, a symbolic and abstract intelligence involving analogic (metaphoric) thought. This visual symbolic system is normally inhibited by left hemisphere verbal systems. The internal orientation of dreams (and ASCs) allows for the expression of this presentational intelligence based on a fusion of visual imagery, spatial orientation, and bodily information. Dreams' predominantly visual (as opposed to verbal) qualities reflect this visuospatial intelligence that uses analogic reasoning organized on the basis of similarity (Hunt, 1989; Hobson and Stickgold, 1994). Dream images reflect the operation of a nonlanguage symbolism that is at the root of all symbolic intelligence (Hunt, 1989, 1995).

In dreaming, right hemisphere presentational capacities dominate due to restrictions on the left hemisphere, resulting in the noted cognitive deficits of dreaming (Blagrove, 1996). Dreams' single-minded awareness reflects an impairment of voluntary attentional mechanisms, critical self-reflective awareness, and the awareness of contradiction (Blagrove, 1996). Ordinary dreams lack conscious awareness and intentionality and generally have amnesia, a failure to transfer dream memory content to waking consciousness.

In contrast, shamanic ASCs reflect conditions more like waking consciousness and reflection and the daydreamer's engagement with fantasy: the ability to exercise conscious control and reconsider scenarios or possibilities. Shamanistic traditions provide technologies for transferring information back into waking consciousness through dream incubation and other ASCs before or during sleep, engagement in ASCs during ordinary periods of sleep (overnight rituals), and stimulation of the sympathetic nervous system and its arousing properties during extremely relaxed states. Ritual activities enhance the transfer between modes of consciousness, integrating self-conscious aspects of identity with processes of the paleomammalian brain and its management of emotions and self. Properties of shamanic ASCs are illustrated in lucid dreams, in which the dreamer is aware of being in a dream (LaBerge, 1985; Gackenbach and LaBerge, 1988). Lucid dreams involve waking faculties such as reason, memory, reflection, and volition, yet also have physiological, experiential, and cognitive characteristics similar to the spontaneous meditative states of yogis and the soul flight of shamanic traditions (Hunt, 1989).

Functions of Shamanic ASCs

Human cognitive capacities evolved through specialized brain-processing modules (Mithen, 1996), leading to an increased fragmentation of consciousness. Shamanism engaged healing ("wholing") by integrating consciousness through rituals that produce integrative brain states. As noted above, shamanic rituals produce such integration across functional levels of the brain (Winkelman, 2000a, 2002b, 2002c). Healing is produced by eliciting paleomammalian brain processes to manipulate emotions, attachments, and sense of self. The ritual manipulation of specialized brain modules for representing self, others, and nature in visual symbols produces metaphoric representations at the core of shamanism:

■   The conceptualization of "others" as embodied in the spirit world (**animism**) and in totemism

■   The construction of self as exemplified in soul flight and the guardian spirit complex

■   The visionary state, a presentational mode (Hunt, 1995) of symbolic expression

Shamanism served a central role in cognitive evolution (Winkelman, 2002a) through

■ Activation of basic brain structures, producing synchronization across levels of the brain

■ Metaphoric (analogic) and visual representations (visions)

■ Socioemotional processes and their psychological and physiological effects on healing

The induction procedures of ASCs have effects on emotions, unconscious mental processes, and identity. The triune brain module (MacLean, 1990, 1993) provides a framework for explicating the functional aspects of ASCs. They enhance the integration of instinctual behavioral responses of the reptilian brain with emotional processes of the paleomammalian brain and the cognitive processes of the neomammalian brain. ASCs involve integrative consciousness, synchronizing behavioral, emotional, and mental levels and evoking emotional mentation processes that manage social identity, bonding, and attachment.

Shamanic universals reflect biological structures of identity and social relations produced through a metaphorical integration of innate processing modules for knowledge about mind, social relations (self and others), and the animal world. Metaphoric representations are reflected in animism, guardian spirits, and the soul journey. Shamanic rituals and activities integrate the functions of **innate modules:** anatomical structures and functional systems of the brain with specific information-processing functions (e.g., the language module and self-recognition module). Other innate modular structures elicited by shamanic practice involve those for processing perceptions of the other, their intentions (mind reading), and animal species (natural history). Shamanism elicits and combines these innate representational processes to produce these metaphoric representations of the identity of self and others, such as the use of animals to represent self (animal powers) and social groups (totemic animals, such as the "bear clan").

These enhanced self and social representations provide adaptive advantages in personal development, social integration, and psychological healing. These are derived from information integration provided in visions and expressed through emotions, facial expressions, behaviors, and gestures. This emotional mentation provokes physiological changes through the meaning for self and interpersonal attachments: for instance, when one is empowered by having "bear power" or feels social inclusion in a bear clan. These socioemotional processes can counter the effects of illness produced through self-doubt, anxiety, fear, and social isolation. Shamanic healing practices involve a holistic imperative, a drive toward more integrated consciousness (Laughlin et al., 1992).

Shamans use symbols and ritual to engage transformative processes, entraining neurological and cognitive structures to restructure the self. These psychodynamic transformations produce integration at psychological, social, affective, and physiological levels. These are based in shamanic projection (unconscious transference of control of individual intentional processes) and role-taking techniques that involve spirit world representations that alter relationships between self and others.

Shamanism also provides resources for intensifying community and intercommunity alliances (Hayden, 1987, 2003). Shamanic ritual intensifies interpersonal bonding, within-group cohesion, and interband alliances through producing a sense of unity and panhuman identity. Such emotional bonds and interband alliances contributed to survival in times of resource scarcity because intense emotional bonding strengthened commitment to others and a willingness to assist them in times of need. This bonding was enhanced by the elicitation of opioid and serotonergic mechanisms through ritual activities.

NEUROGNOSTIC STRUCTURES

Shamanic universals involve innate brain processes, or neurognostic structures, forms of knowledge provided by the biological structures and functions of the organism (Boyer, 1992; d'Aquili and Newburg, 1999; Laughlin et al., 1992; Winkelman, 2000a). These structures underlie ASCs, spirit beliefs, visionary perceptions, soul flight, and death-and-rebirth experiences (Winkelman, 2000a). Innate brain modules of particular relevance to shamanistic healing include automatic information-processing capacities for a knowledge of natural history domains (animal behavior), recognizing self and social others, and an interpersonal psychology for mind-reading others' intentions. The metaphoric integration of the processing capacities of the different innate modules is proposed as the basis for shamanic universals (Winkelman, 2000a, 2002b). Abilities for mind-reading others' intentions, recognizing social others and the self, and a knowledge of animal behavior provided foundations for

- Anthropomorphic thinking: attributing human mental and social characteristics to animals, including animism, and applying human mental models to produce perceptions of spirits

- Guardian spirits: applying the concepts of animals to interpret and differentiate self

- Totemism: applying animal species models to the social domain

Shamanic engagement of these modules is exemplified in shamans' skills in

- Self-management, exemplified in identities developed in animal powers and guardian spirits

- Natural history, or being the master of the game animals

- Social intelligence, as in being the leader of the group and mediator of intergroup relations

These forms of metaphoric thinking created mechanisms for creative thought by providing new ways of processing existing knowledge and forming representations. These metaphoric processes produce cognitive, psychological, and social integration by providing models for conceptualizing self, others, and self-development.

Meaning is constructed through the use of metaphor, particularly analogic models that map relations between systems, allowing for representation of the unknown as something more familiar (Shore, 1996). For example, if someone says, "He is such a snake," your understanding of snakes and their dangerous properties leads you to infer that this person is dangerous. Basic metaphoric processes are involved in the central representations of shamanic thought, as revealed in their relationship to foundational metaphors (Friedrich, 1991). Shamanic universals have bases in these contiguity, modal, and imagistic metaphors that reflect underlying biological structures of representation. The body and its ability to act are the most fundamental of analogic schema (Newton, 1996; Hunt, 1995; Laughlin, 1997), manifesting metaphoric processes in mimesis (full-body imitation) as a natural symbolic system. This body-based reference for experience is exemplified in the shaman's soul journey or soul flight, conceptualized in contemporary cultures as an *out-of-body* experience. The most fundamental of shamanic ASCs both references the body and establishes a perspective or point of view apart from the body. Contiguity metaphors based in the body and animals are at the basis of shamanic thought and are manifested in sympathetic magic, animal powers, and totemism. Imagery metaphors are exemplified in visionary experiences, a use of presentational symbolism (Hunt, 1995) that links different domains of experience through information processing involving images.

This capacity for representation through reference to the body embodied in mimesis evolved before modern human cognition (Donald, 1991). Mimesis derived from the ability to produce intentional representations of events through mimicry and imitation, perhaps beginning with the acting out of successful hunts or other dramatic experiences. The mimetic representational system, the basis of the first human culture, persisted as a communication and representational system after the development of language. Mimesis operates in expressive social interchange, emotional communication, and modeling social roles through facial expressions, gestures, and movements. Mimesis is manifested in rhythmic abilities such as drumming, dancing, and imitative performances. It is still a significant system for symbolic communication today, reflected in the concept of body language.

Animism: Spirits as Self and Other

At the basis of shamanism is animism: the spirit world. These systems of meaning have structures and functions that reflect human psychological, social, and biological needs for concepts of self and socially referenced others. Spirits reflect a personality model and a theory of the fundamental aspects of consciousness. Shamanism uses spirit constructs to represent personal, intrapsychic, and social dynamics. Spirit beliefs produce psychophysiological manipulations through their meanings and attachments, including the management of emotions, construction of relations between self and others, and the use of these systems to alter emotions.

Animism, a universal aspect of human culture and religion, involves the attribution of humans' intentional abilities and other cognitive and self qualities to animals and nonphysical entities. We have a tendency to personify the physical world with the attribution of human characteristics. Storms seem "angry," even through they do not have emotions. **Anthropomorphism,** attributing humanlike mind characteristics to gods, spirits, and nonhuman entities (particularly animals), exemplifies animism. We think our pet cats love us, although such elevated human sentiments are beyond their capabilities. This postulation of unseen humanlike beings—spirits and gods—that motivate the behaviors of the universe reflects the projection of self: qualities of humans and our mental and personal characteristics and desires. This universal cognitive strategy to conceive of the unknown as being like ourselves helps ensure that we respond to the most important contingencies affecting our survival: those with humanlike capabilities (Guthrie, 1993, 1997).

This projection of the self as a model of the unknown other is a basic manifestation of symbolic capabilities (Hunt, 1995) and a universal relational mode based on the grounding of perception of the world through relationships with the environment (Bird-David, 1999). Animistic agents manifested in guardian spirits and sacred others reflect a natural social and relational epistemology derived from social intelligence, the ability to infer the mental states of others. This social intelligence uses a "theory of mind," or mind-reading, an intuitive psychology based in the organism's use of its own mind and feelings to construct a model of others' likely thoughts and behaviors. The world is like us.

Animistic concepts provide a natural symbolic framework for representing the internal psychodynamics of self and other social beings (Winkelman, 2004a). Spirits represent aspects of the person conceptualized in psychology as features of personal and social identity, such as the self, id (unconscious emotional impulses), ego, and superego (moral standards); emotions and drives; social motivations; obsessions; and other psychodynamic processes and complexes. Psychological functions of spirit concepts are exemplified in the guardian spirit complex (Swanson, 1973). Spirits play a fundamental role in representing social relations and in formulating the self. Spirit concepts provide symbolic representations of social groups and their norms, attitudes, values, morals, purposes, motivations, goals, and relations.

Animistic principles are "superpersons" that provide models for identity. They are key to the formation of individual and communal identities in totemism. Totemism and animal spirit identities involve the metaphoric representation of the self and social others with the natural history module. Taxonomic classification schemas for the natural world provide a metaphoric system for the creation of meaning. Totemism involves a metaphoric relationship between the natural history and social domains, where humans and their groups are attributed characteristics from the natural world (Levi-Strauss, 1962). Totemism represents human commonalities and differences through models provided by animal species, which provide characterizations of social and personal identities.

Guardian Spirit Quest The vision quest (or guardian spirit quest) involves seeking spirit relations; it was the most fundamental and widespread religious complex of Native American cultures (Swanson, 1973) and hunter-gatherer societies around the world (Winkelman, 1992a). This involves seeking a personal relationship with a spirit as a central aspect of developing adult skills and competencies. Training for the vision quest traditionally began as young as six or seven years old with instruction on behavior for attracting guardian spirits. Extreme pain—purgatives, prolonged fasting, psychoactive plants, temperature extremes, extensive physical exercise, whipping and scourging the body, and self-inflicted wounds—provoked visionary experiences of the spirit world. The spirits provided powers, often represented in objects symbolizing the power source (e.g., a feather from an eagle). Guardian spirits assist in personal and social choices for adult development and the formation of aspects of one's personal power and identity. For example, eagle power gives one keen eyesight and swiftness; with mouse power, one might be expected to develop the ability to hide inconspicuously and be unobtrusive.

Incorporating animal spirits as part of one's identity reflects a form of self-representation embodied in shamanistic thought, that of the sacred other (Pandian, 1997). This intersection of the spiritual and social worlds involves cultural processes for the production of the symbolic self through incorporation of others. Beliefs about spirit entities can provide projective systems that structure individual psychodynamics and behavior. If one acquires lion power, for instance, one knows what is expected to be personal development goals based on the characteristics of the lion: ferocious, violent, and brave. Spirit identities activate social and self modules, providing alternate forms of personal identity. These alternate identities provide a new point of reference for problem solving and psychosocial adaptation (Waller, 1996; Scheff, 1993). For instance, how might a lion (versus a mouse) solve this problem? Spirit concepts provide the self with different command-control agents that can mediate conflict within a hierarchy of social and personal goals. For instance, one might be inclined to act in one's best interest, but personal identification with membership in the bear clan reminds one to think about the well-being of all bear clan members. Shamanism provides the opportunity to construct and manipulate a variety of self-concepts to produce personal, psychological, and social integration.

Animism, totemism, and guardian spirits are natural symbolic systems derived from our innate capacities; through ritual, they become combined in new ways that allow for differentiation of the self and its development in relationship to others. Differentiation occurs when one encounters one's own special power, such as a lion as an animal ally, and can develop new self-characteristics. When initiated into the bear clan, one has a new identity linked to membership with other bear clan members.

Visionary Experiences and Healing

Central to shamans' activities are internal visions, exemplified in soul flight where intense visual experiences provide a sense of entry into and interaction with the spirit world. Shamanic development focuses on "mental-imagery cultivation" (Noll, 1985) in ASCs, training experiences that allow an individual to develop control over the production of these internal visual experiences. Through practice, a person learns how to use them to enter into interaction with the spirit world. These visionary experiences are natural phenomena of the central nervous system that result from disinhibition in the regulation (suppression) of the visual cortex. This visionary world has adaptive advantages, with these internal images used for analysis, synthesis, diagnosis, future planning, and psychological manipulations. Internal images reflect an innate cognitive capacity for producing representations from the mind's own materials and through its own agency. Imagery employs a substrate of the visual system shared with perceptual information (Baars, 1997).

Imagery plays a role in cognition, integrating different domains of experience and levels of information processing. Mental imagery activates psychophysiological processes at the emotional levels, linking somatic and cognitive levels. Inner images are a form of biological communication reflecting basic principles of neural organization and involving a preverbal symbol system that acts directly on the physiological substrate outside of deliberation and consciousness (Achterberg, 1985). Images play a central role in muscular control, representing goals and recruiting and coordinating a wide range of unconscious biological systems. They also stimulate sympathetic activation and the parasympathetic system's relaxation response. "Imagery seems to be the only conscious modality that can trigger autonomic process" (Baars, 1997, p. 141). Shamans' visionary experiences engage this imagistic capacity, eliciting neurologically based representations of the fundamental forces of life and death, self and others, and the dynamics of emotional and social life.

CULTURE AND HEALTH

Imagery in Catholic Charismatic Healing

In Catholic charismatic healing, internal images play important roles in diagnosis and healing. Images are considered important revelatory information, communication from the body that is embodied and reflected in a "presentational immediacy" in consciousness (e.g., presentational symbolism). Images are evocative and allusive, linking the past and present, self and others, and mind and body in ways that allow for the reconstruction of memories. The repressed dynamics created by trauma are revealed in these images. Retrieval of traumatic memories from the subconscious can heal by releasing emotional blockages. Evoking these memories in the presence of divinity can neutralize the emotions and provide them with new meanings. These images also play a central role in the development of an identity as a charismatic Catholic, which provides the person with healing experiences. This requires a personal relationship with Jesus manifested in visions that reveal spiritual gifts, provide inspiration, and produce a new sense of self. Csordas (1994) considers this to be the "real self," involving "genuine intimacy with a primordial aspect of the self" (p. 157). "The vivid presence of Jesus in imaginal performance is a culturally specific way to . . . provid[e] an ideal other" (p. 158). The images involve a special relationship between memory and self that removes suffering through the creation of a positive sacred self. Imagery reveals the conflicts and the dynamics of the true self that must be addressed to heal these earlier developmental traumas. Images of divinities, particularly Jesus, play roles as "internalized others" that facilitate the resolution of developmental blockages produced by trauma. Csordas characterizes divine images such as Jesus as models that are used in the development of a mature self.

Shamanic Flight as a Body-Based Experience

The shamanic soul journey or flight (also referred to as an out-of-body experience and "astral projection") exemplifies this imagistic symbolic modality. Soul flight is manifested cross-culturally because it is based in innate psychophysiological structures and reflects homologies across symbolic, somatic, and physiological systems (Hunt, 1995; Laughlin, 1997). These soul-flight experiences, in which an individual senses some separation of an aspect of personal identity from one's body, may occur spontaneously in near-death or clinical-death experiences. In these cases, on recovery from a severe injury or temporary cessation of heartbeat or respiration, such people report that they experienced a separation from their body, a sense of floating away from their physical form. It is also easily produced among contemporary people who engage in shamanistic practices. The similarities in deliberate and spontaneous experiences indicate that soul flight reflects innate psychophysiological processes involving innate modular structures of the brain and consciousness.

Soul flight is a symbolic representation of the shaman's transcendence. The flight itself involves a movement into the heavens or the spirit world, reflecting the shaman's transformation to higher levels of consciousness. This concept is reflected in the linguistic roots of ecstasy, from the Greek *ekstasis,* meaning "to stand outside oneself." The shamanic flight also engages the human capacity to take the role of the other toward self. This involves the ordinary psychosocial processes through which we construct a model of our own self that is derived from an awareness of others' perceptions of our self. These perspectives, based on the inferred perceptions of others, assist in the formation of self-representations and provide new forms of self-awareness derived from referencing ourselves to others' views.

Laughlin (1997) assesses the body image as a natural symbolic system, an innate module for organizing both internal and external experiences. This body image develops under sociocultural influences but is largely based in hardwired programs that constitute a neurological foundation for human experience. Body-based principles are the foundation of all knowing (Newton, 1996) and a principal aspect of foundational metaphors and analogic thinking (Friedrich, 1991). Body-based representational systems are universal because they reflect the natural use of the body to understand attributes of the world. Body models provide a symbolic system for all levels of organization, from metabolic levels through self-representation and advanced conceptual functions (Laughlin, 1997).

Body images combine memory, perception, affect, and cognition in an image-based symbolic information system that Hunt (1995) refers to as "presentational" symbolism. A skull reflects a natural presentational symbol of death; it requires no abstract interpretation but visually screams "death" to us. The concept *presentational* refers to the meanings derived from the immediate experience, rather than their symbolic representational forms exemplified in language. This integration of visual image and bodily sensations reflects a capacity for metaphoric representation across sensory modalities that is the foundation of symbolic thought (Hunt, 1995). Presentational symbolism has a greater immediate capacity than verbal activity for presenting information, expressed in the saying "A picture is worth a thousand words." This reflects the ability of the presentational mode to maximize use of the symbolic capacity in the imagistic-intuitive mode, where a single glance at a scene (or picture) can immediately convey an understanding that might take paragraphs to adequately describe in words. These presentational experiences are often considered more real than ordinary reality, reflecting access to integrative consciousness and its enhanced potentials for uniting conscious and unconscious knowing processes. This integration of the unconscious has the power to produce self-transformative experiences and the acquisition of a new identity, exemplified in the shaman's death-and-rebirth experience.

Shamanic Initiatory Crisis: Death and Rebirth

Spirit world interactions that stimulate psychological development are exemplified in a universal aspect of shamanism, the death-and-rebirth experience. Seeking of the shamanic role is often motivated by a psychological crisis characterized by illness or insanity provoked by the spirits who have selected the individual to be a shaman. This crisis generally leads the initiate to experiences interpreted as death. They may occur spontaneously or in cultures where people actively engage in the shamanic vision quest, and this death-rebirth experience occurs in the context of training. In either case, the death-rebirth crisis typically involves a sequence of illness and suffering from attacks by spirits that leads to an experience of bodily death and dismemberment. The dismemberment generally takes place following a descent to the lower world, where spirits, often in animal form, attack and destroy the victim. Subsequently, they reconstruct the pieces, adding their powers to the reborn shaman.

These initiatory experiences have been characterized as involving neurosis, psychosis, and hysteria. This is a misunderstanding, reflecting ethnocentric attributions of pathology to ASCs by using views of normalcy referenced to the rationality of ordinary consciousness. These experiences are not schizophrenic or derived from other pathologies (Noll, 1983) but do involve emotional turmoil and distress that may entail a temporary crisis resembling a brief reactive psychosis (Walsh, 1990). In some cultures, shamanic initiatory experiences are evaluated as pathological, but the general expectation is that they are the basis for important personal development.

The shaman's death-rebirth initiatory crisis involves natural symbolic forms of self-reference and self-development. The death-rebirth phenomenon is manifested cross-culturally because it reflects natural processes of self-transformation that occur under conditions of overwhelming stress and the fragmentation of the ego that results from internal conflict (Walsh, 1990). Shamans are often driven to their profession by a chronic illness or affliction, and its resolution requires that they become new kinds of people—healers—to overcome their own health problems. Consequently, a "death" of their current identity (as a "normal" but ill person) is necessary for a new identity to develop as a healer. The dismemberment experiences they see are "autosymbolic images" reflecting breakdown and disintegration of their own psychological structures and senses of self (Laughlin et al., 1992).

The death-rebirth cycle reflects, first, the fragmentation and, second, reformation of the self. This process of psychological transformation results from the inability of the psyche to maintain its integrity. Conflicts lead to destruction of the ego, experienced symbolically as death; rebirth reflects a psychological reorganization. These reformulations of the self are guided by innate drives toward psychological integration. The threatening and destroying spirits are symbolic representations of aspects of the self that are not useful for the new identity.

Shamanic development involves manipulation of symbolic constructs and neurological structures to restructure the ego, producing changes in attachments, affect, and other psychological processes. Shamanic development transforms the self, producing a restructuring at a new level of identity. Restructuring of the ego is promoted by holistic imperatives toward psychointegration, providing a dramatic alleviation of psychosomatic and emotional problems. This self-transformation produces the widely reputed exceptional health of shamans through their **individuation** and self-actualization.

Shamans as Psychopaths? Despite the similarity between shamanistic ASCs and some pathological states (see Ackerknecht, 1943; Silverman, 1967; Noll, 1983; Siikala, 1978; Hultkrantz, 1978), evidence indicates that shamanic experiences are not pathological. Shamans are generally among the healthiest and best-adjusted members of their culture and are not seen as pathological from the perspectives of their own culture. A central difference is the voluntary nature of the shamanic ASC and the deliberate actions taken to induce it that makes it distinct from the involuntary conditions experienced by a person suffering from a psychopathologic disorder. Differences in characteristics of shamanic states and schizophrenia refute arguments that acute schizophrenia underlies shamanic ASCs (Noll, 1983). Shamanism differs from schizophrenia in the different kinds of experiences and responses, including

- Volition, the willful entry into the ASC

- The shaman's continued social functions and deliberate communication during an ASC

- The shaman's ability to discriminate shamanic experiences from those of everyday life

Even when ASCs include hallucinatory experiences, the experiential qualities of shamanic ASCs differ sharply from those of schizophrenia. Shamanic ASCs involve the expression of positive affective experiences and intensification of emotion, in contrast to the emotional flattening of schizophrenia. The shaman's considerable skill in emotionally manipulating patients contrasts with the schizophrenic's lack of control.

Epilepsy has been attributed to shamanic ASCs because of shaking, tremors, and seizures. Epilepsy refers to disorders characterized by electrical discharge patterns, generalized symptoms of the brain's failure to inhibit normal discharge patterns. Seizure characteristics are found in shamans only during ASC induction and not at other times, rejecting an organic explanation for their presence in shamans. Dissociative disorders such as hysteria and hysterical neurosis often attributed to shamanism have clinical characteristics that do not correspond to shamanic ASCs. For instance, the loss of conscious awareness and amnesia characteristic of hysterical neurosis is not found in shamanic ASCs.

CULTURE AND HEALTH

Healing the Catholic Psyche of Unwanted Others

Catholic charismatic healing involves relationships with "unwanted others," reflected in the movement's concern with demonology and its implications for the self. The characteristics of these evil beings reflect the negative attributes of the person. Demonic spirits are believed to attach to the patient, bonding undesirable behaviors and emotions that must be severed to heal the patient. These evil beings are conceptualized as "persons" and "intelligent entities" whose qualities, reflecting sins and negative emotions, are represented in their names: greed, lust, anger, bitterness, and jealousy. Demonic possession involves a loss of control exhibited in the negative behaviors that the demonic entities produce in a person. These negative aspects are disowned, viewed as not-self, and dissociated from personal identity in the process of attributing one's unwanted behaviors to the effects of the demonic entity. Nonetheless, their effects on the person illustrate a crisis of control, a contested self. The effects of the demonic spirits provide insight into the cultural concerns about afflictions to the self. The nature of one's problem is manifested in the qualities of these demonic spirits, exhibited indirectly in mannerism and mood of the patient, including facial and eye expression and bodily posture.

BASES FOR SHAMANISTIC THERAPIES

The therapeutic mechanisms of shamanistic healing are embodied in the major foci of Eliade's (1964) classic characterization of the shaman as using ecstatic states (ASCs) on behalf of the community and in interaction with the spirit world. ASCs, community, and spirits have mutually reinforcing effects in enhancing health. Shamanic ASCs produce physiological changes, inducing the relaxation response and psychophysiological integration. The spirit world and community provide social support and models for personal development. The spirit world plays a role as sacred others, representing self and aspects of the psyche. Shamanistic therapeutics elicit the psychobiological dynamics of ASCs and community bonding, stimulating neurological responses through enhanced serotonergic action and endogenous opioid release, as described in the following sections.

Physiological Basis of Shamanistic Therapies

Shamanistic healing practices are universal because their therapeutic effects derive from biological mechanisms of ASCs (see Winkelman, 1986a, 1992a, 1996a, 1997, 2000a). Physiological aspects of ASCs—parasympathetic dominance, interhemispheric synchronization, and limbic-frontal integration—have therapeutic effects. These therapeutic effects involve actions of the paleomammalian brain areas that

- Induce synchronized brain waves integrating functional levels of the brain

- Mediate the balance between the sympathetic and parasympathetic divisions of the ANS

- Enhance emotional balance, self-integration, and positive social attachment

These physiological changes facilitate healing through a variety of mechanisms:

- Inducing physiological relaxation and reducing tension, stress, anxiety, and phobic reactions

- Accessing unconscious information and integrating it into consciousness

- Enhancing behavioral-emotional-cognitive integration

- Enhancing the positive emotional aspects of social bonding and affiliation

The parasympathetic dominant state produced by ASCs involves the basic relaxation response of the organism, which has therapeutic value in diseases involving increased sympathetic nervous system activity, such as hypertension and other stress-related conditions. Rapid collapse into a parasympathetic dominant state can have therapeutic effects through the erasure of conditioned responses, inducing dramatic changes in beliefs, and increasing suggestibility and placebo and psychosomatic effects. ASCs activate unconscious processes associated with the paleomammalian brain, making it possible to integrate normally repressed material into the conscious mind. These repressed dynamics are the source of conflicts and self-defeating tendencies that have effects on emotions and physiological responses.

Shamanic ASCs enhance the expression of repressed aspects of the self by both reducing left hemispheric dominance and permitting the expression of right hemispheric and lower brain processes. Shamanic rituals reprogram the emotional dynamics of the lower brain through the material embodied in the chants, songs, and dramatic enactments that change perceptions of self, social relations, and emotions.

Music and Dance as Expressive Therapies Shamanic healing involves expressive therapies such as music, singing, and dance. Expressive activities have a variety of healing effects: "art, music, dance, drama, humor, spirituality, . . . and social rituals can evoke immediate early gene protein cascades to optimize brain growth, mind-body communication, and healing" (Rossi, 2000, p. 198). Singing and chanting, universal aspects of shamanic ritual, reflect a human capacity for music that has deep evolutionary roots (Oubré, 1997) based in innate brain modules (Molino, 2000). Human musical expressions have their progenitors in the calls, expressive systems, and group enactment activities of other primates. These affective vocalizations involve states of high arousal that communicate important information for other members of the species (Geissmann, 2000), including affective states, social contact, interpersonal attraction, and group cohesion.

Music is part of a larger group of cultural activities such as chanting, singing, poetry, dancing, and play that share origins in innate modules that provide rhythm, affective semantics, and melody (Molino, 2000; Donald, 1991). These brain modules provide an expressive system that predates language. Music and dance appear to have coevolved as uniquely human capabilities (Freeman, 2000) based on the common feature of rhythm. These signaling systems are adaptations to enhance social bonding and communication of internal states. Music's adaptive roles include its ability to promote group cohesion and coordination, enhancing synchrony and cooperation among group members, and providing a mechanism for coordinating cognitive and emotional expression (Brown, 2000; Merker, 2000).

BIOCULTURAL INTERACTIONS

"Old-Time Religion" in the Management of African American CVD

Religion is widely recognized for its role in managing psychological and emotional distress; it is also increasingly recognized for its possible roles in managing and preventing disease. Jacobs (2005) illustrates the many mechanisms through which the healing characteristics of the evangelical Protestant churches operate: emotionality, positive prophecy, manifestations of inspiration in prayer, testimonies of healing, uplifting music, inspirational reading of Scriptures, preaching and singing, and a popular engagement (call and response) between the preacher and the congregation. The highly emotional services reinforce a charismatic atmosphere in which religious healing may address physical, psychological, social, and spiritual problems. The role of religious healing in successfully addressing African American hypertension and CVD is illustrated by Koenig, McCullough, and Larson (2001), who state "There is growing evidence that involvement in organized religion can . . . help reduce the negative consequences of stress on blood pressure" (p. 263). Church-based health interventions not only can address CVD and other chronic illness but also are generally successful in changing high-risk behaviors such as being overweight and smoking: "Thus, it appears that church-based weight control and blood pressure programs can have a significant impact on both treatment and prevention of hypertension in African Americans" (p. 263). In *Religion in the Lives of African Americans,* Taylor, Chatters, and Levin (2003) examine the ways in which religion has played a role as a vital coping strategy for African Americans. They review a wide range of empirical literature illustrating the significant role of religion in addressing both psychological and physical health problems. In addition, the ability of religion to address stress, mobilize social support, and provide emotionally uplifting messages means that it is an important ethnomedical resource in combating CVD.

Opioid Release and Emotional Healing Through Community Bonding

The shaman's interaction with spirits is on behalf of a *community,* generally involving participation of the entire local residential group. This community presence enhances healing by reintegrating a patient into the social group. Community participation facilitates therapeutic effects derived from psychobiological influences, social support, and physiological effects derived from the opioid-attachment and immune responses. Ritual groups can produce healing by providing a sense of belonging, euphoria, and omnipotence that reflects activation of the body's own opioids, or endorphins. Shamanic practices involve psychobiologically mediated attachment processes that are based in the social elicitation of endogenous opioid mechanisms associated with maternal-infant bonding (Frecska and Kulcsar, 1989). Opioid release is produced by emotionally charged cultural symbols that are associated during developmental learning with patterns of attachment and their physiological, emotional, and cognitive responses. This linkage of mythological and physiological domains through emotional processes provides a basis for the ritual elicitation of the opioid system. ASC-induction procedures (dancing, exhaustion, pain) can also stimulate opioid release (see Prince, 1982; Winkelman, 1997, 2000a). The endogenous opioids also enhance environmental adaptation, memory, group biological synchronization, pain reduction, tolerance of stress, and immune system functioning.

Social and Emotional Healing Ritual practices heal by meeting fundamental human needs for belonging, comfort, and bonding with others. Rituals integrate and bond people, enhancing social support systems, group identity, and self-development. Community bonding elicits biologically based attachment processes, facilitating adaptive change and healing for individuals and groups. Religious healing practices involve the formation of attachments that meet fundamental needs in the mammalian system (Kirkpatrick, 1997). Attachment bonds that evolved to maintain proximity between infants and caregivers provide a secure basis for the self by inducing feelings of comfort and protection received from a powerful figure. These attachments contribute to emotional development through relationships that influence self-adaptations and behavior toward others, enhancing altruistic behavior modeled on the role of the benevolent helping other.

Shamanistic healing affects emotional processes through confession and forgiveness, restructuring painful memories, resolving conflicts, alleviating repressions, and the expression of unconscious concerns. The explanations provided in shamanistic healing processes typically minimize personal guilt and intrapsychic conflict by attributing causation of problems to external spirits. Shamanic healing may also evoke unpleasant emotions and fearful memories, providing a basis for patients to confront their fears. This mirrors contemporary therapies for the treatment of anxiety through desensitization created by exposure to feared objects. Shamanic treatment of anxiety focuses on inducing vivid images of threatening objects and confronts them with the assistance of the shaman, community, and spirits, who provide support.

ASCs—shamanic, possession, and meditative—all heal by manipulating the emotions, but there are psychological differences in the emotional transformations they produce. The commonalities in their effects on emotions include the use of ritual and psychosocial processes to alter emotional relationships, attachments, and sense of self through incorporating others into one's identity. Shamanistic traditions provide a variety of therapeutic mechanisms for altering emotions. Physiological effects of ASCs activate the limbic brain, which regulates emotions and their integration with memories, self-concepts, and social attachments (MacLean, 1990). ASCs synchronize the frontal cortex with theta brain waves, producing an emotional flooding and reevaluation of memories and affective attachments (Mandell, 1980).

Soul Loss A central shamanic illness is soul loss, which Achterberg (1985) characterizes as an injury to the core or essence of one's being (also see the special feature "Case Study: Shamanic Treatment of Soul Loss"). This injury to one's essence is manifested as despair and disharmony and feelings of loss of meaning in life, of belonging, and of connection with others. Soul loss involves aspects of the self that provide vitality to life (Ingerman, 1991). "Soul" constitutes our vital essence, particularly self-emotions. Soul loss occurs as a consequence of trauma that causes an aspect of one's self to dissociate.

This separated aspect of the self carries with it the impact of the traumatic experiences that are dissociated from the rest of the self. Soul loss early in life can arrest ego and emotional development at the time when the loss occurred. Reintegration of these dissociated aspects of self is central to healing.

Soul recovery involves dramatic enactments of the shaman's battle with terrifying spirits to rescue a patient's soul. Threatening spirit images symbolize the repressed aspects of the self. Shamanic ASCs manage emotional life and self-loss by reintegrating those repressed aspects. Through soul recovery, one regains a valued sense of social self that was alienated through trauma.

Community participation in healing rituals indicates the importance of social relations in retrieving a lost soul. The cross-cultural literature and contemporary shamanic work suggest that healing power is derived from others witnessing the return of the soul. Emotional healing through social bonding is also facilitated by the release of the body's own opioids that enhance attachment and produce a sense of well-being.

The shaman's dramatic struggles with the spirit world engage a conceptual framework representing dissociated aspects of self and emotions. The attribution systems of shamanism provide a self-empowering system in control of the spirits.

Possession Possession ASCs externalize control through concepts of possessing spirits operating outside one's self but acting on one's body and consciousness. Possession ASCs involve dramatic experiences that change emotion-self dynamics by using the possessing spirits to engage alternate selves and prohibited social roles and emotional expressions. Through possession, responsibility for feelings and behaviors is attributed to a spirit entity that controls the body and mind. Possession involves a variety of psychodynamic processes, including dissociation, emotional transactions, and interpersonal and self-transformations (see Chapter Six). Behaviors of the possessed often involve a dramatic enactment of conflictive situations, the expression of repressed desires, or the performance of prohibited behaviors. The spirits' roles shift responsibility from the patient to the other, objectifying emotions and placing responsibility for them within broader social relations. Possession manages emotional problems by exerting social influence and changing relationships by making indirect demands, thus altering power relations. Possessing spirits may require that the patient be treated in certain ways or receive special privileges.

Possession provides adaptive expressive functions, enabling the transformation of emotional dynamics and one's personal identity. Possession changes relations between individuals and groups through the incorporation of various others into the self. It reformulates emotional dynamics by expanding identity and mechanisms of self-expression, using possession performances to assert dominance through the possessing alter egos.

Meditative Detachment Meditation integrates emotions and thoughts and suspends emotional reactions to achieve freedom from suffering. Meditative practices enhance the control of attention to change mental processes and, consequently, emotions. Emotions are changed by the development of a detached observational attitude involving the suspension of evaluative processes. Meditation provides the framework for the development of an "observing self" or "witnessing consciousness" that is capable of observing without reacting (Hunt, 1995). The awareness of feelings developed in meditative forms of consciousness provides a basis for dialectical reasoning and an appreciation for opposing perspectives (Wade, 1996; Winkelman, 2000a). An analysis of Vedic psychology by Alexander, Davies, Dixon, Dillbeck, Drucker, Oetzel, Muehlman, and Orme-Johnson (1990) illustrates that feelings have a role in interconnecting the levels of mind. Mature levels of emotional consciousness provide information to integrate ego, self, intellect, and motivations in intuitive decision-making processes that transcend earlier stages of emotional development. These developments provide a basis for the ability to elicit and suspend emotional processes. These developments are reflected in the experiences of rapture, bliss, and overwhelming love and compassion characteristic of advanced meditators.

Meditation also affects emotions through ASCs that enhance ego regression, promote the release of repressed memories, induce the relaxation response, and produce counterconditioning or desensitization (see Taylor, Murphy, and Donovan, 1997). Meditation reduces stress, fears, and phobias by their occurrence in conjunction with extreme relaxation. Meditation provides a focus on the perceptions, memories, thoughts, sensations, and emotions that arise because of their psychodynamic energy, providing primary material for processing and emotional release. Enhanced awareness of unconscious emotional processes may lead to the compassion, charity, and service characteristic of meditative traditions.

APPLICATIONS

Shamanistic Healing in Catholic Charismatic Healing

Shamanistic healing principles are manifested in the Catholic charismatic movement. Charismatic healing is distinct from shamanism but involves analogous functions involving the self, sacred others, and imaginal transformations (Csordas, 1994). Csordas characterizes Catholic charismatic healing as involving self-processes and emotions that engage themes central to North American culture: personal control, intimacy, and spontaneity. Needs for intimacy are met in personal relationships with Jesus, and spontaneous spiritual experiences of surrendering to the deity provide release from the cultural emphasis on control.

The self and body are involved in charismatic healing processes that link the self, body, and social world with the personal unconscious. Csordas (1994) suggests that bodily self-awareness produced through ritual engagement is interpreted as awareness of the divine. The "otherness" of self that seems "not-me" is a consequence of the autonomic functioning of our bodies that produces an embodied hidden presence.

ASCs are prominent features of charismatic healing, involving falling into a sacred swoon or "resting in the spirit," falling backward to the ground from being overpowered by a divine presence. Someone (a "catcher") is there to break the fall and allow the person to rest comfortably for up to hours in an ASC and in the presence of a divine power. The manifestation of the divine power engages the patient in a person-to-person relationship that is interpreted by Csordas as an intimate preobjective relationship, a nurturing, healing communication and companionship that surpass the capacity of human relations.

Spirit Relations and Self

The action of spirits on the self is reflected in the illness concepts of spirit aggression, the most widespread of all theories of illness (Murdock, 1980). These universal spirit aggression beliefs are a fundamental concern of shamans, who engage in struggles with the spirits to recover the soul stolen from the patient or remedy other afflictions that spirits cause. Spirit illness, soul loss, and possession involve psychological structures representing personal identity and attachments. Spirits are a symbolic system representing psychological complexes and relations with others. Spirits' characteristics and effects provide an externalization of nonverbal and unconscious meanings. The spirit world symbolically represents self, the social world (others), individual psychodynamics, and their interrelationships in a natural symbol system.

These representations of fundamental aspects of the self and others enable spirit experiences to influence emotions and physiology. Ritual manipulates these natural structures through symbolic processes. Spirits represent psychological complexes, organized dynamics of perception, and behavior dissociated from awareness, normal personality, and identity. These dissociated aspects of the personality, as manifested in multiple personality disorders, involve unintegrated aspects of one's own capabilities. Shamanic practices heal through symbolically manipulating these spirit concepts to restructure the interactions among dissociated complexes and between self and others. The ritual elicitation of these unconscious emotional dynamics enables a realignment of the individual with social roles, cultural expectations, and the cosmological order. Shamanic healing practices elicit a holistic imperative (Laughlin et al., 1992), a drive toward psychological integration, through the projection of a more advanced state of development represented in both the shaman and in the spirit world. Shamanic healing integrates conscious and unconscious aspects of the self, transforming identity and one's social relations through symbolically invoking new models for identity provided by the spirits.

Ritual Transformation of the Self The shamans' ability to transform the self through ritual interactions with the spirit world is explained by role theory. Religious healing in general engages role interactions similar to those that people use in interacting with one another but using interactions with a divine other (Holm, 1997) or sacred others (Pandian, 1997). Peters and Price-Williams (1981) show that therapeutic processes are involved in engaging the self in an intense emotional relationship with spirit others, providing means for personal development. One's self is modified by internalizing the identity and expectations represented in the divine other in the same way that ordinary human roles are developed by internalizing the expectations of others. Shamanic use of the spirits for modeling the self is exemplified in the use of animal spirits for self-identification and internal differentiation.

Shamanic models for self link the individual's emotional processes with new social expectations. Ritual dramatization, the enactment of conflict, and a resolution of threats provide a dramatic expression of social relations. Ritual transforms identity by the modeling involved in shamanic ritual enactments, a role-taking manifested in the adoption of various personalities of the spirits. This provides new roles for the patient to internalize and enact, affecting the patient's psychodynamics. Spirits represent personal and social roles, emotions, attachments, repressed complexes, dissociated aspects of identity, and social forces. The shaman's role-taking provides models of social roles, with ritually induced ASCs loosening psychological boundaries to these new social roles. The images of the spirit world play important psychological roles in

- Representing and evoking innate experiences
- Mediating between body, psyche, and society
- Managing intrapsychic and psychosocial dynamics

The ritual engagement with spirits and their manipulations can have therapeutic effects because these spirit concepts represent fundamental aspects of self and others. Spirits can be representations of generic aspects of human emotions and the basic structures of human thought and self. This role of the spirit world in representing aspects of

PRACTITIONER PROFILE

Marlene Dobkin de Rios

Early in her studies, Marlene Dobkin de Rios, Ph.D., was a research affiliate with a Peruvian psychiatrist whose interests were in traditional mestizo healing in Peru, specifically with the psychedelic vine, ayahuasca (various *Banisteropsis* species), used to reverse witchcraft-induced illnesses among Amazonian peasants in Peruvian cities. For more than a decade, Dobkin de Rios conducted research on this topic, publishing widely from an anthropological perspective. With the desire to become a therapist and use skills she had chronicled and observed among shamanic healers in the Peruvian Amazon and coastal areas, she returned to graduate school to study clinical psychology and began to use her Spanish-language skills and knowledge of the culture of the urban poor to treat immigrant clients in southern California. She worked part-time for fifteen years (in addition to teaching duties as professor of anthropology at California State University, Fullerton) at the University of California-Irvine Medical Center, where she was director of counseling in the Burn Center.

As Dobkin de Rios worked with trauma victims suffering from post-traumatic stress disorders subsequent to burn injuries and explosions and then with couples and children who had a variety of psychiatric disorders, she began to use hypnosis and provide culturally resonant interventions. Hypnosis relaxation tapes she prepared for clients were an essential part of shamanic healing: self-soothing techniques to reverse anxiety, despair, depression, and dysfunction. She also used behavior modification techniques similar to those she observed shamanic healers using to promote change in families.

Dobkin de Rios has written about her experiences and medical anthropological perspectives in *Brief Psychotherapy with the Latino Immigrant Client* (2003) and research she conducted on the use of ayahuasca as a religious sacrament in Brazil and New Mexico (Groisman and de Rios, 2007).

the self is exemplified in Csordas's discussion (1994) of the role of spirits such as evil, lust, gluttony, and others addressed in Christian charismatic healing. These spirit representations can be seen as mediating the manifestations of ancient forms of motivation, communication, and representation in ways that facilitate emotional well-being. For instance, one can disown one's own lustful impulses by attributing them to the "Spirit of Lust." Ritual interactions with spirits elicit, mediate, and transform these primordial psychological and cognitive processes related to well-being and attachment. Shamanistic ritual activities provide access to unconscious psychological structures and processes not normally accessible to the conscious ego. Shamanistic ritual induces healing through physiological, psychological, and emotional changes that alter the relationship of the self to the world to achieve a new psychological integration.

SHAMANIC ROOTS IN CONTEMPORARY RELIGIOUS EXPERIENCES AND HEALING

The neurological basis of shamanic practices in the fundamental structures of the human brain and consciousness is shown by the persistence of shamanic features in contemporary religious experiences, pathologies, and healing practices. These experiences reveal the centrality of the shamanic paradigm in human functioning and its continued relevance.

Contemporary Religious Experiences

Contemporary religious experiences are primarily perceptions and sensations of contact with a supernatural agency and the relationship of the individual with that divine other (Stark, 1997). These are perceptions of a presence with volitional characteristics like our self, with intentional, moral, and social characteristics. These contemporary religious experiences can be ordered by degrees of interaction with the divine as (Stark, 1997)

- Confirming: self's awareness of a divine other
- Responsive: divine's awareness of self
- Ecstatic: union of self and a divine other
- Revelation: messages from a divine other
- Control: the self dominated by the divine other

Contact with the divine other through intense emotional experiences of reverence and awe, an experience of the presence of the spirit other, is the essence of animism that underlies shamanism. Responsive experiences involving the self's and divine's mutual awareness (a social inclusion of self with the divine other) is exemplified in shamans' relationships with spirit allies. Shamanism provides the original ecstatic experience, a deeply affective, intimate relationship and union with the divine other.

Shamans' experiences are fundamentally revelatory: acquiring information from the spirit world about causes of illness and procedures for healing. The shaman represents the primordial function of a confidant and messenger of the divine other through revelatory

APPLICATIONS

Shamanism and DSM-IV Spiritual Emergencies

The introduction of spiritual considerations into biomedicine was a direct outgrowth of efforts to make evaluations more culturally sensitive, recognizing religion as a cultural factor in the psychosocial environment. Anthropological perspectives help overcome providers' tendencies to pathologize religious experiences. Mistreatment can result from a failure to understand that beliefs about witches, sorcery, and possession may be cultural beliefs rather than pathologies.

Cultural Components in Spiritual, Religious, and Pathological Experiences

Cultural components of religious and spiritual experiences are of particular relevance to providers because of the potential to confuse them with symptoms of pathology (Turner, Lukoff, Barnhouse, and Lu, 1995). People who have overwhelming spiritual experiences face the risk of being treated as mentally ill and hospitalized or medicated. Providers need to be able to differentiate normative religious experiences from abnormal behaviors. A central concern is how they impact clients' lives, whether they contribute to distressing experiences and problems, or whether they are growth experiences. Characteristics of psychotic episodes—terrifying, extremely intense, and overwhelming abilities of self-care—can be used to distinguish them from religious experiences. Because of similarities between religious experiences and psychological problems, potential psychological problems with religious characteristics need to be understood and differentiated from normative cultural phenomena.

Spiritual Emergencies

An aspect of spirituality and religiosity incorporated into the DSM-IV was the category of "spiritual emergence" and "spiritual emergencies" (see Grof and Grof, 1989; Turner et al., 1995; Walsh, 1990). These experiences may emerge spontaneously or result from deliberate activities such as meditation. Contemporary psychological crises reflected in the DSM-IV category spiritual emergencies include mystical experiences; spirit communication; psychic energies; extrasensory perceptions such as clairvoyance and telepathy; spontaneous shamanic journeys or out-of-body experiences; past-life memories; possession; death-and-rebirth experiences; and "psychic opening," an experience of psychic abilities.

The shamanic paradigm provides a framework for addressing these experiences as natural manifestations of consciousness and as developmental opportunities rather than pathologies. Just as the shamanic initiatory crisis provides the opportunity for a transformational development, the symptoms of emotional disturbance, hallucinations, and traumatic spirit attacks can be interpreted as symbolic communications that provide information for personal growth.

These spiritual emergencies can be managed by integrating the principles of shamanic healing into counseling and psychotherapy (Krippner and Welch, 1992). Spirit communication, out-of-body experiences, and dismemberment experiences can be more effectively managed within the per-spectives of shamanism than with those of psychology. Shamanistic procedures provide alternative treatment approaches, substituting for traditional psychiatric drugs that repress these experiences with ritual opportunities to develop control and to understand them. Control over these changes of consciousness allows for the replacement of distressing intrusions with experiences mediated by healing symbol systems. The classic shamanic vision quest involves processes for self-empowerment. A similar approach underlies contemporary shamanic counseling and its training of clients to make a shamanic journey on their own to acquire or restore their personal power. This active aspect of shamanic journeying induces a sense of mastery and control.

Addressing Spirituality as Cultural Competence

The ability to address spirituality in healing relationships is part of cultural competency (Fukuyama and Sevig, 1999). Cultural self-awareness of one's own religious beliefs and values and how they affect perceptions of clients is necessary for cultural competence in healing relationships. Providers need to understand when differences between their own and their client's religious predilections result in conflicts, dictating that clients be referred to other providers (Fukuyama and Sevig, 1999). Caregivers must be able to differentiate clients' religious behaviors that are culturally appropriate from those that are personally detrimental, assessing spiritual experiences in the overall context of the person's life. Providers should have an empathic and practical understanding of the role of reli-gion in culture and clients' lives and be able to engage these cultural belief systems as resources that can assist in coping and healing processes.

Cultural evaluations of religious and spiritual experiences are essential for cultural compe-tency because inappropriate responses by providers (psychotropic medication, pathological attri-butions) can undermine their transformational potential. But this is not to treat all spiritual experiences as paths to personal growth. Assessment of a client's personal and social context may suggest a process of grounding that moderates the unfolding of the spiritual experience within the developing capabilities of the person to manage the experience. Other issues may need to be addressed before engaging in spiritual exploration. Severe mental illnesses such as psychoses are contraindications for engagement in spiritual experiences and development.

The importance of spiritual experiences for providers as a part of cultural competency devel-opment is suggested by Fukuyama and Sevig (1999). They indicate that the development of spirit-uality can help one become multiculturally competent, providing a philosophical stance that can be used to inform and guide one's behavior. Multiculturalism and spirituality share universal char-acteristics and qualities—connectedness, compassion, relationships outside of self, social justice, management of ambiguity, and detachment—that reinforce an ethos of tolerance toward cultural differences.

experiences in visual and intuitive modalities, as exemplified in the soul journey. The divine control of the self ranges from mutual awareness through the union of self with a divine other and possession of the self. The control of self by the divine other exemplified in possession is part of the broader shamanistic paradigm rather than classic shamanism. Possession involves an evil and terrorizing religious experience, where the divine other controls one's thoughts and behaviors.

These experiences of supernatural control have roots in shamanic initiatory crises, but their fullest developments are in practices associated with mediums and possession. They are also found in contemporary psychological disorders, as described in the special feature "Applications: Shamanism and DSM-IV Spiritual Emergencies."

Shamanic Techniques in Contemporary Psychotherapy

Principles of shamanic healing are employed in psychotherapy, some of them explicitly derived from shamanism (see Achterberg, 1985; Gagan, 1998; Perkins, 1997; Dobkin de Rios, 2001, 2002). Hypnosis and Freudian psychotherapy approaches reflect the use of shamanic principles without an explicit recognition of their roots. Freud's psychotherapeutic approach is based on having clients lie down, relax (regress), and free-associate with the material that emerges from their preconscious and unconscious or from recalled dreams. Dreams and free association provide access to material not ordinarily available to consciousness.

Journeying and Power Animals in Attachment Dynamics Gagan (1998) employs shamanic journeying to provide surrogate entities for bonding experiences, reflecting general concepts about spirits in personal development. Well-being is related to the development of attachment. Gagan suggests that attachment development creates a false self that involves identifications to please caretakers, producing dissociation from aspects of the self of which they disapprove. This begins a psychological abandonment of the true self that manifests later in life in anger, frustration, and blockage of access to one's creative potentials. Part of healing involves a resolution of the division between the true and false self.

Shamanic journeying can heal these developmental traumas and reestablish contact with one's true self. Power animals can nurture the traumatized self and provide experiences of merging and unity with others. Journeying allows a reframing of early traumas, particularly those that are still dissociated. Animal powers can provide help in managing these traumas and reactivating lost potentials. Journey time spent with power animals provides a context for feeling safe. Power animals encountered in shamanic journeying may be recovered as manifestations of "lost souls," dissociated aspects of self, or deeply embedded memories from the unconscious. Incorporating power animals can provide healing through their integration into the self, bringing qualities and characteristics that help address shortcomings, particularly deficits in personality development (Gagan, 1998).

Visions as Psychobiological Communication ASCs also aid the emergence of primary process thinking and visual symbolic experiences. This allows for the manifestation of emotional and social dynamics understood at pre-egoic levels where developmental

CULTURE AND HEALTH

Divine Relationships in Catholic Charismatic Healing

In charismatic Catholic healing, similar dynamics of visual symbols and their power are manifested. Imagery reveals the conflicts and the dynamics of the true self that must be addressed to heal these earlier developmental traumas. Divinities play a role as internalized others that facilitate the resolution of developmental blockages produced by trauma. Csordas (1994) characterizes divine images, and Jesus in particular, as an "internal transitional object" that serves as a "developmental way station" that leads to a mature relationship (pp. 155–156). The divine entity provides protection and power that aids patients in their confrontation with traumatic memories. A predominant theme in charismatic healing is related to the lack of intimacy or failure in intimacy, often stemming from childhood or marital relations. The divine embrace with Jesus substitutes for absent or lost parental or spousal intimacy, providing an enduring relation of interpersonal intimacy.

blockages occurred and enhances the management of social and personal attachments and emotions. Journeying facilitates the transfer of unconscious material into consciousness, an awareness of one's own psychodynamics. Achterberg (1985) analyzes the shaman's imagery as a preverbal process that permits the imagination to act directly on the physical substrate (tissues, organs, and cells). Images can also change behaviors, exerting influences on the muscles and autonomic nervous system and coordinating a wide range of unconscious systems to achieve goals. Threatening images can evoke the fight-or-flight response and stimulate the sympathetic system whereas pleasant images can stimulate the parasympathetic nervous system and evoke the relaxation response. Achterberg (1985) characterizes shamanic transpersonal imagery as using universal symbols reflecting the collective unconscious (neurognostic structures). Visions link personal experiences with natural symbols of the cosmos, mind, and the unconscious, providing therapeutic mechanisms for manipulation of the psyche and body.

Containment and Release Gagan (1998) uses shamanic journeying to provide clients with processes of containment, a protective space for manifesting feelings that provides security and unleashes the potential for transformation. Shamanic journeying can address negative human emotions, particularly manifestations and repressions of aggression. Journeying provides a mechanism for identifying sources of repressed anger and symbolically reengaging the context in visions that enable one to make more appropriate responses. It can provide a therapeutic release or discharge of repressed aggressive tendencies that would be destructive if expressed in interpersonal relations. Journeying experiences permit their expression in a context that contributes to empowerment. This release of emotional blockages forms when one who was oppressed by others can provide therapeutic processes that mend developmental wounds and allow one to proceed to new levels.

Unfolding Unconscious Potentials Shamanism engages the holistic imperative, an inherent tendency for the organism to seek psychological integration and growth (Laughlin et al., 1992). These holistic impulses are reflected in visions that integrate the unconscious emotional life into consciousness. Visionary experiences can be diagnostic, providing content and structure reflective of a client's current needs for psychological growth. Visions reflect repressed energies, unresolved conflicts, and developmental dynamics, often manifested in archetypal images that Gagan (1998) considers particularly powerful tools because they link back into earlier trauma and forward into the next developmental stage. Jung characterized shamanic images as archetypal motifs, natural symbols that enable the unconscious to connect an individual's natural or biological basis with developmental goals. The collective unconscious embodied in the spirit world provides a matrix for engaging and releasing archetypal energies. Rituals channel energy from the biological to psychological levels, from the unconscious to the conscious. Shamanic visionary activities provide mechanisms for a reconnection with this archetypal ground. The psychotherapeutic processes that incorporate these foundational shamanic images (archetypes) heal by connecting the psyche with its ancient natural roots and energy for healing, producing a sense of wholeness and connectedness.

Individuation: Self-Integration Gagan (1998) points out that journeying reveals wisdom inherent in the unconscious, presenting information beyond a client's current level of development. The visionary revelations may be retained for later processing as the client's psychological integration proceeds. The symbolic emergence of unconscious material allows for individuation (producing a psychologically whole and integrated consciousness) to occur outside of conscious awareness. Journeying accelerates development by symbolic elevation of this embedded material into personal consciousness where it can transform self-awareness.

Shape-Shifting Shamans' ability to transform into an animal has been applied to personal transformation as a process of shape-shifting (Perkins, 1997). Shape-shifting is concerned with changing into the self that we want to be, producing a paradigm shift in our personal and social nature. These include changes in our attitudes and behaviors, our perceptions and appearance, and our health and personal relationships. Perkins characterizes shape-shifting as focusing personal energy (or spirit) and intent to achieve our goals. Shape-shifting engages the capacity for dreaming and our personal intent to change thought patterns to alter affect, attitudes, character, and action. The use of animal identities can help this shape-shifting, providing an external model with desired characteristics for the person to emulate and internalize into personal identity.

Summary Shamanic practices engage a variety of healing processes, including dream work, self-expression, unconscious association, personal integration, and self-transformation. The journeying process, however, is not appropriate for all clients or at all stages of development. Gagan (1998) points out the importance of assessing the clients' level of functioning to determine if they are ready for shamanic experiences. She suggests that noncandidates include people in acute grief, those with frequent dissociative experiences, and clients with psychotic symptoms. Other people may find journeying incompatible with personal beliefs,

APPLICATIONS

Applying Shamanic Potentials in Psychotherapy with Latinos

Dobkin de Rios (2002, 2003) has integrated shamanistic healing principles into her psychothera-peutic practices, based on her study of healers in Peru and around the world. She found that shamanic methods could be used to reinforce mainstream counseling methods. Aspects of the Latino cultural background make counseling techniques such as hypnosis, behavioral modifica-tion, and cognitive restructuring particularly powerful when used in a shamanic context. Dobkin de Rios uses hypnosis as a tool for inducing an ASC and treating a variety of conditions associ-ated with stress, anxiety, depression, and post-traumatic stress disorder. Personal empowerment is a key shamanic concept that she engages, using symbols provided by powerful animals, espe-cially the eagle, to provide a focus for empowerment and a sense of personal control. She (2003) also employs a play therapy that she calls "magical realism" to address state-dependent emo-tional memories formed by childhood trauma. Mutual story-telling is first used to recreate the traumatized emotional state and memory. Dobkin de Rios then calls on cultural superheroes to help a child reexperience the event with a different outcome. This enables the child to reprocess the event, reducing anxiety and contributing to mastery of the traumatizing experience. The analogies to the shamanic ritual encounter with the spirit world are apparent: dramatic story-telling, encounters with feared circumstances, and addressing them with the assistance of super-natural powers. These mechanisms for behavior modification and personal empowerment provide models for clients to emulate in later social encounters. Dobkin de Rios also uses tech-niques of cognitive restructuring by employing cultural proverbs that remind clients to focus new attitudes on their problems, changing irrational beliefs and negative self-talk.

particularly religious orientations. The therapist must play a role in the containment process, balancing cognitive and emotional dynamics and the appropriate timing of interventions.

ASC Therapy for Drug Rehabilitation

McPeake, Kennedy, and Gordon (1991) point out that substance abuse rehabilitation pro-grams need to incorporate the important benefits of ASCs to avoid relapse. They attribute the failure of treatment programs to the absence of practices for teaching addicts to address their basic needs by achieving ASCs through nondrug means. McPeake and coworkers (1991) point to the voluminous literature documenting the benefits of natural ASCs and the central role in Alcoholics Anonymous (AA) of a new state of consciousness to replace the self-destructive pursuit of drug states. Training in inducing ASCs can enhance the spiritual awakening considered essential to recovery in AA. They propose an altered state of con-sciousness therapy approach as a natural complement to the AA Twelve-Step recovery pro-gram. The ASC therapy approach induces positive mental attitudes, provides consciousness of a power greater than one's self, meets human needs to alter consciousness, and provides a path for personal growth and development associated with transcendental needs.

APPLICATIONS

Meditation and Shamanism in Substance Abuse Rehabilitation

There has been a reinvention of shamanism in modern Western societies and its application in treatments for modern health problems; one of the areas is in the rehabilitation of substance abuse (McPeake et al., 1991; Jilek, 1994; Rioux, 1996; Winkelman, 2001b, 2003a, 2004c). These applications are in part inspired by the cross-cultural use of shamanistic practices for treating substance abuse (Heggenhougen, 1997; Jilek, 1994). These approaches typically include a number of common features:

- The use of plants containing indole alkaloids for detoxification and managing drug craving
- Physical and psychological purification through purging and confession
- Use of traditional cultural procedures for the induction of ASCs
- Rituals to provoke emotional and psychodynamic release
- Provision of support systems through ritual groups and collective therapies
- Helping client achieve social reintegration

The rituals generally induce a process of self-transformation involving a death-rebirth experience to produce a newer, more positive self-image. In Asia these healing practices are often incorporated within meditative traditions. Meditative traditions have also been used in the United States as drug rehabilitation programs.

Meditation in the Treatment of Addiction

The Transcendental Meditation (TM) program has been widely used for the treatment of addiction; these treatments have undergone systematic clinical evaluation and meta-analyses of their effectiveness (O'Connell and Alexander, 1994; Gelderloos, Walton, Orme-Johnson, and Alexander, 1991). TM has a substantial effect in reducing addiction. Studies on both user and addict populations show that TM has had substantial success and that the treatment effects of TM are greater than those associated with conventional drug rehabilitation approaches. The mechanisms by which TM successfully treats addictions include its effects on psychological, social, and physiological levels. TM enhances self-esteem, stress management, coping, physiological balance, and spirituality. The physiological mechanisms through which TM can address addictions involve neuroendocrine systems (Walton and Levitzky, 1994). TM reduces addiction through enhancing the functioning of the serotonin neurotransmitter system. Enhancement of serotonin levels, which have been depleted by chronic substance abuse, provides relief from stress and reestablishes a homeostatic balance. The enhanced neuroendocrine balance produces relaxation, personal contentment, and mood elevation, reducing the need for drug-induced tension relief.

Rioux (1996) illustrates how shamanic healing techniques can play a role in holistic addiction counseling. Shamanism's focus on ASCs and inner realities can play a role in developing a sense of harmony and self-wholeness. The shamanic ASCs provide a link between inner and outer realities, utilizing a form of *seeing* that enables the inner-world perspectives to operate on the outer world to produce harmony and wholeness. Shamanic ASCs facilitate

TM's effects in addiction treatment also involve spiritual factors (Alexander, Robinson, Orme-Johnson, Schneider, and Walton, 1994), addressing spiritual problems, such as a soul loss that involves subtle aspects of one's personal existence and connectedness with others. TM affects addiction by integrating the individual—"body, mind, spirit, social interaction, and environment" (Alexander et al., 1994, p. 18). It produces a restful alertness, pleasant experiences, and an ASC that provides what "substance users are looking for: relief from distress, increased self-esteem, enhancement of well being and self-efficacy, and a sense of personal power and meaning in life" (Gelderloos et al., 1991, p. 317).

Sacred Plants as Substance Abuse Treatments

In the Americas, a number of shamanistic traditions have addressed addiction through the use of sacred plants (Schultes and Hofmann, 1979): hallucinogens, psychedelics, or psychointegrators (Winkelman, 1996a, 2007a; see also Winkelman and Roberts, Chapters 1–6, 2007a, Volume 2). The use of these substances for drug rehabilitation is exemplified in the Native American church or peyote religion. The peyote ritual combines peyote, which contains indole alkaloids, with a variety of other psychotherapeutic modalities (see Aberle, 1966; Wiedman, 1990; Calabrese, 1997, 2007). Sanchez-Ramos and Mash (1996) review the research on the treatment of drug dependence with ibogaine from Africa, which is being used in addict communities in the United States and Europe to provide treatment for opiate and stimulant dependence (also see Alper, Lotsof, Frenken, Luciano, and Bastiaans, 1999, 2000). Reformulated traditional ayahuasca rituals are being used to rehabilitate cocaine paste (base) addicts in the Peruvian Amazon (Mabit, Giove, and Vega, 1996). These plant medicines may have their primary effects in reducing addiction by their intervention in the serotonergic neurotransmitter system (Winkelman, 1996a, 2001a; also see Winkelman, 2007a, and Winkelman and Roberts, 2007a [Volume 2], for a review of recent studies).

Although there is limited clinical assessment of the effectiveness of these substances because they have been banned from human research and psychotherapeutic practice for more than thirty years, evidence suggests that they are effective in treating alcoholism, addictions, and a range of other conditions (e.g., see Bliss, 1988; Yensen, 1985, 1996; Passie, 1997; Winkelman and Roberts, 2007a, Volume 1). These substances are unlikely to be used in contemporary treatment programs for political rather than medical reasons (Grob and Bravo, 1996; Winkelman and Roberts, 2007b). There are, however, nondrug means of achieving similar ASCs with comparable physiological and psychodynamic effects that may also make them effective tools for treating addiction.

recovery from addiction through transforming consciousness and through specific healing techniques: those empowering clients by teaching them to journey to achieve wholeness on their own. Power animals or other guardian spirits conceptualized as metaphoric healing energies mediate these interactions. This contact with the power animals provides an expansion on the AA's Twelve-Step concept of a higher power and has a direct healing effect.

Other important aspects of the shamanic practice include focusing intention on one's purpose, empowering, dreaming, and spending journey time in special places that provide restful healing. These practices free one from ego-bound emotions and balance conflicting internal energies. Work through dreaming helps achieve the sense of wholeness considered to be lacking in addicts by opening them to the multidimensional shamanic universe. This broader perspective can enhance self-esteem by providing experiences of the connectedness with patterns of meaning beyond the egoic self. This opens up different levels of reality to clients and makes possible holistic counseling through a biopsychosociospiritual approach.

"Drumming Out Drugs"

Winkelman (2003a, 2004c) describes shamanic interventions in substance abuse rehabilitation programs often referred to as "Drumming out Drugs!" Evidence suggests that drumming can enhance recovery and that it has some specific psychophysiological effects that have therapeutic efficacy in addiction recovery. Drumming acts like other ASCs in producing physiological changes that can enhance the recovery process. Listening to drumming induces the relaxation response and elicits pleasurable experiences by restoring balance in the opioid and serotonergic neurotransmitter systems. Drumming also facilitates an emergence of preconscious dynamics that can produce a release of emotional trauma, contributing to a reintegration of self. Social and personal relations that help meet psychodynamic needs for self-awareness, insight, and psychological integration also help. Community drumming meets social needs for connectedness with others and interpersonal support and can counter the sense of isolation and alienation addicts feel. Winkelman (2003) characterizes drumming circles as a secular approach to accessing higher power and spiritual experiences, providing a nondenominational means of applying spiritual perspectives to addiction.

Programs that have incorporated drumming circles indicated they have important roles as complementary addiction therapy and may be particularly appropriate for clients suffering repeated relapse. Winkelman (2001b) also outlines ways in which shamanism can be applied to substance abuse rehabilitation (see the special feature "Applications: Meditation and Shamanism in Substance Abuse Rehabilitation"). The documented physiological effects of drumming and the reported positive effects of drumming experiences attested to by providers and clients provide compelling rationale for the use of this valuable resource in addiction recovery.

CHAPTER SUMMARY

Eliade's classic (1964 [published originally in 1951 in French]) characterization of the shaman as entering ecstasy to communicate with the spirit world on behalf of the community referenced three primordial and contemporary aspects of biologically based healing processes. Ecstasy, or ASC, involves physiologically induced changes of consciousness providing psychophysiological integration. The spirit world is a symbolic system for representing and constructing cultural aspects of the self. The community enhances immune system functioning, elicits healing responses, and provides social support. A variety of aspects of shamanism such as the soul journey, death-rebirth experiences, and animal allies are manifestations of innate processing modules. Shamanic practices utilize these innate modules to elicit fundamental psychological functions and to integrate these processes to produce metaphoric representations of the self and others. These representations provide mechanisms for self-development and therapeutic manipulations of psychological processes. These ASCs, spirit world constructs, and community relations remain an essential component of healing that are increasingly missing in therapeutic relationships today. Shamanism manipulates innate structures of the brain-mind that provide healing responses by connecting with deep structures of human consciousness and psyche, prelinguistic symbolic systems that still mediate human experience. These are engaged by the physiological dynamics of ASCs, symbolic healing processes, and by establishing relations with spirit beings that represent aspects of the personal unconscious and personal and social relations. The basis of shamanic healing practices in innate biosocial processes makes them relevant for contemporary use.

KEY TERMS

Animism

Anthropomorphism

Endogenous opioids

Individuation

Innate modules

Mimesis

Neurognostic structures

Opioids

Parasympathetic nervous system

Psychointegrators

REM sleep

Serotonin neural pathways

Shaman

Shamanistic healer

Soul journey (flight)

Triune

SELF-ASSESSMENT 10.1. SPIRITUAL EXPERIENCES AND HEALING

Have you or someone you know well ever been treated by a spiritual healer? What was the condition treated?

How was the condition treated?

What was the outcome?

Have you or someone you know well ever had a spiritual experience? What was it like?

How did the spiritual experience affect your health and psychological well-being? Your social relations with others?

Have you ever felt that a spiritual relationship affected your health? How?

ADDITIONAL RESOURCES

Books

Katz, R. 1999. *The straight path of the spirit: Ancestral wisdom and healing traditions in Fiji.* Rochester, Vt.: Park Street Press.

Katz, R., M. Biesele, and V. St. Denis. 1997. *Healing makes our hearts happy: Spirituality and cultural transformations among the Ju!'hoansi.* Rochester, Vt.: Inner Traditions.

McClenon, J. 2002. *Wondrous healing: Shamanism, human evolution, and the origin of religion*. DeKalb: Northern Illinois University Press.

Rayburn, C. A., and L. J. Richmond, eds. 2002. Theobiology: Interfacing theology, biology, and other sciences for deeper understanding. *American Behavioral Scientist*, 45(12):entire issue.

Web Site

Foundation for Shamanic Studies: http://www.shamanism.org

NOTES

1. A number of the sections of this chapter are excerpted from Winkelman (2000a), where more complete references are provided.

2. These different modes of consciousness do not have a single specific anatomical center for their elicitation. Their systemic functional nature provides multiple mechanisms for inducing their operation. This is attested to not only in the multiple control circuits for the sleep-waking cycle control and dreaming (Koella, 1985) but also in the multiple mechanisms that induce ASCs and the integrative mode of consciousness (Mandell, 1980; Winkelman, 1986a, 1992a, 2000a).

3. Primary research sources for the following information are available in Winkelman (1992a, 1997, 2000a).

4. For instance, Aberle (1966), Dobkin de Rios (1984), Furst (1976), Harner (1973), Schultes and Hofmann (1979), Schultes and Winkelman (1996), Wasson (1980), Wasson, Cowan, Cowan, and Rhodes (1974); and Wasson, Kramrisch, Ott, and Ruck (1986).

5. The dream is characterized by a cessation of serotonin and norepinephrine activity. The serotonergic system has an inhibitory or gating role in the activity of the cholinergic system, which is responsible for inducing REM sleep. The role of serotonergic pathways in integrative consciousness suggests that the differences with respect to dreams reflect their lack of integrative serotonergic influences linking emotional and cognitive systems, a characteristic of shamanic practices.

GLOSSARY

Acculturation. Change that occurs as a consequence of contact with another culture.

ACTH. Adrenocorticotropic hormone.

Adaptations. Physiological and behavioral adjustments to an environment.

Advocacy. Action on behalf of communities to help ensure their access to needed resources and services.

AIDS. Acquired immunodeficiency syndrome.

Altered states of consciousness. Generally involves an enhancement of the brain's slow wave patterns (alpha and theta).

Alternative medicine. A global term used to refer to healing traditions in Western cultures that are viewed as an alternative to biomedical care.

AMA. American Medical Association.

Animism. A belief in spirits.

ANS. Autonomic nervous system.

Anthropomorphism. Attributing humanlike qualities to gods, spirits, animals, and other entities.

ASC. Altered state of consciousness.

Assimilation. Culture loss due to contact with another culture.

Biomedicine. Refers to the Western societies' healing traditions based upon the practices of physicians (M.D.s) and scientific medicine; also known as allopathic medicine.

Biopsychosocial model. A systems approach to health that addresses not only biological factors but also psychosocial factors, patients' social context, and their relationships to the health care system. Refers to the interaction among biological, social, and psychological dimensions of a person; generally implies that the psychological and social dimensions have a causal relation with the distribution of biological conditions.

Biosocialization. Socialization processes that have permanent effects on biological development.

Blended family. A family formed by the combination of two unrelated families by the marriage of two people, each with a prior family.

CAM. Complementary or alternative medicine.

Capitalist medicine. A system in which health care is purchased by consumers.

Care. The assistance necessary for recovery from illness and maintaining well-being and health in culturally meaningful ways.

CCLE. Center for Cognitive Liberty and Ethics.

CDC. Centers for Disease Control and Prevention.

CIA. Central Intelligence Agency.

Cline. Frequency of a genetic form across a geographical area, based on genetic drift and gene flow.

Community empowerment. "[T]he group's belief in its capability to succeed in future actions."

Complementary medicine. A conceptualization of popular (lay), ethnomedical (folk), and nonbiomedical practices that view these resources as being used as a *complement* to rather than a replacement for biomedical treatment; implies the simultaneous use of multiple health sectors and remedies.

Compliance. Refers to patients adopting medical advice for treatment of their conditions.

Confounding variables. Causes of disease that are related to, but are not caused by, risk factors.

Constructivist perspective. A social science perspective that considers the basis of human experience of reality to derive from human assumptions and activities.

Contextualization. Determination of life circumstances and the economic and political forces that play a role in shaping individual exposure to disease through the social and cultural factors that place groups of people at risk.

Contributory factors. Conditions in the external environment that increase the likelihood or effects of a medical condition, such as a lack of adequate nutrition contributing to susceptibility to infection.

Critical medical anthropology. An approach to the study of health that emphasizes the economic and political impacts on health and the role of biomedicine as an institutional and ideological power that affects health and disease.

Cultural awareness. A personal awareness of the effects of cultural differences on behavior and health care. Awareness constitutes the beginning of intercultural adaptation and effectiveness. It involves a self-awareness of one's own cultural values and their influences on one's behavior.

Cultural competence. The ability to identify with, effectively relate to, and work with another cultural group using culturally relevant communication skills, motivational strategies, and organizational approaches based on their expectations and perspectives. A culturally competent individual is capable of using knowledge of cultural patterns to understand priorities, communicate empathy and acceptance, be responsive to individual and community needs, and work effectively with cultural groups to develop culturally relevant interventions.

Cultural defense. A legal analysis of culpability based on assessments of the cultural influences on mens rea, the state of mind of a defendant when performing what is considered a crime.

Cultural proficiency. The ability to train others in cross-cultural competence.

Cultural relativism. Understanding behavior relative to cultural context.

Cultural-responsiveness. A nursing concept of cultural skills that involves the ability to respond in appropriate ways to a patient's cultural care needs.

Cultural sensitivity. An ability to establish relationships with members of other cultures with culturally appropriate behavior and care; involves awareness of relevant cultural differences and the ability to accommodate to them through appropriate adaptations.

Cultural systems model. A perspective that considers cultures to comprise a number of interacting subsystems, particularly material (infrastructure), social (interpersonal), and ideological (mental) systems.

Culture. Shared patterns of group behavior acquired through intergenerational learning; knowledge and behavior shared by a group.

Culture-bound syndrome. An ethnomedical syndrome generally without correspondence to conditions recognized by biomedicine.

Curandero. (Mexican origin) An ethnomedical practitioner, meaning "one who cures"; it is a general term applied to virtually any ethnomedical practitioner.

Cure. The removal of the physical effects of a disease or injury.

CVD. Cardiovascular disease.

DEA. Drug Enforcement Agency.

Depersonalization. A split in consciousness between the participating self and observing self; defined as "an experience of being detached from and an outside observer of one's mental processes of body. . . . may include: feelings of dizziness, floating, or giddiness, a feeling of the self being 'dead,' a loss of affective responsiveness, and a feeling of calm detachment" (Castillo, 1991, p. 2).

Determinant. Scientifically established to be the greatest or most proximal causes of a disease.

Diagnostic and Statistical Manual of Mental Disorders (DSM). A classification schema for mental illness developed in American psychiatry and biomedicine. It lists conditions presumed universally relevant to the classification of illness. The fourth edition is DSM-IV.

Directly contributing factors. Conditions that have a role in the chain of causation of a malady by affecting the extent of a health determinant or risk factor; for example, factors such as a mother's drug use, weight, and nutritional status that affect low birth weight and high neonatal mortality.

Disease. A health malady defined as an abnormal condition of the organism that involves an organic impairment of normal physiological functioning.

Dissociative disorder. A situation where a split-off part of the personality temporarily controls the entire field of consciousnes; these disorders typically involve some loss of consciousness or some loss of integration of perception, motor function, memory, cognition, and sense of self or personal identity.

Distal causes. Factors that lead to an initiation of a disease but that are far removed from the physical manifestations of the disease, usually modified behaviors.

Double-blind clinical trial. A clinical evaluation procedure in which neither physician nor patient knows who is receiving the active medication and who is receiving a control placebo; this provides a basis for establishing the pharmacological effects of a drug beyond the placebo effect.

DSM. See *Diagnostic and Statistical Manual of Mental Disorders.*

Ecology. The total physical and sociocultural environments. The environment has three major aspects: physical (abiotic), biotic, and cultural.

Emic. The insiders' or culture's perspectives.

Endogenous healing responses. Natural healing responses of the body, not only the physical healing processes but also those that include psychological components, such as the relaxation response, placebo effects, and psychological integration.

Endogenous opiates. Natural substances of the body (i.e., enkephalins and endorphins) that are the basis for the effects of the opiate drugs (heroin, morphine) and their ability to produce the experiences of pleasure.

Entheogens. "God-containing plants": plants used in religious practices.

Entrainment. The habitual association of symbols and neural networks that enables symbols to elicit and control physiological processes entrained with the same neural networks.

Epidemiology. An interdisciplinary study of the distribution of deaths, diseases, and other health conditions and the associated behavioral, dietary, social, environmental, and other factors that may explain their causes.

Ethnicity. A socially recognized group in a society that maintains identity differences on the basis of cultural or social differences.

Ethnography. A written account describing a culture; a process of studying other cultures that is focused on acquiring an emic perspective through participant observation and other methods.

Ethnomedicine. Cultural medicine; technically applies to all healing practices but is generally used in contrast to biomedicine.

Etic. A transcultural or cross-cultural framework for interpreting culture and behavior.

Etiology. Cause of a disease.

Explanatory model. A patient's perspective on the nature of his or her health problem, including its causes, likely course of development, and appropriate treatments.

Extended family. Three or more generations: for example, grandparents, parents, and children.

FDA. Food and Drug Administration.

Folk healing. Refers to nonprofessional healing specialists, cultural healing practitioners and practices of most cultures, and a variety of forms of healing that are institutionalized in cultural traditions but not generally part of an official or professional medical system.

General adaptation syndrome. The common physiological response to stress, which involves three main stages: (1) stress or alarm reaction of the body; (2) resistance with a new adaptation at an increased level of pituitary or adrenal activity; and (3) exhaustion from resource depletion, leading to disease or death.

General cultural competence. Knowledge of the ways culture in general affects intergroup interactions, and an ability to apply cultural knowledge, cultural resources (translators, interpreters), and intercultural skills to resolve the difficulties presented by cultural differences.

Genotype. The genetic code of a species.

Heal. Resolving the problems of illness and sickness, rather than the cure of disease.

Health. A positive state of physical, emotional, mental, personal, and spiritual well-being, a condition of balance of an individual with nature and his or her social world (based on World Health Organization conceptualization).

Health behavior. Activities that affect health either beneficially or negatively.

Health beliefs model. A public health approach to health behaviors based on a consideration of the many factors that affect people's awareness of causes of health problems and the possible resources for ameliorating them.

Heterozygous. A location on a gene that has two different kinds of a DNA sequence (alleles); a different allele is contributed by each parent.

HIV. Human immunodeficiency virus.

HMO. Health maintenance organization.

Homozygous. A location on a gene that has two identical copies (alleles) of a DNA sequence; the same gene is contributed by both parents.

Iatrogenic. Diseases or other adverse effects occurring as a consequence of medical intervention.

ICD. International Classification of Diseases.

Ideology. Beliefs and philosophies; typically a doctrine about political behavior. *See* Superstructure.

Idioms of distress. A culturally patterned way of presenting distress and illness; a metaphoric language in which the symptoms constitute a symbolic system that expresses the relationship of patients to others in their interpersonal and social worlds.

Illness. A concept of health maladies that focuses on the personal experience of suffering.

Incidence. The number or rate of new cases of a specific disease during a specific period.

Indigenous psychology. Cultural views, assumptions, and metaphors about the nature of the person, including how to relate to others and the world.

Indirectly contributing factors. Conditions that are less proximal to health outcomes but contribute to them by effects on directly contributing factors, such as how community practices that affect access to food stamps indirectly contribute to infant mortality through influencing mothers' nutritional status.

Individuation. Processes producing a psychologically whole and integrated consciousness.

Infrastructure. Cultural institutions that regulate production and reproduction: production involves energy-extraction procedures; reproduction refers to cultural influences on copulation, fertility, birth, and the population growth patterns.

Innate modules. Anatomical structures and functional systems of the brain with specific information-processing functions (e.g., a language module, a self module).

IOM. Institute of Medicine.

Kin. People who are related by biology or social relations (e.g., marriage); kinship involves the extensions of family structures into broader networks of relations.

Lay. Nonprofessional practices of health care based in remedies from home and community networks. *See* Popular sector.

Macrolevel. Approaches that focus on societal institutions, such as politics or the economy.

MADD. Mothers Against Drunk Driving.

Malady. A general term used to include disease, illness, sickness, and other health problems that are problematic for people's well-being; an umbrella reference for illness, sickness, and disease.

Matrilocal family. A family system organized around residence with mother and mother's kin.

Meaning. The significance and implications of circumstances for a person.

Medicalization. A process by which life conditions are brought under the purview of medical care (e.g., making a disease of alcoholism or homosexuality and providing treatments).

Medical pluralism. The existence of several different medical systems within a society.

Microlevel. Approaches that focus on the domain of interpersonal relations, such as direct interactions between physician and patient.

Midwife. A person who specializes in the delivery of babies without the professional training and designation of nursing or biomedicine.

Mimesis. The ability to consciously reproduce intentional representations of the structures of events through mimicry and imitation.

Morbidity. An assessment of disease, injury, and disability.

Mortality. Death; the rate of death from specific causes.

NAC. See Native American church.

Native American church. A syncretic religious healing tradition of Native Americans based on a blend of ancient peyote rituals and Christianity.

Natural selection. A process and mechanism by which genetic characteristics most adaptive for current circumstances are more likely to occur in subsequent generations of a population; natural selection enables those members of a species with the best genetically determined physiological and behavioral capacities for adapting to their immediate environment to increase their chances of survival and reproduction.

Necessary cause. Cause that is required to be present to cause disease.

Neomammalian brain (telencephalon or neocortical structures). Aspects of the brain that resulted from hominid encephalization and provided the basis for advanced symbolic processes and language.

Neurognostic structures. Basic forms of knowledge provided by the biological structures and functions of an organism.

NIH. National Institutes of Health.

Nocebo effects. Generally conceptualized as negative placebo effects; "the causation of sickness (or death) by expectations of sickness (or death) and by associated emotional states" (Hahn, 1997, p. 607).

Noncompliance. Patients' failure to comply with medical recommendations.

Nosologies. Systems for the scientific and medical classification of disease conditions.

Nuclear family. Family comprising spouses and their children.

OCD. Obsessive-compulsive disorder.

Opioids. The body's natural opiate substances. *See* Endogenous opiates.

Paleomammalian brain (limbic system). Primitive mammalian brain or "emotional brain" that mediates sex; eating and drinking; fighting or self-defense; emotions; social relations, bonding, and attachment; and the sense of self that provides the basis for beliefs, certainty, and convictions.

Partera. Mexican midwife.

Participant observation. A method of studying culture by direct participation in everyday life.

Patient empowerment. Acquiring the ability to understand and affect the allocation of health resources.

Patrilineal extended family. Extended family structure organized around multigenerational descent in the male line.

Personality. The overall organization and dynamics of the psychological processes that provide stability for individual behavior, encompassing cultural concepts of the person and symbolic, mental, emotional, behavioral, and social capacities as well as beliefs, dispositions, drives, perceptions, cognition, and memory.

Peyote religion. *See* Native American church.

Phenotype. The physical appearance of an organism, the manifestations of its genetic potentials in its adaptation to the environment.

Placebos. Inert substances without biochemical characteristics for evoking physiological responses but that nonetheless produce measurable physiological or psychological changes (or both).

Popular sector. Healing practices that are part of general cultural knowledge; primarily focused on what one's family and community do for health care and in response to illness and disease.

Possession. A cultural interpretation involving the control of a person by spirits. Possession takes many forms and interpretations and may mean an altered state of consciousness; explain changes in behavior and appearances; or provide a mechanism for expressing unconscious material, normative expectations, psychosocial relations, and interpersonal conflicts.

Possession trances. An altered state of consciousness believed to involve changes in personality, consciousness, or awareness that are explained by a belief in an external spirit or power that takes over and controls the person and his or her body and experiences.

Prevalence. The relative number or percentage of cases of a condition in a population at a time, assessing all of the cases of disease at a particular time.

Professional sector. Official and legally sanctioned medical care services; the professional sphere differs cross-culturally, reflecting the effects of culture and politics on health systems; biomedicine is the dominant representative of the professional sector cross-culturally.

Protective factors. Factors that reduce disease risks, such as good hygiene.

Protomentation. Thought processes that regulate the daily master behavioral routines and subroutines; emotional mentation influences behavior on the basis of information subjectively manifested as affects.

Proximal cause. Biological changes that lead to a diseased state, the most direct causes of a disease, that are medically treated.

Psychocultural adaptations. The development of psychobiological capacities in culturally specific ways.

Psychogenic. Caused by psychological factors. *See* Somatization.

Psychointegrators. Substances that affect brain-wave integration through effects on serotonergic neurotransmission; also called hallucinogens, psychedelics.

Psychoneuroimmunology. The investigation of the interaction among the central nervous system, the endocrine system, and the immune system (Lyon, 1993), particularly symbolic tuning between the nervous and immune systems (Varela, 1997). This illustrates the ability of symbols, expectations, stress, and social relations to affect the immune response through the ways in which thought and feeling interact with the body.

Psychophysiological symbolism. Refers to the effects of symbols on physiological processes.

Psychosomatic disorders. The effects of psychological dynamics such as thought and feeling on the body.

Race. A concept historically developed to represent genetically distinct groups of humans having unique biological traits; such populations do not exist. Race is a misconception about the basis of human differences that are better reflected in the concept of ethnicity.

Rapid assessment, response, and evaluation (RARE). An ethnographic approach that is based in collaboration with community leaders, incorporation of community resources in assessment of problems, and development and implementation of solutions.

Rates. The relative frequency of a condition, such as a disease, in a population.

Religious experiences. Religious experiences are differentiated from spiritual experiences in being associated with behaviors and beliefs related to specific institutions and traditions whereas spiritual experiences are conceptualized as a personal experience in relationship to a transcendent being.

REM [rapid eye movement] sleep. The period during which dream activity occurs.

Reptilian brain (R complex). An ancient part of the brain based in the upper spinal cord, portions of the mesencephalon (midbrain), diencephalon (thalamus-hypothalamus), and basal ganglia; it regulates organic functions such as metabolism, digestion, and respiration and coordinates behavior, including reproduction and self-preservation.

Risk factors. Conditions found to be associated with the presence of disease and death; these may reflect direct or indirect contributory factors in a causal web, or they may reflect noncausal associations with other primary causal factors.

Roles. The responsibilities and behavioral expectations associated with a status or position.

Self. A social organism's representation of the organism for the organism and others.

Serotonin neural pathway. A key neurotransmitter system involved in the integration of brain processes and the modulation of the functions of other neurotransmitter systems.

Shaman. A spiritual healing potential that emerged during human evolution and was found in hunter-gatherer societies worldwide.

Shamanistic healer. A healing practitioner who uses altered states of consciousness as the basis for training and professional functions involving community healing rituals.

Sickness. The socially induced aspect of a malady.

Sick role. Cultural, social, and interpersonal expectations regarding the behavior of a person suffering a malady.

Socialization. Experiences that teach how to behave as members of society.

Socialized medicine. A political system in which health care is provided by the government as a public right.

Social networks. A person-centered web of social ties that link people.

Social support. Aid in the form of social interaction that can reduce patient stress and increase support and effectiveness of treatment through personal relationships; includes relations with others that are protective, reducing the deleterious effects of stress through aid; refines the social network concept by determining what assistance is actually or potentially available from the network; has numerous functional dimensions, including emotional, expressive, instrumental, material, financial, informational, and appraisal.

Sociogenic diseases. Conditions that have their roots in social causes as a consequence of lifestyle, behavior, diet, activity, and other factors that increase risks.

Sociosomatic. Social effects on individual physiological responses.

Somatization. A group (family) of **somatoform disorders**; a process by which psychological conflict is transformed into bodily symptoms; and a process or style of clinical presentation of symptoms in which somatic conditions take precedence over emotional or psychological concerns. It involves a language of distress in which somatic or bodily complaints are reflective of psychological dynamics and concerns and a person's psychological relationship to his or her social world, including the social dimensions of suffering or the intrapsychic dynamics of guilt, shame, or self-inflicted punishment.

Somatoform disorders. Psychiatric illnesses with bodily symptoms as central features; in earlier periods, these types of mental illness were often referred to as hysteria.

Soul journey. Also known as shamanic flight, an experience in which some aspect of the self (soul, spirit) is thought to depart the body and travel to other places in ordinary or nonordinary reality.

Spiritual experiences. Differentiated from religious responses in being a transcendent and personal relationship with a higher being rather than associated with behaviors related to specific institutions.

Stakeholders. People and groups with interests and involvements in specific health outcomes.

Status. At position within a social network (e.g., different types of positions in a family).

STD. Sexually transmitted disease.

Sufficient cause. Cause that alone results in a disease.

Superstructure. The abstract essence of culture, the mental and symbolic forms of a culture; a central aspect is the worldview, the broad organizing frameworks and principles for understanding and relating to the universe.

Symbolic healing. Method using myth to associate mind, meaning, and structures in the brain to evoke a healing response.

Symbolic penetration. The effects of a symbolically elicited neural system on other physical systems; allows meaning to influence biological processes.

Taxon. A basic biologically determined integrated behavioral response of the body.

Total drug effect. Includes the nonpharmacological factors that are responsible for variation in individual responses to drugs, including the placebo effect and other social, interpersonal, and personal factors.

Transcultural. The perspectives of many cultures.

Triangulation. Using several sources of information.

Triune brain. Three anatomically distinct systems that provide behavioral, emotional, and cognitive functions through the reptilian brain or R complex, paleomammalian brain (limbic system), and the neomammalian brain (neocortical structures), respectively.

Unconventional medicine. Medical practices not generally accepted by biomedicine; a synonym for alternative and complementary medicine.

WHO. World Health Organization.

REFERENCES

Aberle, D. 1966. *The peyote religion among the Navaho.* Chicago: Aldine.

Achterberg, J. 1985. *Imagery in healing: Shamanism and modern medicine.* Boston: New Science Library/Shambhala.

Ackerknecht, E. H. 1943. Psychopathology, primitive medicine, and primitive culture. *Bulletin of the History of Medicine* 14:30–67.

Aghajanian, G. 1994. Serotonin and the action of LSD in the brain. *Psychiatric Annals* 24(3):137–141.

Alcalay, R., A. Ghee, and S. Scrimshaw. 1993. Designing prenatal care messages for low-income Mexican women. *Public Health Reports* 108(3 May-Jun):354–362.

Aldrich, K. 1999. *The medical interview: Gateway to the doctor-patient relationship.* London: Taylor & Francis.

Alexander, C., J. Davies, C. Dixon, M. Dillbeck, S. Drucker, R. Oetzel, J. Muehlman, and D. Orme-Johnson. 1990. Growth of higher stages of consciousness: The Vedic psychology of human development. In *Higher stages of human development: Perspectives on adult growth,* eds. C. Alexander and E. Langer, 286–341. New York: Oxford University Press.

Alexander, C., P. Robinson, D. Orme-Johnson, R. Schneider, and K. Walton. 1994. The effects of transcendental meditation compared to other methods of relaxation and meditation in reducing risks factors, morbidity, and mortality. *Homeostasis* 35(4–5): 243–264.

Alper, K., H. Lotsof, G. Frenken, D. Luciano, and J. Bastiaans. 1999. Treatment of acute opioid withdrawal with ibogaine. *American Journal on Addictions* 8(3):234–242.

Alper, K., H. Lotsof, G. Frenken, D. Luciano, and J. Bastiaans. 2000. Ibogaine in acute opioid withdrawal. An open label case series. *Annals of the New York Academy of Sciences* 909:257–259.

American Psychiatric Association. 1952. *Diagnostic and statistical manual of mental disorders.* 1st ed. (DSM-I). Washington, D.C.: American Psychiatric Press.

American Psychiatric Association. 1968. *Diagnostic and statistical manual of mental disorders.* 2nd ed. (DSM-II). Washington, D.C.: American Psychiatric Press.

American Psychiatric Association. 1980. *Diagnostic and statistical manual of mental disorders.* 3rd ed. (DSM-III). Washington, D.C.: American Psychiatric Press.

American Psychiatric Association. 1994. *Diagnostic and statistical manual of mental disorders.* 4th ed. (DSM-IV). Washington, D.C.: American Psychiatric Press.

American Psychiatric Association. 2000. *Diagnostic and statistical manual of mental disorders.* 4th ed., text rev. (DSM-IV-TR). Washington, D.C.: American Psychiatric Press.

American Public Health Association (APHA), Association of Schools of Public Health, Association of State and Territorial Health Officials, National Association of County Health Officials, United States Conference of Local Health Officers, Department of Health and Human Services, Public Health Service, Centers for Disease Control. 1991. *Healthy communities 2000: Model standards.* 3rd ed. Washington, D.C.: APHA.

Ames, G., and C. Janes. 1987. Heavy and problem drinking in an American blue-collar population. *Social Science and Medicine* 25:949–960.

Ames, G., and C. Janes. 1990. Drinking, social networks, and the workplace. In *Alcohol problem intervention in the workplace,* ed. P. Roman, 95–112. New York: Quorum Books.

Ames, G., and C. Janes. 1992. A cultural approach to conceptualizaing alcohol and the workplace. *Alcohol, Health and Research World* 16(2):102–112.

Ames, G., W. Delaney, and C. Janes. 1992. Obstacles to effective alcohol policy in the workplace: A case study. *British Journal of Addiction* 87:91–105.

Anderson, R. 1987. The treatment of musculoskeletal disorders by a Mexican bonesetter (*sobador*). *Social Science and Medicine* 24(1):43–46.

Andritzky, W. 1989a. Sociopsychotherapeutic Functions of Ayahuasca Healing in Amazonia. *Journal of Psychoactive Drugs* 21(1): 77–89.

Armstrong, D. 2007. Pfizer is sued over Lipitor marketing. *Wall Street Journal,* December 20, B5.

Asante, M. 1984. The African American mode of transcendence. *Journal of Transpersonal Psychology* 16:167–177.

Ashbrok, J., ed. 1993. *Brain, culture, and the human spirit: Essays from an emergent evolutionary perspective.* Lanham, Md.: University Press of America.

Averill, J. 1996. An analysis of psychophysiological symbolism and its influence on theories of emotion. In *The emotions: Social, cultural and biological dimensions,* eds. R. Harre and W. Parrott, 204–228. Thousand Oaks, Calif.: Sage.

Baars, B. J. 1997. *In the theater of consciousness.* New York: Oxford University Press.

Baer, H. 1981a. Prophets and advisors in black spiritual churches: Therapy, palliative or opiate? *Culture, Medicine and Psychiatry* 5:145–170.

Baer, H. 1981b. The organizational rejuvenation of osteopathy as a reflection of the decline of professional dominance in medicine. *Social Science and Medicine* 15(a):701–712.

Baer, H. 1982. On the political economy of health. *Medical Anthropology Newsletter* 14(1):1–17.

Baer, H. 1984. *The black spiritual movement: A religious response to racism.* Knoxville: University of Tennessee Press.

Baer, H. 1988. *Recreating utopia in the desert: A sectarian challenge to modern Mormonism.* Albany: State University of New York Press.

Baer, H. 1990. Kerr McKee and the NRC: From Indian country to Silkwood to Gore. *Social Science and Medicine* 30:237–248.

Baer, H. 1997a. Partisan observation in the formation of a faculty union: The challenge of organizing in a southern urban university. In *Practicing anthropology in the South,* ed. J. Wallace, 133–141. Athens: University of Georgia Press.

Baer, H. 1997b. Introduction to symposium: Ongoing studies in critical medical anthropology. *Social Science and Medicine* 44(10):1563–1573.

Baer, H. 1998. *Crumbling walls and tarnished ideals: An ethnography of East Germany before and after unification.* Lanham, Md.: University Press of America.

Baer, H. 2001. *Biomedicine and Alternative healing systems in America: Issues of class, race, ethnicity, and gender.* Madison: University of Wisconsin Press.

Baer, H. 2004. Toward an integrative medicine: Merging alternative therapies with biomedicine. Lanham, Md.: Altamira Press.

Baer, H., and C. Hughes. 1987. Institutional factors in the implementation of a health care program in rural Utah towns. In *Encounters with biomedicine: Case studies in medical anthropology,* ed. H. Baer, 29–42. New York: Gordon & Breach.

Baer, H., J. Johnsen, and M. Singer, eds. 1986. Towards a critical medical anthropology. Special Issue of *Social Science and Medicine* 23(2).

Baer, H., and M. Singer. 1992. *African-American religion in the twentieth century.* Knoxville: University of Tennessee Press.

Baer, H., M. Singer, and J. Johnsen. 1986. Introduction toward a critical medical anthropology. *Social Science and Medicine* 23(2):95–98.

Baer, H., M. Singer, and I. Susser. 1997. *Medical anthropology and the world system: A critical perspective.* Westport, Conn.: Bergin & Garvey.

Baer, R., and M. Bustillo. 1993. Susto and mal de ojo among Florida farmworkers: Emic and etic perspectives. *Medical Anthropology Quarterly* 7(1):90–100.

Baer, R., and M. Bustillo. 1998. Caida de mollera among children of Mexican migrant workers: Implications for the study of folk illnesses. *Medical Anthropology Quarterly* 12(2):241–249.

Bailey, E. 2004. African Americans. In *Encyclopedia of medical anthropology,* ed. C. Ember and M. Ember, 545–557. New York: Kluwer/Plenum.

Bandlamudi, L. 1994. Dialogics of understanding self/culture. *Ethos* (22):160–193.

Bannerman, R., J. Burton, and C. Wen-Chieh, eds. 1983. *Traditional medicine and health care coverage.* Geneva: World Health Organization.

Barnes, L., and S. Sered. 2005. *Religion and healing in America.* New York: Oxford University Press.

Bartlett, H. 2003. Working definition of social work practice. *Research on Social Work Practice* 13(3):267–270. Originally published in *Social Work* 3(2):5–8.

Bates, M. S. 1987. Ethnicity and pain, a biocultural model. *Social Science and Medicine* 24:47–50.

Bates, M. S. 1996. *Biocultural dimensions of chronic pain: Implications for treatment of multiethnic populations.* Albany: State University of New York Press.

Bates, M. S., and W. T. Edwards. 1998. Ethnic variation in the chronic pain experience. In *Understanding and applying medical anthropology,* ed. P. Brown. Mountain View, Calif.: Mayfield. Originally published in *Ethnicity and Disease* 1992; 2(1):63–83.

Bates, M. S., and L. Rankin-Hill. 1994. Control, culture and chronic pain. *Social Science and Medicine* 39(5):629–645.

Bates, M. S., L. Rankin-Hill, M. Sanchez-Ayendez, and R. Mendez-Bryan. 1995. A cross-cultural comparison of adaptation to chronic pain among Anglo-Americans and native Puerto Ricans. *Medical Anthropology* 16:141–173.

Baum, A., and J. Garofalo. 2000. Biochemistry of emotions. In *Encyclopedia of human emotions,* eds. D. Levinson, J. Ponzetti, and P. Jorgensen, 101–105. New York: Macmillan.

Becker, M. 1974. *The health beliefs model and personal health behavior.* Thorofare, N.J.: SLACK.

Beebe, J. 2001. *Rapid assessment process: An introduction.* Walnut Creek, Calif.: AltaMira Press.

Benedetti, F., and M. Amanzio. 1997. The neurobiology of placebo analgesia: From endogenous opioids to cholecystokinin. *Progress in Neurobiology* 51:109–125.

Benedict, R. 1923. *The concept of the guardian spirit in North America.* New York: American Anthropological Association.

Bennett, M. 1993. Toward ethnorelativism: A developmental model of intercultural sensitivity. In *Education for the intercultural experience,* ed. M. Paige, 21–71. Yarmouth, Me.: Intercultural Press.

Bennett, P., P. LeCompte, M. Miller, and N. Rushforth. 1976. Epidemiological studies of diabetes in the Pima Indians. *Hormonal Research* 32:333–376.

Benyshek, D., C. Johnston, and J. Martin. 2004. Post-natal diet determines insulin resistance in fetally malnourished rats (F_1) but diet does not modify the insulin resistance of their offspring (F_2). *Life Sciences* 74:3033–3041.

Benyshek, D., C. Johnston, and J. Martin, 2006. Glucose metabolism is altered in the adequately nourished grand offspring $(F_3$ generation) of rats malnourished during gestation and perinatal life. *Diabetologia* 49:1117–1119.

Benyshek, D., J. Martin, and C. Johnston. 2001. A reconsideration of the origins of the type 2 diabetes epidemic among Native Americans and the implications for intervention policy. *Medical Anthropology* 20(1):25–63.

Berkman, L. 1981. Physical health and the social environment: A social epidemiological perspective. In *The relevance of social science for medicine,* ed. L. Eisenberg and A. Kleinman, 51–75. Dordrecht, Holland: D. Reidel.

Berkman, L. 1983. *Health and ways of living: The Alameda County study.* New York: Oxford University Press.

Berkman, L. 1984. Assessing the physical health effects of social networks and social support. *American Review of Public Health* 5:413–432.

Berkman, L. 1985. The relationship of social networks and social support to morbidity and mortality. In *Social support and health,* eds. S. Cohen and S. Syme, 241–262. New York: Academic Press.

Berkman, L., and I. Kawachi. 2000. *Social epidemiology.* New York: Oxford University Press.

Bird-David, N. 1999. "Animism" revisited: Personhood, environment, and relational epistemology. *Current Anthropology* 40:67–91.

Blagrove, M. 1996. Problems with the cognitive psychological modeling of dreaming. *Journal of Mind and Behavior* 17(2):99–134.

Bliatout, B. 1983. *Hmong sudden unexpected nocturnal death: A cultural study.* Portland, Ore.: Sparkle Enterprise.

Bliss, K. 1988. LSD and psychotherapy. *Contemporary Drug Problems* Winter, 519–563.

Blum, H. 1983. *Expanding health care horizons from a general systems concept of health to a national health policy.* Oakland, Calif.: Third Party.

Blumhagen, D. 1979. The doctor's white coat: The image of the physician in modern America. *Annals of Internal Medicine* 91:111–116.

Bock, P. 1988. *Rethinking psychological anthropology.* New York: Freeman.

Boddy, J. 1994. Spirit possession revisited: Beyond instrumentality. *Annual Review of Anthropology* 23:407–434.

Boire, R. 2007. Psychedelic medicine and the law. In *Psychedelic medicine,* vol. 1, eds. M. Winkelman and T. Roberts, 217–232. Westport, Conn.: Praeger.

Bolton, M., and B. Wilson. 2005. The influence of race on heart failure in African-American women. *MEDSURG Nursing* 14(1):8–16.

Boone, M. 1991. Policy and praxis in the 1990s: Anthropology and the domestic health policy arena. In *Training manual in applied medical anthropology,* ed. C. Hill, 23–53. Washington, D.C.: American Anthropology Association.

Bourgeault, I., C. Benoit, and R. Davis-Floyd, eds. 2002. *Reconceiving midwives: The new Canadian model of care.* Ann Arbor: University of Michigan Press.

Bourguignon, E. 1976a. *Possession.* San Francisco: Chandler & Sharp.

Bourguignon, E. 1976b. Spirit possession beliefs and social structure. In *The realm of the extra-human ideas and actions,* ed. A. Bhardati. The Hague: Mouton.

Bourguignon, E., and T. Evascu. 1977. Altered states of consciousness within a general evolutionary perspective: A holocultural analysis. *Behavior Science Research* 12(3):197–216.

Bowser, B., E. Quimby, and M. Singer, eds. 2007. *When communities assess their AIDS epidemics: Results of rapid assessment of HIV/AIDS in eleven U.S. cities.* Lanham, Md.: Lexington Books.

Boyer, P. 1992. *The naturalness of religious ideas.* Berkeley: University of California Press.

Bravo, G., and C. Grob. 1989. Shamans, sacraments and psychiatrists. *Journal of Psychoactive Drugs* 21(1):123–128.

Brenner, H. 1973. *Mental illness and the economy.* Cambridge, Mass.: Harvard University Press.

Brindis, C. 1992. Adolescent pregnancy prevention for Hispanic youth: The role of schools, families, and communities. *Journal of School Health* 62(7):345–351.

Brody, H. 1973. The systems view of man: Implications for medicine, science and ethics. *Perspectives in Biology and Medicine* Autumn, 71–91.

Brody, H. 1987. *Stories of sickness.* New Haven, Conn.: Yale University Press.

Brody, H. 2000. *The placebo response: How you can release the body's inner pharmacy for better health.* New York: HarperCollins.

Brown, P., M. Inhorn, and D. Smith. 1996. Disease, ecology and human behavior. In *Handbook of medical anthropology contemporary theory and method,* eds. C. Sargent and T. Johnson, 183–218. Westport, Conn.: Greenwood Press.

Brown, S. 2000. The "musilanguage" model of music. In *The origins of music,* eds. N. Wallin, B. Merker, and S. Brown, 271–300. Cambridge, Mass.: MIT Press.

Browner, C., B. Ortiz de Montellano, and A. Rubel. 1988. A methodology for cross-cultural ethnomedical research. *Current Anthropology* 29(5):681–702.

Browner, C., and C. Sargent. 1996. Anthropology and studies of human reproduction. In *Handbook of medical anthropology contemporary theory and method,* eds. C. Sargent and T. Johnson, 219–234. Westport, Conn.: Greenwood Press.

Brownlee, A. T. 1978. *Community, culture and care: A cross-cultural guide for health workers.* St. Louis: Mosby.

Brues, A. 1977. *People and races.* Prospect Heights, Ill.: Waveland Press.

Burgess, C., A. O'Donohoe, and M. Gill. 2000. Agony and ecstasy: A review of MDMA effects and toxicity. *European Psychiatry* 15(5):287–94.

Burns, K. 1999. *Forensic anthropology training manual.* Upper Saddle River, N.J.: Prentice Hall.

Byrd, R. 1988. Positive therapeutic effects of intercessory prayer in coronary care unit population. *Southern Medical Journal* 81:826–829.

Calabrese, J. 1997. Spiritual healing and human development in the Native American church: Toward a cultural psychiatry of peyote. *Psychoanalytic Review* 84(2):237–255.

Calabrese, J. 2007. The therapeutic use of peyote in the Native American church. In *Psychedelic medicine,* vol. 2, eds. M. Winkelman and T. Roberts, 29–42. Westport, Conn.: Praeger.

Callahan, G. 2006. Eating dirt: Emerging infectious diseases. In *Health and healing in comparative perspective,* ed. E. Whitaker, 467–474. Upper Saddle River, N.J.: Pearson.

Callaway, J., and C. Grob. 1998. Ayahuasca preparations and serotonin reuptake inhibitors: A potential combination for severe adverse interactions. *Journal of Psychoactive Drugs* 30(4):367–369.

Cannon, W. 1942. "Voodoo" death. *American Anthropologist* 44(2):169–181.

Cannon, W. 2002. "Voodoo" death. *American Journal of Public Health* 92(10):1592–1596.

Cassidy, C. 1996. Social and cultural context of complementary and alternative medicine systems. In *Fundamentals of complementary and alternative medicine,* ed. M. Micozzi, 9–34. New York: Churchill Livingstone.

Castillo, R. 1985. The transpersonal psychology of Pata–jali's Yoga-Sûtra (Book I: Samâdhi): A translation and interpretation. *Journal of Mind and Behavior* 6: 391–417.

Castillo, R. 1990. Depersonalization and meditation. *Psychiatry* 53:158–168.

Castillo, R. 1991a. Divided consciousness and enlightenment in Hindu Yogis. *Anthropology of Consciousness* 2(3–4):1–6.

Castillo, R. 1991b. Culture, trance and mental illness: Divided consciousness in South Asia. Doctoral dissertation, Harvard University.

Castillo, R. 1992a. Cultural considerations for trance and possession disorder in DSM-IV. *Transcultural Psychiatric Research Review* 29:333–337.

Castillo, R. 1992b. Cultural considerations for the dissociative disorders in DSM-IV. In *Cultural proposals for DSM-IV,* ed. J. Mezzich and A. Kleinman et al., 138–143. Pittsburgh: University of Pittsburgh.

Castillo, R. 1993. Comments on DSM-IV drafts of the dissociative disorders. In *Revised cultural proposals for DSM-IV,* ed. J. Mezzich and A. Kleinman et al., 90–104. Pittsburgh: University of Pittsburgh.

Castillo, R. 1994a. Spirit possession in South Asia, dissociation or hysteria? Part 1: Theoretical background. *Culture, Medicine and Psychiatry* 18(1):1–21.

Castillo, R. 1994b. Spirit possession in South Asia, dissociation or hysteria? Part 2: Case histories. *Culture, Medicine and Psychiatry* 18(2):141–162.

Castillo, R. 1994c. The impact of culture on dissociation: On enhancing the cultural suitability of DSM-IV. In *Cultural issues and DSM-IV: Support papers,* ed. J. Mezzich and A. Kleinman et al., 149–158. Pittsburgh: University of Pittsburgh.

Castillo, R. 1995. Culture, trance and the mind-brain. *Anthropology of Consciousness* 6(1):17–34.

Castillo, R. 1997a. *Culture and mental illness: A client-centered approach.* Pacific Grove, Calif.: Brooks/Cole.

Castillo, R. 1997b. Dissociation. In *Culture and psychopathology: A guide to clinical assessment,* eds. W. S. Tseng and J. Streltzer, 101–123. New York: Brunner/Mazel.

Castillo, R. 1997c. Impact of culture on dissociation: Enhancing the cultural suitability of DSM-IV. In *DSM-IV Sourcebook,* vol. 3, eds. T. Widiger, A. Frances, H. Pincus, R. Ross, M. B. First, and W. Davis, 943–949. Washington, D.C.: American Psychiatric Press.

Castillo, R. 1998a. *Meanings of madness.* Pacific Grove, Calif.: Brooks/Cole.

Castillo, R. 1998b. Yoga in India: Mental health perspectives. In *Proceedings of the second Pan-Asia Pacific Conference on mental health,* eds. S. Yucan and X-S. Chen, 363–369. Beijing: China Association for Mental Health.

Castillo, R. 1999. Unrecognized dissociation in psychotic outpatients and implications of ethnicity. *Journal of Nervous and Mental Disease* 187(12):751–754.

Castillo, R. 2001. Lessons from folk healing practices. In *Culture and psychotherapy: A guide to clinical practice,* eds. W. Tseng and J. Streltzer, 81–101. Washington, D.C.: American Psychiatric Press.

Castro, F. 1998. Cultural competence in clinical psychology: Assessment, clinical intervention, and research. In *Comprehensive clinical psychology,* eds. S. Bellack and M. Hersen, 127–140. Oxford, U.K.: Pergamon.

Chambers, E. 1985. *Applied anthropology: A practical guide.* Englewood Cliffs, N.J.: Prentice-Hall.

Chaplin, S. 1997. Somatization. In *Culture and psychopathology,* eds. W-S. Tseng and J. Streltzer, 67–86. New York: Brunner/Mazel.

Chassin, M. R., R. W. Galvin, and National Roundtable on Health Care Quality. 1998. The urgent need to improve health care quality. *Journal of the American Medical Association* 280:1000–1005.

Chavez, L. 1984. Doctors, curanderos and brujas: Health care delivery and Mexican immigrants in San Diego. *Medical Anthropology Quarterly* 15(2):31–37.

Chrisman, N. 1974. Middle-class communities: The fraternal order of badgers. *Ethos* 2(4):356–376.

Chrisman, N. 1977. The health seeking process: An approach to the natural history of illness. *Culture, Medicine and Psychiatry* 1(4):351–377.

Chrisman, N. 1981. Ethnic persistence in an urban setting. *Ethnicity* 8:256–292.

Chrisman, N. 1985. Alcoholism: Illness or disease? In *The American experience with alcohol: Contrasting cultural perspectives,* eds. L. Bennett and G. Ames, 7–21. New York: Plenum Press.

Chrisman, N. 1998. Faculty infrastructure for cultural competence education. *Journal of Nursing Education* 37(1):45–48.

Chrisman, N. 2005. Community building for health. In *Community building in the twenty-first century,* ed. S. Hyland, 167–190. Santa Fe: School of American Research Press.

Chrisman, N. 2007. Extending cultural competence through systems change: Academic, hospital, and community partnerships. *Journal of Transcultural Nursing* 18(1):68–76.

Chrisman, N., and J. Backyard. 1998. Cultural change: Diversity workshops at the institution level. *Journal of Multicultural Nursing and Health* 4(1):6–10.

Chrisman, N., and T. Johnson. 1990. Clinically applied anthropology. In *Medical anthropology: Contemporary theory and method,* eds. T. Johnson and C. Sargent, 93–113. New York: Praeger.

Chrisman, N., and T. Johnson. 1996. Clinically applied anthropology. In *Medical anthropology: Contemporary theory and method,* eds. C. Sargent and T. Johnson, 88–113. New York: Praeger.

Chrisman, N., and T. Maretzki, eds. 1982. *Clinically applied anthropology: Anthropologists in health settings.* Boston: Reidel.

Chrisman, N., and P. Schultz. 1997. Transforming health care through cultural competence training. In *Cultural diversity in nursing: Issues, strategies and outcomes,* ed. J. Dienemann, 70–79. Washington, D.C.: American Academy of Nursing.

Chrisman, N., C. Strickland, K. Powell, M. Squeoch, and M. Yallup. 1999. Participatory action research with the Yakima Indian nation. *Human Organization* 58(2):34–140.

Chrisman, N., and M. Thomas, eds. 1982. *Clinically applied anthropology.* Dordrecht, Holland: Reidel.

Chrisman, N., and P. Zimmer. 2000. Cultural competence in primary care. In *Adult primary care,* eds. P. Meredith and N. Horan, 65–75. Philadelphia: Saunders.

Cohen, S., and S. Syme, eds. 1985. Social support and health. Orlando, Fla.: Academic Press.

Csordas, T. 1983. The rhetoric of healing in ritual healing. *Culture, Medicine and Psychiatry* 7:333–375.

Csordas, T. 1994. *The sacred self: A cultural phenomenology of charismatic healing.* Berkeley: University of California Press.

Culhane-Pera, K., D. Vawter, P. Xiong, B. Babbitt, and M. Solberg. 2003. *Healing by heart: Clinical and ethical case stories of Hmong families and western providers.* Nashville: Vanderbilt University Press.

Czaplicka, M. A. 1914. *Aboriginal Siberia: A study in social anthropology.* Oxford, U.K.: Oxford University Press.

d'Aquili, E., and A. Newburg. 1999. *The mystical mind: Probing the biology of religious experience.* Minneapolis: Fortress Press.

Davis-Floyd, R. 1992. *Birth as an American rite of passage.* Berkeley: University of California Press.

Davis-Floyd, R. 1994. The technocratic body: American childbirth as cultural expression. *Social Science and Medicine* 38(8):1125–1140.

Davis-Floyd, R. 1998a. The ups, downs, and interlinkages of nurse- and direct-entry midwifery: Status, practice, and education. In *Getting an education: Paths to becoming a midwife,* eds. J. Tritten and J. Southern, 67–118. Eugene, Ore.: Midwifery Today.

Davis-Floyd, R. 1998b. Types of midwifery training: An anthropological overview. In *Getting an education: Paths to becoming a midwife,* eds. J. Tritten and J. Southern, 119–133. Eugene, Ore.: Midwifery Today.

Davis-Floyd, R. 2000. Global issues in midwifery: Mutual accommodation or biomedical hegemony? *Midwifery Today* March, 12–16, 68–69.

Davis-Floyd, R. 2001. *La partera profesional*: Articulating identity and cultural space for a new kind of midwife in Mexico. *Medical Anthropology* 20(3):85–243.

Davis-Floyd, R. 2003. Home birth emergencies in the U.S. and Mexico: The trouble with transport. In *Reproduction gone awry,* eds. G. Jenkins and M. Inhorn. Special issue of *Social Science and Medicine* 56(9):1913–1931.

Davis-Floyd, R. 2004. Consuming childbirth: The qualified commodification of midwifery care. In *Consuming motherhood,* eds. D. Wozniak, L. Layne, and J. Taylor. New Brunswick, N.J.: Rutgers University Press.

Davis-Floyd, R., and S. Arvidson, eds. 1997. *Intuition: The inside story.* New York: Routledge.

Davis-Floyd, R., L. Barclay, B. A. Daviss, and J. Tritten, eds. 2008. *Birth models that work.* Berkeley: University of California Press.

Davis-Floyd, R., and K. Cox. 2002. *Space stories: Oral histories from the pioneers of the American space program.* New York: Routledge.

Davis-Floyd, R., and E. Davis. 1996. Intuition as authoritative knowledge in midwifery and home birth. *Medical Anthropology Quarterly* 10(2):237–269.

Davis-Floyd, R., and J. Dumit, eds. 1998. *Cyborg babies: From techno-sex to techno-tots.* New York: Routledge.

Davis-Floyd, R., and C. B. Johnson. 2006. *Mainstreaming midwives: The politics of change.* New York: Routledge.

Davis-Floyd, R., S. L. Pigg, and S. Cosminsky. 2001. Daughters of time: The shifting identities of contemporary midwives. *Medical Anthropology* 20(3):185–243.

Davis-Floyd, R., and C. Sargent, eds. 1997. *Childbirth and authoritative knowledge: Cross-cultural perspectives.* Berkeley: University of California Press.

Davis-Floyd, R., and G. St. John. 1998. *From doctor to healer: The transformative journey.* New Brunswick, N.J.: Rutgers University Press.

Delbanco, T. L. 1992. Enriching the doctor-patient relationship by inviting the patient's perspective. *Annals of Internal Medicine* 116(5):414–418.

Delgado, P., and F. Moreno. 1998. Hallucinogens, serotonin, and obsessive-compulsive disorder. *Journal of Psychoactive Drugs* 30(4):359–366.

Denniston, G., and M. Milos, eds. 1997. *Sexual mutilations: A human tragedy.* New York: Plenum.

Diamond, J. 2006. The double puzzle of diabetes. In *Health and healing in comparative perspective,* ed. E. Whitaker, 449–457. Upper Saddle River, N.J.: Pearson.

Dobkin de Rios, M. 1984. *Hallucinogens: Cross-cultural perspectives.* Albuquerque: University of New Mexico.

Dobkin de Rios, M. 2000. *Brief psychotherapy with the Latino immigrant client.* New York: Haworth Press.

Dobkin de Rios, M. 2001. *Brief psychotherapy with the Latino immigrant client.* New York: Haworth Press.

Dobkin de Rios, M. 2002. What we can learn from shamanic healing: Brief psychotherapy with Latino immigrant clients. *American Journal of Public Health* 92:1576–1578.

Dobkin de Rios, M., and D. Smith. 1977. Drug use and abuse in cross-cultural perspective. *Human Organization* 36(1):14–21.

Donald, M. 1991. *Origins of the modern mind.* Cambridge, Mass.: Harvard University Press.

Dougherty, M., and T. Tripp-Reimer. 1985. The interface of nursing and anthropology. *Annual Review of Anthropology* 14:219–241.

Douglas, J. G. 2002. Hypertension in African Americans. *Postgraduate Medicine* 112(4):24–26.

Dow, J. W. 1986. Universal aspects of symbolic healing: A theoretical synthesis. *American Anthropologist* 88:56–69.

Dressler, W. W. 1994. Cross-cultural differences and social influences in social support and cardiovascular disease. In *Social support and cardiovascular disease,* eds. S. Shumaker and S. Czajkowski, 167–192. New York: Plenum.

Dressler, W. W. 1996. Culture, stress, and disease. In *Handbook of medical anthropology: Contemporary theory and method,* eds. C. Sargent and T. Johnson, 252–271. Westport, Conn.: Greenwood Press.

Dressler, W. W., M. C. Balieiro, and J. E. Dos Santos. 1998. Culture, socioeconomic status, and physical and mental health in Brazil. *Medical Anthropology Quarterly* 12(4):424–446.

Dressler, W. W., J. R. Bindon, and Y. H. Neggers. 1998. Culture, socioeconomic status, and coronary heart disease risk factors in an African American community. *Journal of Behavioral Medicine* 21(6):527–544.

Dressler, W. W., A. Mata, A. Chavez, F. E. Viteri, and P. Gallagher. 1986. Social support and arterial pressure in a central Mexican community. *Psychosomatic Medicine* 48(5):338–350.

Dressler, W. W., F. E. Viteri, A. Chavez, G. A. Grell, and J. E. Dos Santos. 1991. Comparative research in social epidemiology: Measurement issues. *Ethnicity and Disease* 1:379–393.

Dubisch, J., and M. Winkelman, eds. 2005. *Pilgrimages and healing.* Tucson: University of Arizona Press.

Dundes-Renteln, A. 2004. *The cultural defense.* New York: Oxford University Press.

Dunn, F., and C. Janes. 1986. Introduction: Medical anthropology and epidemiology. In *Anthropology and epidemiology,* eds. C. Janes, R. Stall, and S. Guifford, 3–34. Dordrecht, Holland: Reidel.

Durch, J., L. Bailey, and M. Stoto, eds. 1997. *Improving health in the community: A role for performance monitoring.* Washington, D.C.: National Academy Press.

Eaton, S., M. Shostak, and M. Konner. 1988. *The paleolithic prescription.* New York: HarperCollins.

Eisenberg, D. M., R. C. Kessler, C. Foster, F. E. Norlock, D. Calkins, and T. L. Delbanco. 1993. Unconventional medicine in the United States: Prevalence, costs, and patterns of use. *New England Journal of Medicine* 328(4):246–252.

Eisenberg, D. M., R. B. Davis, S. L. Ettner, S. Appel, S. Wilkey, M. Van Rompay, and R. C. Kessler. 1998. Trends in alternative medicine use in the United States, 1990–1997: Results of a follow-up national survey. *Journal of the American Medical Association* 280:1569–1575.

Eisenberg, L. 1977. Disease and illness. *Culture, Medicine and Psychiatry* 1:9–23.

Ekman, P. 1972. Universals and cultural differences in facial expressions of emotion. In *Nebraska symposium on motivation,* ed. J. Cold, 207–283. Lincoln: University of Nebraska Press.

Ekman, P. 1973. *Darwin and facial expression: A century of research in review.* New York: Academic Press.

Ekman, P. 1982. *Emotion in the human face.* New York: Cambridge University Press.

Ekman, P. 1986. A new pancultural expression of emotion. *Motivation and Emotion* (10):159–168.

Ekman, P. 2003. *Emotions inside out: 130 years after Darwin's expression of the emotions in man and animals.* New York: New York Academy of Sciences.

Eliade, M. 1964. *Shamanism: Archaic techniques of ecstasy.* New York: Pantheon Books.

Eliade, M. 1974. *Gods, goddesses and myths of creation.* New York: HarperCollins.

Engel, G. 1977. The need for a new medical model: A challenge for biomedicine. *Science* 196(4286):129–136.

Engel, G. 1980. The clinical application of the biopsychosocial model. *American Journal of Psychiatry* 125(5):535–544.

Erickson, P. 2008. *Ethnomedicine.* Long Grove, Ill.: Waveland Press.

Etkin, N., ed. 1986. *Plants in indigenous medicine and diet: Biobehavioral approaches.* New York: Gordon & Breach.

Etkin, N. 1991. The behavioral dimensions of malaria control: Guidelines for culturally sensitive and microecologically germane policies. In *Malaria and development in Africa: A cross-sectoral approach,* ed. AAAS SubSaharan Africa Program, 59–69. Washington D.C.: American Association for the Advancement of Science.

Etkin, N., ed. 1994a. *Eating on the wild side: The pharmacologic, ecologic, and social implications of using nonculti-gens.* Tucson: University of Arizona Press.

Etkin, N. 1994b. The negotiation of "side" effects in Hausa (Northern Nigeria) therapeutics. In *Medicines: Meanings and contexts,* eds. N. Etkin and M. Tan, 17–32. Amsterdam: University of Amsterdam.

Etkin, N. 1996. Ethnopharmacology: The conjunction of medical ethnography and the biology of therapeutic action. In *Medical anthropology: Contemporary theory and method,* eds. C. Sargent and T. Johnson, 169–209. New York: Praeger.

Etkin, N. 1997a. Plants as antimalarial drugs: Relation to G6PD deficiency and evolutionary implications. In *Adaptation to malaria: The interaction of biology and culture,* eds. L. Greene and M. Danubio, 139–176. New York: Gordon & Breach.

Etkin, N. 1997b. Antimalarial plants used by Hausa in Northern Nigeria. *Tropical Doctor* 27(S1):12–16.

Etkin, N., J. Mahoney, M. W. Forsthoefel, J. R. Eckman, J. D. McSwigan, R. F. Gillum, and J. W. Eaton. 1982. Racial differences in hypertension-associated red cell sodium permeability. *Nature* 297:588–589.

Etkin, N., and P. Ross. 1982. Food as medicine and medicine as food: An adaptive framework for the interpretation of plant utilization among the Hausa of Northern Nigeria. *Social Science and Medicine* 16:1559–1573.

Etkin, N., and P. Ross. 1997. Malaria, medicine and meals: A biobehavioral perspective. In *The anthropology of medicine,* eds. L. Romanucci-Ross, D. Moerman, and L. Tancredi, 169–209. New York: Praeger.

Etkin, N., P. Ross, and I. Muazzamu. 1999. The rational basis of "irrational" drug use: Pharmaceuticals in the context of "development." In *Anthropology in public and international health,* ed. R. Hahn, 165–181. Oxford, U.K.: Oxford University Press.

Evans, R. G., and G. L. Stoddart. 1994. Producing health, consuming health care. In *Why are some people healthy and others not? The determinants of health populations,* eds. R. G. Evans, M. L. Baker, and T. R. Marmor, 27–66. New York: Aldine DeGruter.

Evans-Pritchard, E. 1937. *Witchcraft, oracles and magic among the Azande.* Philadelphia: Clarendon.

Fábrega, H. 1997. *Evolution of sickness and healing.* Los Angeles: University of California Press.

Fackelmann, K. 1991. The African gene? *Science news* 140(16):254.

Fadiman, A. 1997. *The spirit catches you and you fall down: A Hmong child, her American doctors, and the collision of two cultures.* New York: Farrar, Strauss, & Giroux.

Faldon, J. 2005. *Negotiating the holistic turn.* Albany: State University of New York Press.

Fallon, S., and M. Enig. 2007. Dangers of statin drugs: What you haven't been told about popular cholesterol-lowering medicines. http://www.westonaprice.org/moderndiseases/statin.html.

Feldman, D. 1986. Anthropology, AIDS, and Africa. *Medical Anthropology Quarterly* 17(2):38–40.

Finkler, K. 1974. *Un estudio comparativo de la economia de dos communidades de Mexico.* Mexico City: Instituto Nacional Indigenists SEPINI Series.

Finkler, K. 1980. Non-medical treatments and their outcomes, part I. *Culture, Medicine and Psychiatry* (4):301–340.

Finkler, K. 1981a. Dissident religious movements in the service of women's power. *Journal of Sex Roles* (7):481–495.

Finkler, K. 1981b. A comparative study of health care seekers: Or, why do some people go to doctors rather than to spiritualist healers? *Medical Anthropology* (4):383–424.

Finkler, K. 1981c. Non-medical treatments and their outcomes, part II. *Culture, Medicine and Psychiatry* (5):65–103.

Finkler, K. 1983. Dissident sectarian movements: The Catholic Church and social class in Mexico. *Comparative Studies in Society and History* 25(2):277–305.

Finkler, K. 1984. The nonsharing of medical knowledge among spiritualist healers and their patients: A contribution to the study of intra-cultural diversity and practitioner-patient relationship. *Medical Anthropology* 3:95–209.

Finkler, K. 1985a. *Spiritualist healers in Mexico.* South Hadley, Mass.: Bergin & Garvey.

Finkler, K. 1985b. Symptomatic differences between the sexes in rural Mexico. *Culture, Medicine and Psychiatry* 9:27–57.

Finkler, K. 1987. Spiritualist healing outcomes and the status quo: A micro and macro analysis. *Social Compass* 34(4):381–396.

Finkler, K. 1989. The universality of nerves. In *Gender, health and illness,* eds. D. Davis and S. Low, 79–88. Health Care for Women International Publication. New York: Hemisphere.

Finkler, K. 1991. *Physicians at work, patients in pain: Biomedical practice and patients' responses in Mexico.* Boulder, Colo.: Westview.

Finkler, K. 1994a. Sacred and biomedical healing compared. *Medical Anthropology Quarter* 8(2):179–198.

Finkler, K. 1994b. El cuidada de la salud: Un problema de relaciones de poder. In *La antropologia medica en Mexico,* ed. R. Campos, 202–221. Mexico City: Universidad Autonomia Metropolitana.

Finkler, K. 1994c. *Women in pain*. Philadelphia: University of Pennsylvania Press.

Finkler, K. 1996. Factors influencing perceived recovery in Mexico. *Social Science and Medicine* 42(2):199–207.

Finkler, K. 1997. Gender, domestic violence and sickness in Mexico. *Social Science and Medicine* 45:1147–1160.

Finkler, K. 2000a. *Experiencing the new genetics: Family and kinship on the medical frontier.* Philadelphia: University of Pennsylvania Press.

Finkler, K. 2000b. Diffusion reconsidered: Variation and transformation in biomedical practice, a case study from Mexico. *Medical Anthropology* 18(1):1–39.

Fitzgerald, M. 2000. Critical thinking 101: The basics of evaluating information. *Knowledge Quest* 29(2):13–20.

Flaherty, G. 1992. *Shamanism and the eighteenth century.* Princeton, N.J.: Princeton University Press.

Flaten, A., T. Simonsen, and H. Olsen. 1999. Drug-related information generates placebo and nocebo responses that modify the drug response. *Psychosomatic Medicine* 61:250–255.

Foster, G., and B. Anderson. 1978. *Medical anthropology.* New York: Wiley.

Fowler, S., and M. Mumford, eds. 1995–1999. *Intercultural sourcebook: Cross-cultural training methods,* vol. 1 and 2. Yarmouth, Me.: Intercultural Press.

Frank, A. 1995a. *At the will of the body: Reflections on illness.* Boston: Houghton Mifflin.

Frank, A. 1995b. *The wounded storyteller: Body, illness, and ethics.* Chicago: University of Chicago Press.

Frazer, J. 1900. *The golden bough: A study in magic and religion.* New York: Macmillan.

Frecska, E. 2007. Therapeutic guidelines: Dangers and contra-indications in therapeutic applications of hallucinogens. In: *Psychedelic medicine,* vol. 1, eds. M. Winkelman and T. Roberts, 69–95. Westport, Conn.: Praeger.

Frecska, E., and Z. Kulcsar. 1989. Social bonding in the modulation of the physiology of ritual trance. *Ethos* 17(1):70–87.

Freeman, W. 2000. A neurobiological role of music in social bonding. In *The origins of music,* eds. N. Wallin, B. Merker, and S. Brown, 411–424. Cambridge, Mass.: MIT Press.

Friedrich, P. 1991. Polytrophy. In *Beyond metaphor: The theory of tropes in anthropology,* ed. J. Fernandez, 17–55. Stanford, Calif.: Stanford University Press.

Fukuyama, M., and T. Sevig. 1999. *Integrating spirituality into multicultural counseling.* Thousand Oaks, Calif.: Sage.

Fuller, R. 2005. Subtle energies and the American metaphysical tradition. In *Religion and healing in America,* eds. L. Barnes and S. Sered, 375–386. New York: Oxford University Press.

Furin, J. 1997. "You have to be your own doctor": Sociocultural influence on alternative therapy use among gay men with AIDS in West Hollywood. *Medical Anthropology Quarterly* 11(4):498–504.

Furst, P., ed. 1976. *Hallucinogens and culture.* San Francisco: Chandler & Sharp.

Gackenbach, J., and S. LaBerge, eds. 1988. *Conscious mind, sleeping brain: New perspectives on lucid dreaming.* New York: Plenum Press.

Gagan, J. 1998. *Journeying where shamanism and psychology meet.* Santa Fe: Rio Chama.

Gaines, A., and R. Davis-Floyd. 2004. Biomedicine. In *Encyclopedia of medical anthropology,* eds. C. Ember and M. Ember, 95–108. New York: Kluwer /Plenum.

Galloway, A., T. Woltanski, and W. Grant, eds. 1993. *Bibliography for the forensic application of anthropology.* Knoxville: University of Tennessee.

Garrity, T. 1974. Psychic death: Behavioral types and psychological parallels. *Omega* 5(3):207–215.

Geissmann, T. 2000. Gibbon songs and human music from an evolutionary perspective. In *The origins of music,* eds. N. Wallin, B. Merker, and S. Brown, 103–123. Cambridge, Mass.: MIT Press.

Gelderloos, P., K. G. Walton, D. W. Orme-Johnson, and C. N. Alexander. 1991. Effectiveness of the transcendental meditation program in preventing and treating substance misuse: A review. *International Journal of the Addictions* 26:293–325.

Gevitz, N., ed. 1988. *Other healers' unorthodox medicine in America.* Baltimore: John Hopkins University Press.

Gilbert, M. J. 1989. Policymaking roles for applied anthropologists: Personally ensuring that your research is used. In *Making our research useful: Case studies in the utilization of anthropological knowledge,* eds. J. Van Willigen, B. Rylko-Bauer, and A. McElroy, 71–88. Boulder, Colo.: Westview Press.

Gilbert, M. J., ed. 2002. The principles and recommended standards for the cultural competence education of health care professionals. Available at: http://www.calendow.org.

Gilbert, M. J., N. Tashima, and C. C. Fishman. 1991. Ethics and practicing anthropologists' dialogue with the larger world: Considerations in the formulation of ethical guidelines for practicing anthropologists. In *Ethics and the profession of anthropology,* ed. C. Fluehr-Lobban, 198–210. Philadelphia: University of Pennsylvania Press.

Gilbert, M. J., and L. Collins. 1997. Ethnic variations in women and men's drinking. In *Individual and social perspectives gender and alcohol,* eds. R. Wilsnack and S. Wilsnack, 357–378. New Brunswick, N.J.: Rutgers Center of Alcohol Studies.

Goldman, R. 1997. *Circumcision: The hidden trauma.* Boston: Vanguard.

Good, B. 1994. *Medicine, rationality, and experience: An anthropological perspective.* Cambridge, Mass.: Cambridge University Press.

Good, B., and M. Good. 1981. The meanings of symptoms. In *The relevance of social sciences for medicines,* eds. L. Eisenberg and A. Kleinman, 165–196. Dordrecht, Holland: Reidel.

Good, M., B. Good, P. Brodwin, and A. Kleinman, eds. 1992. *Pain as human experience: Anthropology studies.* Berkeley: University of California Press.

Goodman, A. 1997. Bred in the bone? *The Sciences* March/April, 20–25.

Goodman, A., and T. Leatherman eds. 1998. *Building a new biocultural synthesis: Political economy perspectives on human biology.* Ann Arbor: University of Michigan Press.

Goodman, F. 1988. *How about demons? Possession and exorcism in the modern world.* Bloomington and Indianapolis: Indiana University Press.

Goodman, R., A. Wandersman, M. Chinman, P. Imm, and E. Morrisey. 1996. An ecological assessment of community-based interventions for prevention and health promotion: Approaches to measuring community coalitions. *American Journal of Community Psychology* 24:33–61.

Graham, R. 1990. *Physiological psychology.* Belmont, Calif.: Wadsworth.

Green, E. C., ed. 1986. *Practicing development anthropology.* Boulder, Colo., and Oxford, U.K.: Westview Press.

Green, E. C. 1987. Anthropology and the planning of health education strategies in Swaziland. In *Anthropological praxis: Translating knowledge into action,* eds. B. Wulff and S. Fiske, 15–25. Boulder, Colo., and Oxford, U.K.: Westview Press.

Green, E. C. 1988a. Can collaborative programs between biomedical and indigenous health practitioners succeed? *Social Science and Medicine* 27(11):1125–1130.

Green, E. C. 1988b. A consumer intercept study of oral contraceptive users in the Dominican Republic. *Studies in Family Planning* 19(2):109–117.

Green, E. C. 1992. Evaluating the response of Swazi traditional leaders to development workshops. *Human Organization* 53(4):379–388.

Green, E. C. 1994. *AIDS and STDs in Africa: Bridging the gap between traditional healers and modern medicine.* Boulder, Colo., and Oxford, U.K.: Westview Press.

Green, E. C. 1996. *Indigenous healers and the African state.* New York: Pact.

Green, E. C. 1997. Purity, pollution and the invisible snake in Southern Africa. *Medical Anthropology* 17(2):83–100.

Green, E. C. 1999a. *Indigenous theories of contagious disease.* Lanham, Md.: Rowman & Littlefield.

Green, E. C. 1999b. The involvement of African traditional healers in the prevention of AIDS and STDs. In *Anthropology in public health: Bridging differences in culture and society,* ed. R. Hahn, 63–83. New York: Oxford University Press.

Green, E. C. 2001. Can qualitative research produce reliable quantitative findings? *Field Methods* 13(1):3–19.

Green, E. C. 2003. *Rethinking AIDS prevention.* Westport, Conn.: Praeger.

Green, E. C., D. T. Halperin, V. Nantulya, and J. A. Hogle. 2006. Uganda's HIV prevention success: The role of sexual behavior change and the national response. *AIDS and Behavior* 10(4):335–346.

Green, E. C., A. Jurg, and A. Dgedge. 1994. The snake in the stomach: Child diarrhea in central Mozambique. *Medical Anthropology Quarterly* 8(1):4–24.

Green, E. C., and K. Witte. 2006. Fear arousal, sexual behavior change and AIDS prevention. *Journal of Health Communication* 11:245–259.

Greer, G., and R. Tolbert. 1998. A method of conducting therapeutic sessions with MDMA. *Journal of Psychoactive Drugs* 30(4):371–379.

Grisbaum, G., and D. Ubelaker. 2001. An analysis of forensic anthropology cases submitted to the Smithsonian Institute by the Federal Bureau of Investigation from 1962 to 1994. *Smithsonian Contributions to Anthropology* 45.

Grob, C., and G. Bravo. 1996. Human research with hallucinogens: Past lessons and current trends. In *Sacred plants, consciousness and healing. Yearbook of cross-cultural medicine and psychotherapy, 5,* eds. M. Winkelman and W. Andritzky, 129–142. Berlin: Verlag.

Grof, S. 1975. *Realms of the unconscious: Observations from LSD research.* New York: Viking Press.

Grof, S. 1980. *LSD psychotherapy.* Pomona, Calif.: Hunter House.

Grof, S. 1992. *The holotropic mind.* San Francisco: HarperCollins.

Grof, S., and C. Grof. 1989. S*piritual emergency: When personal transformation becomes a crisis.* New York: Putnam.

Groisman, A., and M. Dobkin de Rios. 2007. Ayahuasca, the U.S. Supreme Court, and the UDV-U.S. Government Case. In: *Psychedelic medicine,* vol. 1, eds. M. Winkelman and T. Roberts, 271–298. Westport, Conn.: Praeger.

Gropper, R. 1996. *Culture and the clinical encounter: An intercultural sensitizer for the health professions.* Yarmouth, Me.: Intercultural Press.

Guthrie, S. 1993. *Faces in the clouds: A new theory of religion.* New York: Oxford University Press.

Guthrie, S. 1997. The origin of an illusion. In *Anthropology of religion: A handbook,* ed. S. Glazier, 489–504. Westport, Conn.: Greenwood Press.

Haglund, W., and M. Sorg, eds. 1996. *Forensic taphonomy: The postmortem fate of human remains.* Boca Raton, Fla.: CRC Press.

Hahn, R. 1995. *Sickness and healing: An anthropological perspective.* New Haven, Conn.: Yale University Press.

Hahn, R. 1997. The nocebo phenomenon: Concept, evidence, and implications for public health. *Preventive Medicine* 26:607–611.

Hahn, R., and A. Gaines. 1985. *Physicians of western medicine: Anthropological approaches to theory and practice.* Boston: Reidel.

Halifax, J. 1979. *Shamanic voices.* New York: Dutton.

Halpern, J., and H. Pope. 1999. Do hallucinogens cause residual neuropsychological toxicity? *Drug and Alcohol Dependence* 53(3):247–256.

Hammerschlag, C. 1988. *The dancing healers.* San Francisco: HarperCollins.

Harner, M. ed. 1973. *Hallucinogens and shamanism.* New York: Oxford University Press.

Harner, M. 1990. *The way of the shaman.* San Francisco: HarperCollins.

Harrington, A., ed. 1997. *The placebo effect: An interdisciplinary exploration.* Cambridge, Mass.: Harvard University Press:.

Harris, M. 1988. Theoretical principles of cultural materialism. In *High points in anthropology,* eds. P. Bohannan and M. Glazer, 377–403. New York: McGraw-Hill.

Harvard Law Review. 1986. Notes: The cultural defense in criminal law. *Harvard Law Review* 99(6):1293–1311.

Harwood, A., ed. 1981. *Ethnicity and medical care.* Cambridge, Mass.: Harvard University Press.

Hayden, B. 1987. Alliances and ritual ecstasy: Human responses to resource stress. *Journal for the Scientific Study of Religion* 26(1):81–91.

Hayden, B. 2003. *Shamans, sorcerers, and saints: A prehistory of religion.* Washington, D.C.: Smithsonian Books.

Heaney, C., and B. Israel. 2002. *Social networks and social support. Health behavior and health education: Theory, research, and practice,* 3rd ed. San Francisco: Jossey-Bass.

Heath, D. B. 2000. *Drinking occasions: Comparative perspectives on alcohol and culture.* International Center for Alcohol Policies, Series on Alcohol in Society. New York: Routledge.

Heelas, P. 1981. Introduction: Indigenous psychologies. In *Indigenous psychologies,* eds. P. Heelas and A. Lock, 3–18. London: Academic Press.

Heelas, P., and A. Lock. 1981. *Indigenous psychologies.* London: Academic Press.

Heggenhougen, C. 1997. *Reaching new highs: Alternative therapies for drug addicts.* Northvale, N.J.: Aronson.

Helman, C. 1985. *Culture, health and illness.* Worcester: Billing & Sons.

Helman, C. 1994. *Culture, health and illness.* Oxford: Butterworth Heinemann.

Helman, C. 2001. *Culture, health, and illness.* London: Oxford University Press.

Henderson, J., and K. Adour. 1981. Comanche ghost sickness: A biocultural perspective. *Medical Anthropology* 5:195–205.

Herdt, G. 1987. *Guardians of the flutes.* New York: Columbia University Press.

Hess, D. J. 1999. *Evaluating alternative cancer therapies: A guide to the science and politics of an emerging medical field.* New Brunswick, N.J.: Rutgers University Press.

Heurtin-Roberts, S. 1993. High-pertension: The use of chronic folk illness for personal adaptation. *Social Science and Medicine* 37:285–295.

Hill, P. 1997. Toward an attitude process model of religious experience. In *The psychology of religion,* eds. B. Spilka and D. N. McIntosh, 184–193. Boulder, Colo.: Westview Press.

Hinton, A. 1999a. *Biocultural approaches to emotions.* New York: Cambridge University Press.

Hinton, A. 1999b. Introduction. In *Biocultural approaches to emotions,* ed. A. Hinton, 1–37. New York: Cambridge University Press.

Hirsch, M. 2004. A biopsychosocial perspective on cross-cultural healing. In *Handbook of culture, therapy, and healing,* eds. U. Gielen, J. Fish, and J. Draguns, 83–99. Mahwah, N.J.: Erlbaum.

Hobson, J. 1992. Sleep and dreaming: Induction and mediation of REM sleep by cholinergic mechanisms. *Current Opinion in Neurobiology* 2:759–763.

Hobson, J., and R. Stickgold. 1994. Dreaming: A neurocognitive approach. *Consciousness and Cognition* 3:1–15.

Hogan, M. 2007. *The four skills of cultural diversity competence: A process for understanding and practice.* 3rd ed. Pacific Grove, Calif.: Brooks/Cole-Thomson.

Hogan-Garcia, M. 2003. *The four skills of cultural diversity competence.* Pacific Grove, Calif.: Wadsworth-Brooks/Cole.

Holden, P., and J. Littlewood, eds. 1991. *Anthropology and nursing.* London: Routledge.

Holm, N. 1997. An integrated role theory for the psychology of religion: Concepts and perspectives. In *The psychology of religion,* eds. B. Spilka and D. N. McIntosh, 73–84. Boulder, Colo.: Westview Press.

Hughes, C. 1985. Culture-bound or construct bound? In *The culture bound syndromes: Folk illnesses of psychiatric and anthropological interest,* eds. R. Simons and C. Hughes, 3–24. Dordrecht, Holland: Reidel.

Hultkrantz, A. 1978. Ecological and phenomenological aspects of shamanism. In *Shamanism in Siberia,* eds. V. Dioszegi and M. Hoppal, 27–58. Budapest: Akademiai Kiado.

Hunt, H. 1989. *The multiplicity of dreams: Memory, imagination, and consciousness.* New Haven, Conn., and London: Yale University Press.

Hunt, H. 1995. *On the nature of consciousness.* New Haven, Conn., and London: Yale University Press.

Ingerman, S. 1991. *Soul retrieval.* San Francisco: HarperCollins.

Institute of Medicine. 2005. *Complementary and alternative medicine in the United States.* Washington, D.C.: National Academic Press.

Izard, C. 1971. *The face of emotion.* New York: Appleton-Century-Crofts.

Izard, C. 1980. Cross-cultural perspectives on emotion and emotion communication. In *Handbook of cross-cultural psychology* .vol. 3, chap. 5, eds. H. Triandis and W. Lonner, 185–221. Boston: Allyn & Bacon.

Jacobs, C. 2005. Rituals of healing in African American spiritual churches. In *Religion and healing in America,* eds. L. Barnes and S. Sared, 333–342. New York: Oxford University Press.

Janes, C. 1986. Migration and hypertension: An ethnography of disease risk in an urban Samoan community. In *Anthropology and epidemiology: Interdisciplinary approaches to the study of human health and disease,* eds. C. Janes, R. Stall, and S. Gifford, 175–211. Dordrecht, Holland: Reidel.

Janes, C. 1990a. Gender, stress and health: The Samoan case. *Medical Anthropology* 12:217–248.

Janes, C. 1990b. Migration, social change and health: A Samoan community in urban California. Stanford, Calif.: Stanford University Press.

Janes, C. 1995. The transformations of Tibetan medicine. *Medical Anthropology Quarterly* 9(1):6–39.

Janes, C. 1999a. The health transition and the crisis of traditional medicine: The case of Tibet. *Social Science and Medicine* 48:1803–1820.

Janes, C. 1999b. Imagined lives, suffering and the work of culture: The embodied discourses of conflict in modern Tibet. *Medical Anthropology Quarterly* 13(4):391–412.

Janes, C. 2000. Tibetan medicine at the crossroads: Radical modernity and the social organization of traditional medicine in the Tibet autonomous region, China. In *Healing power and modernity in Asian societies,* eds. G. Samuel and L. Connor. London and Westport, Conn.: Bergin & Garvey.

Janes, C., and G. Ames. 1989. Men, blue-collar work and drinking: Alcohol use in an industrial subculture. *Culture, Medicine and Psychiatry* 13:245–274.

Janes, C., and A. Genevieve. 1992. Ethnographic explanations for the clustering of attendance, injury and health problems in a heavy machinery assembly plant. *Journal of Occupational Medicine* 34: 993–1003.

Janes, C., and A. Genevieve. 1993. The workplace. In *Recent developments in alcoholism,* ed. M. Galanter, 123–141. New York: Plenum Press.

Janes, C., and I. G. Pawson. 1986. Migration and biocultural adaptation: Samoans in urban California. *Social Science and Medicine* 22:821–834.

Janes, C., R. Stall, and S. Gifford, eds. 1986. *Anthropology and epidemiology: Interdisciplinary approaches to the study of human health and disease.* Dordrecht, Holland: Reidel.

Jilek, W. 1982. *Indian healing: Shamanistic ceremonialism in the Pacific Northwest today.* Baline, Wash.: Hancock House.

Jilek, W. 1994. Traditional healing and the prevention and treatment of alcohol and drug abuse. *Transcultural Psychiatric Research Review* 31:219–258.

Johnson, T. 1991. Anthropologists in medical education: Ethnographic prescriptions. In *Training manual in applied medical anthropology,* ed. C. Hill, 125–160. Washington, D.C.: American Anthropology Association.

Johnston, F., ed. 1987. *Nutritional anthropology.* New York: Liss.

Jones, D. 1972. *Sanapia, Comanche medicine woman.* New York: Holt, Rinehart and Winston.

Jordan, B. 1993. *Birth in four cultures.* 4th ed., revised and updated by R. Davis-Floyd. Prospect Heights, Ill.: Waveland Press.

Joseph, J. 1980. *Social affiliation, risk factor status, and coronary heart disease: A cross-sectional study of Japanese-American men.* Doctoral dissertation, University of California, Berkeley.

Joseph, J., and S. Syme. 1981. Risk factor status, social isolation, and CHD. Paper presented at the 21st Conference on Cardiovascular Disease Epidemiology, San Antonio, American Heart Association.

Jung, C. G. 1934–1954. *The archetypes and the collective unconscious.* 1981. 2nd ed. Collected works. Princeton, N.J.: Bollingen

Kadish, S. 1987. Excusing crime. *California Law Review* 75(1):257–289.

Kasdan, M. L., K. Lewis, A. Bruner, and A. L. Johnson. 1999. The nocebo effect: Do no harm. *Journal of the Southern Orthopaedic Association* 8:108–113.

Katz, P. 1981. Ritual in the operating room. *Ethnology* 20:247–257.

Katz. P. 1999. *The scalpel's edge: The culture of surgeons.* Needham Heights, Mass.: Allyn & Bacon.

Kawachi, I., and L. Berkman, eds. 2003. *Neighborhoods and health.* New York: Oxford University Press.

Kay, M. 1996. *Healing with plants in the American and Mexican west.* Tucson: University of Arizona Press.

Kelsey, J., A. Whittemore, A. Evans, and W. D. Thompson. 1996. *Methods in observational epidemiology.* New York: Oxford University Press.

Kenny, M. 1978. Latah: The symbolism of a putative mental disorder. *Culture, Medicine and Psychiatry* 2:209–231.

Kenny, M. 1985. Paradox lost: The Latah problem revisited. In *The culture bound syndromes: Folk illnesses of psychiatric and anthropological interest,* eds. R. Simons and C. Hughes, 63–76. Dordrecht, Holland: Reidel.

Kim, V., and J. Berry. 1993. *Indigenous psychologies.* Newbury Park, Calif.: Sage.

Kirkpatrick, L. 1997. An attachment-theory approach to psychology of religion. In *The psychology of religion,* eds. B. Spilka and D. N. McIntosh. Boulder, Colo.: Westview Press.

Kirmayer, L. 1993. Healing and the invention of metaphor: The effectiveness of symbols revisited. *Culture, Medicine and Psychiatry* 17:161–195.

Kirmayer, L. 2003. Reflections on embodiment. In *Social and cultural lives of immune systems,* ed. J. Wilce, 282–302. New York: Routledge.

Kirmayer, L, T.H.T. Dao, and A. Smith. 1998. Somatization and psychologization. In *Clinical methods in transcultural psychiatry,* ed. S. Okpaku, 233–265. Washington, D.C.: American Psychiatric Press.

Kirsch, I. 1997. Specifying nonspecifics: Psychological mechanisms of placebo effects. In *The placebo effect: An interdisciplinary exploration,* ed. A. Harrington, 166–186. Cambridge, Mass.: Harvard University Press.

Kleinman, A. 1973a. Medicine's symbolic reality: On a central problem in the philosophy of medicine. *Inquiry* 16:206–213.

Kleinman, A. 1973b. Toward a comparative study of medical systems: An integrated approach to the study of the relationship of medicine and culture. *Social Science and Medicine* 1:55–65

Kleinman, A. 1980. *Patients and healers in the context of culture: An exploration of the borderland between anthropology, medicine, and psychiatry.* Berkeley: University of California.

Kleinman, A. 1982. The teaching of clinically applied medical anthropology on a psychiatric consultation-liaison service. In *Clinically applied anthropology: Anthropologists in health science settings,* eds. N. Chrisman and T. Maretzki, 83–115. Boston: Reidel.

Kleinman, A. 1988a. *Rethinking psychiatry: From cultural category to personal experience.* New York: Free Press.

Kleinman, A. 1988b. *The illness narratives: Suffering, healing and the human condition.* New York: Basic Books.

Kleinman, A., and B. Good, eds. 1985. *Culture and depression.* Berkeley: University of California Press.

Kleinman, A., L. Eisenberg, and B. Good. 1978. Culture, illness, and care: Clinical lessons from anthropologic and cross-cultural research. *Annals of Internal Medicine* 88(2):251–258.

Koella, W. 1985. Organization of sleep. In *Brain mechanisms of sleep,* eds. D. McGinty, R. Drucker-Colin, A. Morrison, and P.L. Parmeggioni. New York: Raven Press.

Koenig, H. 2004. Religion, spirituality, and medicine: Research findings and implications for clinical practice. *Southern Medical Journal* 97(12):1194–1200.

Koenig, H., J. Hays, D. Larson, L. George, H. Cohen, M. McCullough, K. Meador, and D. Blazer. 1999. Does religious attendance prolong survival? A six-year follow-up study of 3,968 older adults. *Journal of Gerontology, Series A* (54):370–377.

Koenig, H., M. McCullough, and D. Larson. 2001. *Handbook of religion and health.* Oxford, U.K.: Oxford University Press.

Kohls, R., and H. Brussow. 1995. *Training know-how for cross-cultural and diversity trainers.* Duncanville, Tex.: Adult Learning Systems.

Kohls, R., and J. Knight. 1994. *Developing intercultural awareness: A cross-cultural training handbook,* 2nd ed. Yarmouth, Me.: Intercultural Press.

Koopman, S., S. Eisenthal, and J. Stoekle. 1984. Ethnicity in the reported pain, emotional distress, and requests of medical patients. *Social Science and Medicine* 18(6):487–490.

Koss, J. 1980. The therapist-spiritist training project in Puerto Rico: An experiment to relate the traditional healing system to the public health system. *Social Science and Medicine* 14B: 255–266.

Kramer, B. 1996. American Indians. In *Culture and nursing care,* eds. J. Lipson, S. Dibble, and P. Manarik, 11–22. San Francisco: University of California-San Francisco Nursing Press.

Krieger, N. 1994. Epidemiology and the web of causation: Has anyone seen the spider? *Social Science and Medicine* 39:887–903.

Krieger, N. 1999. Sticky webs, hungry spiders, buzzing flies, and fractal metaphors: On the misleading juxtaposition of "risk factors" versus "social epidemiology." *Journal of the Epidemiology of Community Health* 52:608–611.

Krippner, S. 1987. Cross-cultural approaches to multiple personality disorder: Practices in Brazilian spiritism. *Ethos* 15(3):273–295.

Krippner, S., and P. Welch. 1992. *Spiritual dimensions of healing: From native shamanism to contemporary health care.* New York: Irvington.

Kristjansson, K., A. Manolescu, A. Kristinsson, T. Hardarson, H. Knudsen, S. Ingason, G. Thorleifsson, M. Frigge, A. Kong, J. Gulcher, and K. Stefansson. 2002. Linkage of essential hypertension to chromosome 18q. *Hypertension* 39:1044–1049.

Kunitz, S. 2006. Life-course observations of alcohol use among Navajo Indians: Natural history or career? *Medical Anthropology Quarterly* 20(3):279–296.

La Barre, W. 1972. Hallucinogens and the shamanic origins of religion. In *Flesh of the gods,* ed. P. Furst, 261–278. New York: Praeger.

LaBerge, S. 1985. *Lucid dreaming.* Los Angeles: Tarcher.

Lasker, R., and The Committee on Medicine and Public Health. 1997. *Medicine and public health: The power of collaboration.* New York: New York Academy of Medicine.

Laughlin, C. 1997. Body, brain, and behavior: The neuroanthropology of the body image. *Anthropology of Consciousness* 8(2–3):49–68.

Laughlin, C., J. McManus, and E. d'Aquili. 1992. *Brain, symbol and experience: Toward a neurophenomenology of consciousness.* New York: Columbia University Press.

Leary, T. 1997. *Psychedelic prayers and other meditations.* Berkeley, Calif.: Ronin.

LeDoux, J. 1995. Emotion: Clues from the brain. *Annual Review of Psychology* 46:209–235.

Lefley, H. 1984. Delivering mental health services across cultures. In *Mental health services: The cross-cultural context,* eds. P. Pedersen, N. Sartorius, and A. Marsella. Beverly Hills, Calif.: Sage.

Leininger, M. 1970. *Nursing and anthropology: Two worlds to blend.* New York: Wiley.

Leininger, M. 1973. Witchcraft practices and psychocultural therapy with urban U.S. families. *Human Organization* 32(1):73–83.

Leininger, M. 1976. Two strange health tribes: The Gnisrun and Enicidem in the United States. *Human Organization* 35(3):253–261.

Leininger, M., ed. 1991. *Culture care diversity and universality.* New York: National League for Nursing.

Leininger, M. 1995. *Transcultural nursing: Concepts, theories, research, and practices.* New York: McGraw-Hill.

Lester, D. 1972. Voodoo death: Some thoughts on an old phenomenon. *American Anthropologist* 76:818–823.

Levenson, R. W. 1992. Autonomic nervous system differences among emotions. *Psychological Sciences* 3:23–27.

Levin, J. 1994. Religion and health: Is there an association, is it valid, and is it causal? *Social Science and Medicine* 38(11):1475–1482.

Levin, J. 2001. *God, faith, and health: Exploring the spirituality-healing connection.* Hoboken, N.J.: Wiley.

Levin, J., and H. Vanderpool. 1989. Is religion therapeutically significant for hypertension? *Social Science and Medicine* 29:69–78.

LeVine, R. 1974. *Culture and personality.* New York: Aldine.

Levi-Strauss, C. 1962. *Totemism.* Boston: Beacon.

Levi-Strauss, C. 1963. The effectiveness of symbols. In *Structural anthropology.* New York: Basic Books.

Lilienfeld, A., and D. Lilienfeld. 1980. *Foundations of epidemiology.* 2nd ed. New York: Oxford University Press.

Link, B. G., and J. Phalen. 1995. Social conditions as fundamental causes of disease. *Journal of Health and Social Behavior.* Special Issue:80–94.

Livingstone, F. 1958. Anthropological implications of sickle cell gene distribution in West Africa. *American Anthropologist* 60:533–562.

Lock, A. 1981a. Universals in human conception. In *Indigenous psychologies*, eds. P. Heelas and A. Lock, 19–36. London: Academic Press.

Lock, A. 1981b. Indigenous psychology and human nature: A psychological perspective. In *Indigenous psychologies*, eds. P. Heelas and A. Lock, 183–204. London: Academic Press.

Loewe, R. 2004. Illness narratives. In *The encyclopedia of medical anthropology: Health and illness in the world's cultures*, eds. C. Ember and M. Ember, 42–49. New York: Kluwer /Plenum.

Lyman, J. 1986. Cultural defense: Viable doctrine of wishful thinking. *Criminal Justice Journal* 9:87–117.

Lynch, J. W., G. A. Kaplan, and S J. Shema. 1997. Cumulative impact of sustained economic hardship on physical, cognitive, psychological, and social functioning. *New England Journal of Medicine* 337(26):1889–1895.

Lyon, M. 1993. Psychoneuroimmunology: The problem of the situatedness of illness and the conceptualization of healing. *Culture, Medicine and Psychiatry* 17:77–97.

Lyon, M. 2003. "Immune" to emotion: The relative absence of emotion in PNI and its centrality to everything else. In *Social and cultural lives of immune systems*, ed. J. Wilce, 82–101. New York: Routledge.

Mabit, J., R. Giove, and J. Vega. 1996. *Takiwasi*: The use of Amazonian shamanism to rehabilitate drug addicts. In *Sacred plants, consciousness, and healing: Yearbook of cross-cultural medicine and psychotherapy, 5*, eds. M. Winkelman and W. Andritzky, 257–285. Berlin: Verlag.

MacLean, P. 1990. *The triune brain in evolution*. New York: Plenum.

MacLean, P. 1993. On the evolution of three mentalities. In *Brain, culture, and the human spirit: Essays from an emergent evolutionary perspective*, ed. J. Ashbrok. Lanham, Md.: University Press of America.

Malinowski, B. 1954. *Magic, science, and religion*. New York: Anchor.

Maloney, C., ed. 1976. *The evil eye*. New York: Columbia University Press.

Mandell, A. 1980. Toward a psychobiology of transcendence: God in the brain. In *The psychobiology of consciousness*, eds. D. Davidson and R. Davidson, 379–464. New York: Plenum.

Mandell, A. 1985. Interhemispheric fusion. *Journal of Psychoactive Drugs* 17(4):257–266.

Marmot, M. G., and S. L. Syme. 1976. Acculturation and coronary heart disease in Japanese-Americans. *American Journal of Epidemiology* 104:225–247.

Martin, J. F., C. S. Johnston, C. T. Han, and D. C. Benyshek. 2000. Nutritional origins of insulin resistance: A rat model for diabetes-prone human populations. *Journal of Nutrition* 130:741–744.

Marwick, M., ed. 1970. *Witchcraft and sorcery*. Baltimore: Penguin.

Mattingly, C. 1998. *Healing dramas and clinical plots: The narrative structure of experience*. Cambridge, U.K.: Cambridge University Press.

Mattingly, C., and L. Garro, eds. 2000. *Narrative and the cultural construction of illness and healing*. Berkeley: University of California Press.

Mausner, J., and S. Kramer. 1985. *Epidemiology: An introductory text*. Philadelphia: Saunders.

May, P. 1994. The epidemiology of alcohol abuse among American Indians: The mythical and real properties. *American Indian Culture and Research Journal* 18(2):121–143.

McClain, C., ed. 1989. *Women as healers*. New Brunswick, N.J.: Rutgers University Press.

McClenon, J. 1997. Shamanic healing, human evolution, and the origin of religion. *Journal for the Scientific Study of Religion* 36(3):345–354.

McClenon, J. 2002. *Wondrous healing: Shamanism, human evolution and the origin of religion*. De Kalb: Northern Illinois University Press.

McCombie, S. 1987. Folk flu and viral syndrome. *Social Science and Medicine* 25(9):987–993.

McCombie, S. 1999. Folk flu and viral syndrome. In *Anthropology and public health*, ed. R. Hahn, 27–43. Oxford: Oxford University Press.

McDermott, R. 2006. Ethics, epidemiology, and the thrifty gene. In *Health and healing in a comparative perspective*, ed. E. Whitaker, 459–466. Upper Saddle River, N.J.: Pearson.

McElroy, A., and P. Townsend. 1985. *Medical anthropology in ecological perspective*. Boulder, Colo.: Westview Press.

McElroy, A., and P. Townsend, eds. 1996. *Medical anthropology in ecological perspective*. Boulder, Colo.: Westview Press.

McGuire, M. 1988. *Ritual healing in suburban America*. New Brunswick, N.J.: Rutgers University Press.

McKay, B., and L. Musil. 2005. The "spiritual healing project." In *Religion and healing in America*, eds. L. Barnes and S. Sered, 49–58. New York: Oxford University Press.

McKee, J. 1988. *Holistic health and the critique of Western medicine*. Social Science and Medicine 26(8): 775–84.

McKinlay, J., and L. Marceau. 2000. Public health matters: To boldly go. *American Journal of Public Health* 90(1):25–33.

McPeake, J. D., B. Kennedy, and S. Gordon. 1991. Altered states of consciousness therapy: A missing component in alcohol and drug rehabilitation treatment. *Journal of Substance Abuse Treatment* 8:75–82.

Meaney, F. J. 2004. Mental retardation. In *Encyclopedia of medical anthropology,* eds. C. Ember and M. Ember, 493–505. New York: Kluwer /Plenum.

Mechanic, D. 1962. The concept of illness behavior. In *Concepts of health and disease,* eds. A. Caplan, H. Engelhardt Jr., and J. McCartney, 485–492. Menlo Park, Calif.: Addison-Wesley.

Meleis, A. 1992. Community participation and involvement: Theoretical and empirical issues. *Health Services Management Research* 5:5–16.

Melzack, R., and P. D. Wall. 1983. *The challenge of pain.* New York: Basic Books.

Mercer, J. 1973. *Labeling the mentally retarded.* Berkeley: University of California Press.

Merker, B. 2000. Synchronous chorusing and human origins. In *The origins of music,* eds. N. Wallin, B. Merker, and S. Brown, 315–327. Cambridge, Mass.: MIT Press.

Metzner, R. 1998. Hallucinogenic drugs and plants in psychotherapy and shamanism. *Journal of Psychoactive Drugs* 30(4):333–341.

Micozzi, M. *Fundamentals of complementary and alternative medicine.* Philadelphia: Churchill Livingstone.

Middleton, J., and E. Winter, eds. 1963. *Witchcraft and sorcery in East Africa.* London: Routledge.

Mishler, E. 1981. The social construction of illness. In *Social contexts of health illness and patient care,* eds. E. Mishler, L. Amarasingham, S. Hauser, S. Osherson, N. Waxler, and R. Liem, 141–168. Cambridge, U.K.: Cambridge University Press.

Mithen, S. 1996. *The prehistory of the mind: A search for the origins of art, religion and science.* London: Thames & Hudson.

Moerman, D. 1983. Physiology and symbols: The anthropological implications of the placebo effect. In *The anthropology of medicine,* eds. L. Románucci-Ross, D. Moerman, and L. Tancredi, 240–253. New York: Praeger.

Moerman, D. 2000. Cultural variations in the placebo effect: Ulcers, anxiety, and blood pressure. *Medical Anthropology Quarterly* 14(1):51–72.

Moerman, D. 2002. *Meaning, medicine and the "placebo effect."* Cambridge, U.K.: Cambridge University Press.

Molino, J. 2000. Toward an evolutionary theory of music. In *The origins of music,* eds. N. Wallin, B. Merker, and S. Brown, 165–176. Cambridge, Mass.: MIT Press.

Montgomery, G., and I. Kirsch. 1997. Classical conditioning and the placebo effect. *Pain* 72:107–113.

Moore, L., P. Van Arsdale, J. Glittenberg, and R. Aldrich. 1980. *The biocultural basis of health: Expanding views of medical anthropology.* Prospect Heights, Ill.: Waveland Press.

Moore, P., and J. T. Hepworth. 1994. Use of perinatal and infant health services by Mexican-American medicaid enrollees. *Journal of the American Medical Association* 272(4):297–304.

Moran, E. 1979. *Human adaptability: An introduction to ecological anthropology.* Boulder, Colo.: Westview Press.

Morris, W. 1981. *American heritage dictionary of the English language.* Boston: Houghton Mifflin.

Morsy, S. 1979. The missing link in medical anthropology: the political economy of health. *Reviews in Anthropology* 6: 349–363.

Morsy, S. 1996. Political economy in medical anthropology. In *Handbook of medical anthropology,* ed. C. Sargent and T. Johnson, 21–40. Westport, CT: Greenwood Press.

Morsy, S. 1996. Political economy in medical anthropology. In *Handbook of medical anthropology,* eds. C. Sargent and T. Johnson, 21–40. Westport, Conn.: Greenwood Press.

Munroe, R., and R. Munroe. 1975. *Cross-cultural human development.* Monterey, Calif.: Brooks/Cole.

Murdock, G. 1980. *Theories of illness: A world survey.* Pittsburgh: University of Pittsburgh.

National Center for Health Statistics. 2000. *Healthy people, 2010.* Washington, D.C.: Department of Health and Human Services.

National Committee for Quality Assurance (NCQA). 1993. *Health plan employer data and information set and user's manual: Version 2.0* (HEDIS 2.0). Washington, D.C.: NCQA.

Neel, J. 1999. The thrifty genotype in 1998. *Nutrition Reviews* 57(5PartII):S2-S9.

Nemeroff, C., and P. Rozin. 2000. The makings of the magical mind. In *Imagining the impossible: Magical, scientific, and religious thinking in children,* eds. K. S. Rosengren, C. N. Johnson, and P. L. Harris, 1–34. New York: Cambridge University Press.

Ness, R. 1985. The *old hag* phenomenon as sleep paralysis: A biocultural interpretation. In *The culture bound syndromes: Folk illnesses of psychiatric and anthropological interest,* eds. R. Simons and C. Hughes, 123–145. Dordrecht, Holland: Reidel.

Newham, P. 1994. *The singing cure.* Boston: Shambhala.

Newton, N. 1996. *Foundations of understanding.* Philadelphia: Benjamins.

Ng, F., ed. 2003. *Hmong American concepts of health, healing, and conventional medicine.* New York: Routledge.

Nichter, M. 1984. Project community diagnosis: Participatory research as a first step toward community involvement in primary health care. *Social Science and Medicine* 19(3):237–252.

Noll, R. 1983. Shamanism and schizophrenia: A state-specific approach to the schizophrenia metaphor of shamanic states. *American Ethnologist* 10(3):443–459.

Northridge, M. E., and R. Mack. 2002. Integrating ethnomedicine into public health. *American Journal of Public Health* 92(10):1561.

O'Connell, D., and C. Alexander, eds. 1994. *Self-recovery: Treating addictions using transcendental meditation and Maharishi ayur-veda.* New York: Haworth Press.

O'Connor B. 1995. *Healing traditions: Alternative medicine and the health professions.* Philadelphia: University of Pennsylvania Press.

O'Connor, J. 1978. *The young drinkers: A cross-national study of social and cultural influences.* London: Tavistock.

Office of Minority Health, U.S. Department of Health and Human Services. 2000. National standards for culturally and linguistically appropriate services (CLAS) in health care. *Federal Register* 65(247):80865–80879.

Osis, R. 2005. Cult of the saints. In *Religion and healing in America,* eds. L. Barnes and S. Sered, 29–48. New York: Oxford University Press.

Oubré, A. 1997. *Instinct and revelation reflections on the origins of numinous perception.* Amsterdam: Gordon & Breach.

Pandian, J. 1997. The sacred integration of the cultural self: An anthropological approach to the study of religion. In *The anthropology of religion,* ed. S. Glazier. Westport, Conn.: Greenwood Press.

Paniagua, F. 2005. *Assessing and treating culturally diverse clients: A practical guide.* Thousand Oaks, Calif.: Sage.

Panksepp, J. 1998. *Affective neuroscience: The foundations of human and animal emotions.* New York: Oxford University Press.

Panksepp, J. 2000. Affective consciousness and the instinctual motor system: The neural sources of sadness and joy. In *The caldron of consciousness: Motivation, affect and self-organization,* eds. R. Ellis and M. Newton, 231–244. Amsterdam: Benjamins.

Papademetriou, V. 2004. Cardiovascular risk assessment and triptans. *Headache: Journal of Head & Face Pain* 44: S31–S39.

Parrott, A., E. Sisk, and J. Turner. 2000. Psychobiological problems in heavy "ecstasy" (MDMA) polydrug users. *Drug & Alcohol Dependence* 60(1):105–110.

Parsons, T. 1951. *The social system.* Glencoe, Ill.: Free Press.

Passie, T. 1997. *Psycholytic and psychedelic therapy research 1931–1995: A complete international bibliography.* Hannover, Germany: Laurentius.

Patel, M. 1987. Evaluation of holistic medicine. *Social Science and Medicine* 24(2):169–175.

Pawluch, D., R. Cain, and J. Gillet. 2000. Lay constructions of HIV and complementary therapy use. *Social Science and Medicine* 51:251–264.

Payer, L. 1996. *Medicine and culture.* New York: Holt.

Pearson, M. 1988. What does distance matter? Leprosy control in West Nepal. *Social Science and Medicine* 26(1):25–36.

Perkins, J. 1997. Shapeshifting shamanic techniques for global and personal transformation. Rochester, Vt.: Destiny.

Pennebaker, J. 2003. Telling stories: The health benefits of disclosure. In *Social and cultural lives of immune systems,* ed. J. Wilce Jr., 1–16. London: Routledge.

Peters, L. 1989. Shamanism: Phenomenology of a spiritual discipline. *Journal of Transpersonal Psychology* 21(2):115–137.

Peters, L., and D. Price-Williams. 1981. Towards an experiential analysis of shamanism. *American Ethnologist* 7:398–418.

Phinney, J. 1996. *When we talk about American ethnic groups, what do we mean?* Los Angeles: California State University.

Poland, M. 1985. Importance of cross-training and research strategies in clinical medicine. *Medical Anthropology Quarterly* 16(3):61–63.

Pope, G. 2000. *The biological bases of human behavior.* Boston: Allyn & Bacon.

Press, I. 1982. Witch doctor's legacy: Some anthropological implications for the practice of clinical medicine. In *Clinically applied anthropology: anthropologists in health science settings,* eds. N. Chrisman and T. Maretzki, 179–198. Culture, Illness, and Healing, vol. 5. Boston: Reidel.

Press, I. 1985. Speaking hospital administrations' language: Strategies for anthropological entree in the clinical setting. *Medical Anthropology Quarterly* 16(3):67–69.

Press, I. 1997. The quality movement in U.S. health care: Implications for anthropology. *Human Organization* 56(1):1–8.

Prince, R. 1982. Shamans and endorphins. *Ethos* 10(4):409.

Prince, R., S. Okpaku, and L. Merkel. 1998. Transcultural psychiatry. In *Methods in transcultural psychiatry*, ed. S. Okpaku, 3–17. Washington, D.C.: American Psychiatric Press.

Purnell, L. and B. Paulanka, eds. 2003. *Transcultural health care: A culturally competent approach.* Philadelphia: Davis.

Quandt, S. 1996. Nutrition in medical anthropology. In *Handbook of medical anthropology contemporary theory and method*, eds. C. Sargent and T. Johnson, 272–289. Westport, Conn.: Greenwood Press.

Rätsch, C. 2001. *Marijuana medicine: A world tour of the healing and visionary powers of cannabis.* Rochester, Vt.: Healing Arts Press.

Rätsch, C. 2005. *The encyclopedia of psychoactive plants: Ethnopharmacology and its applications.* Trans. J. Baker. Rochester, Vt.: Park Street Press. Originally published *Enzyklopädie der psychoaktiven Pflanzen.* (Aarau, Switzerland: AT Verlag, 1998).

Rhine, S. 1998. *Bone voyage: A journey in forensic anthropology.* Albuquerque: University of New Mexico Press.

Rioux, D. 1996. Shamanic healing techniques: Toward holistic addiction counseling. *Alcoholism Treatment Quarterly* 14(1):59–69.

Ritenbaugh, C. 1982. New approaches to old problems: Interactions of culture and nutrition. In *Clinically applied anthropology*, eds. N. Chrisman and T. Maretzki, 141–178. Dordrecht, Holland: Reidel.

Roberts, J. 1976. Belief in the evil eye in world perspective. In *The evil eye,* ed. C. Maloney. New York: Columbia University Press.

Robins, L., J. Helzer, and D. Davis, 1975. Narcotic use in Southeast Asia and afterward: An interview study of 898 Vietnam returnees. *Archives of General Psychiatry* 32(8):955–961.

Romero-Daza, N. 1994a. Migrant labor, multiple sexual partners, and sexually transmitted diseases: The makings for an AIDS epidemic in rural Lesotho. Doctoral dissertation, State University of New York at Buffalo.

Romero-Daza, N. 1994b. Multiple sexual partners, migrant labor, and sexually transmitted diseases, the makings for an epidemic. Knowledge and beliefs about AIDS among women in highland Lesotho. *Human Organization* 53:192–205.

Romero-Daza, N., and D. Himmelgreen. 1998. More than money for your labor: Migration and the political economy of AIDS in Lesotho. In *The political economy of AIDS,* ed. M. Singer, 185–204. Critical Approaches in Health Social Sciences Series. New York: Baywood Press.

Romero-Daza, N., D. Himmelgreen, R. Perez-Escamilla, S. Segura-Millan, and M. Singer. 1999. Food habits of drug using Puerto Rican women in inner city Hartford. *Medical Anthropology* 18:281–298.

Romero-Daza, N., M. Weeks, and M. Singer. 1999. Much more than HIV: The reality of life on the streets for drug-using sex workers in inner city Hartford. *International Quarterly of Community Health Education* 18(1):107–119.

Rosaldo, M. 1983. The shame of headhunters and the autonomy of the self. *Ethos* 11(3):135.

Rossi, E. L. 2000. In search of a deep psychobiology of hypnosis: Visionary hypotheses for a new millennium. *American Journal of Clinical Hypnosis* 42(3–4):178–207.

Rubel, A., and M. Hass. 1990. Ethnomedicine. In *Medical anthropology contemporary theory and method*, eds. T. Johnson and C. Sargent, 115–131. New York: Praeger.

Rubel, A., J. O'Nell, and R. Collado. 1984. *Susto, a folk illness.* Berkeley: University of California Press.

Rubel, A., J. O'Nell, and R. Collado. 1985. The folk illness called susto. In *The culture bound syndromes: Folk illnesses of psychiatric and anthropological interest*, eds. R. Simons and C. C. Hughes, 333–350. Dordrecht, Holland: Reidel.

Rubinstein, R., and S. Lane 1990. International health and development. In *Medical anthropology contemporary theory and method*, eds. T. Johnson and C. Sargent, 366–390. New York: Praeger.

Rush, J. 1996. *Clinical anthropology: An application of anthropological concepts within clinical settings.* Westport, Conn.: Praeger.

Russell, J. A. 1994. Is there universal recognition of emotion from facial expression? A review of cross-cultural studies. *Psychological Bulletin* 115(1):102–141.

Russo, C. J., E. Melista, J. Cui, A. L. DeStefano, G. L. Bakris, A. J. Manolis, H. Gavras, and C. T. Baldwin. 2005. Association of NEDD4L ubiquitin ligase with essential hypertension. *Hypertension* 46(3):488–491.

Sallis J., and N. Owen. 1998. Ecological models. In *Health behavior and health education*, eds. K. Glanz, M. Lewis, and B. Rimer, 403–424. San Francisco: Jossey-Bass.

Sanchez-Ramos, J., and D. Mash. 1996. Pharmacotherapy of drug dependence with ibogaine. In *Sacred plants, consciousness, and healing: Yearbook of cross-cultural medicine and psychotherapy, 5*, eds. M. Winkelman and W. Andritzky, 353–367. Berlin: Verlag.

Sargent, C., and T. Johnson, eds. 1996. *Handbook of medical anthropology contemporary theory and method*. Westport, Conn.: Greenwood Press.

Scheff, T. 1993. Toward a social psychological theory of mind and consciousness. *Social Research* 60(1):171–195.

Schensul, J., and M. LeCompte. 1999. *The ethnographer's toolkit*. Walnut Creek, Calif.: AltaMira Press.

Scheper-Hughes, N., ed. 1987. *Child survival: Anthropological perspectives on the treatment and maltreatment of children*. Dordrecht, Holland/Boston: Reidel.

Scheper-Hughes, N. 1990. Three positions for a critically applied medical anthropology. *Social Science and Medicine* 30(2):189–197.

Scheper-Hughes, N. 1992. *Death without weeping: The violence of everyday life in Brazil*. Berkeley: University of California Press.

Scheper-Hughes, N., and M. Lock. 1987. The mindful body: A prolegomenon to future work in medical anthropology. *Medical Anthropology Quarterly* 1(3):6.

Scherer, K. R. 1994. Toward a concept of "modal emotions." In *The nature of emotion: Fundamental questions*, eds. P. Ekman and R. Davidson, 25–31. London: Oxford University Press.

Scherer, K. 2000a. Universality of emotional expression. In *Encyclopedia of human emotions*, eds. D. Levinson, J. Ponzetti, and P. Jorgensen, 669–674. New York: Macmillan.

Scherer, K. 2000b. Cross-cultural patterns. In *Encyclopedia of human emotions*, eds. D. Levinson, J. Ponzetti, and P. Jorgensen, 147–156. New York: Macmillan.

Schlomann, P., and J. Schmitke. 2007. Lay beliefs about hypertension: An interpretive synthesis of the qualitative research. *Journal of the American Academy of Nurse Practitioners* 19(7):358–367.

Schoenberg, N. 1997. A convergence of health beliefs: An "ethnography of adherence" of African-American rural elders with hypertension. *Human Organization* 56(2):174–181.

Schultes, R., and A. Hofmann. 1979. *Plants of the gods origins of hallucinogenic use*. New York: McGraw-Hill. (Reprinted 1992 by Healing Arts Press, Rochester, Vt.).

Schultes, R., and M. Winkelman. 1996. The principal American hallucinogenic plants and their bioactive and therapeutic properties. In *Sacred plants, consciousness, and healing: Yearbook of cross-cultural medicine and psychotherapy, 5.*, eds. M. Winkelman and W. Andritzky, 205–239. Berlin: Verlag.

Scrimshaw, N., M. Carballo, and L. Ramos. 1991. The AIDS rapid anthropological assessment procedures: A tool for health education planning and evaluation. *Health Education Quarterly* 18(1):111–123.

Seelye, N., ed. 1996. *Experiential activities for intercultural learning*. Yarmouth, Me.: Intercultural Press.

Selye, H. 1956. *The stress of life*. New York: McGraw-Hill.

Selye, H. 1976. *Stress in health and disease*. Boston: Butterworths.

Sered, S. 2005. Exile, illness, and gender in Israeli pilgrimage narratives. In *Pilgrimage and healing*, eds. J. Dubisch and M. Winkelman, 69–90. Tucson: University of Arizona Press.

Shapiro, A., and E. Shapiro. 1997. *The powerful placebo from ancient priest to modern physician*. Baltimore: Johns Hopkins University Press.

Sheybani, M. 1987. Cultural defense: One person's culture in another's crime. *Loyola Los Angeles International and Comparative Law Journal* 9:751–783.

Shiloh, A. 1977. Therapeutic anthropology: The anthropologist as private practitioner. *American Anthropologist* 79:443–445.

Shore, B. 1996. *Culture in mind cognition: Culture and the problem of meaning*. New York: Oxford University Press.

Siegel, R. 1990. *Intoxication: Life in pursuit of artificial paradise*. New York: Dutton.

Siikala, A. 1978. The rite technique of Siberian shaman. In *Folklore fellows communication 220*. Helsinki: Soumalainen Tiedeskaremia Academia.

Silverman, J. 1967. Shamans and acute schizophrenia. *American Anthropologist* 69:21–31.

Simons, R. 1996. *Boo! Culture, experience, and the startle reflex*. New York: Oxford University Press.

Simons, R., and C. Hughes, eds. 1985. *The culture bound syndromes: Folk illnesses of psychiatric and anthropological interest*. Dordrecht, Holland: Reidel.

Singer, M. 1989a. The coming age of critical medical anthropology. *Social Science and Medicine* 28(11):1193–1203.

Singer, M. 1989b. The limitations of medical ecology: The concept of adaptation in the context of social stratification and social transformation. *Medical Anthropology* 10:223–234.

Singer, M. 1990. Reinventing medical anthropology: Toward a critical realignment. *Social Science and Medicine* 30(2):179–187.

Singer, M. 1992. AIDS and US ethnic minorities: The crisis and alternative anthropological responses. *Human Organization* 51(1):89–95.

Singer, M. 1997. *The political economy of AIDS*. Amityville, N.Y.: Baywood.

Singer, M. 2006. *The face of social suffering: The life history of a street drug addict*. Long Grove, Ill.: Waveland Press.

Singer, M. 2008. *Drugging the poor: Legal and illegal drugs and social inequality*. Long Grove, Ill.: Waveland Press.

Singer, M., and H. Baer. 1995. *Critical medical anthropology*. Amityville, N.Y.: Baywood.

Singer, M., and H. Baer. 2007. *Introducing medical anthropology: A discipline in action*. Lanham, Md.: AltaMira Press.

Singer, M., F. Valentin, H. Baer, and Z. Jia. 1992. Why does Juan Garcia have a drinking problem? The perspective of critical medical anthropology. In *Understanding and applying medical anthropology*, ed. P. Brown, 286–302. Mountain View, Calif.: Mayfield.

Sloan, R., E. Bagiella, and T. Powell. 1999. Religion, spirituality and medicine. *Lancet* 353:664–667.

Smith, C. 1995. The lived experience of staying healthy in rural African American families. *Nursing Spring Quarterly* 8(1):17–21.

Smithies, J., and G. Webster. 1998. Community involvement in health from passive recipients to active participants. Aldershot, U.K.: Ashgate.

Snow, L. 1983. Traditional health beliefs and practices among lower class Black Americans. *Western Journal of Medicine* 139(6):820–828.

Snow, L. 1993. *Walkin' over medicine*. Boulder, Colo.: Westview Press.

Spector, R. 1991. *Cultural diversity in health and illness*. Norwalk, Conn.: Appleton & Lange.

Spiegel, H. 1997. Nocebo: The power of suggestibility. *Preventive Medicine* 26:616–621.

Spilka, B., and D. McIntosh, eds. 1997. *The psychology of religion: Theoretical approaches*. Boulder, Colo.: Westview Press.

Spiro, M. 1993. Is the western concept of self "peculiar" within the context of world cultures? *Ethos* 21(2):107–153.

Stark, R. 1997. A taxonomy of religious experience. In *The psychology of religion: Theoretical approaches,* eds. B. Spilka and D. McIntosh. Boulder, Colo.: Westview Press.

Starr, P. 1982. *The social transformation of American medicine*. New York: Basic Books.

Stewart, T. 1979. *Essentials of forensic anthropology*. Springfield, Ill.: Charles C. Thomas.

Stimson, G., C. Fitch, and T. Rhodes, eds. 1998. *The rapid assessment and response guide on injecting drug use (IDU-RAR)*. Geneva: World Health Organization Program on Substance Abuse.

Stimson, G., C. Fitch, and T. Rhodes, eds. 1999. *The rapid assessment and response guide on psychoactive substance use and prevention (PSUP-RAR) (draft version)*. Geneva: World Health Organization Program on Substance Abuse and UNAIDS, UNDCP, UNICEF.

Strawbridge, W. J., R. D. Cohen, S. J. Shema, and G. A. Kaplan. 1997. Frequent attendance at religious services and mortality over 28 years. *American Journal of Public Health* 87(6):957–961.

Strecher, V. J. and Rosenstock, I. M. (eds) (1997) The Health Belief Model. Jossey-Bass, San Francisco, CA.

Suchman, E. 1965. Stages of illness and medical care. *Journal of Health and Human Behavior* 6(3):114.

Swanson, G. 1973. The search for a guardian spirit: The process of empowerment in simpler societies. *Ethnology* 12:359–378.

Taylor, E., M. Murphy, and S. Donovan. 1997. *The physical and psychological effects of meditation: A review of contemporary research with a comprehensive bibliography: 1931–1996*. Sausalito, Calif.: Institute of Noetic Sciences.

Taylor, R., L. Chatters, and J. Levin. 2003. *Religion in the lives of African Americans: Social, psychological, and health perspectives*. Thousand Oaks, Calif.: Sage.

Tobin, J., and J. Friedman. 1983. Spirits, shamans, and nightmare death: Survivor stress in a Hmong refugee. *American Journal of Orthopsychiatry* 53(3):439–448.

Tom-Orme, L. 1988. Chronic disease and the social matrix: A Native American diabetes intervention. *Recent Advances in Nursing* 22:89–109.

Tom-Orme, L. 2006. Research and American Indian/Alaska Native health: A nursing perspective. *Journal of Transcultural Nursing* 17(3):261–265.

Trevathan, W. 1999. Evolutionary obstetrics. In *Evolutionary medicine,* eds. W. Trevathan, E. Smith, and J. McKenna, 183–207. New York: Oxford University Press.

Trevathan, W., E. Smith, and J. McKenna, eds. 1999. *Evolutionary medicine.* New York: Oxford University Press.

Trevathan, W., E. Smith, and J. McKenna, eds. 2008. *Evolutionary medicine and health: New perspectives.* New York: Oxford University Press.

Trivieri, L. 2001. *Guide to holistic health.* New York: Wiley.

Trostle, J., and J. Sommerfield. 1996. Medical anthropology and epidemiology. *Annual Review of Anthropology* 25:253–274.

Trotter, R., and J. Chavira. 1997. *Curanderismo Mexican American folk healing.* Athens.: University of Georgia Press.

Trotter, R., and R. Needle. 2000a. *RARE project RARE community guide.* Washington, D.C.: Department of Health and Human Services. Office of Public Health and Science, Office of HIV/AIDS Policy.

Trotter, R., and R. Needle. 2000b. *RARE project field assessment training methods workbook.* Washington, D.C.: Department of Health and Human Services. Office of Public Health and Science, Office of HIV/AIDS Policy.

Turner R., D. Lukoff, R. Barnhouse, and F. Lu. 1995. Religious or spiritual problem: A culturally sensitive diagnostic category in the DSM-IV. *Journal of Nervous and Mental Disorders* 183(7):435–444.

Twaddle, A. 1973. Illness and deviance. *Social Science and Medicine* 7:751–762.

Twaddle, A. 1981. Sickness and the sickness career: Some implications. In *The relevance of social science for medicine,* eds. L. Eisenberg and A. Kleinman, 111–133. Dordrecht, Holland: Reidel.

Ulijaszek, S., and S. Strickland. 1993. *Nutritional anthropology.* London: Smith-Gordon.

U.S. Department of Health and Human Services. 1991. *Healthy people 2000: National health promotion and disease prevention objectives.* DHHS Pub. No. (PHS) 91–50212. Washington, D.C.: Office of the Assistant Secretary for Health.

Valle, J., and R. Prince. 1989. Religious experiences as self-healing mechanisms. In *Altered states of consciousness and mental health: A cross-cultural perspective,* ed. C.A. Ward. Newbury Park, Calif.: Sage.

Varela, F. 1997. The body's self. In *Healing emotions,* ed. D. Goleman. Boston: Shambhala.

Wade, J. 1996. *Changes of mind: A holonomic theory of the evolution of consciousness.* Albany: State University of New York Press.

Waid, W., ed. 1984. *Sociophysiology.* New York: Springer-Verlag.

Waitzkin, H. 1979. Medicine, superstructure and micropolitics. *Social Science and Medicine* 13A:601–609.

Waitzkin, H. 1991. *The politics of medical encounters: How patients and doctors deal with social problems.* New Haven, Conn.: Yale University Press.

Waitzkin, H. 2001. At *the front lines of medicine: How the health care system alienates doctors and mistreats patients . . . and what we can do about it.* Lanham, Md.: Rowman & Littlefield.

Walker, E., ed. 1970. *Systems of North American witchcraft and sorcery.* Moscow: University of Idaho.

Waller, M. 1996. Organization theory and the origins of consciousness. *Journal of Social and Evolutionary Systems* 19(1):17–30.

Wallerstein, E. 1980. *Circumcision: An American health fallacy.* New York: Springer.

Walsh, R. 1990. *The spirit of shamanism.* Los Angeles: Tarcher.

Walton, K., and D. Levitsky. 1994. A neuroendocrine mechanism for the reduction of drug use and addictions by transcendental meditation. In *Self-recovery: Treating addictions using transcendental meditation and Maharishi ayur-veda,* eds. D. O'Connell and C. Alexander, 89–117. New York: Haworth Press.

Ward, C. 1989. The cross-cultural study of altered states of consciousness and mental health. In *Altered states of consciousness and mental health. A cross-cultural perspective,* ed. C. Ward. Newbury Park, Calif.: Sage.

Wardwell, W. I. 1992. *Chiropractic: History and evolution of a new profession.* St. Louis: Mosby Year Book.

Wardwell, W. I. 1994. Alternative medicine in the United States. *Social Science and Medicine* 38(8):1061–1068.

Wasson, R. 1980. *The wondrous mushroom: Mycolatry in Mesoamerica.* New York: McGraw-Hill.

Wasson, R., C. Cowan, F. Cowan, and W. Rhodes. 1974. *Maria Sabina and her Mazatec mushroom velada.* New York: Harcourt Brace.

Wasson, R., S. Kramrisch, J. Ott, and C. Ruck. 1986. *Persephone's quest: Entheogens and the origins of religion.* New Haven, Conn.: Yale University Press.

Waterston, A. 1997. Anthropological research and the politics of HIV prevention: Towards a critique of politics and priorities in the age of AIDS. *Social Science and Medicine* 44(9):1381–1391.

Waxler, N. 1981. Learning to be a leper: A case study in the social construction of illness. In *Social contexts of health, illness and patient care,* eds. E. Mishler, L. Amarasingham, S. Hauser, S. Osherson, N. Waxler, and R. Liem, 169–194. Cambridge, U.K.: Cambridge University Press.

Weathersbee, T. 2007. Black children more likely to be stricken by obesity. *Tennessee Tribune,* July 5–July 11, B8.

Weeks, W. H., P. B. Pedersen, and R. W. Brislin, eds. 1986. *A manual of structured experiences for cross-cultural learning.* Washington, D.C.: Society for Intercultural Education, Training and Research.

Weidman, H. 1985. Stylistic aspects of clinical anthropology. *Medical Anthropology Quarterly* 16(3):63–64.

Weisenfeld, S. 1967. Sickle-cell trait in human biological and cultural evolution. *Science* 157:1134–1140.

Whaley, B. B. ed. 2000. *Explaining illness: Research, theory, and practice.* Mahwah, N.J.: Erlbaum.

Whiteford, L., and L. Manderson, eds. 2000. *Globalization and health: Global health policies and local realities: The fallacy of the level playing field.* Boulder, Colo.: Rienner.

Whiteford, L., and L. Nixon. 1999. Comparative health systems: Emerging convergences and globalization. In *The handbook of social studies in health and medicine,* eds. G. L. Albrecht, R. Fitzpatrick, and S. Scrimshaw. London: Sage.

Whiteford, L., and M. Poland. 1989. *New approaches to human reproduction: Social and ethical dimensions.* Boulder, Colo.: Westview Press.

Whiting, B., and J. Whiting. 1975. *Children of six cultures: A psychocultural analysis.* Cambridge, Mass.: Harvard University Press.

Wiedman, D. 1990a. Big and little moon peyotism as health care delivery systems. *Medical Anthropology* 12(4):371–387.

Wiedman, D. 1990b. University accreditation: Academic subcultural and organizational responses to directed change. In *Cross-cultural management and organizational culture,* ed. T. Hamada and A. Jordan, 227–246. Williamsburg, Va.: Studies in Third World Societies.

Wiedman, D. 1992. Effects on academic culture of shifts from oral to written traditions: The case of university accreditation. *Human Organization* 51(4):398–407.

Wiedman, D. 1998. Effective strategic planning roles for anthropologists. *Practicing Anthropology* 20(1):36–39.

Wiedman, D. 2000a. "Best practices" compared to strategic management and total quality management: A new paradigm or an incremental change in management culture. *High Plains Applied Anthropology* 20(2):146–152.

Wiedman, D. 2000b. Directing organizational cultural change through strategic planning and leadership. In *Careers in anthropology; Profiles of practitioner anthropologists,* ed. P. Sabloff, 99–103. NAPA Bulletin 20. Washington, D.C.: American Anthropological Association.

Wilce, J., ed. 2003. *Social and cultural lives of immune systems.* New York: Routledge.

Wilce, J., and L. Price. 2003. Metaphors our bodyminds live by. In *Social and cultural lives of immune systems,* ed. J. Wilce, 50–81. New York: Routledge.

Wiley, A. 1992. Adaptation and the biocultural paradigm in medical anthropology: A critical review. *Medical Anthropology Quarterly* 6(3):216–236.

Williams, G., and R. Nesse. 1991. The dawn of Darwinian medicine. *Quarterly Review of Biology* 46(1):1–22.

Winkelman, M. 1985. A cross-cultural study of magico-religious practitioners. Doctoral dissertation, University of California, Irvine. Ann Arbor, Mich.: University Microfilms.

Winkelman, M. 1986a. Trance states: A theoretical model and cross-cultural analysis. *Ethos* 14(2):174–203.

Winkelman, M. 1986b. Magico-religious practitioner types and socioeconomic conditions. *Behavior Science Research* 20:17–46.

Winkelman, M. 1989. Ethnobotanical treatments of diabetes in Baja California Norte. *Medical Anthropology* 11:255–268.

Winkelman, M. 1990. Shaman and other "magico-religious" healers: A cross-cultural study of their origins, nature, and social transformations. *Ethos* 18:308–352.

Winkelman, M. 1991. Physiological, social and functional aspects of drug and non-drug altered states of consciousness. In *Yearbook of cross-cultural medicine and psychotherapy,* 1, ed. W. Andritzky, 183–198. Berlin: Verlag.

Winkelman, M. 1992a. Shamans, priests, and witches: A cross-cultural study of magico-religious practitioners. *Anthropological Research Papers #44.* Tempe: Arizona State University.

Winkelman, M. 1992b. *Properties of Piman (O'odham) medicinal plants for the treatment of diabetes. Native seeds search monograph #1.* Tucson: Native Seeds Search.

Winkelman, M. 1994. Cultural shock and adaptation. *Journal of Counseling and Development* 73:121–126.

Winkelman, M. 1996a. Psychointegrator plants: Their roles in human culture and health. In *Sacred plants, consciousness, and healing. Yearbook of cross-cultural medicine and psychotherapy,* 5, eds. M. Winkelman and W. Andritzky, 9–53. Berlin: Verlag.

Winkelman, M. 1996b. Cultural factors in criminal defense proceedings. *Human Organization* 55(2):154–159.

Winkelman, M. 1997. Altered states of consciousness and religious behavior. In *Anthropology of religion: A handbook of method and theory,* ed. S. Glazier. Westport, Conn.: Greenwood Press.

Winkelman, M. 1998. *Ethnic relations in the US: A sociohistorical cultural systems approach.* Dubuque, Iowa.: Eddie Bowers.

Winkelman, M. 1999. *Ethnic sensitivity in social work.* Dubuque, Iowa.: Eddie Bowers.

Winkelman, M. 2000a. Shamanism: The neural ecology of consciousness and healing. Westport, Conn.: Bergin & Garvey.

Winkelman, M. 2000b. Altered states of consciousness. In *Encyclopedia of human emotions,* ed. D. Levinson, 32–38. New York: Macmillan.

Winkelman, M. 2001a. Psychointegrators: Multidisciplinary perspectives on the therapeutic effects of hallucinogens. *Complementary Health Practice Review* 6(3):219–237.

Winkelman, M. 2001b. Alternative and complementary medicine approaches to substance abuse: A shamanic perspective. *International Journal of Drug Policy* 12:337–351.

Winkelman, M. 2001c. Ethnicity and psychocultural models. In *Cultural diversity in the United States,* eds. I. Susser and T. Patterson, 281–301. Boston: Blackwell.

Winkelman, M. 2002a. Shamanism and cognitive evolution. *Cambridge Archaeological Journal* 12(1):71–101.

Winkelman, M. 2002b. Shamanic universals and evolutionary psychology. *Journal of Ritual Studies* 16(2):63–76.

Winkelman, M. 2002c. Shamanism as neurotheology and evolutionary psychology. *American Behavioral Scientist* 45(12):1875–1887.

Winkelman, M. 2003. Complementary therapy for addiction: "Drumming out drugs." *American Journal of Public Health* 93(4):647–651.

Winkelman, M. 2004a. Spirits as human nature and the fundamental structures of consciousness. In *From shaman to scientist: Essays on humanity's search for spirits,* ed. J. Houran, 59–96. Lanham, Md.: Scarecrow Press.

Winkelman, M. 2004b. Shamanism as the original neurotheology. *Zygon* 39(1):193–217.

Winkelman, M. 2004c. Spirituality and the healing of addictions: A shamanic drumming approach. In *Religion and healing in America,* eds. L. Barnes and S. Sered, 455–470. New York: Oxford University Press.

Winkelman, M. 2005. *Cultural awareness, sensitivity, and competence.* Peosta, Iowa.: Eddie Bowers.

Winkelman, M. 2006a. *American ethnic history.* Dubuque, Iowa.: Kendal Hunt.

Winkelman, M. 2006b. Cross-cultural assessments of shamanism as a biogenetic foundation for religion. In *Where God and science meet: How brain and evolutionary studies alter our understanding of religion,* ed. P. McNamara, 139–159. Westport, Conn.: Praeger.

Winkelman, M. 2006c. Shamanism: A biogenetic perspective. In *Science, religion, and society: An encyclopedia of history, culture, and controversy* (2-vol. set) eds. A. Eisen and G. Laderman. Armonk, N.Y.: Sharpe.

Winkelman, M. 2007a. Therapeutic bases of psychedelic medicines: Psychointegrative effects. In: *Psychedelic medicine,* vol. 1, eds. M. Winkelman and T. Roberts, 1–19. Westport, Conn.: Praeger/Greenwood Press.

Winkelman, M. 2007b. Shamanic guidelines for psychedelic medicines. In: *Psychedelic medicine,* vol. 2, eds. M. Winkelman and T. Roberts, 143–168. Westport, Conn.: Praeger/Greenwood Press.

Winkelman, M. 2008. Cross-cultural and biogenetic perspectives on the origins of shamanism. In *Belief in the past: Theory and the archaeology of religion,* eds. D. S. Whitley and K. Hays-Gilpin. Walnut Creek, Calif.: Left Coast Press [forthcoming].

Winkelman, M., and W. Andritzky, eds. 1996. *Sacred plants, consciousness and healing. Yearbook of cross-cultural medicine and psychotherapy,* 5. Berlin: Verlag.

Winkelman, M., and B. K. Bletzer. 2005. Drugs and modernization. In *A companion to psychological anthropology: Modernity and psychocultural change,* eds. C. Casey and R. Edgerton, 337–357. Oxford: Blackwell.

Winkelman, M., and J. Dubisch. 2005. The anthropology of pilgrimage. In *Pilgrimages and healing,* eds. J. Dubisch and M. Winkelman, ix–xxxvi. Tucson: University of Arizona Press.

Winkelman, M., and P. Peek, eds. 2004. *Divination and healing: Potent vision.* Tucson: University of Arizona Press.

Winkelman, M., and T. Roberts, eds. 2007a. *Psychedelic medicine: New evidence for hallucinogenic substances as treatments,* vols. 1 and 2. Westport, Conn.: Praeger/Greenwood Press.

Winkelman, M., and T. Roberts. 2007b. Conclusions: Guidelines for implementing the use of psychedelic medicines. In *Psychedelic medicine: New evidence for hallucinogenic substances as treatments,* vol. 2, eds. M. Winkelman and T. Roberts, 271–298. Westport, Conn.: Praeger/Greenwood Press.

Winkelman, M., and D. White. 1987. A cross-cultural study of magico-religious practitioners and trance states: Data base. In *Human relations area files research series in quantitative cross-cultural data,* vol. 3D, eds. D. Levinson and R. Wagner. New Haven, Conn.: HRAF Press.

Winkelman, M., and C. Winkelman. 1991. Shamanistic healers and their therapies. In *Yearbook of cross-cultural medicine and psychotherapy,* 1, ed. W. Andritzky. Berlin: Verlag.

Winson, J. 1985. *Brain and psyche: The biology of the unconscious.* Garden City, N.J.: Anchor Press/Doubleday.

Winson, J. 1990. The meaning of dreams. *Scientific American* November, 86–96.

World Health Organization. 1992. *Health promotion and chronic disease.* Geneva: WHO Regional Publications.

World Health Organization. 2000. *International classification of diseases: Revision 9th: Clinical modification,* 5th, vols. 1 and 2: Millennium edition. U.S. Department of Health and Human Services.

Wright, I. 1992. Anthropology and capital case litigation. In *Double vision: Anthropologists at law,* ed. Randy Kandal, 29–42. NAPA Bulletin II. Washington, D.C.: American Anthropological Association.

Wright, P. 1989. The shamanic state of consciousness. In Theme issue on "Shamanism and altered states of consciousness in the cross-cultural perspective," eds. M. De Rios and M. Winkelman. *Journal of Psychoactive Drugs* 21(1):25–34.

Yensen, R. 1985. LSD and psychotherapy. *Journal of Psychoactive Drugs* 17(4):267–277.

Yensen, R. 1996. From shamans and mystics to scientists and psychotherapists. In *Sacred plants, consciousness and healing. Yearbook of cross-cultural medicine and psychotherapy,* 5, eds. M. Winkelman and W. Andritzky, 109–128. Berlin: Verlag.

Xiong, P, C. Numrich, C. Youngyuan Wu, D. Yang, and G. Plotnikoff. 2005. Hmong shamanism. In *Religion and healing in America,* eds. L. Barnes and S. Sered, 439–454. New York: Oxford University Press.

Zborowski, M. 1969. *People in pain.* San Francisco: Jossey-Bass.

Zola, I. 1966. Culture and symptoms: An analysis of patients' presenting complaints. *American Sociological Review* 31:615–630.

Zola, I. 1973. Pathways to the doctor: From person to patient. *Social Science and Medicine* 7:677–689.

Zuckerman, D., S. Kasl, and A. Ostfeld. 1984. Psychosocial predictors of mortality among the elderly poor: The role of religion, well-being, and social contacts. *American Journal of Epidemiology* 119:419–423.

NAME INDEX

SUBJECT INDEX

Community health assessment
  adapting community and cultural
    factors in, 149
  APEX model steps on, 147–148
  of community health
    involvement, 149–150
  formative evaluations of,
    150–151
  implementing model standards
    for, 148
  outcome evaluations of, 151–153
  process evaluations of, 151
  RARE used for, 149–160
  See also Assessment
Community health coalitions
  MADD (Mothers Against Drunk
    Driving), 330–331
  processes for building, 330–331
  public policy and development
    of, 327, 330
Community Health Improvement
  Process (CHIP), 148
Community morbidity surveys, 102
Community Oriented Primary
  Care, 147
Compassion, 96
Complementary or alternative medi-
  cine. *See* CAM (complementary
  or alternative medicine)
*Complementary and Alternative
  Medicine in the United States*
  (IOM), 179
Conduct disorder, 210
Confounding, 269
Confounding variables, 268
Consciousness
  ASCs in the integrative mode of,
    393–398
  dreams and shamanic, 398–399
  integrative modes of, 392–393
  See also ASC (altered state of
    consciousness); Shamanistic
    ASC (altered state of
    consciousness)
Construction model, 24
Constructive marginality, 90
Constructivist perspectives, 55–57
Contagion theory, 242–245, 376
Containment processes, 421
Contextualization, 308
Contributory factors (or causes)
  definition of, 48
  iatrogenic (medically caused)
    illness, 184
  natural disease, 236–238
  personalistic theories of
    supernatural, 239–243

See also Disease causation; Risk
  factors
Critical medical anthropology
  drinking problems from
    perspective of, 318–319
  on macrolevel social effects on
    clinical health, 315–324
  political economy approaches to
    health and, 296–306
  on public policy and community
    involvement, 324–333
  on social conditions as causes of
    disease/health, 306–311
  on social networks and support,
    312–315
Cross-cultural adaptation
  concepts of culture context of,
    92–93
  using culture to care for patients/
    providers, 109–117
  description of, 89
  interpersonal skills for
    intercultural relations, 95–98
  medical anthropology specialty
    applications of, 98–109
  types of effective, 93–94
  See also Cultural sensitivity
Cross-cultural competence levels
  adaptation (cultural
    sensitivity), 89
  cultural awareness and
    acceptance, 88
  cultural competence, 89
  cultural proficiency, 90
  description of, 87
  ethnocentrism, 88
  integration, 89–90
  marginalization and
    biculturalism, 89
  universalism, 88
  See also Cultural competence
Cross-cultural differences
  between Hmong and
    biomedicine, 4, 37
  in conceptions of the body,
    174–176
  on genital cutting, 56
  health care adaptations to, 84–85
  as legal defense in courtroom,
    104–105
  mental retardation as social
    classification and, 51, 52
  Mexican *caida de mollera* belief,
    8, 9, 62
  Native American religious
    beliefs, 17
  in pain responses, 170–173

in sick role, 66, 68
  somatoform disorders and, 45,
    46–48
  See also Culture/cultures; Racial/
    ethnicity differences
Cross-cultural ethnomedical
  syndromes
  description of, 236
  natural disease causation and,
    236–238
  personalistic theories of
    supernatural causation,
    239–243
Cuban health care system, 13
"Cues to action," 76
"Cult of the saints," 144
Cultural acceptance, 88
Cultural adaptation
  disease in ecological context and,
    266–267
  overview of, 264–265
Cultural analysis
  macrolevel approach to, 8
  macrolevel psychedelics use
    effects, 364–365
  macrolevel social effects of
    clinical care and health,
    315–324
  microlevel approach to, 8
  microlevel psychedelics use
    effects, 365
Cultural attribution (or cultural
  relativism), 87, 92, 94
Cultural awareness, 10, 84, 86, 88
Cultural characterizations, 92–93
Cultural communication style,
  96–98
Cultural competence
  caida de mollera
    understanding as, 9
  in clinically applied
    anthropology, 86–91
  definition of, 9, 86, 89
  general, 87
  importance of, 8–9
  model of, 125
  organizational, 90–91
  practitioner development of,
    328–329
  self-assessments of, 28–33,
    117–120
  socialization processes of, 10
  See also Cross-cultural
    competence levels;
    Intercultural relationship skills
"Cultural consonance in lifestyle,"
  356–357

472 Subject Index

Schizophrenia
  comparing shamanism to, 408
  cultural factors in, 211
  diagnosis of, 44
Scientific presumptions of
    medicine, 50, 52, 54
Self
  animism spirits as, 402–404
  definition of, 214
  immune system as coterminous
    with the, 374
  indigenous psychology on
    personality and, 210–216
  religion and "sacred," 213–214
  "self-reference criteria" on, 94
  shaman ritual transformation of
    the, 415–417
  spirit relations and, 415
  status, role, and, 214–216
  See also Personality
Self-assessments
  on cultural competence, 28–33,
    117–120
  cultural systems framework for,
    161–162
  on disease, illness, and sick role
    experiences, 80–81
  on ecological assessment of
    disease causation, 293
  on indigenous psychology,
    246–247
  on political-economic effects on
    health, 334
  of psychobiological dynamics of
    stress/well-being, 382–383
  on spiritual experiences and
    healing, 427
  on various health sector
    practices, 200–202
  See also Assessment
Self-care (Mexican American),
    176–177
Self-efficacy, 76
"Self-reference criteria," 94
Serotonin neural pathways, 387
SES (socio-economic-status)
  Alameda County Longitudinal
    Study (1997) on, 309, 349
  "cultural consonance in lifestyle"
    relationship to, 356–357
  CVD relationship to, 357
  disease causation and, 306–309
  poor health caused by
    lower, 309
  See also Status
Shamanism: Archaic Techniques of
    Ecstasy (Eliade), 387

Shamanism
  contemporary religious
    experiences and healing roots
    of, 417–426
  as cross-cultural phenomenon,
    390–392
  origins and practices of, 386–387
  self-assessment on, 427
  significance and core of, 387, 389
  soul loss treatment by, 388
Shamanistic ASC (altered state of
    consciousness)
  animism role in, 399–400,
    402–404
  as cross-cultural shaman
    characteristic, 390, 391
  death-and-rebirth experience,
    407–408
  dreams and, 398–399
  functions of, 399–401
  healing response role of,
    283–284
  meditative, 394, 413–414
  minimized by new societies, 392
  neurognostic structures and,
    401–408
  physiological model of, 394–398,
    409–410
  possession, 393–394, 413
  psychoactive plants used to
    induce, 395, 398
  as psychopathic experience, 408
  rhythmic auditory stimulation
    and, 395
  rituals associated with, 386–387
  soul journey as, 389, 402,
    406–407, 420–422
  substance abuse rehabilitation
    using, 423–426
  visionary experiences and healing
    through, 404–405, 420–422
  See also ASC modes;
    Consciousness
Shamanistic healers
  cross-cultural characteristics of,
    390–391
  description of, 140, 386
  evolution of, 392
  individuation and self-
    actualization of, 408, 422
  as link between spirit world and
    community, 387, 389
  physical healing by, 391
  as psychopaths, 408
  shape-shifting by, 422
  soul journey of, 389, 402,
    406–407, 420–422

universal characteristics of, 389,
    391–392
Shamanistic practices
  Catholic charismatic healing
    manifestation of, 414
  death-and-rebirth experience,
    407–408
  DSM-IV spiritual emergencies
    and, 418–419
  integrative mode of
    consciousness in, 392–401
  neurognostic structures of,
    401–409
  overview of, 386–387
  soul journey, 389, 402, 406–407
  soul recovery, 388, 412–413
  therapeutic bases of, 409–417
Shamans, 386
Shape-shifting, 422
Sick role
  African Americans and the, 68
  assumption of, 67
  cultural and social acceptance
    of, 68–70
  definition of, 65
  expansion of the, 65–67
  Mexican American culture, 66
  primary, secondary, and tertiary
    gains of, 69
  self-assessment on experience
    of, 80–81
  See also Patient role
Sickle cell anemia, 254–255
Sickness
  characteristics of, 60–62
  comparing illness to, 60
  cult of the saints and medically
    induced, 144
  definition of, 36
  evolution of sickness-and-healing
    responses to, 282–285
  explanatory model on experience
    of, 38, 74–79
  health beliefs model on
    experience of, 38, 75–78
  sequences in experiences of,
    67–68
  as social process, 68–70
  See also Diseases; Illness;
    Maladies
Sickness career, 68–70
Sickness-and-healing responses
  foundations for innate healing
    capacities, 284–285
  origins of, 282–283
  shamanism as, 283–284
"Six-hour mental retardation," 51